Pathology of Bone and Joint Neoplasms

OTHER MONOGRAPHS IN THE SERIES MAJOR PROBLEMS IN PATHOLOGY

VIRGINIA A. LIVOLSI, M.D.
Series Editor

Published

Azzopardi: *Problems in Breast Pathology*

Frable: *Fine Needle Aspiration Biopsy*

Wigglesworth: *Perinatal Pathology,* 2/ed

Katzenstein: *Katzenstein and Askin's Surgical Pathology of Non-Neoplastic Lung Disease,* 3/ed

Finegold: *Pathology of Neoplasia in Children and Adolescents*

Wolf and Neiman: *Disorders of the Spleen*

Fu and Regan: *Pathology of the Uterine Cervix, Vagina, and Vulva*

LiVolsi: *Surgical Pathology of the Thyroid*

Virmani, Atkinson, and Fenoglio: *Cardiovascular Pathology*

Whitehead: *Mucosal Biopsy of the Gastrointestinal Tract,* 5/ed

Mackay, Lukeman, and Ordonez: *Tumors of the Lung*

Ellis, Auclair, and Gnepp: *Surgical Pathology of the Salivary Glands*

Nash and Said: *Pathology of AIDS and HIV Infection*

Lloyd: *Surgical Pathology of the Pituitary Gland*

Henson and Albores-Saavedra: *Pathology of Incipient Neoplasia,* 2/ed

Taylor and Cote: *Immunomicroscopy,* 2/ed

Lack: *Pathology of Adrenal and Extra-Adrenal Paraganglia*

Jaffe: *Surgical Pathology of Lymph Nodes and Related Organs,* 2/ed

Striker, Striker, and d'Agati: *The Renal Biopsy,* 3/ed

Isaacs, Jr: *Tumors of the Fetus and Newborn*

Foster and Bostwick: *Pathology of the Prostate*

Carter and Patchefsky: *Tumors and Tumor-like Lesions of the Lung*

Forthcoming

Owen and Kelly: *Surgical Pathology of the Gallbladder, Bile Ducts, and Pancreas*

Kao: *Surgical Pathology of the Skin and Mucocutaneous Junction*

Fu: *Pathology of the Uterine Cervix, Vagina, and Vulva,* 2/ed

Weidner: *Surgical Pathology of the Breast*

LiVolsi: *Pathology of the Thyroid,* 2/ed

Neiman and Orazi: *Disorders of the Spleen,* 2/ed

MPP

37

TIMOTHY R. HELLIWELL, M.D., MRCPath
Reader in Pathology
Department of Pathology
The University of Liverpool
Liverpool, UK

Pathology of Bone and Joint Neoplasms

Volume 37 in the Series
MAJOR PROBLEMS IN PATHOLOGY

W.B. SAUNDERS COMPANY
A Division of Harcourt Brace & Company
PHILADELPHIA LONDON TORONTO MONTREAL SYDNEY TOKYO

W.B. SAUNDERS COMPANY
A Division of Harcourt Brace & Company

The Curtis Center
Independence Square West
Philadelphia, Pennsylvania 19106

Library of Congress Cataloging-in-Publication Data

Pathology of bone and joint neoplasms / [edited by] Timothy R. Helliwell.—1st ed.

p. cm.—(Major problems in pathology: v. 37)
Includes bibliographical references.

ISBN 0–7216–6439–3

1. Bones—Cancer. 2. Joints—Cancer. I. Helliwell, Timothy R. II. Series.

[DNLM: 1. Bone Neoplasms—pathology. 2. Joint Diseases—pathology.
W1 MA492X v.37 1999/WE 258 P297 1999]

RC280.B6P38 1999

616.99′271—dc21

DNLM/DLC 97–48343

PATHOLOGY OF BONE AND JOINT NEOPLASMS ISBN 0–7216–6439–3

Printed in the United States of America.

Last digit is the print number: 9 8 7 6 5 4 3 2 1

Study the past and be aware of the modern;
then you may become a teacher

Confucius

Contributors

NICHOLAS A. ATHANASOU, PhD, MRCPath

Reader in Orthopaedic Pathology, University of Oxford; Consultant Osteoarticular Pathologist, Nuffield Orthopaedic Centre, Oxford, U.K.

Cell and Organ Culture in the Understanding of Bone and Its Neoplasms

DR. NICOLA BALDINI

Laboratorio di Ricerca Oncologica, Istituti Ortopedici Rizzoli, Bologna, Italy

Assessment of the Effects of Treatment on Bone Neoplasms

JULIA A. BRIDGE, M.D.

Associate Professor, Rehabilitation and Genetic Medicine, University of Nebraska Medical Center, Omaha, Nebraska

Cytogenetic Analysis of Bone and Joint Neoplasms

DR. H. CHRISTIANSEN

Senior Physician, Universitäts-Krankenhaus Eppendorf, Kinder- und Poliklinik, Abt. für Pädiatr. Hamatologie und Onkologie, Hamburg, Germany

Molecular Markers in the Evaluation of Bone Neoplasms

DR. ALAN J. DARBY, FRCPath

Consultant Histopathologist, Department of Pathology, Robert Jones and Agnes Hunt Orthopaedic Hospital, Shropshire, U.K.

Vascular Neoplasms of Bone

DR. A. MARK DAVIES, FRCR

Consultant Radiologist, M.R.I. Centre, The Royal Orthopaedic NHS Trust, Birmingham, U.K.

Imaging Studies in Bone Neoplasia

KENNETH DEVANEY, M.D.

The University of Michigan, Department of Pathology, Ann Arbor, Michigan

Benign Fibro-Osseous Lesions of Bone

PROF. LESLIE G. DODD, M.D.

Assistant Professor; Chief, Section of Cytopathology, Department of Pathology, Duke University Medical Center, Durham, North Carolina

Fine Needle Aspiration of Bone and Joint Neoplasms

PROF. ANTHONY J. FREEMONT, M.D., FRCPath

Professor of Osteoarticular Pathology, Department of Osteoarticular Pathology, University of Manchester, Manchester, U.K.

Bone Development, Structure, and Turnover

TIMOTHY R. HELLIWELL, M.D., MRCPath

Reader in Pathology, Department of Pathology, The University of Liverpool, Royal Liverpool University Hospital, Liverpool, U.K.
Classification and Diagnosis of Bone Neoplasms; Central Cartilaginous Neoplasms of Bone; Tumors and Tumor-Like Lesions of Joints and Juxta-Articular Bone

DR. HARMUT KABISCH

Senior Physician, Universitäts-Krankenhaus Eppendorf, Kinder- und Poliklinik, Abt. für Pädiatr. Hamatologie und Onkologie, Hamburg, Germany
Molecular Markers in the Evaluation of Bone Neoplasms

SCOTT E. KILPATRICK, M.D.

Assistant Professor of Pathology, Department of Pathology and Laboratory Medicine, University of North Carolina at Chapel Hill; Surgical Pathologist and Cytopathologist, University of North Carolina Hospitals, Chapel Hill, North Carolina
Spindle Cell Lesions of Bone

PROF. LESTER J. LAYFIELD, M.D.

Director of Surgical Pathology, Head of Fine Needle Aspiration Service, Department of Pathology, University of Utah, Salt Lake City, Utah
Fine Needle Aspiration of Bone and Joint Neoplasms

DR. DAVID C. MANGHAM, MRCPath

Honorary Senior Lecturer, University of Birmingham; U.K. Consultant Pathologist, Department of Musculoskeletal Pathology, Royal Orthopaedic Hospital, Birmingham, U.K.
Giant Cell Tumor of Bone and Giant Cell–Containing Lesions of Bone

CHARLOTTE ORNDAL, M.D., PhD

Rehabilitation and Genetic Medicine, University of Nebraska Medical Center, Omaha, Nebraska
Cytogenetic Analysis of Bone and Joint Neoplasms

ELIZABETH J. PERLMAN, M.D.

Associate Professor, Pathology and Pediatrics, Department of Pathology, The Johns Hopkins Hospital, Baltimore, Maryland
Ewing's Sarcoma, Lymphoma, and Langerhans' Cell Proliferations

PIERO PICCI, M.D.

Director, Laboratorio di Ricerca Oncologica, Istituti Ortopedici Rizzoli, Bologna, Italy
Assessment of the Effects of Treatment on Bone Neoplasms

DR. JEAN A.S. PRINGLE, FRCS

Department of Morbid Anatomy, Institute of Orthopaedics, Royal National Orthopaedic Hospital, Middlesex, U.K.
Bone-Forming Neoplasms Arising Within Bone

DR. ROBIN P. REID, MRCPath

Senior Lecturer in Osteoarticular Pathology, Department of Pathology, Western General Infirmary, Glasgow, U.K.
Bone Neoplasms and Tumor-Like Lesions on the Bone Surface

DR. DAVID A. RITCHIE, FRCR

Honorary Clinical Lecturer, Consultant Radiologist, Radiology Department, Royal Liverpool University Hospitals, Liverpool, U.K.
Imaging Studies in Bone Neoplasia; Tumors and Tumor-Like Lesions of Joints and Juxta-Articular Bone

JONATHAN R. SALISBURY, M.D., MRCPath

Reader in Histopathology, Department of Histopathology, Kings College School of Medicine and Dentistry; Clinical Director for Histopathology and Honorary Consultant Histopathologist, Kings College Hospital, London, U.K.
Bone Neoplasms Containing Epithelial and Epithelioid Cells

DR. R. BARBARA SCHOLZ

Universitäts-Krankenhaus Eppendorf, Kinder- und Poliklinik, Abt. für Pädiatr. Hamatologie und Onkologie, Hamburg, Germany
Molecular Markers in the Evaluation of Bone Neoplasms

DR. K. KRISHNAN UNNI

Professor and Consultant in Pathology, Mayo Graduate School of Medicine, Mayo Clinic, Rochester, Minnesota
Spindle Cell Lesions of Bone

DR. KURT WINKLER

Emeritus Director, Universitäts-Krankenhaus Eppendorf, Kinder- und Poliklinik, Abt. für Pädiatr. Hamatologie und Onkologie, Hamburg, Germany
Molecular Markers in the Evaluation of Bone Neoplasms

Foreword

This volume in the Major Problems in Pathology series covers in detail diagnostic pathology of bones and joints and related orthopedic lesions. Dr. Helliwell has gathered an international group of experts in orthopedic pathology who have contributed their diagnostic acumen to this volume. This book promises to guide the reader through the often confusing area of reactive and neoplastic bone lesions encountered by the surgical pathologist. Chapters devoted to cell culture, cytogenetics, molecular changes, and fine needle aspiration biopsy characterize this "up-to-the-minute" monograph.

VIRGINIA A. LIVOLSI, M.D.
Philadelphia, PA
Series Editor

NOTICE

Pathology is an ever-changing field. Standard safety precautions must be followed, but as new research and clinical experience broaden our knowledge, changes in treatment and drug therapy become necessary or appropriate. Readers are advised to check the product information currently provided by the manufacturer of each drug to be administered to verify the recommended dose, the method and duration of administration, and the contraindications. It is the responsibility of the treating physician, relying on experience and knowledge of the patient, to determine dosages and the best treatment for the patient. Neither the publisher nor the editor assumes any responsibility for any injury and/or damage to persons or property.

THE PUBLISHER

Preface

This book provides practical guidance for the diagnosis of both common and uncommon bone and joint neoplasms and an appreciation of the scientific foundations on which the knowledge of the nature of these neoplasms will develop. It is not a comprehensive text but concentrates on discussion of those areas in which diagnostic difficulties may occur. Advances in the understanding of the biology of bones and joints and of their neoplasms will lead to changes in the management of these tumors and improve the chances of survival for those patients who currently suffer and die from disseminated malignant disease. The paradigm for these developments is the treatment of osteosarcoma and Ewing's sarcoma where, over the last 30 years, amputation and radiotherapy have largely been superseded by limb-sparing surgery and chemotherapy, leading to major improvements in patient survival and preservation of function. In parallel with the improvements in the management of bone tumors, imaging and laboratory diagnostic techniques have become more sophisticated; for example, the identification of specific cellular components by immunocytochemical methods allows the histopathologist to resolve relatively easily some of the diagnostic problems that troubled pathologists earlier this century. As knowledge of the molecular and genetic changes in bone and joint neoplasms increases, its application to the diagnostic arena will become essential.

This is primarily a book for the surgical histopathologist and cytopathologist who is faced with making diagnostic decisions for patients with suspected bone or joint neoplasms. The book should also appeal to the orthopedic surgeon and radiologist who, in order to assess and treat patients appropriately, must be sufficiently informed about the probems of the pathologist's work to appreciate the potential and the limitations of each facet of the diagnostic process. In turn, pathologists reporting on osteoarticular specimens must have insight into the benefits and limitations of imaging studies in order to be able to engage in a constructive dialogue with their radiological and surgical colleagues on the nature of a particular diagnostic problem. A difficulty for many pathologists is their lack of expertise in imaging techniques, and the appropriate level of radiological expertise may not be available to help them. Most chapters emphasize the idea that the pathologist should have access to the radiological images when making a diagnosis. This is essential for many tumors where the imaging studies provide the best representation of the gross pathology and invasive behavior of a neoplasm.

For the trainee pathologist the nomenclature of bone tumors may be confusing, and information on the basic principles of terminology and the historical recognition of diagnostic entities is therefore helpful. In many cases, the diagnosis is facilitated by knowing which bone lesions are most likely in a particular clinical or radiological situation. The trainee also needs to know where the diagnostic pitfalls lie so that they may be avoided.

The rarity of some osteoarticular tumors means that many patients are referred to specialist centers for management if a primary bone tumor is suspected clinically. Nevertheless, all pathologists will eventually be faced with a diagnostic problem that was clinically unsuspected. Some common lesions may occasionally cause problems because of atypical features or the development of complications; for example, malignancy in osteochondroma. Even if the pathologist cannot make a definitive diagnosis, then it is important that the clinical, imaging, and pathological information be acquired in such a way as to facilitate the patient's diagnosis and management at a referral center. A referring pathologist should send both histological and radiological material. This book should not discourage the referral of cases to expert pathologists, and indeed, non–expert pathologists should be careful not to exceed the boundaries of their own knowledge as this can lead to clinical disaster. Expert opinion should be available to confirm a suspected diagnosis that may be unusual or that may imply a complex therapeutic protocol; such opinion is frequently sought to provide moral and practical support for the diagnosis made by the referring pathologist.

I am grateful to the many experts who have agreed to place their experience and views on the interpretation of diagnostic problems within the context of this volume. This should be invaluable information for the non–expert pathologist who needs to appreciate how a diagnosis is made so as to be able to explain and justify to the local surgeon and patient the fine judgments that an expert makes. The non–expert should also appreciate the limitations of knowledge of the prediction of behavior of particular types of neoplasm.

The first section of this book provides the practicing pathologist with an understanding of the molecular biology of the cells in normal bone and an appreciation of the principles of the laboratory techniques, such as cell and tissue culture, cytogenetics, and molecular biology, that can be applied to the study of osteoarticular tumors. The second section emphasizes the important contributions that radiology and fine needle aspiration cytology can make to the diagnosis of bone and joint neoplasms; this section includes a chapter on the interpretation of bone specimens in relation to the treatment that the patient has received or will receive. The chapters in the main section have been defined partly on the basis of histological features that are common to certain neoplasms and partly on the features of neoplasms that affect particular anatomic sites. The authors discuss in detail their approaches to the diagnostic problems that occur with particular groups of lesions as they might present to the diagnostic pathologist. The reader will appreciate that the extent of the discussion varies with the nature of the topic and the personalities of the authors, but in each situation I hope that practical guidance is provided. Many diagnostic entities are referred to in several chapters but I have not tried to avoid all repetition as different presentations often create different differential diagnostic issues that need to be addressed separately. Hopefully, contradictions have been avoided, and the extensive cross-referencing should allow the reader to move between chapters with ease.

I must thank George Meachim, who stimulated my interest in osteoarticular pathology, and the several Professors in Orthopaedic Surgery in Liverpool who encouraged my interest to develop over the last 15 years. I am also grateful to my colleagues in the British Bone Tumour Panel who have helped me to refine this interest, particularly to those who were kind enough to allow me to coerce them into contributing to this book. Thanks also go to David Ritchie, Consultant Radiologist in Liverpool, who has not only contributed to two excellent chapters but who has also encouraged me to use consistent radiological terminology throughout the book.

T. R. Helliwell

Contents

Color section follows Table of Contents

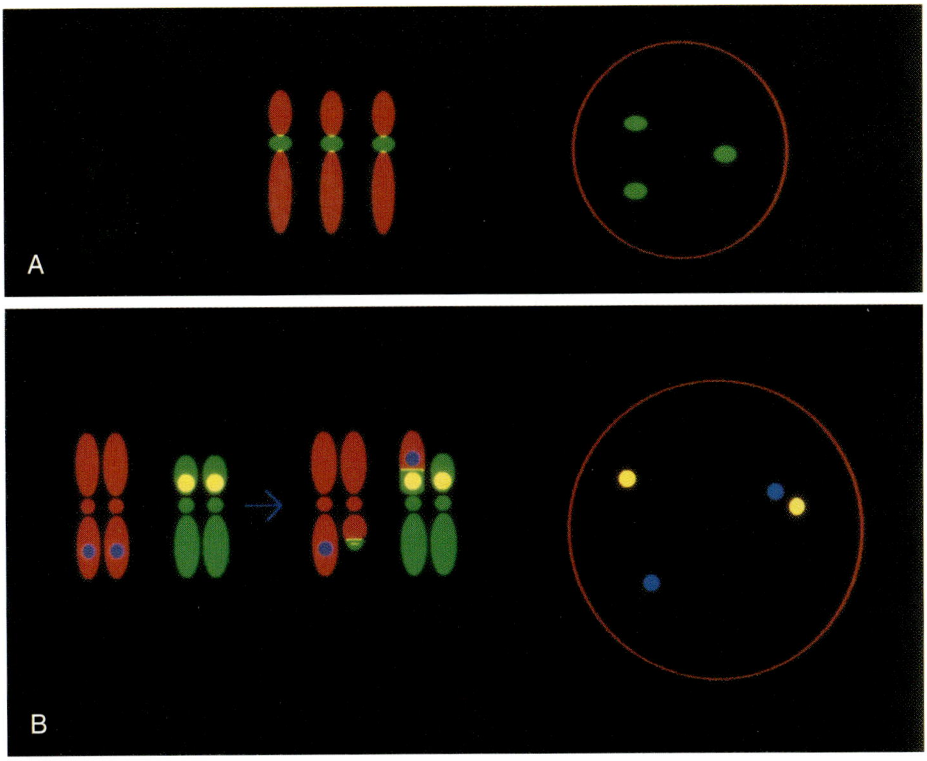

Figure 4–2. Fluorescence in situ hybridization (FISH). *A,* Schematic representation of FISH with a centromere specific probe (labeled in green). Three green signals are seen in an interphase cell demonstrating trisomy *(right). B,* Schematic representation of the detection of a reciprocal translocation utilizing FISH with breakpoint flanking probes (yellow and blue signals). In the interphase cell, the two different colored probes will lie in close proximity *(right)* to each other if a rearrangement has occurred and may be visualized as a third color; for example, a green and red probe may create a yellow signal.

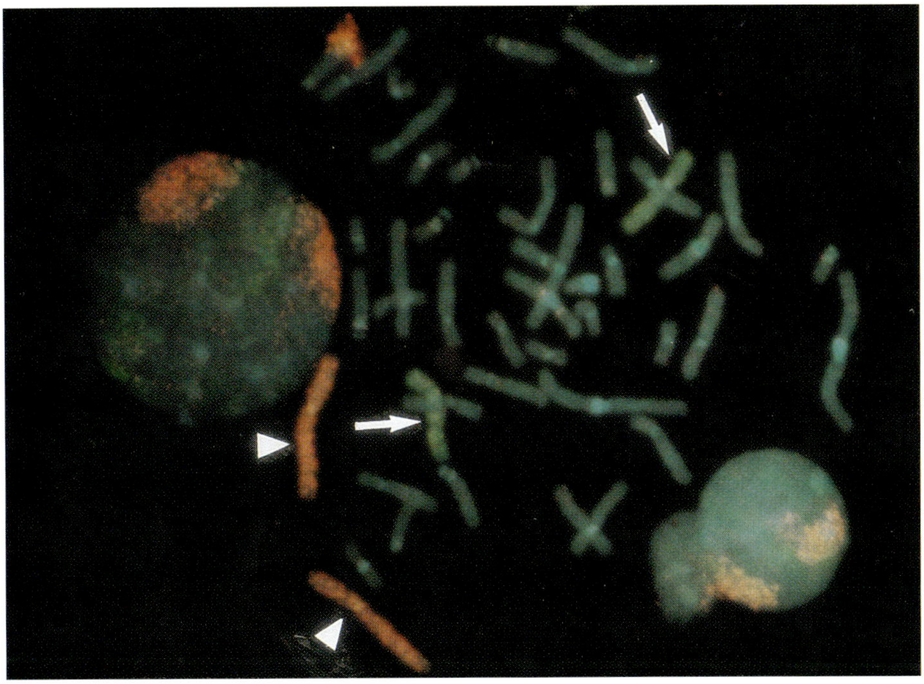

Figure 4–3. Multicolor FISH with chromosomal paint probes for specific identification of chromosomes 2 (spectrum orange, *arrowheads*) and 7 (spectrum green, *arrows*), performed on karyotypically normal male peripheral blood lymphocytes. The remaining nonprobed chromosomes are counterstained with DAPI (4,6-diamino-2-phenylindolhydrochloride, blue). These probes can be used to define or uncover various structural abnormalities.

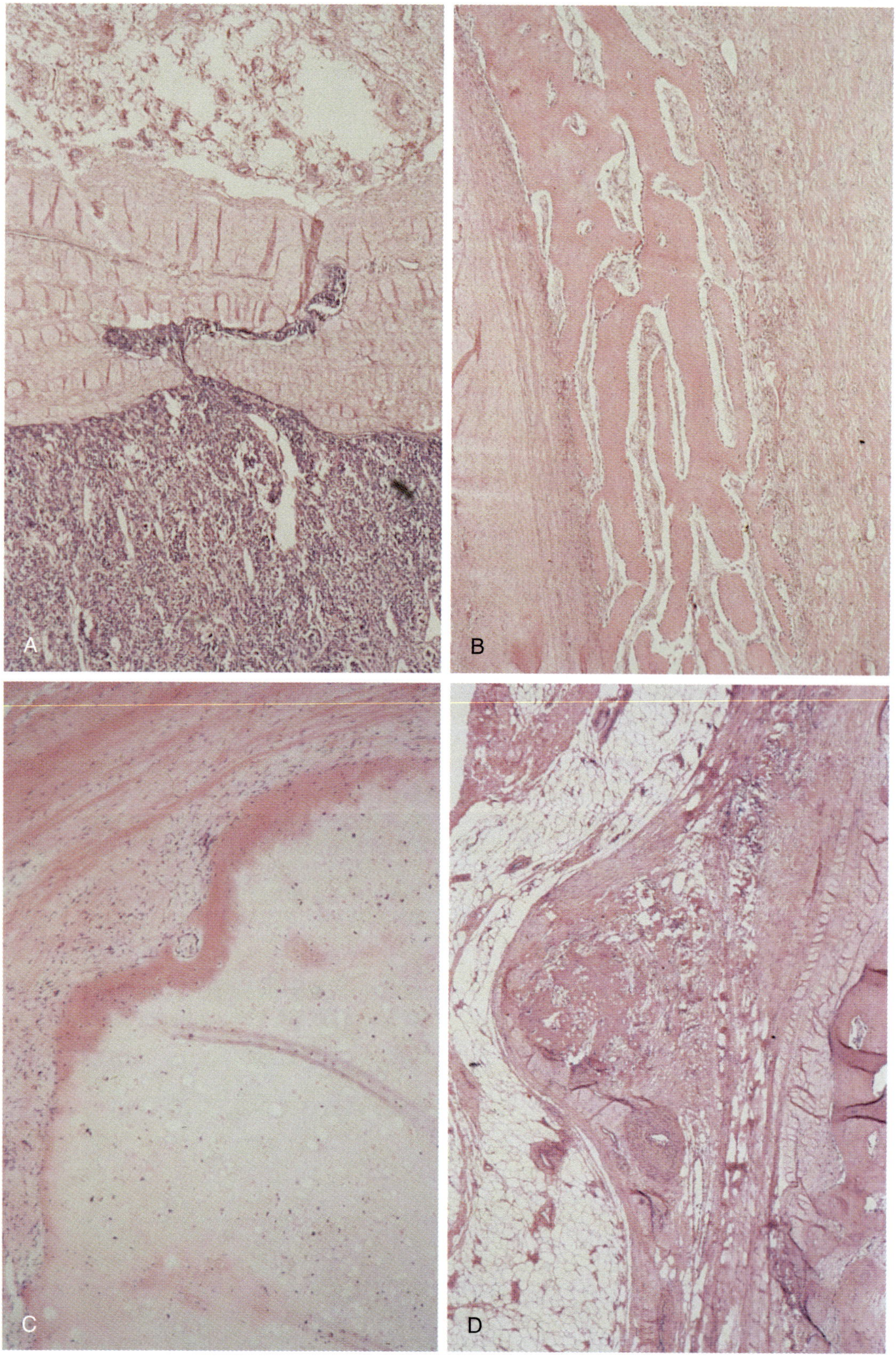

Figure 8–3. Osteosarcoma before (A) and after (B,C,D) chemotherapy. *A,* In untreated tumors, the reactive pseudocapsule is often penetrated by finger-like projections. *B,* When the tumoral cells are destroyed by chemotherapy *(right),* the pseudocapsule matures and becomes a true capsule. Mature bone trabeculations, probably associated with the periosteum, may be seen. *C,* Cartilaginous tumor lobules ossify peripherally. *D,* Satellite nodules, when present, appear to be encapsulated.

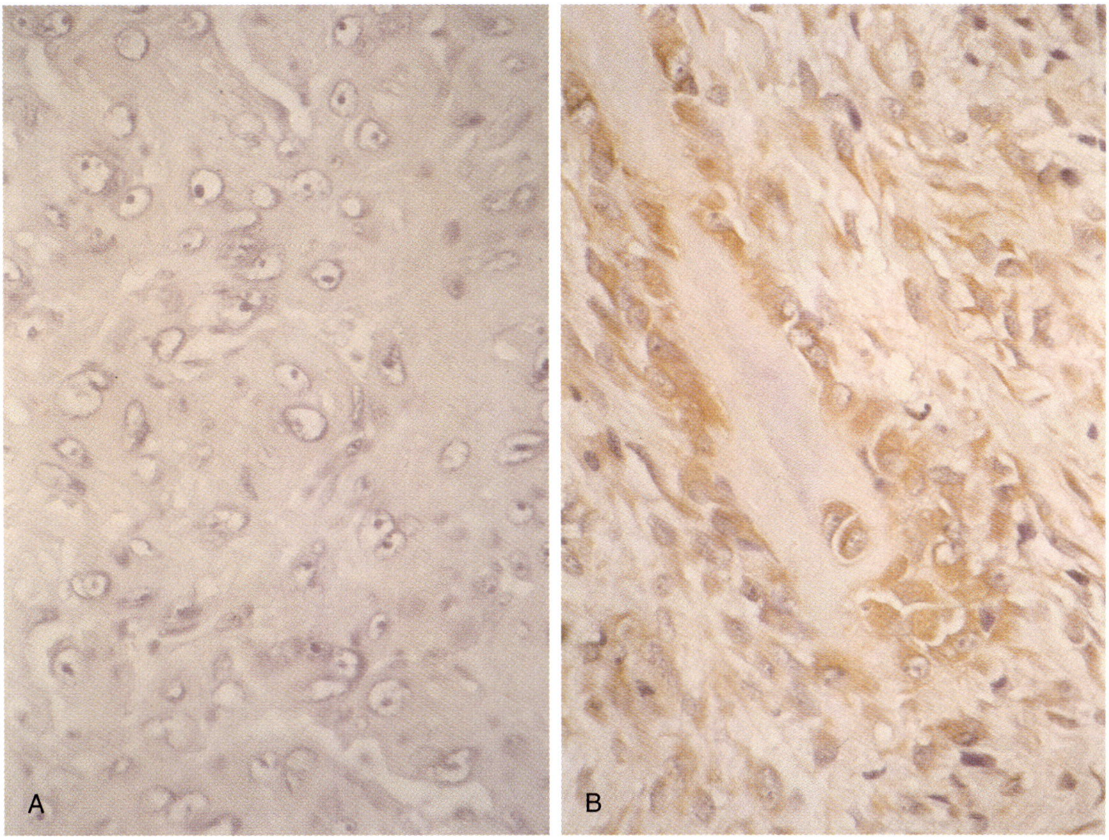

Figure 8–6. Different patterns of P-glycoprotein immunoreactivity in human osteosarcoma. *A,* In this osteosarcoma the malignant cells do not show detectable labeling for the P-glycoprotein. *B,* In a different osteosarcoma, there is strong cytoplasmic labeling in most malignant cells for P-glycoprotein. (Avidin-peroxidase immunostaining using JSB-1 monoclonal antibody at 1:20 dilution.)

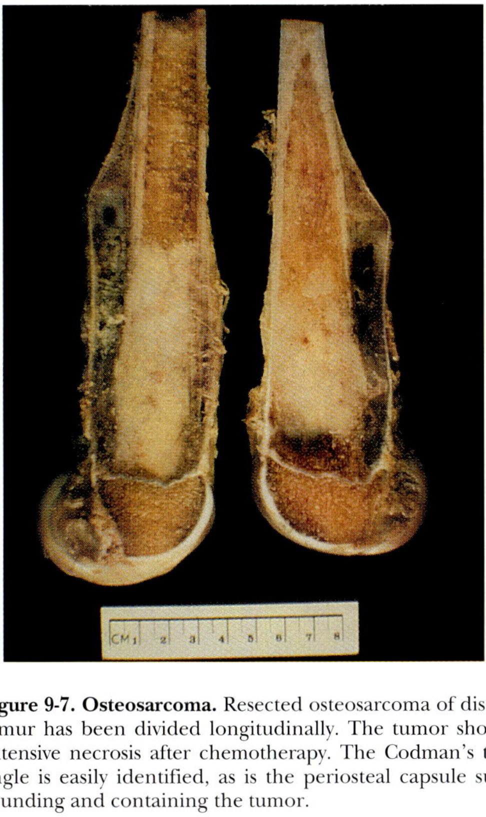

Figure 9-7. Osteosarcoma. Resected osteosarcoma of distal femur has been divided longitudinally. The tumor shows extensive necrosis after chemotherapy. The Codman's triangle is easily identified, as is the periosteal capsule surrounding and containing the tumor.

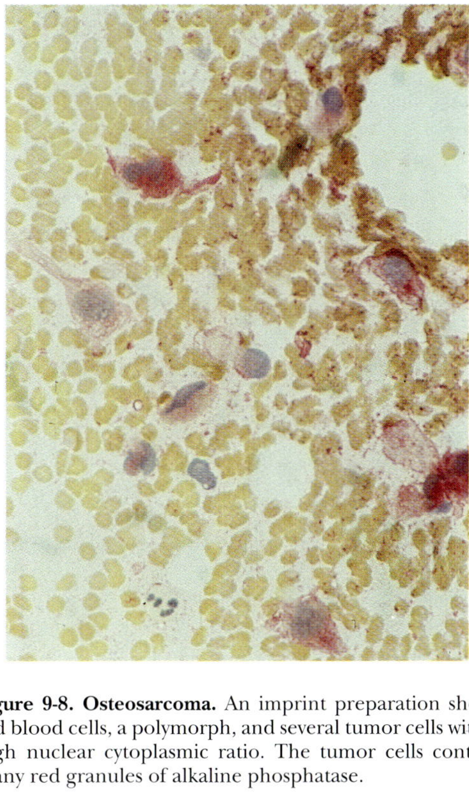

Figure 9-8. Osteosarcoma. An imprint preparation shows red blood cells, a polymorph, and several tumor cells with a high nuclear cytoplasmic ratio. The tumor cells contain many red granules of alkaline phosphatase.

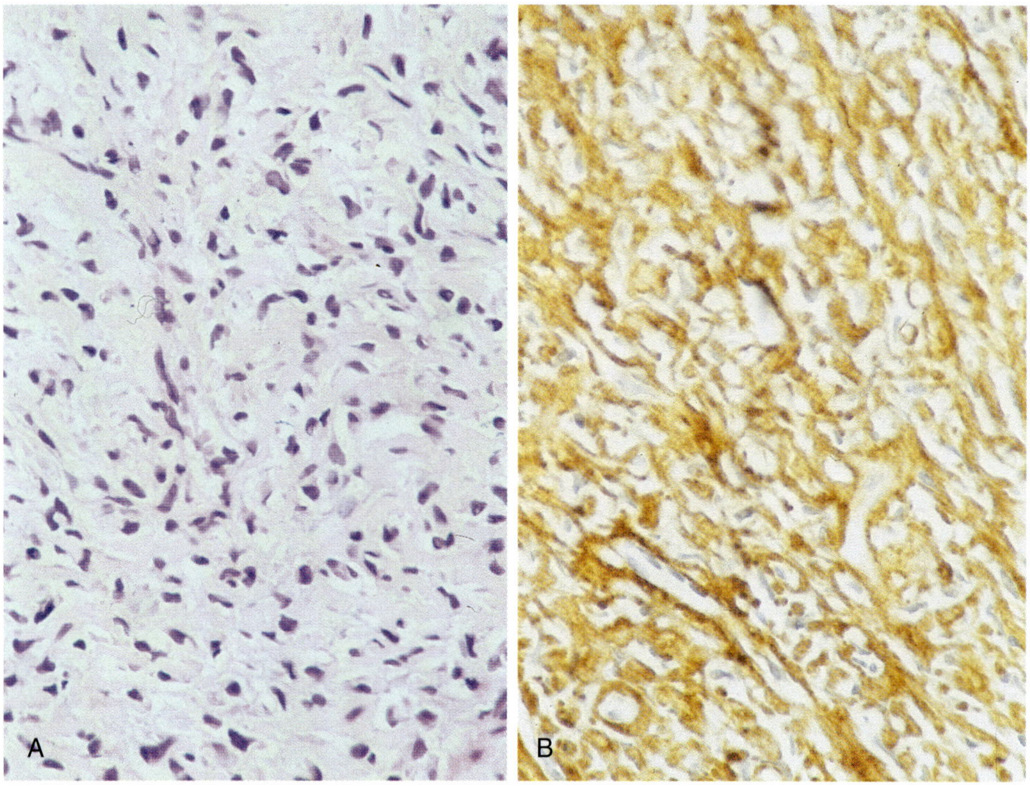

Figure 9–9. Osteosarcoma. *A,* Osteosarcoma of the spine shows delicate strands of possible tumor osteoid. *B,* Immunohistochemical labeling for vimentin highlights the branching trabecular pattern of the matrix.

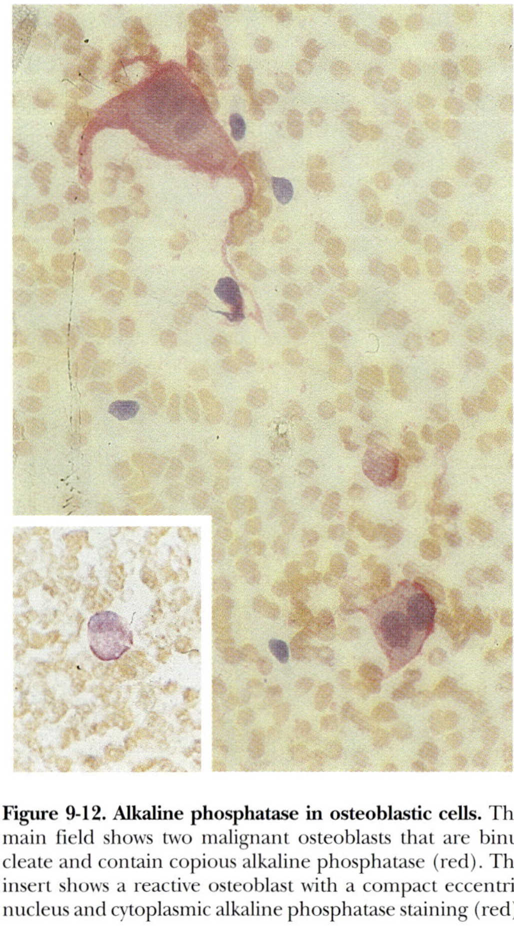

Figure 9-12. Alkaline phosphatase in osteoblastic cells. The main field shows two malignant osteoblasts that are binucleate and contain copious alkaline phosphatase (red). The insert shows a reactive osteoblast with a compact eccentric nucleus and cytoplasmic alkaline phosphatase staining (red).

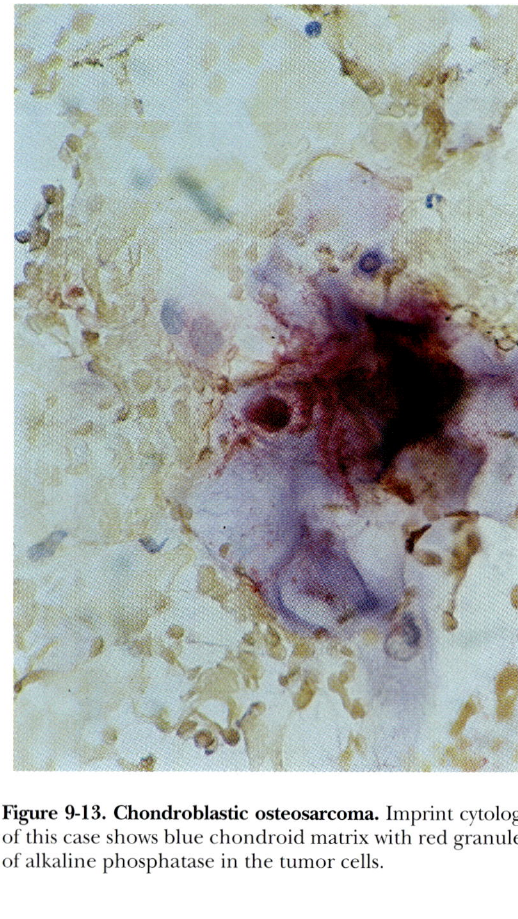

Figure 9-13. Chondroblastic osteosarcoma. Imprint cytology of this case shows blue chondroid matrix with red granules of alkaline phosphatase in the tumor cells.

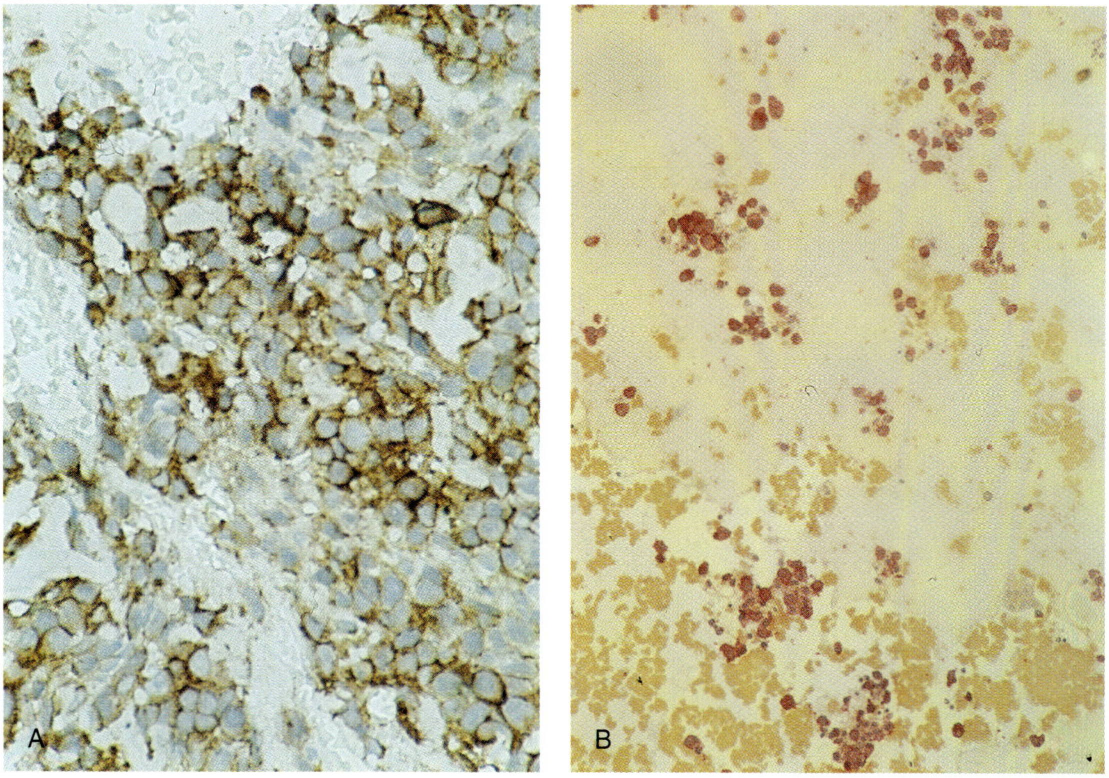

Figure 9–18. Small cell osteosarcoma. *A,* The neoplastic cells show intense membrane labeling for CD99 (*MIC2* antibody). *B,* Imprint preparation shows the small malignant cells contain copious alkaline phosphatase.

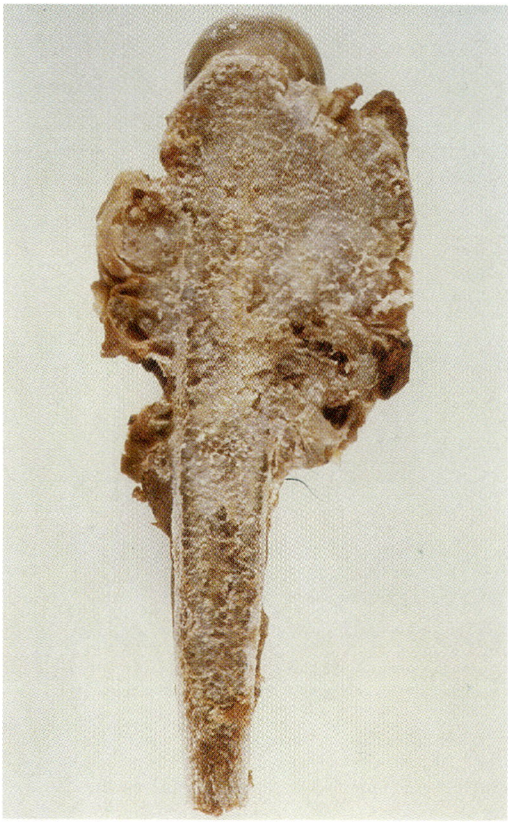

Figure 10–2. Macroscopic appearance of chondrosarcoma. Blue-gray nodules of cartilage, with yellow specks of calcification, are present centrally and extend out of the bone into soft tissues.

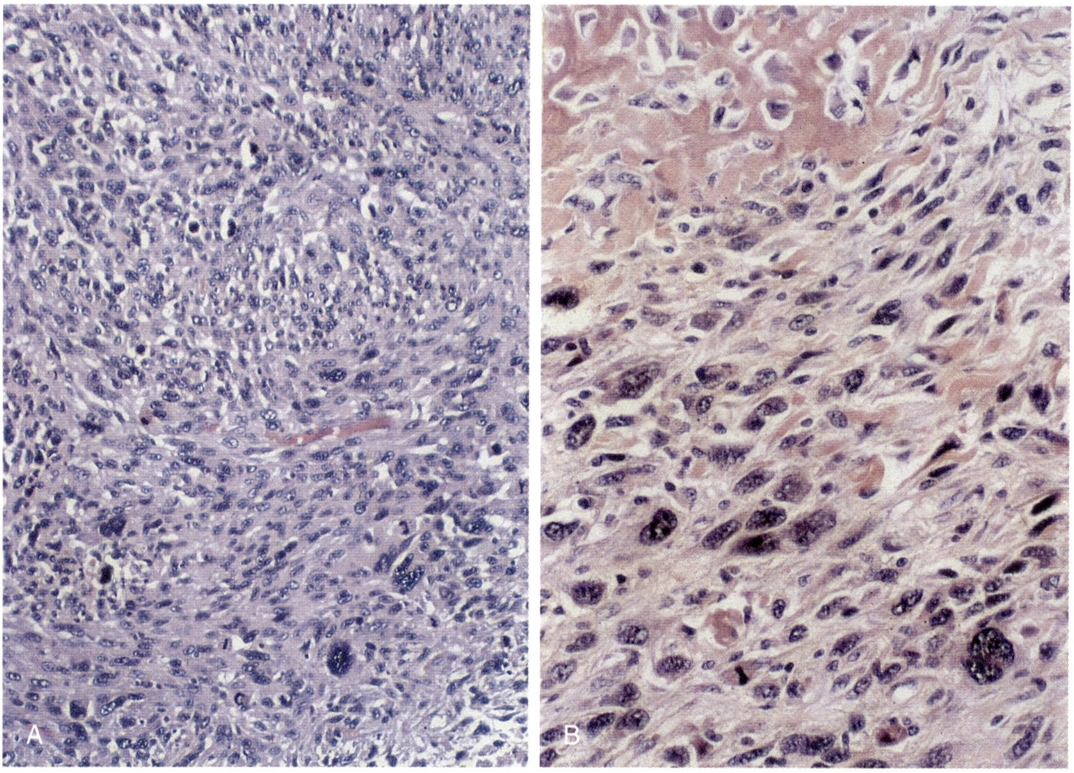

Figure 12–9. Malignant fibrous histiocytoma of bone. *A,* Classic case with markedly anaplastic spindle cells. *B,* Malignant fibrous histiocytoma-like osteosarcoma. The presence of osteoid production by the tumor cells *(upper left)* excludes the diagnosis of malignant fibrous histiocytoma.

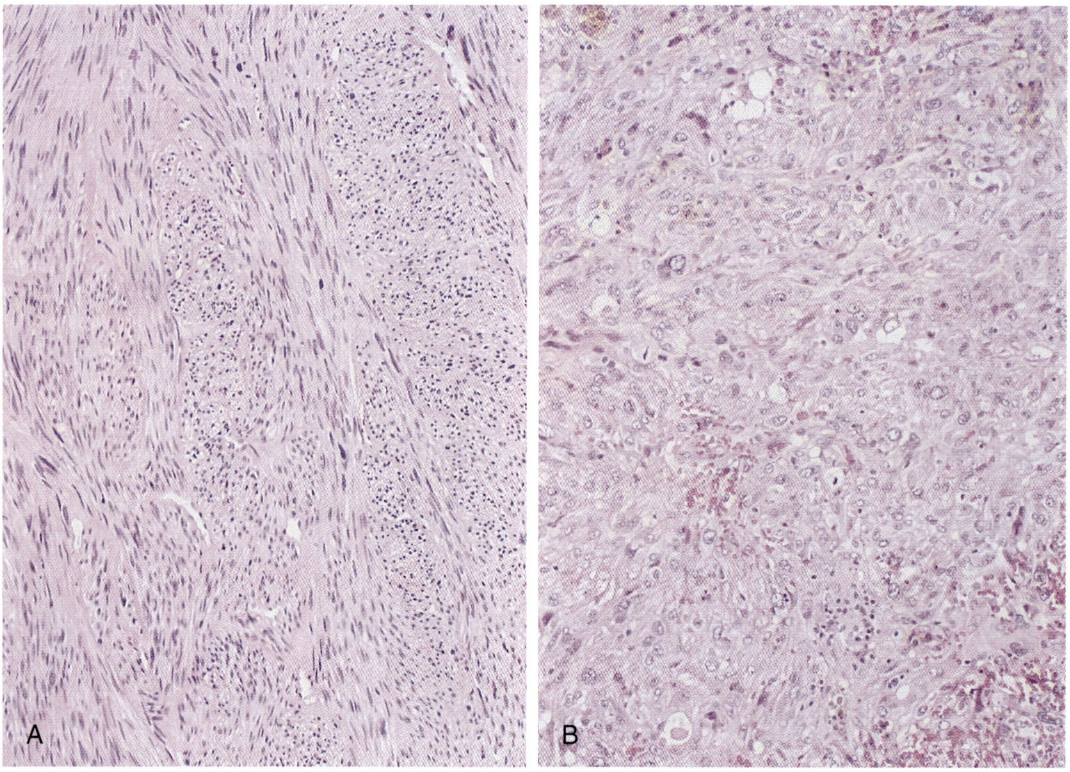

Figure 12–12. Leiomyosarcoma. *A,* Case with intersecting fascicles of spindle cells containing cigar-shaped nuclei and tapering eosinophilic cytoplasm. *B,* Occasional cases may show more obvious nuclear anaplasia resembling malignant fibrous histiocytoma. Immunohistochemical staining for α-smooth muscle actin is needed to make this distinction.

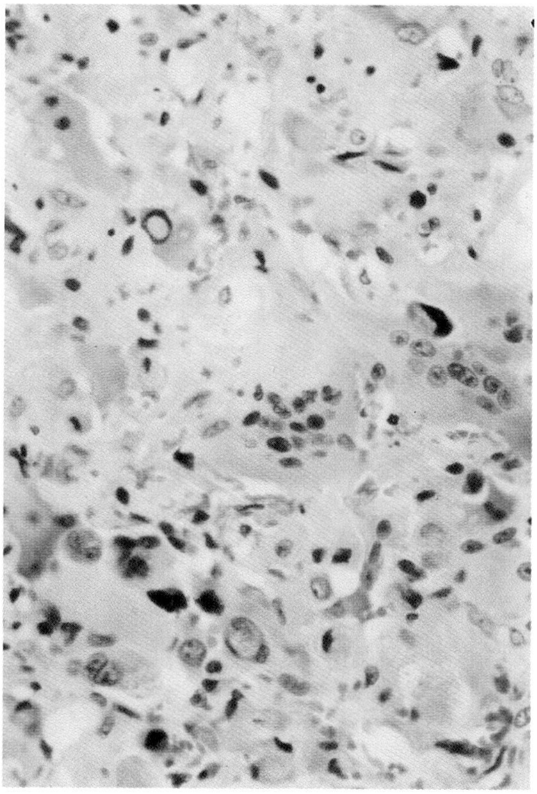

Figure 15–6. Area of giant cell tumor of bone showing degenerate nuclear features of the stromal cells. The nuclei show vacuolization, smudged chromatin, and hyperchromatism. No mitoses are present in this area of the tumor. The importance in recognizing this change is in the distinction from the nuclear pleomorphism of malignancy.

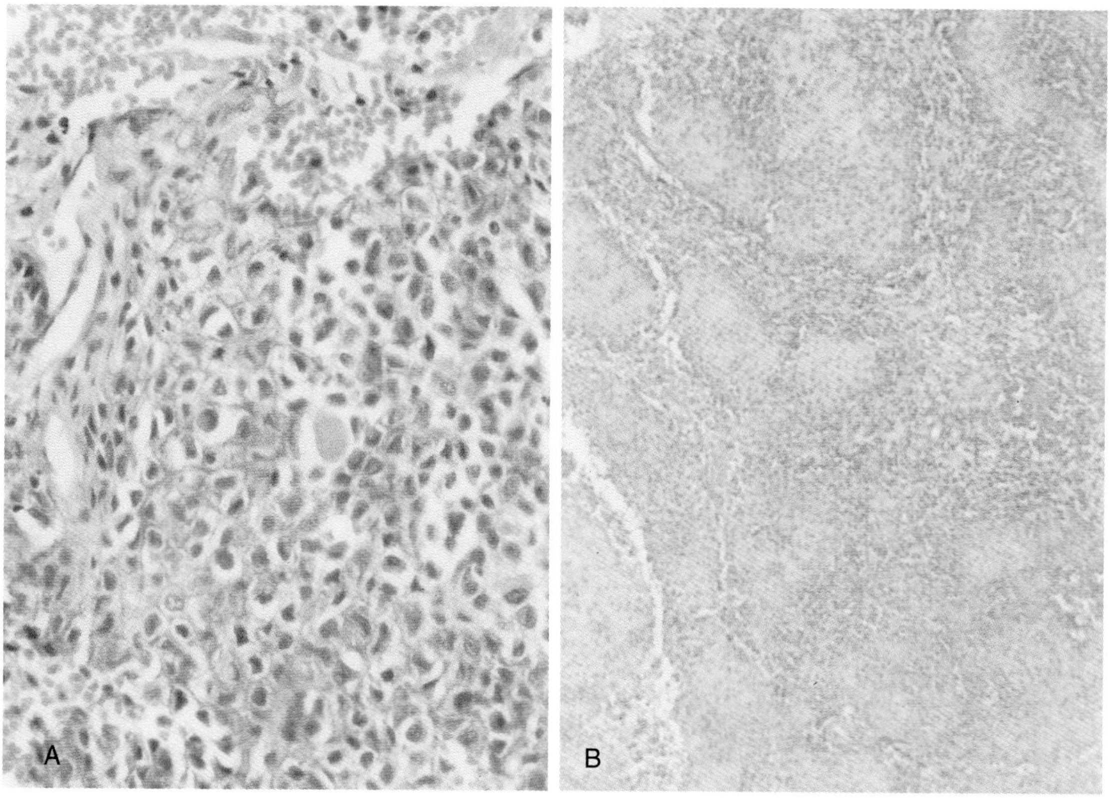

Figure 15–10. Chondroblastoma. *A,* Cellular area composed of polygonal cells with so-called "chicken-wire" calcification caused by mineralization of reticulin fibers around the individual tumor cells. An area of pink chondroid is present at the edge of the field. *B,* Low-power view showing the typical lobularity of chondroblastoma due to alternating areas of pink chondroid and cellular tumor. Osteoclast-like giant cells are present, especially around lobules of pink chondroid.

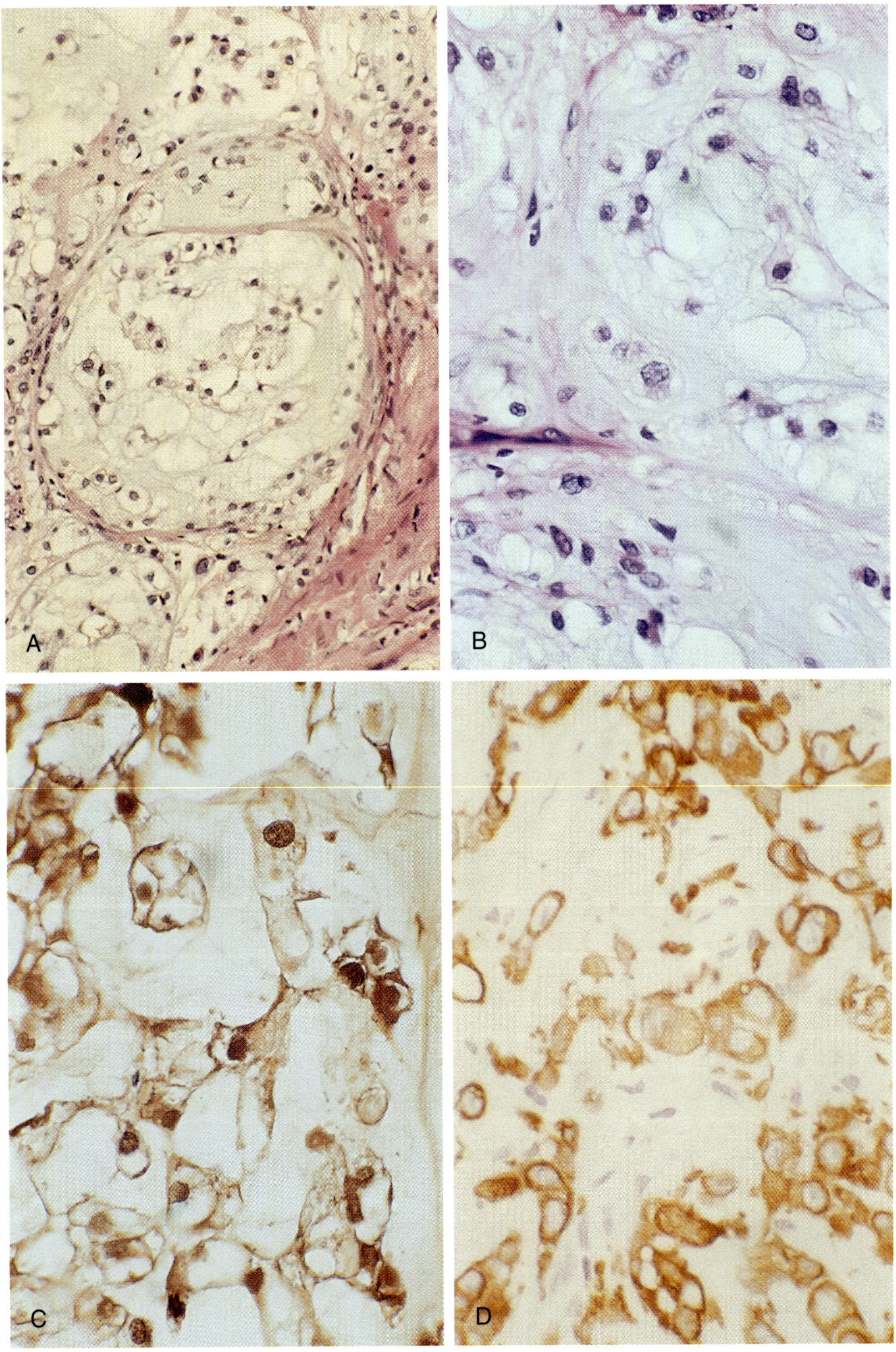

Figure 17–8. Chordoma. *A,* Low-power view of a typical chordoma showing the lobulated arrangement, with clusters of tumor cells surrounded by abundant extracellular mucin. *B,* High-power view of a typical chordoma. The clusters contain physaliphorous cells with numerous intracellular vacuoles. *C,* The nuclei and cytoplasm of the tumor cells stain strongly for S-100 protein. (Immunoperoxidase.) *D,* The cytoplasm of the tumor cells stains strongly for cytokeratins (Immunoperoxidase using CAM 5.2 as the primary antibody, hematoxylin counterstain.)

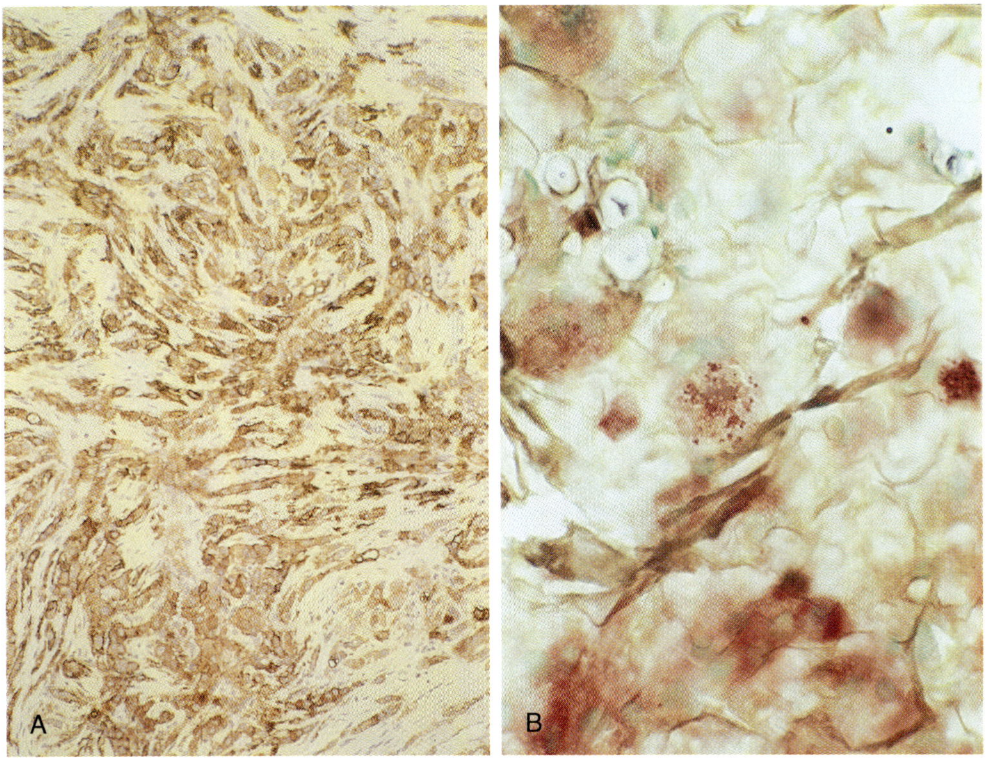

Figure 17–9. Chordoma. *A,* The cytoplasm, and especially the cell and vacuole membranes, stains for epithelial membrane antigen. (Immunopero using HMFG-2 as the primary antibody, hematoxylin counterstains.) *B,* Touch preparation stained for α-naphthyl acetate esterase showing positivity in the cell cytoplasm. (Simultaneous capture technique using hexazonium pararosaniline.)

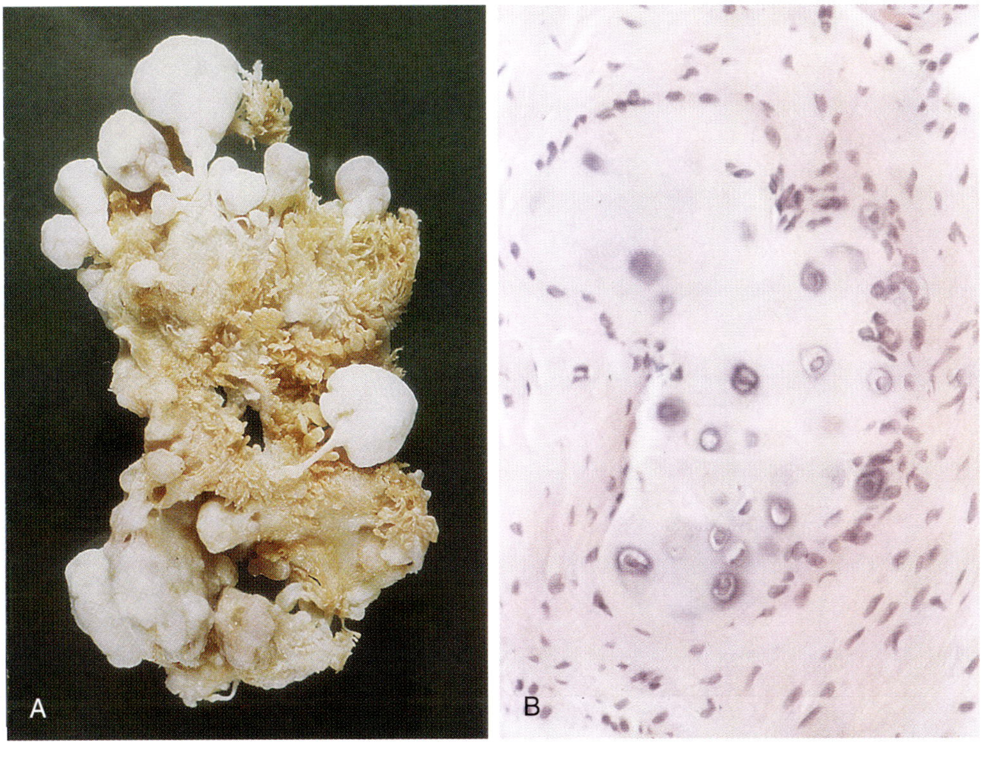

Figure 18–2. Synovial chondromatosis. *A,* Macroscopic appearance of typical synovial chondromatosis with pale cartilaginous nodules projecting from the synovial surface. *B,* A small chondroid nodule in synovial tissue is one of the earliest manifestations of synovial chondromatosis.

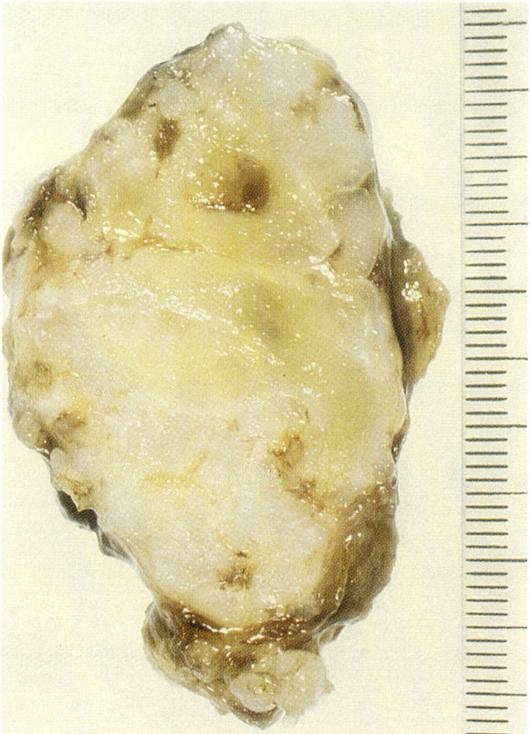

Figure 18–4. Massive synovial chondromatosis. Macroscopic appearance of a lesion of the shoulder that is up to 50 mm in diameter in this aspect.

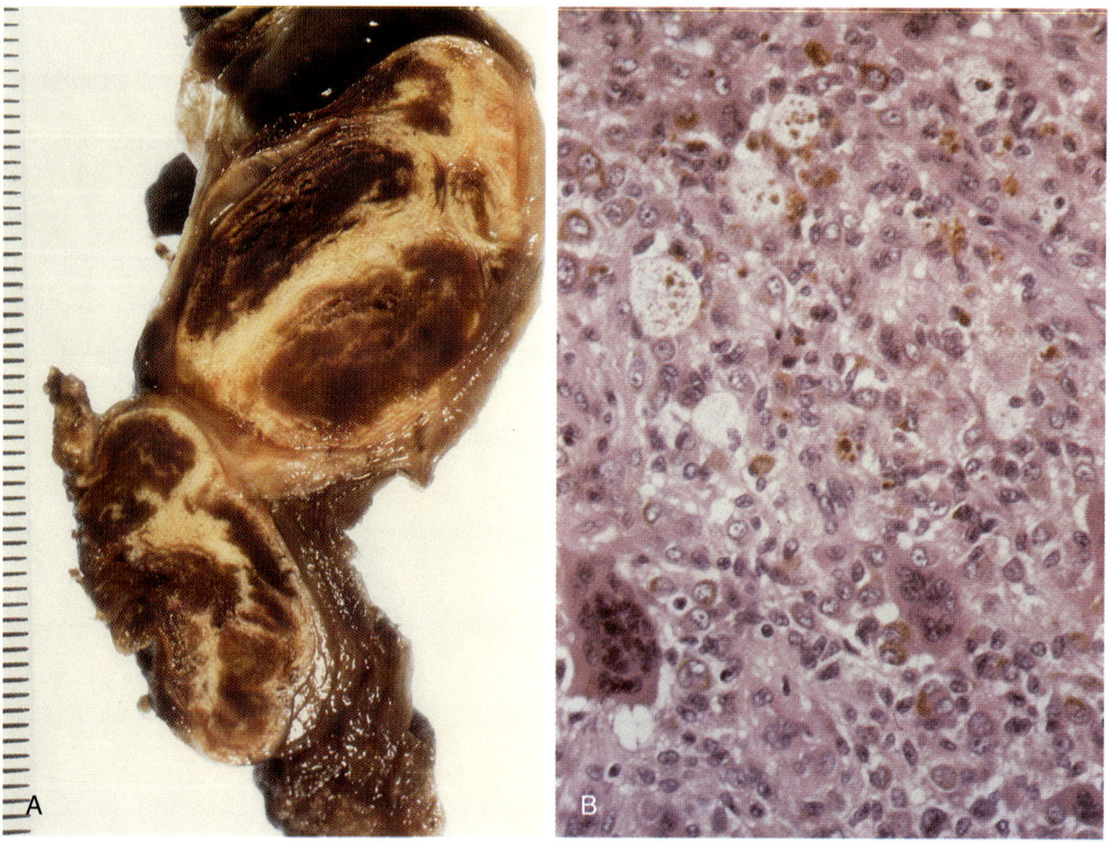

Figure 18–7. Pigmented villonodular synovitis of the elbow. *A,* Macroscopic appearance of predominantly nodular PVNS of the elbow showing the characteristic golden-brown and yellow coloration. *B,* Fibrohistiocytic mononuclear cells contain hemosiderin granules. Two osteoclast-like multinucleate cells are present.

Chapter

1

CLASSIFICATION AND DIAGNOSIS OF BONE NEOPLASMS

TIMOTHY R. HELLIWELL

CLASSIFICATION OF BONE NEOPLASIA

A system for the classification of neoplasia should do the following:

- Describe in unambiguous terms the clinical and pathologic appearances of a neoplasm and the range of appearances that are acceptable for this diagnosis.
- Provide a framework around which therapeutic approaches can be constructed.
- Offer the patient accurate prognostic information about his or her disease.
- Facilitate communication on the best ways in which specific conditions can be diagnosed and treated, both within a single institution and between institutions.

To a large extent, classification requires the labeling of a neoplasm, with the label defining both treatment and prognosis. Many bone neoplasms have a sufficiently characteristic clinical, radiologic, and pathologic appearance to make diagnosis straightforward but, in some instances, classification may be difficult when lesions show a range of appearances that appear to cross diagnostic boundaries. In such cases, even experts will only provide an opinion on the basis that they do not know precisely what label to place on a lesion but they know how it is likely to behave.

Ideally, a diagnostic label should describe a clinicopathologic entity that can be defined in etiologic and molecular genetic terms, with a precise histopathologic correlation and for which there is a specific and effective method of treatment. The rarity of most primary bone neoplasms means that etiologic factors are often not known. For a few neoplasms, particularly Ewing's sarcoma, lymphoma, and osteosarcoma, chemotherapy is specifically designed to optimize the chance of curing the patient and histopathologic methods are important in determining the treatment option. For other neoplasms, this goal has yet to be achieved, and surgery remains the main therapeutic option.

WORLD HEALTH ORGANIZATION CLASSIFICATION OF BONE TUMORS

The most widely accepted classification is that of the World Health Organization (Table 1–1), which was first published in 1972 and revised in 1993.[1] This framework is based on the apparent lines of tissue differentiation and avoids theoretical histogenetic controversies. Histologic criteria, including immunohistochemical studies, and observed patterns of biologic behavior separate primary neoplasms occurring within bone into those forming bone, cartilage, or vessels; giant cell tumor; neoplasms that affect primarily the bone marrow;

Table 1–1. World Health Organization Histologic Classification of Primary Bone Neoplasms and Tumor-like Lesions

Bone-Forming Tumors
Benign
- Osteoma
- Osteoid osteoma
- Osteoblastoma

Intermediate
Aggressive (malignant) osteoblastoma

Malignant
Central osteosarcoma
- Conventional central osteosarcoma
- Telangiectatic osteosarcoma
- Intraosseous well-differentiated (low-grade) osteosarcoma
- Round (small) cell osteosarcoma

Surface osteosarcoma
- Parosteal (juxtacortical) osteosarcoma
- Periosteal osteosarcoma
- High-grade surface osteosarcoma

Cartilage-Forming Tumors
Benign
- Chondroma
  - Enchondroma
  - Periosteal (juxtacortical) chondroma
- Osteochondroma
- Chondroblastoma
- Chondromyxoid fibroma

Malignant
- Typical central chondrosarcoma
- Juxtacortical (periosteal) chondrosarcoma
- Mesenchymal chondrosarcoma
- Dedifferentiated chondrosarcoma
- Clear cell chondrosarcoma
- Malignant chondroblastoma

Giant Cell Tumor

Marrow Tumors (Round Cell Tumors)
Ewing's sarcoma
Primitive neuroectodermal tumor of bone
Malignant lymphoma of bone
Myeloma

Vascular Tumors
Benign
- Hemangioma
- Lymphangioma
- Glomus tumor (glomangioma)

Intermediate or Indeterminate
- Hemangioendothelioma
- Hemangiopericytoma

Malignant
- Angiosarcoma
- Malignant hemangiopericytoma

Other Connective Tissue Tumors
Benign
- Benign fibrous histiocytoma
- Lipoma

Intermediate
- Desmoplastic fibroma

Malignant
- Fibrosarcoma
- Malignant fibrous histiocytoma
- Liposarcoma
- Malignant mesenchymoma
- Leiomyosarcoma
- Undifferentiated sarcoma

Other Tumors
Chordoma
Adamantinoma of long bones
Neurilemoma and neurofibroma

Unclassified Tumors

Tumor-like Lesions
Solitary (simple or unicameral) bone cyst
Aneurysmal bone cyst
Juxta-articular bone cyst (intraosseous ganglion)
Metaphyseal fibrous defect (nonossifying fibroma)
Eosinophilic granuloma (Langerhans' cell histiocytosis)
Fibrous dysplasia and fibro-osseous dysplasia
Myositis ossificans (heterotopic ossification)
Brown tumor of hyperparathyroidism
Intraosseous epidermal cyst
Giant cell (reparative) granuloma

Modified from Schajowitz F: Histological Typing of Bone Tumours. 2nd ed. Berlin, Springer-Verlag, 1993.

and a miscellaneous group of connective tissue, notochordal, and epithelial neoplasms. The classification also recognizes a category of tumor-like lesions that are important to consider in the differential diagnosis of bone tumors.

All primary bone tumors (with the exception of multiple myeloma) are uncommon or rare, and their incidence at a particular institution will depend on the referral pattern of patients and whether clinical or surgical biopsy cases are considered. To provide a general guide as to the relative incidence of different primary bone neoplasms, data from the Mayo Clinic series are used in the following section.[2] In this biopsy series of 7975 primary bone neoplasms, malignant neoplasms were 2.4 times more frequent than benign neoplasms.

The benign bone-forming neoplasms osteoid osteoma and osteoblastoma (together comprising 5% of all primary osseous neoplasms) are recognized as closely related histologic entities, and the category of aggressive osteoblastoma has been introduced to describe a rare, clinically locally aggressive osteoblastic lesion with characteristic histologic features but that does not show the degree of cytologic atypia associated with osteosarcoma and does not metastasize.

Osteosarcoma is now the preferred term (replacing osteogenic sarcoma) for a malignant tumor in which there is bone or osteoid formation by the malignant cells. Osteosarcoma accounts for 30% of malignant bone neoplasms and is divided into central (medullary) and surface (peripheral) osteosarcoma. Each group includes a range of diseases with different biologic behaviors and which may show differing responses to chemotherapy.

Cartilage-forming neoplasms are divided into benign (chondroma, osteochondroma, chondroblastoma, chondromyxoid fibroma) and malignant (chondrosarcoma) groups, and new entities included in the 1993 revision include dedifferentiated chondrosarcoma (in which low-grade and anaplastic components are juxtaposed) and clear cell chondrosarcoma (a low-grade malignancy with a typical epiphyseal location). Osteochondromas account for 9.3% and chondromas for 3.6% of all bone neoplasms, whereas chondrosarcomas account for 20% of all malignant bone neoplasms.

Giant cell tumor of bone (7% of all bone neoplasms) forms a separate group in recognition of its uncertain histogenesis and biologic behavior.

The group of "marrow tumors" includes neoplasms of diverse phenotype that collectively fall into the differential diagnosis of round cell tumors. Immunohistochemical and molecular genetic investigations of these lesions have greatly facilitated the distinction between the Ewing's sarcoma/primitive neuroectodermal tumor type, lymphomas, and multiple myeloma. Multiple myeloma (excluding nonsurgical cases) accounts for 14% of the malignant primary bone neoplasms, and Ewing's sarcoma accounts for 9% of malignancies.

The classification acknowledges that, as in similar lesions of soft tissues, the criteria for the distinction between benign, intermediate, and malignant vascular tumors are not satisfactorily defined, although these are rare tumors in surgical series, accounting for 2.5% of all primary bone neoplasms.

In the group of fibrous neoplasms, the 1993 classification includes benign and malignant fibrous histiocytomas, defined using similar criteria to those used in soft tissue pathology. Many tumors now regarded as malignant fibrous histiocytoma would have formerly been diagnosed as fibrosarcoma, malignant giant cell tumor, or unclassified sarcoma. Fibrosarcoma and malignant fibrous histiocytoma together account for 6% of malignant primary bone neoplasms.

HISTORICAL ASPECTS OF THE CLASSIFICATION OF BONE TUMORS

Primary bone neoplasms are uncommon, but a few cases have been described in archaeologic material. Despite the problems of defining the true nature of diseases in ancient bone, examples of osteochondromas are described in skeletons from Europe and Egypt, dating back as far as 3000 to 2000 BC.[3] A putative osteoid osteoma has been described in a 7th-century Anglo-Saxon femur,[4] and it has been suggested that a humerus from a 140 million-year-old dinosaur may contain a chondrosarcoma.[5]

It is salutary to realize that many of the diagnostic problems that face the modern pathologist are a reflection of the difficulties encountered by previous generations in developing a satisfactory system for the classification of bone tumors. Lessons can therefore be learned from the ways in which the current classification has evolved. The main characteristics of many bone neoplasms were defined during the early 19th century, when it was possible to observe the natural history of many neoplasms. What we now regard as the likely progression of a disease is heavily modified by advances in health service provision that allow the early diagnosis and treatment of these diseases.

Developments over the past two centuries have involved (1) changing fashions and refinements in the semantics of diagnostic terminology; (2) the gradual recognition of new subgroups of tumors as a result of cumulative experience and astute observation; and (3) improvements in diagnostic techniques through the use of electron microscopy, immunohistochemistry, and molecular genetic technology. Some nomenclature has become outdated as knowledge has advanced but is retained as a clinically useful label (e.g., giant cell tumor of bone).

The term *sarcoma* was introduced by Abernethy in 1804 to describe tumors that had a "firm and fleshy feel" and only came to be associated with malignancies of the connective tissues in the mid-19th century by Virchow.[6] Boyer, in 1805, described two types of tumor in bone: osteosarcoma, in which bone was converted to flesh, and "spina ventosa" (literally bag of wind), which was a hemorrhagic dilation of bone that may represent the first description of the giant cell tumor.[6]

Sir Astley Cooper, surgeon to Guy's Hospital in London, clearly described, in 1818, the essential characteristics of what we now know as osteosarcoma and chondrosarcoma in his essay "Exostosis."[7] He separated the range of tumors that arise within bones into periosteal and medullary groups. Cartilaginous tumors are recognized as undergoing ossification, and the lesion termed *cartilaginous exostosis* is clearly a chondrosarcoma. A group of fungus tumors with a softer structure than cartilage and containing bone spicules, which were malignant, most frequent in the femur of younger persons, and metastasized, is reminiscent of osteosarcoma. Cooper attributed the development of "fungous" tumors to "depending upon a peculiar state of constitution and action of vessels."

Sir James Paget recognized many types of bone tumors in his *Lectures on Surgical Pathology* in 1853,[8] which combined clinical and histologic descriptions of what would now be defined as enchondroma, osteochondroma, enchondromatosis of the hands, synovial chondromatosis, chondrosarcoma, multiple hereditary osteochondromas, myositis ossificans, giant cell tumor, and osteosarcoma. He also recognized that "osteoid cancer" could contain a mixture of fibrous, osseous, and cartilaginous material, with spicules of calcified tissue surrounded by cancer cells; and he noted that this type of cancer usually showed rapid growth and was often fatal within 6 months of diagnosis.

The first detailed report of the clinical pathology of bone malignancies is credited to Gross in 1879,[9] who also recognized the importance of the site of a lesion within the bone, the nature of the tumor cells (small or large, osteoid cell, round cell, spindle cell, or giant cell), and the nature of the tumor matrix (ossifying or chondroid) in the classification of bone sarcomas.

Bone-Forming Neoplasms

During the 19th century and the early part of the 20th century, the term *osteogenic sarcoma* was used to describe any malignancy that arose in bone, and there was considerable debate as to whether the terms *osteogenic sarcoma* and *osteosarcoma* should be used to describe tumors derived from bone, tumors producing bone, or tumors derived from cells with the potential to produce bone.[10, 11] This semantic difficulty has now been set aside, and *osteosarcoma* is now the accepted term for a malignant, bone (osteoid)-forming neoplasm.

The proportion of primary bone neoplasms that deserve the label "osteosarcoma" has decreased as cartilaginous tumors, giant cell tumors, and others were recognized as distinct biologic entities with a different behavior from the classic osteosarcoma. Benign bone-forming neoplasms, other than the osteoma of the nasal sinuses, became accepted as specific entities with the description of osteoid osteoma by Jaffe in 1935,[12] although isolated cases had been described previously, some being interpreted as examples of chronic osteomyelitis. Osteoblastoma was described independently in 1956 by Lichtenstein and Jaffe[13, 14] and distinguished from osteosarcoma by its less aggressive behavior. Parosteal osteosarcoma was first described as parosteal osteoma by Geschickter and Copeland in 1951,[15] who recognized that these slow-growing, bone-forming lesions on the surface of bone often demonstrated a malignant, metastatic phenotype if not widely excised.

Cartilaginous Neoplasms

Benign cartilaginous neoplasms had been described in the 19th century (see earlier) with the hereditary form of multiple enchondromas described by Paget and definitively by Ollier[16, 17] and their association with soft tissue angiomas by Maffucci.[18]

The classification of bone sarcomas devised by the Bone Sarcoma Registry of the American College of Surgeons in 1928 recognized the main groups of bone malignancy as being osteogenic sarcoma (with subtypes), giant cell tumors, endothelioma (Ewing's sarcoma), and myeloma (marrow-derived tumors).[11] Chondrosarcoma was described as a biologic entity in 1930,[19] and in 1931 Geschickter and Copeland proposed a classification based on the cartilaginous embryology of bone that, although it had many problems, emphasized the need to include a separate category for cartilaginous tumors.[11] The revised American College of Surgeons classification of 1939 provided for chondroma and chondrosarcoma as separate groups from the osteogenic neoplasms.

The cytologic criteria for the distinction of benign from malignant cartilaginous neoplasms were clearly defined by Lichtenstein and Jaffe,[20] and the relevance of these criteria to the diagnosis and management of cartilaginous tumors was reinforced by Barnes and Catto.[21] Rare types of chondrosarcoma such as the mesenchymal chondrosarcoma were not defined until 1959,[22] in a paper that reviews the overlap of diagnostic criteria for atypical chondroid lesions.

Giant Cell Tumor of Bone

The history of the nomenclature of giant cell tumor of bone has been reviewed by McCarthy.[6] Paget, in 1853, described this tumor as "myeloma" in recognition that its soft, reddish brown appearance resembled bone marrow.[8] *Giant cell sarcoma* was a term used by Gross in 1879[9] and probably included examples of both giant cell tumor and of high-grade malignancies containing multinucleate cells. The clinical concept and conservative management of "myeloid sarcoma" was formulated by Bloodgood in 1910, who recognized that it was not a lesion likely to metastasize and suggested the term *giant cell tumor.*[23] Stewart, in 1922,[24] recognized that the multinucleate cells in this tumor were osteoclasts and suggested the term *osteoclast sarcoma,* which was later modified to *osteoclastoma.* These reports recognized that the giant cell tumor had a wide range of behavior, making the term *sarcoma* appropriate for some cases but not for others. During the 1930s and 1940s, careful clinical, radiologic, and pathologic studies were able to remove from the category of giant cell tumors lesions that had particular characteristics (the so-called giant cell variants). Thus, Codman, in 1931, described the "epiphyseal chondromatous giant cell tumor,"[25] later renamed chondroblastoma by Jaffe and Lichtenstein in 1942,[26] and chondromyxoid fibroma was separated from other giant cell–containing lesions in 1948.[27] The defining features of a true giant cell tumor were enunciated by Jaffe et al. in 1940.[28] The term *giant cell tumor* is retained even though the multinucleate giant cells are not the neoplastic elements of this lesion (see Chapter 15).

Fibrous Neoplasms and Tumor-like Lesions

The recognition of a group of fibrous neoplasms gradually evolved from the changes attributed in the 19th century to hyperparathyroid bone disease (osteitis fibrosa).[23] Periosteal desmoid was described by Kimmelsteil and Rapp in 1951,[29] and desmoplastic fibroma was described by Jaffe in 1958.[30] *Malignant fibrous histiocytoma* was a term coined in the 1960s to describe an aggressive soft tissue sarcoma that in tissue culture produced cells resembling both fibroblasts and histiocytes. Although variously considered to be the most common soft tissue sarcoma, and a distinctly uncommon sarcoma, the term has been retained to describe a pleomorphic spindle cell tumor with a storiform growth pattern that shows no other signs of specific differentiation. Similar lesions have been described in bone.[31, 32] Many tumors now regarded as malignant fibrous histiocytoma would have formerly been diagnosed as fibrosarcoma, malignant giant cell tumor, or unclassified sarcoma—it is not yet clear whether this change in diagnostic fashion has any significant meaning in terms of describing the biologic behavior of an aggressive group of poorly differentiated neoplasms.

Ewing's Sarcoma and Lymphoma

Lucke is credited with the first description in 1866 of the disease that we now know as Ewing's sarcoma (cited by Huvos[33]), with other cases described in the 19th and early 20th centuries under the name of endotheliome. Ewing, in 1921 and 1924, drew attention to this primary malignant bone tumor that he designated "diffuse endothelioma" or "endothelial myeloma."[34, 35] The histologic features of Ewing's sarcoma can be clearly delineated from those of other similar round cell tumors.[36] There was controversy regarding the histogenesis of this sarcoma until the recognition of cytogenetic and molecular abnormalities similar to primitive neuroectodermal tumors (see Chapter 14).

Malignant lymphoma arising in bones was described by Weiland in 1901,[37] with reliable and consistent separation of reticulum cell sarcoma from Ewing's sarcoma described by Oberling in 1928 and 1932.[38, 39]

Vascular Neoplasms

Hemangioma was first described in the English literature in 1845 by Toynbee.[40] Many of the earliest descriptions of malignant vascular tumors of bone appear to be unreliable and are examples of metastatic carcinomas, Ewing's sarcoma, or hemangioma.[41] Kolodny, in 1926, provided the first adequate description of hemangioendothelioma of bone,[42] whereas Thomas, in 1942 (who excluded Ewing's endothelioma from the vascular neoplasms),[43] and Stout, in 1943,[44] provided the basis of the modern classification. Even so, by comparison with the developments in the classification of vascular neoplasms in the soft tissues, the classification of osseous vascular neoplasms has remained confused. There appears to be a good argument for adopting the nomenclature of the soft tissue vascular neoplasms in bone pathology so that the relatively small numbers of cases can be sensibly categorized (see Chapter 16).

Aneurysmal bone cyst was described in the earlier literature of the 20th century[45] but was first clearly defined by Jaffe and Lichtenstein in 1942,[46] who separated this disease from the simple unicameral bone cyst, giant cell tumor, and sarcomas.

Adamantinoma

Adamantinoma is an enigmatic neoplasm typically located in the tibia. Although this was the term used to describe this lesion as long ago as 1913,[47] by virtue of its resemblance to similar lesions (ameloblastomas) in the jaw, doubts as to its histogenesis have led to changes in terminology, including a malignant angioblastoma[48] and dermal inclusion tumor of bone.[49] The term *adamantinoma* is now established as a defining label, regardless of the precise histogenesis.

A DIAGNOSTIC STRATEGY FOR THE DIAGNOSIS OF BONE NEOPLASMS

All the contributors to this book emphasize that it is essential to combine clinical, radiologic, and microscopic observations when approaching the diagnosis of bone neoplasms. Although this approach may appear daunting to the trainee pathologist, radiologist, oncologist, or surgeon, it is a strategy that has been proved by experience as the best way to avoid clinical disasters.

Those involved in the diagnosis and management of patients with bone neoplasms must recognize the complementary nature of the information that is obtained from radiographs, histologic studies, and clinical features and to have the humility to accept that their initial opinions, reached in isolation, may need to be modified in the light of the additional information that others provide. Experience in these fields is essential to ensure the optimal management for patients, and many of the problems that are referred to experts arise as much from a lack of radiologic osteoarticular expertise as from histopathologic inexperience.

The contributions required from the different disciplines will vary depending on the nature of the lesion. The combination of the age of the patient, the site, and radiologic appearance are sufficient in some instances to provide a sufficiently accurate diagnosis for management. In some situations (e.g., osteochondroma, metaphyseal fibrous cortical defect), no treatment may be required unless complications develop, whereas in other cases (e.g., an epiphyseal lesion in a long bone that may be a giant cell tumor or a chondroblastoma), the initial treatment by thorough curettage may be unaffected by the precise histologic diagnosis. However, in those situations in which radical surgery or chemotherapy is being considered, cytologic or histologic examination of the lesion is mandatory before treatment is begun.

There is a twilight zone of lesions that show minimal histologic atypia (e.g., some borderline chondroid lesions and parosteal bone-forming lesions) and that tend to recur locally and may eventually metastasize if they are not widely excised. An accurate interpretation of the radiologic appearances and an appreciation of the growth pattern are essential to reach the correct diagnosis and thus to avoid problems with recurrent tumor and eventual metastasis.

Once an initial impression of the tumor is obtained, the histopathologist should be able to discuss the differential diagnosis with his or her radiologic and clinical colleagues. If one assumes that both radiologist and pathologist have reasonable expertise in osteoarticular work, the following scenarios may emerge:[50]

- If the primary radiologic and histological diagnoses are the same, the possibility of error is small.
- If the primary histologic diagnosis matches one of the radiologic differential diagnoses, then the histologic diagnosis is probably safe.

- If the histologic diagnosis was not considered by the radiologist (owing to the rarity of the disease), the radiologic information should be re-evaluated.
- If the radiologic and histologic diagnoses are incompatible, then the histologic material should be re-evaluated to assess whether it is likely to be adequate and representative of the whole lesion and whether more tissue should be examined (more blocks or rebiopsy).

Clinical Aspects of Diagnosis

A patient with a bone neoplasm usually presents with nonspecific symptoms of pain and interference with normal function. Swelling of the tissues may or may not be noticed. Clinical examination is also often not diagnostic, although the presence of a soft tissue mass and raised local tissue temperature are suggestive of an aggressive malignancy.

The age of the patient is probably the most important clinical clue to the clinicoradiologic diagnosis, because most bone neoplasms develop within a 20- to 30-year age range (Table 1–2). In patients older than 40 years of age, the most likely diagnoses are metastatic carcinoma or multiple myeloma and clearly an appropriate clinical history should be obtained and investigations undertaken.

Table 1–2. Age Range of Peak Incidence of Bone Tumors

Peak Age Incidence (Years)	Tumor Type
0–10	Neuroblastoma
5–20	Simple bone cyst
	Nonossifying fibroma
	Ewing's sarcoma
10–25	Chondroblastoma
	Osteochondroma
	Osteoblastoma
	Osteosarcoma (conventional)
10–35	Osteoid osteoma
	Aneurysmal bone cyst
	Chondromyxoid fibroma
25–45	Giant cell tumor
	Primary lymphoma of bone
30–60	Chondroma (5–50)
	Hemangioma
	Malignant fibrous histiocytoma
	Parosteal osteosarcoma
	Chondrosarcoma
40–80	Myeloma
	Metastasis
	Chordoma
60–65	Osteosarcoma (Paget's associated)

Biochemical investigations should include serum calcium level and alkaline phosphatase level, both as indicators of a destructive bone lesion and to exclude hyperparathyroid bone disease or Paget's disease. Measurement of immunoglobulins and protein electrophoresis is required if myeloma is suggested, and prostate-specific antigen levels should be determined if there may be prostatic disease.

Radiologic Aspects of Diagnosis

The radiologic diagnosis of bone neoplasia is discussed in detail in Chapter 6. The radiologist should be aware of the clinical presentation of a lesion and, on the basis of the radiologic investigations, will be able to offer a provisional diagnosis or differential diagnosis. Plain radiographs are the most informative diagnostic investigation, providing details of the precise site within the bone, the nature of any calcific matrix within the tumor, and the nature of the interface between a tumor and the surrounding bone that is determined by the balance between the destructive tendency of the tumor and the vigor of the reaction of the bone to the presence of the tumor. Radiographs and other imaging investigations also provide information on the transgression of compartmental boundaries.

It is important to perform imaging studies before biopsy, even if metastatic disease or myeloma are suspected. Occasionally, the eventual diagnosis will be that of an unsuspected primary bone neoplasm, the management of which may depend critically on the way in which diagnostic information was obtained. Imaging studies may be impossible to accurately interpret if they are performed after a biopsy.

The Role of the Biopsy in Diagnosis

Once the clinical and radiologic data have been combined, a biopsy might be considered to obtain a tissue diagnosis. Before biopsy it is important to consider whether a localized bone lesion might be due to a non-neoplastic disorder, such as trauma (stress fracture or myositis ossificans), metabolic bone disease, bone infarction or infection, or a primary synovial disease affecting juxta-articular bone. If these conditions are consciously excluded, major errors of management will usually be avoided.

A biopsy should always be undertaken with the possible surgical options for definitive treatment in mind, and any biopsy site placed so that, if necessary, it can be excised at a later date without compromising tissue compartments or affecting the nature of limb-sparing surgery.[51] Biopsy samples should, in general, be taken through muscles rather than along fascial or intermuscular planes and should avoid major neurovascular bundles.

The method used (fine-needle aspiration, needle core, or open biopsy) to obtain diagnostic tissue depends, in part, on the nature of the clinical problem, but the general principle should be to obtain sufficient viable tissue to ensure that a diagnosis can be made while also minimizing the risk of potential complications. The method chosen obviously depends on the expertise of the pathologist in interpreting small fine-needle aspirates or needle core samples. Because the lesion may not be neoplastic, tissue should always be sent for microbiologic investigation.

If a soft tissue mass is present adjacent to a bone lesion, then a biopsy of the bone should be avoided, so as to minimize the possibility of precipitating a pathologic fracture and the likelihood of hemorrhage. It is also helpful to the pathologist if the interface between tumor and normal tissue can be sampled, especially in cartilaginous tumors.

Needle core or fine-needle aspiration biopsies are preferred in many situations, because they minimize the risk of complications and, if multiple samples are obtained from a lesion, the problems of sampling variation are reduced. The small size of these tissue samples reduces the flexibility of the pathologist in the range of tests that can be performed, and it may not be possible to perform cytogenetic studies, some molecular studies, or flow cytometry, for example, in these cases. Nevertheless, the sophistication of immunohistochemical and molecular genetic tests means that it is possible to obtain a diagnosis on such samples in 70 to 80% of cases.[52, 53] Fine-needle aspiration biopsies are more limited by the relative inaccessibility of calcified tissues to this technique and the problem of obtaining adequate material from cystic or necrotic lesions (see Chapter 7), but for the diagnosis of metastatic carcinoma or multiple myeloma this is often the method of choice. Low-grade cartilaginous or osseous malignancies are more easily diagnosed by open biopsy in which sampling problems can be avoided and the tissue architecture retained.[54]

When embarking on the diagnostic process, it may be pragmatic in most situations to try to make the diagnosis on small tissue samples and reserve open biopsy for the lesions in which needle biopsy is inadequate. In cases in which it is imperative to obtain an accurate diagnosis as rapidly as possible, open biopsy may be indicated to be sure of obtaining diagnostic material.

Tissue Handling

The macroscopic assessment of a specimen is important and should be undertaken with knowledge of the clinical and radiologic appearances, particularly for resection specimens. Macroscopic photography and specimen radiography are often invaluable in recording information and helping to interpret histologic information. The appropriate selection of tissue blocks from resection specimens is essential to reaching a diagnosis rapidly and economically. Whenever possible, tissue blocks should be taken perpendicular to normal tissue or to periosteum to demonstrate the interface between lesional and normal tissues.

Few pathologists have the necessary experience to provide a definitive diagnosis on bone neoplasms on the basis of a frozen section. This is because the quality of the histologic detail in frozen sections is inferior to that obtained after processing to paraffin wax and thin sectioning. The use of this technique will therefore vary between institutions, although generally frozen sections may be used to confirm that neoplastic tissue has been obtained at the biopsy even if a definitive diagnosis will have to be deferred until paraffin sections have been examined.

The diagnosis of many bone tumors can be made from the soft tissues included with a biopsy specimen. Calcified tissues need to be demineralized before they can be processed and sectioned by placing the tissue into acidic solution. For tissues requiring rapid decalcification, 5% or 10% nitric acid can be used; and this method, if carefully controlled,[55] provides good results without interference with routine or immunohistochemical stains. Slower decalcification can be achieved using 20% formic acid in 10% formalin or ethylenediaminetetraacetic acid. Whatever method is used, it is essential to avoid overexposure of the tissue to the acid, either by weighing the tissue, specimen radiography, or chemically using the ammonium chloride test.[55]

Histologic Assessment

For the histopathologist, the first practical consideration of the diagnosis of a bone neoplasm will result from the microscopic examination of the tissues.

At low magnification, it is useful to assess the following:

- Overall tissue architecture, including the relationship between lesional tissue and the surrounding bone, noting, in particular, whether there are any reactive changes.
- Cellular pattern—whether the tumor is composed of sheets of cells or has a lobular pattern; are areas of necrosis or hemorrhage present?
- Matrix production—a general impression is gained as to whether the tissue is forming bone or cartilage or whether it is nonspecific spindle celled or round cell tissue without matrix production; the presence of many multinucleate giant cells will also be obvious at low magnification.

At higher magnification, the presence or nature of matrix production may become more obvious, but it is the cytologic features of the cells that will be of most concern. The identification of cell types is achieved by observing the following:

- Morphology of the cells—size and shape of nuclei and cytoplasm.
- Cell function—matrix production, phagocytosis, alkaline phosphatase activity.
- Antigenic profile by immunohistochemistry.

Histologic Features of Bony and Cartilaginous Matrix

Osteoblastic tissue is that in which the component cells have the potential to form osteoid (collagenous tissue that tends to calcify). Osteoid formation occurs in normal tissue as well as in reactive and neoplastic situations. The pattern in which the collagen is laid down can be determined by polarizing microscopy and may provide a clue as to the nature of the disease. Lamellar bone is normal, whereas woven bone can be reactive or neoplastic. In general, the greater the degree of organization of the bone into trabeculae, the less malignant the tissue. It is also helpful to consider the nature of the cells between the bone trabeculae; in reactive bone, vascular granulation tissue occupies the space between the osteoblasts forming bone trabeculae, whereas in (malignant) neoplasms this region is often occupied by neoplastic cells.

Chondroid tissue is that in which the component cells have the ability to form cartilage. This type of matrix may be recognized by metachromatic staining with dyes such as toluidine blue. Depending on the type of hematoxylin used, chondroid matrix may appear very pale (Harris's hematoxylin) or may have a basophilic hue (Ehrlich's hematoxylin).

Histochemistry and Immunohistochemistry

Alkaline phosphatase is an enzyme that is essential for the mineralization of normal bone by osteoblasts. The histochemical demonstration of alkaline phosphatase in frozen sections or cytologic imprints of the neoplastic cells therefore provides a marker of osteoblastic lineage.

The many and varied uses of immunohistochemical techniques are described in the following chapters, and only a few general points are considered here. Although there have been major advances in the development of monoclonal antibodies to particular tissue antigens, and in the sensitivity of the methods to detect antibody binding to tissue sections, it is essential to realize that the optimal immunohistochemical labeling of tissue sections or cytologic preparations may be impossible if the tissue has not been optimally handled before labeling is attempted. Different antigenic epitopes have different degrees of sensitivity to the time of tissue fixation, the nature of decalcification protocols, and the methods of tissue processing, including lipid extraction. Each laboratory therefore needs to define the appropriate methods for the identification of each antigen and to include both positive and negative control sections along with those under test. For many tumors it is usually possible to select a tissue block that includes normal tissue alongside the tumor, and this will provide an in-built control for many of the variables. Antigen-retrieval techniques including the use of microwave heating or pressure cooking of sections have improved the sensitivity of immunohistochemical methods for antigens that were previously difficult to identify in paraffin sections. It is important to realize that the diagnostic and prognostic significance of the detection of very low levels of antigens may differ from that of high levels and that cross-reactions between antibodies and epitopes on other (nonspecific) proteins that have a low binding affinity may be recognized by these techniques. The use of appropriate control tissues is essential for the accurate interpretation of these methods.

A diagnosis should never be made on the basis of labeling with a single antibody, because these are very rarely specific for one cell type. Neoplastic tissues often show unexpected antigen expression, which may be greater in the field of mesenchymal neoplasms owing to the phenotypic plasticity of normal mesenchymal tissues. An example of unexpected antigen expression is cytokeratin expression in chondroblastomas and some osteosarcomas.[56, 57] The results of immunohistochemical labeling studies should always be expressed in terms of the antigenic profile of a tumor (i.e., the balance of positive and negative results). In the differential diagnosis of Ewing's sarcoma, lymphoma, and rhabdomyosarcoma, for example, *MIC2* (CD99), CD45, and desmin should be included in the panel (see Chapter 14). Immunohistochemical results must always be interpreted in the light of the morphologic appearances on hematoxylin and eosin–stained sections and the clinical and radiologic findings. If there are major differences between the immunohistochemical pattern of antigen expression and the diagnostic opinions derived from the other modalities, then all studies should be carefully re-evaluated.

The use of immunohistochemical investigations as prognostic markers for bone neoplasms has received relatively little attention, mainly owing to the rarity of most neoplasms. The potential value of the detection of expression of the multidrug resistance gene in bone sarcomas is considered in detail in Chapter 8. The identification of cell cycle–related markers such as proliferating cell nuclear antigen and the Ki67-detected antigen appears to be related to the grade of osteosarcoma and chondrosarcoma, but it is not yet clear whether their expression is an independent prognostic variable.[57, 58] Other proliferation-related markers such as DNA ploidy and silver-stained nucleolar organizer regions may provide grade-related information in osteosarcomas and chondrosarcomas.[59–61]

Histologic Grading of Bone Tumors

The Enneking system for the staging of musculoskeletal neoplasms (see later) uses a combined clinical, radiologic, and histologic assessment to define the grade of a neoplasm. The histopathologist will provide a histologic grade based on the cytologic features of the neoplasm, although it is important to be aware of the limitations of this method in isolation, particularly for cartilaginous neoplasms.

Most histologic grading systems are based on the work of Broders, who originally classified squamous carcinomas of the lips[62] but later applied his principles to other neoplasms,[63] relating the grade of a tumor to prognosis. Broders based his grading on the degree of cellularity, the degree of pleomorphism, mitotic activity, and evidence of invasion and necrosis. Details of the grading of specific bone neoplasms are provided in the following chapters and are summarized elsewhere.[64]

Histopathologists tend not to formally evaluate each feature in isolation but base the grade on a subjective amalgamation of the various features. The degree of nuclear atypia (pleomorphism, hyperchromasia) determines the grade for bone tumors, because the presence of necrosis and hemorrhage and, to a lesser extent, mitotic activity cannot be reliably determined on small biopsy fragments that are increasingly used to determine the diagnosis and pre-resection treatment. The separation into different grades on an arbitrary three- or four-point scale may please the surgeon or oncologist with its apparent precision, but it is a highly subjective process largely based on an experience of the range of cytologic degrees of malignancy that are possible for a particular neoplasm.

Grading has a limited application in bone neoplasia. Benign neoplasms are not graded; and of the malignant neoplasms, only those that show variations in their appearances between tumors are graded. Thus, all Ewing's sarcomas are regarded as high-grade (poorly differentiated) malignancies. Giant cell tumors are not graded histologically because this is not of prognostic value.[65]

Classic osteosarcomas are Grade 3 or 4 (on a four-point scale), whereas parosteal osteosarcomas are Grade 1 and periosteal osteosarcomas are usually Grade 1 or 2. The histologic grade is generally uniform throughout a particular tumor. If areas of high-grade tumor occur in an otherwise typical low-grade tumor, the tumor is described as showing dedifferentiation. This terminology, although accepted as a clinical diagnosis, is unlikely to be correct in terms of the biology of these tumors in which daughter clones of cells are considered to show divergent differentiation into different histologic patterns.[66]

Chondrosarcomas are graded on a three-point scale (see Chapter 10). Because there is often variation in the histologic pattern from area to area within a single tumor, examination of all the tissue in a biopsy is essential to provide a grade that describes the most aggressive pattern in a tumor.

Histologic grading of fibrosarcomas (see Chapter 12) and of angiosarcomas (see Chapter 16) is also useful.

MANAGEMENT AND STAGING OF NEOPLASMS

Historically, the management of malignant bone neoplasms involved radical surgery, with amputation regarded as the optimal treatment in many cases. Advances in the use of radiotherapy and chemotherapy for the treatment of sarcomas over the past three decades have led to the development of more sophisticated surgical options, such as limb-sparing bone resection and prosthetic or allograft replacement as the main methods to achieving local disease control. The decision as to which method of surgery should be employed is determined partly by the radiologic definition of the extent of spread of a lesion (stage) and partly by the histologic type and grade of the neoplasm. The accurate staging and grading of neoplasms is essential for the meaningful comparison of treatment regimens, and a variety of staging systems have been developed.

The detailed management of patients with osteoarticular neoplasms is beyond the scope of this chapter,[67] but the basic principles of staging and treatment are important considerations for the pathologist who reports such tumors. The most commonly used system for the staging of skeletal neoplasms is that devised by Enneking at the University of Florida, evaluated by the Musculoskeletal Tumour Society and subsequently adopted by the American Joint Committee for Cancer Staging and End Results Reporting.[67, 68] The American Joint Committee system is derived from knowledge of the evolution of musculoskeletal neoplasms and stratifies neoplasms by grade, anatomic site, and metastasis.

Grading in the American Joint Committee System

The grade is an assessment of the biologic aggressiveness of a neoplasm determined from a combination of histologic, radiologic, and clinical features. Details of histologic aspects of grading are described in the previous section, and radiologic features are presented in Chapter 6. The following is a summary of the features used to grade neoplasms in the American Joint Committee system:

- G0 (benign)—cytologically benign, well-differentiated neoplasm with a low to moderate cell-to-matrix ratio; radiologically Lodwick Grade IA, IB, or IC and clearly demarcated from the surrounding tissue; clinically has a distinct capsule with no metastases and a variable growth rate.
- G1 (low grade malignant)—cytologically Broders' Grade 1 or 2, with few mitoses, moderate differentiation, and distinct matrix production; radiologically Lodwick Grade II with indolent invasive features; clinically grows slowly with spread beyond any capsular zone and with uncommon distant metastasis.
- G2 (high grade malignant)—cytologically Broders' Grade 2, 3, or 4 with frequent mitoses, poor differentiation, and sparse and immature matrix; radiologically Lodwick Grade III with a destructive and invasive pattern; clinically these neoplasms grow rapidly, produce symptoms, show growth beyond any capsule, and often show distant metastases.

The behavior of G0 lesions and the distinction of G0 from G1 lesions are often difficult to predict from histologic features alone, and radiologic criteria are important. The distinction between G1 and G2 neoplasms is mainly based on cytologic features, and radiologic features are mainly confirmatory. Although some osteoarticular neoplasms often show a preponderance of lesions as either G1 (parosteal osteosarcoma, secondary chondrosarcoma, chordoma, adamantinoma) or G2 (classic osteosarcoma, Paget's sarcoma, malignant fibrous histiocytoma), exceptions occur, and each lesion must be assessed on its own characteristics.

Anatomic Site

The anatomic site has a direct relationship to the choice of surgical procedure and the prognosis. The staging category is determined by clinical and imaging studies:

- T0—the lesion remains within its capsule and does not extend beyond the borders of its compartment of origin.
- T1—the lesion has extracapsular extensions (in continuity or as satellite nodules), but both the lesion and the surrounding reactive zone are contained within an anatomic compartment bounded by natural barriers to tumor extension (cortical bone, articular cartilage, joint capsule, periosteum). For bones and joints, the compartments are intraosseous, intra-articular, and parosseous (the latter is a potential compartment for lesions arising on the surface of bone that have not invaded either the underlying cortical bone or the adjacent soft tissue).
- T2—lesions extending beyond their compartmental boundaries, either by spread from a previous intracompartmental lesion or by transmission after trauma or surgical intervention.

Metastasis

Unlike staging systems for carcinomas in which metastases are stratified according to whether they occur in regional lymph nodes or distant sites, for sarcomas the involvement of nodes or distant organs has the same prognostic importance:

- M0—no evidence of regional or distant metastasis.
- M1—metastasis present.

The main staging categories are summarized in Table 1–3. Some lesions tend to cluster at particular stages (e.g., classic osteosarcomas tend to be stage IIB at presentation), whereas others show a more even spread of stages at presentation (e.g., giant cell tumor of bone).

Table 1–3. Main Staging Categories of Bone Neoplasms

Stage	Grade	Site	Metastasis
IA	G1	T1	M0
IB	G1	T2	M0
IIA	G2	T1	M0
IIB	G2	T2	M0
IIIA	G1–2	T1	M1
IIIB	G1–2	T2	M1

From Enneking WF: A system of staging musculoskeletal neoplasms. Clin Orthop Rel Res 204:9,1986.

Staging and Surgical Treatment

It is important that the pathologist can communicate effectively with the surgeon and describe the adequacy of local excision of a tumor (see Chapter 8). Surgical margins can be described as *intracapsular* (or intralesional), in which the plane of dissection is within the lesion and tumor is present at the margin; *marginal,* in which the plane of dissection is within the reactive pseudocapsule of the tumor and reactive tissue and/or microsatellites of tumor are present histologically; *wide,* in which the plane of dissection is within normal tissue beyond the reactive zone (this may leave skip-lesions in situ); or *radical,* in which the plane of dissection is outside the tissue compartment containing the tumor.

REFERENCES

1. Schajowitz F: Histological typing of bone tumours. 2nd ed. Berlin, Springer-Verlag, 1993.
2. Unni KK: Introduction and scope of study. *In* Dahlin's Bone Tumors: General Aspects and Data on 11,087 Cases. 5th ed. Philadelphia, Lippincott-Raven, 1996, p 1.
3. Chamberlain AT, Rogers S, Romanowski AJ: Osteochondroma in a British Neolithic skeleton. Br J Hosp Med 47:51, 1992.
4. Wells C: A pathological Anglo-Saxon femur. Br J Radiol 38:393, 1965.
5. Newman ME: Fossil tumour creates interest in prehistoric cancers. J Natl Cancer Inst 83:1289, 1991.
6. McCarthy EF: Giant cell tumor of bone: An historical perspective. Clin Orthop Rel Res 153:14, 1980.
7. Cooper A: Exostosis. *In* Cooper A, Travers B (eds): Surgical essays. 3rd ed. London, Cox & Son, 1818, p 155.
8. Paget J: Tumours. *In* Lectures on Surgical Pathology. London, Longman, Brown, Green & Longmans, 1853, p 171.
9. Gross SW: Sarcoma of the long bones: Based upon a study of one hundred and sixty five cases. Am J Med Sci 78:17, 1879.
10. Kolodny A: Bone sarcoma: The primary malignant tumors of bone and the giant cell tumor. Surg Gynecol Obstet 44(suppl 1):1, 1927.
11. Ewing J: A review of the classification of bone tumors. Surg Gynecol Obstet 68:971, 1939.

12. Jaffe HL: Osteoid osteoma: A benign osteoblastic tumor composed of osteoid and atypical bone. Arch Surg 31:709, 1935.
13. Lichtenstein L: Benign osteoblastoma: A category of osteoid and bone forming tumors other than classical osteoid osteoma which may be mistaken for giant cell tumor or osteogenic sarcoma. Cancer 9:1044, 1956.
14. Jaffe HL: Benign osteoblastoma. Bull Hosp Jt Dis 17:141, 1956.
15. Geschickter CF, Copeland MM: Parosteal osteoma of bone: A new entity. Ann Surg 133:790, 1951.
16. Ollier M: Exostoses osteogeniques multiples. Lyon Med 88:484, 1889.
17. Ollier M: Dyschondroplasie. Lyon Med 93:23, 1900.
18. Maffucci A: Di un caso di encondroma ed angioma multiple: Contribuzione alla genesi embrionale dei tumori. Mov Med Chir 13:399, 1881.
19. Phemister DB: Chondrosarcoma of bone. Surg Gynecol Obstet 50:216, 1930.
20. Lichtenstein L, Jaffe HL: Chondrosarcoma of bone. Am J Pathol 19:553, 1943.
21. Barnes R, Catto M: Chondrosarcoma of bone. J Bone Joint Surg 48B:729, 1966.
22. Lichtenstein L, Bernstein D: Unusual benign and malignant chondroid tumours of bone. Cancer 12:1142, 1959.
23. Bloodgood JC: Benign bone cysts, osteitis fibrosa, giant cell sarcoma and bone aneurism of the long pipe bones: A clinical and pathological study with the conclusion that conservative treatment is justifiable. Ann Surg 52:145, 1910.
24. Stewart MJ: The histogenesis of myeloid sarcoma. Lancet 2:1106, 1922.
25. Codman EA: Epiphyseal chondromatous giant cell tumours of the upper end of the humerus. Surg Gynecol Obstet 52:543, 1931.
26. Jaffe HL, Lichtenstein L: Benign chondroblastoma of bone: A reinterpretation of the so-called calcifying or chondromatous giant cell tumor. Am J Pathol 18:969, 1942.
27. Jaffe HL, Lichtenstein L: Chondromyxoid fibroma of bone: A distinctive benign tumour likely to be mistaken especially for chondrosarcoma. Arch Pathol 45:541, 1948.
28. Jaffe HL, Lichtenstein L, Portis RB: Giant cell tumor of bone: Its pathologic appearance, grading, supposed variants and treatment. Arch Pathol 30:993, 1940.
29. Kimmelsteil P, Rapp IH: Cortical defect due to periosteal desmoids. Bull Hosp Jt Dis 12:286, 1951.
30. Jaffe HL: Desmoplastic fibroma. *In* Tumors and Tumorous Conditions of the Bones and Joints. Philadelphia, Lea & Febiger, 1958, p 629.
31. Huvos AG: Primary malignant fibrous histiocytoma of bone: Clinicopathologic study of 18 patients. NY State J Med 76:552, 1976.
32. Dahlin DC, Unni KK, Matsuno T: Malignant (fibrous) histiocytoma of bone—fact or fancy? Cancer 39:1508, 1977.
33. Huvos AG: Ewing's sarcoma. *In* Bone Tumors: Diagnosis, Treatment and Prognosis. Philadelphia, WB Saunders, 1979, p 322.
34. Ewing J: Diffuse endothelioma of bone. Proc NY Pathol Soc 21:17, 1921.
35. Ewing J: Further report on endothelial myeloma of bone. Proc NY Pathol Soc 24:93, 1924.
36. Ball J, Freedman L, Sissons HA: Malignant round cell tumours of bone: An analytical histological study from the Cancer Research Campaign's Bone Tumour Panel. Br J Cancer 36:254, 1977.
37. Wieland E: Studien uber das primar multipel auftretende lymphosarcom der knochen. Virchows Arch [A] Pathol Anat 166:103, 1901.
38. Oberling C: Les réticulosarcomes et les reticuloendotheliosarcomes de la moelle osseuse (sarcomes d'Ewing). Bull Assoc Fr Cancer 17:259, 1928.
39. Oberling C, Raileanu C: Nouvelles recherches sur les réticulosarcomes de la moelle osseuse (sarcomes d'Ewing). Bull Assoc Fr Cancer 21:333, 1932.
40. Toynbee J: An account of two vascular tumours developed in the substance of bone. Lancet 2:676, 1845.
41. Huvos AG: Angiosarcoma of bone. *In* Bone Tumours: Diagnosis, Treatment and Prognosis. Philadelphia, WB Saunders, 1979, p 358.
42. Kolodny A: Angio-endothelioma of bone. Arch Surg 12:854, 1926.
43. Thomas A: Vascular tumors of bone: A pathological and clinical study of twenty-seven cases. Surg Gynecol Obstet 74:777, 1942.
44. Stout AP: Hemangio-endothelioma: A tumour of blood vessels featuring vascular endothelial cells. Ann Surg 118:445, 1943.
45. Gaylord HR: On the pathology of so-called bone aneurisms. Ann Surg 37:834, 1903.
46. Jaffe HL, Lichtenstein L: Solitary unicameral bone cyst: With emphasis on the roentgen picture, the pathologic appearance and the pathogenesis. Arch Surg 44:1004, 1942.
47. Fischer B: Uber ein primares adamantinom der tibia. Frankf Z Pathol 12:422, 1913.
48. Changus GW, Speed JS, Stewart FW: Malignant angioblastoma of bone: A reappraisal of adamantinoma of long bone. Cancer 10:540, 1957.
49. Lichtenstein L: Dermal inclusion tumor of bone. *In* Bone Tumors. 4th ed. p 343. St. Louis, CV Mosby, 1972, p 343.
50. Stoker D: Imaging procedures in orthopaedic pathology. *In* Salisbury JR, Woods CG, Byers PD (eds): Diseases of Bones and Joints. London, Chapman & Hall Medical, 1994, p 40.
51. Mankin HJ: Biopsy of neoplasms of bone and soft tissues: A rational approach. *In* Uhthoff HK (ed): Current Concepts of Diagnosis and Treatment of Bone and Soft Tissue Tumors. Berlin, Springer-Verlag, 1984, p 33.
52. Dollahite HA, Tatum L, Moinuddin SM, et al: Aspiration biopsy of primary neoplasms of bone. J Bone Joint Surg 71A:1166, 1989.
53. Kreicbergs A, Bauer HCF, Brosjo O, et al: Cytological diagnosis of bone tumours. J Bone Joint Surg 78B:258, 1996.
54. Ayala AG, Ro JY, Fanning CV, et al: Core needle biopsy and fine-needle aspiration in the diagnosis of bone and soft-tissue lesions. Hematol Oncol Clin North Am 9:633, 1995.
55. Mawhinney WHB, Richardson E, Malcolm AJ: Control of rapid nitric acid decalcification. J Clin Pathol 37:1409, 1984.
56. Hasegawa T, Hirose T, Kudo E, et al: Immunophenotypic heterogeneity in osteosarcomas. Hum Pathol 22:583, 1991.
57. Hasegawa T, Seki K, Yang P, et al: Differentiation and proliferative activity in benign and malignant cartilage tumors of bone. Hum Pathol 26:838, 1995.
58. Scotlandi K, Serra M, Manara C, et al: Clinical relevance of Ki-67 expression in bone tumors. Cancer 75:806, 1995.
59. Adler CP, Herget GW, Neuburger M: Cartilaginous

tumors. Prognostic applications of cytophotometric DNA analysis. Cancer 76:1176, 1995.
60. Clohisy JC, Schajowitz F, Vaziri DM, et al: Assessment of argyrophilic nucleolar organiser region quantification in benign and malignant bone tumors. Clin Orthop Rel Res 310:229, 1995.
61. Coughlan B, Feliz A, Ishida T, et al: p53 expression and DNA ploidy of cartilage lesions. Hum Pathol 26:620, 1995.
62. Broders AC: Squamous cell epithelioma of the lip. JAMA 75:656, 1920.
63. Broders AC: The microscopic grading of cancer. *In* Pack GT, Livingston EM (eds): Treatment of Cancer and Allied Disorders, p 19. New York, Paul B. Hoeber, 1946.
64. Inwards CY, Unni KK: Classification and grading of bone sarcomas. Hematol Oncol Clin North Am 9:545, 1995.
65. McDonald DJ, Sim FH, McLeod RA, et al: Giant cell tumor of bone. J Bone Joint Surg 68A:235, 1986.
66. Johnson S, Tetu B, Ayala AG, et al: Chondrosarcoma with additional mesenchymal component (dedifferentiated chondrosarcoma): I. A clinicopathologic study of 26 cases. Cancer 58:278, 1986.
67. Enneking WF: A system of staging musculoskeletal neoplasms. Clin Orthop Rel Res 204:9, 1986.
68. Enneking WF, Spanier SS, Goodman MA: A system for the surgical staging of musculoskeletal sarcoma. Clin Orthop Rel Res 153:106, 1980.

Chapter

2

BONE DEVELOPMENT, STRUCTURE, AND TURNOVER

ANTHONY J. FREEMONT

Bone is an unusual tissue in that during adult life it retains the capacity to alter its shape and structure in response to changes in its environment. In overall structural terms, a bone is well suited to the functional needs of support, protection, and calcium storage,[1] consisting of a mineralized matrix distributed as a dense outer shell, or cortex, and variable numbers of internal struts, or trabeculae. This distribution of bony substance has very important consequences in terms of the physiology and pathology of the individual bones, but to truly understand bone and its diseases requires a much greater and more detailed knowledge of bone as a tissue. This chapter discusses some of the more important aspects of the molecular biology, cell-cell and cell-matrix interactions, and functions of bone.

BONE TYPES

Bones are classified into four types: (1) flat bones, e.g., bones of the skull; (2) long bones, e.g., major limb bones; (3) short bones, e.g., carpus and tarsus; and (4) pneumatic bones, i.e., bones containing air sinuses. There is a fifth type, irregular bones, in which the features of two or more of the other four types are combined. The functions of all these bones are to give form or structure to the body, to provide support, leverage, and protection, and to afford muscle attachments. In addition, bones are a vital reserve of minerals, particularly calcium and magnesium. To facilitate these various functions, the major characteristics of bones are that they are hard, strong, and light. The general structure giving rise to these characteristics is much the same whatever the type of bone.

GENERAL STRUCTURE OF A BONE

Bones consist of an outer shell or cortex in which the majority (>90%) of the tissue is bone matrix. This surrounds a region filled with marrow and variable numbers of interconnecting bone spicules called *trabeculae* (Fig. 2–1). The region is referred to as *trabecular* or *cancellous* bone. The proportion of the trabecular bone volume occupied by bone matrix is very variable. It may be as little as 1 to 2%, even in normal bone, and rarely exceeds 20%. The remaining tissue is bone marrow, which has two components: hematopoietic marrow, where rapid cell turnover and production of all blood cell lineages is occurring, and bone marrow stroma, which consists predominantly of adipocytes together with a few multipotential connective tissue stem cells. Adipocytes are derived from the stromal stem cells, which are also precursors of other connective tissue cells, notably, in normal bone, osteoblasts.

Although the macroscopic examination of a transected bone shows the presence of two

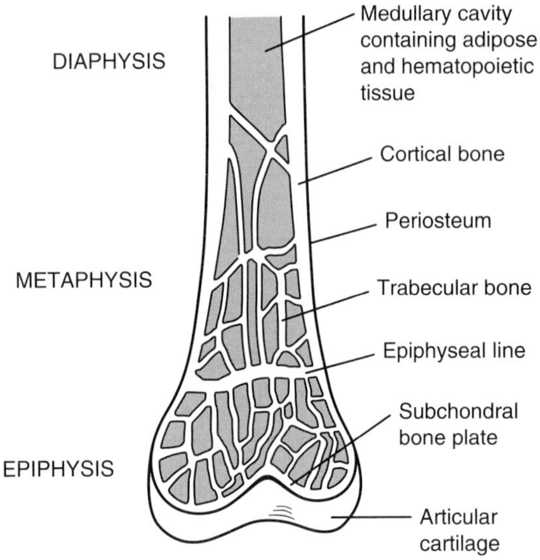

Figure 2–1. Longitudinal section of a long bone, illustrating the main anatomic elements.

types of bone (cortical and trabecular), a more discriminating examination and studies of bone metabolism show four different types of bone (Fig. 2–2). The outer 20% of the cortex consists of concentric shells of bone deposited by the cells of the periosteum. The periosteum consists of two layers of cells, the inner or *cambial* layer having osteoproductive potential. Periosteal bone consists almost entirely of matrix (>99%) and can be recognized by the orientation of its collagen lamellae (see later discussion), which run parallel to the outer surface of the bone. The remainder, and deeper part, of the cortex consists of interlocking complete and partial columns and spindle-shaped composite structures, which consist of a central blood vessel lying in a canal (the haversian canal) surrounded by bone. In this bone, the collagen lamellae are arranged circumferentially around the canal. This part of the cortex is said to be *haversian* bone.[2] Through the action of osteoclasts and osteoblasts (see later discussion), as periosteal bone is deposited on one surface of the cortex, it is changed into haversian bone from below. Thus, the thickness of the periosteal bone remains constant despite its continued production, or apposition. By the same token, the haversian bone should become thicker as periosteal bone is "haversianalized," but this is not necessarily the case, because this bone is being removed and restructured from the marrow, or endosteal, surface.

At the interface between trabecular and haversian bone is a layer of subcortical bone. The matrix in this area contributes little to the volume of the bone, but in cellular terms this is an area of high bioactivity. In particular, it is the site of active remodeling of the inner portion of the cortex.

The trabeculae are like girders of bone crossing the marrow cavity (Fig. 2–3), and they form a meshwork of bone spicules within the bone, acting as braces and struts with their major orientation determined by the regular load acting on the bone. Within the trabeculae, the collagen lamellae run along the long axis. The surfaces of the trabeculae are sites of appreciable bone cell activity.

The distribution of bone matrix and the orientation of the collagen lamellae (see later discussion) in these four components allows bone to be strong and light and to have a sufficiently large surface area for cells to act without interfering with the bone's strength.

BONE MATRIX

In bone, as in most connective tissues, the matrix occupies a greater volume than the

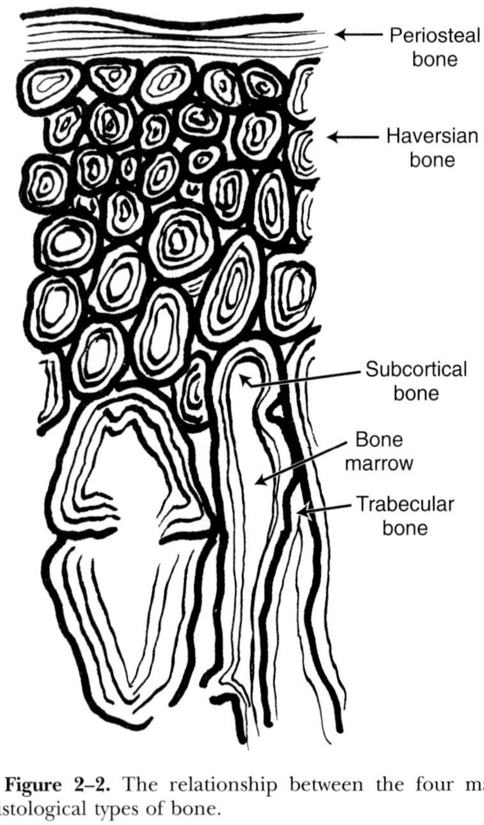

Figure 2–2. The relationship between the four main histological types of bone.

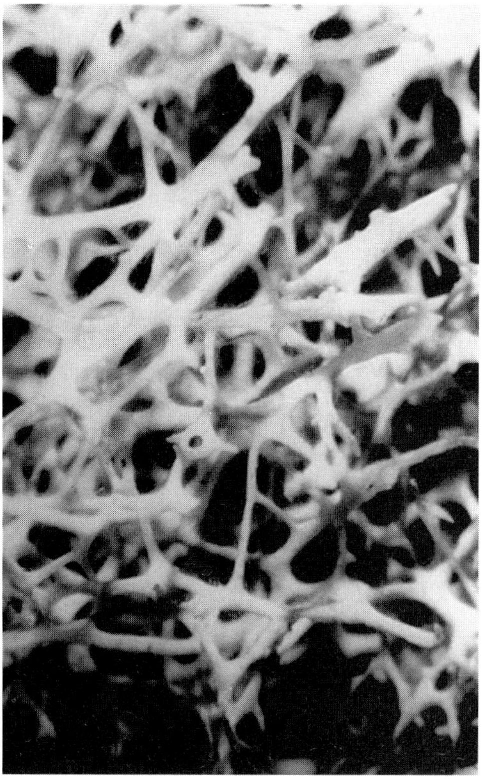

Figure 2–3. The structure of trabecular bone.

cells (Fig. 2–4). In addition to water, which accounts for about 20% of the weight of bone tissue, the matrix has major organic and inorganic components. The organic part of the matrix is 30% to 40% of the dry weight, with type I collagen being by far the most abundant component (90–95%).[3, 4] In addition, there are noncollagenous proteins[5, 6] and complex nonprotein components including saccharides and lipids. The noncollagen matrix macromolecules include the bone-Gla protein osteocalcin,[7] the glycoprotein osteonectin, and the two sialoproteins, bone sialoprotein[8] (BSP) and osteopontin.[9–11] All four are regulators of the process of matrix mineralization (see later discussion), BSP by acting as a crystal nucleator and the others by regulating the rate of mineralization[12] and the size of the crystals.[13] In addition, all but osteonectin have a regulatory function in bone turnover[14, 15] through effects on the formation,[16] or adhesion, or both, of bone cells.[17] Bone also contains latent cytokines and growth factors, notably the members of the transforming growth factor-β (TGF-β) superfamily,[18–20] which are involved with the structural integrity of the bone and the control of bone cell function. Together, the organic molecules form the nonmineralized matrix of bone known as *osteoid.* The final matrix component is a salt of calcium and phosphorus, which in its crystal structure most closely resembles that of hydroxyapatite[21] and accounts for between 60 and 70% of the dry weight of bone matrix.

At both the macroscopic and microscopic levels, bone is a highly organized structure. The complex, molded shapes of individual bones and the relative distributions of cortical and trabecular bone attest to this. Even the orientation of the trabeculae, which at first appears random, is, on closer inspection, seen to be predominantly along the line of the

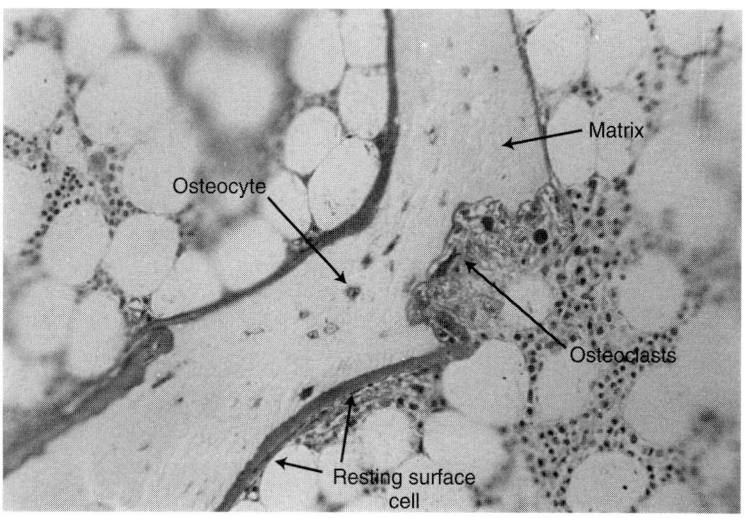

Figure 2–4. Micrograph showing the relationship between bone cells and matrix. The only "permanent" cells in bone are the osteocytes and resting surface cells. Bone-remodeling cells (as exemplified here by osteoclasts) are transient and work on bone surfaces. (Toluidine blue.)

most constant force acting on the bone. At the microscopic and functional levels, both cortical and trabecular bone is arranged into a series of "packets" that interlock with one another, each formed by, and populated with, a highly coordinated group of cells. Even at the molecular level, there is a truly remarkable degree of structural organization, epitomized by the lamellar arrays of collagen fibers. Each lamella represents a thin raft of collagen fibrils in which the long axes of the individual fibrils are oriented in the same direction. The alternating light and dark bands seen when the bone is viewed between crossed polarizers (Fig. 2–5) are the result of the long axes of the collagen fibers of alternating rafts being set at 90 degrees to one another. Each bone unit therefore represents a collagen fiber laminate not dissimilar in structure to plywood or a modern laminated resin. As a consequence of its structure, and like its manufactured counterparts, the material of bone is itself both light and strong.

It is important to recognize that this degree of organization is no accident but is rather a function of the cells that control the synthesis and breakdown of bone. In turn, it is implicit that there must be a degree of control of the site and the nature of bone cell activity that is specifically directed toward the functional requirements of the bone tissue.[22]

BONE CELLS

There are four classical bone cells: the osteoclast, the osteoblast, the osteocyte, and the resting surface cell.[23, 24] The osteocyte and the resting surface cell are derived from the osteoblast.[25]

The Osteoblast

The osteoblast is the cell that manufactures bone, being responsible for the synthesis of collagen and the noncollagenous proteins of bone, the orderly organization of collagen, and the mineralization of osteoid. The osteoblast is characterized by the expression of genes required for the synthesis of alkaline phosphatase, type I collagen (Fig. 2–6), bone-Gla protein osteocalcin, osteonectin, osteopontin, and many cytokines, as well as factors—as yet undetermined—that affect its site of action and relationship to other osteoblasts. Typical osteoblasts are transient cells that work focally on bone surfaces. They function as part of a short-lived consortium with neighboring osteoblasts to form seams of osteoid characteristically many times longer than the diameter of individual cells. These cells will only deposit osteoid on pre-existing mineralized surfaces (Fig. 2–7), most commonly bone in the adult and calcified cartilage in the growing ends of long bones in children. Made up of alternating lamellae of collagen, these seams reach a predetermined thickness (usually less than four lamellae), and then mineralization commences at the interface between the osteoid and the mineralized substrate of bone or cartilage.[18, 26] This surface is the mineralization, or calcification, front (Fig. 2–8). Mineralization

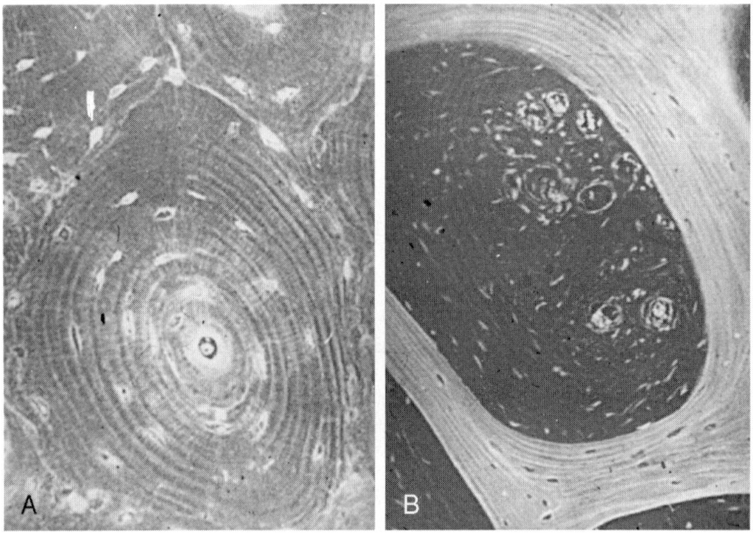

Figures 2–5. Polarizing micrographs showing the lamellar structure of haversian systems.

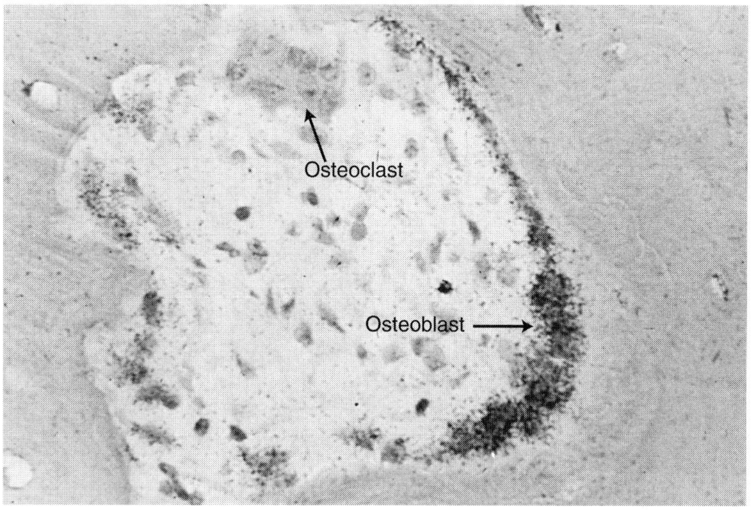

Figure 2–6. In situ hybridization study of bone showing the distribution of type I collagen mRNA.

will occur only if there are adequate supplies of calcium and phosphate in the extracellular fluid; these supplies are in turn dependent on the presence of parathyroid hormone and 1,25 dihydroxy vitamin D_3 (1,25$(OH)_2D_3$). It is believed that osteoblasts entrapped in osteoid produce intracellular membrane–bound structures called *matrix vesicles.*[27] Cytoplasmic vesicles are rich in sulfate and sodium, but, as the vesicles are ejected from the cell, there is a rapid exchange of calcium and phosphate for the sodium and sulfate. The extracellular matrix vesicles act as discrete foci about which the crystal lattice of bone is established by inorganic chemical reactions. Matrix mineralization can be detected in bone biopsies if the patient is given the drug tetracycline prior to biopsy. Tetracycline is a fluorochrome taken up onto the surface of bone at sites of active mineralization, where its presence can be demonstrated by viewing unstained sections of bone in ultraviolet light (Fig. 2–9).[28, 29] The method by which tetracycline is bound to bone is not entirely understood; however, as tetracycline fluorescence is lost during tissue decalcification, it is probable that it binds to the mineral crystal lattice in a manner similar to the way in which it chelates free ions outside bone.

There is incontrovertible evidence that the

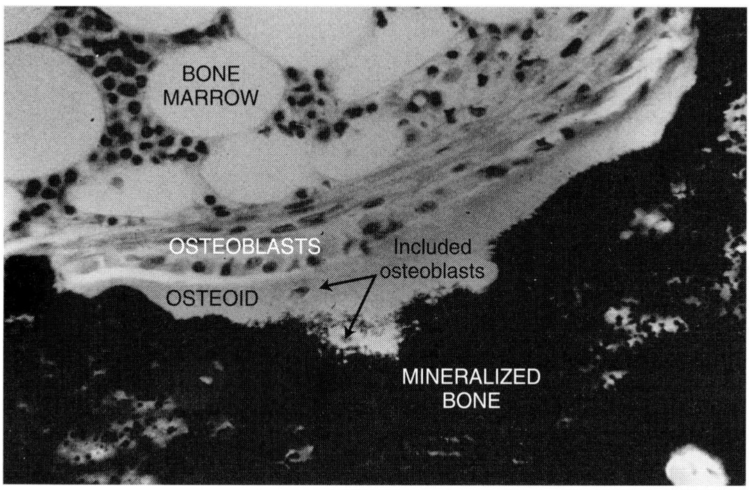

Figure 2–7. Osteoblasts synthesizing and mineralizing osteoid on a bone surface. The patient has hyperparathyroidism, and bone deposition is greater than in normal bone. (Von Kossa.)

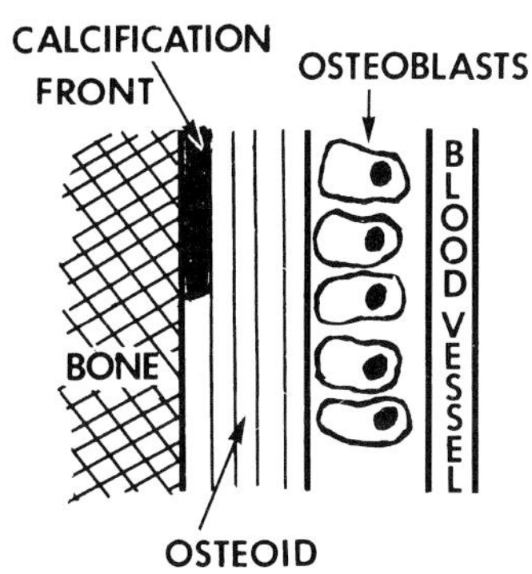

Figure 2–8. Diagramatic representation of osteoblast function.

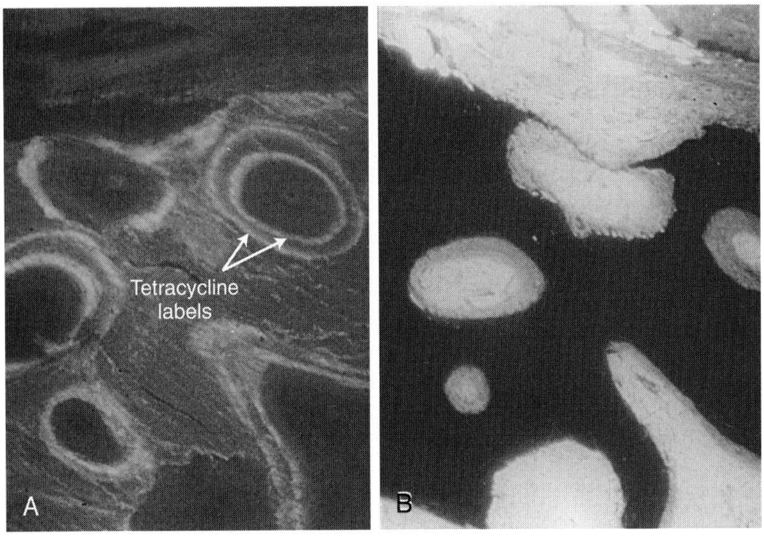

Figure 2–9. Tetracycline label in bone. The patient was given two doses of tetracycline separated by an interval of 10 days. *A*, Unstained section viewed in ultraviolet light; *B*, serial von Kossa-stained sections.

osteoblast is functionally determined toward maintaining the integrity of the matrix of bone. In recent years, it has become apparent that osteoblasts produce local factors controlling bone cell activity.[30–32] These are discussed in more detail in the next sections.

The Osteocyte

The osteocyte is characterized by its site within bone and its shape, which, in many ways, is similar to that of a spiny sea urchin. During osteoid formation, some osteoblasts become incarcerated within the newly formed bone matrix, to become osteocytes (see Fig. 2–7). Osteocytes are a poorly understood group of cells. Their most characteristic feature, in correctly stained sections, is that, although their cell bodies are apparently separated from one another within the bone matrix, the cells are linked by a complex, interconnecting, three-dimensional network of thin, cytoplasmic processes that not only connect osteocytes with one another but also connect them with bone surfaces and the cells thereon (Fig. 2–10). The cell bodies of the osteocytes lie in holes in the bone called *lacunae*, and their cytoplasmic processes run in fine channels called *canaliculi*. Within lacunae and canaliculi, osteocytes are surrounded by extracellular fluid. Ion exchange occurs be-

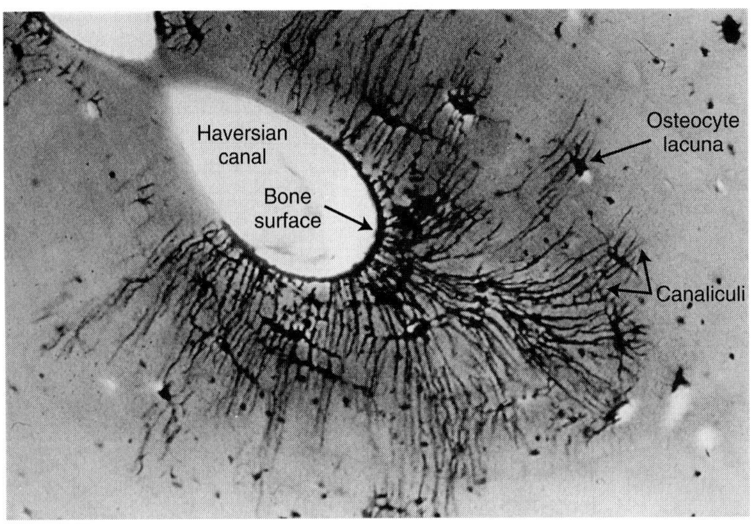

Figure 2–10. Permeation-stained section of haversian bone showing osteocyte lacunae and canaliculi and their relationship to bone surfaces.

tween the crystal lattice of the bone matrix and the extracellular fluid (ECF) around osteocytes.

Much excitement has been generated lately about the potential role of the osteocyte in the maintenance of the structure of bone. An exponentially increased number of studies of osteocyte function indicates that the three-dimensional network of osteocyte cell processes acts as a finely tuned mechanoreceptor, capable of sensing microdistortions in bone matrix and translating these directly, or via passage of information from one osteocyte to another, into signals that influence the activity of bone surface cells (osteoblasts, osteoclasts, and resting surface cells).[33] Currently, the best data indicate that cyclical, rather than constant, load is needed to stimulate these cells and that this can cause a rapid and significant increase in osteoblastic bone formation. Prostanoids[34] and the cytokine, insulin-like growth factor, have been implicated as the chemical mediators synthesized during this process. Data are also now being produced that indicate that, as the main nontransient cell in bone, osteocytes may be the target of certain bone regulatory hormones.[35]

The Resting Surface Cell

The osteoblast may also differentiate into a flat cell lying on the surface of bone; this is known as the *resting surface cell.* It is characterized by being pavemented onto the bone, from which it is separated by a very thin layer of nonmineralized fibrous tissue that completely covers all viable nonresorbing bone surfaces in much the same way as the thin plastic covering of vacuum-packed goods conforms to their surface (Fig. 2–11). It is believed that the integrity of this fine fibrous tissue layer is maintained by the resting surface cell and functions to prevent osteoclasts gaining access to the mineralized bone. It has been suggested that the resting surface cells have the ability to secrete collagenases, which can remove the surface layer of fibrous tissue, and in this manner control and facilitate the access of osteoclasts to the bone surface and their engagement in bone resorption (Fig. 2–12). Whether the resting surface cells can "dedifferentiate" into active osteoblasts in vivo is unknown, but bone explants devoid of marrow can be the source of "osteoblast-like" cells in tissue culture systems.

The Osteoclast

The fourth type of bone cell is the osteoclast.[36, 37] This cell is characterized by its expression of tartrate-resistant acid phosphatase, its multinucleation (Fig. 2–13), its ability to erode mineralized surfaces, and its expression of calcitonin receptors.[38–40] The osteoclast adheres to the surface of bone all around its periphery much like a sucker. This effectively creates a sealed space under the cell into which the osteoclast is able to secrete products that lower the pH of the microenvironment at the bone surface and decalcify the bone,[41] and others that digest the collagen framework of bone matrix (Fig. 2–14).[42] The osteoclast forms by fusion of mononuclear precursors, and it is possible that continuous recruitment of new mononuclear cells into the syncytium is necessary to prevent destruction of the cell by the low pH and high calcium concentration in the space beneath the osteoclast. Even so, the osteoclast is very short-lived and represents a transient bone cell that is inactivated and removed by the process of apoptosis.[43] By the decalcification and breakdown of osteoid, the osteoclast is able to excavate a saucer-shaped depression on the surface of trabecular, subcortical, and periosteal bone (see Fig. 2–14) and tunnels into cortical bone (Fig. 2–15).[44] The concerted effort of several osteoclasts either side by side or acting sequentially at the same site leads to the excavation of larger quantities of bone. Removal of bone in this way has two main purposes: first, it allows bone modeling and remodeling (see following discussion) to occur, and second, it liberates calcium from the bone to add to the calcium pool within the extracellular fluid.

THE CONTROL OF BONE CELL ACTIVITY

Bone Modeling and Remodeling

Throughout life, bone matrix is being continuously replaced and its gross and molecular structure and orientation are being altered.[45] This process is mediated by osteoclasts, osteoblasts, and osteoblast-derived cells working in "teams" or "units." These teams may work in two ways.[46]

In the first case, the osteoclasts resorb bone and the resulting hole is filled with new bone and osteocytes. This has two consequences: the

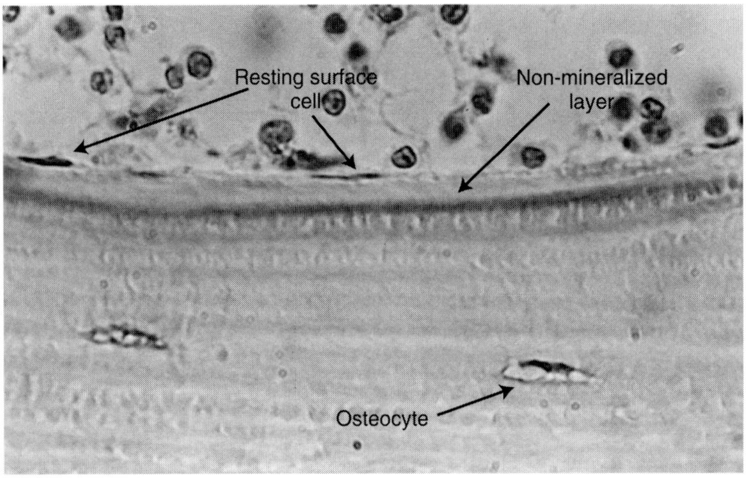

Figure 2–11. Resting surface cells on a bone surface.

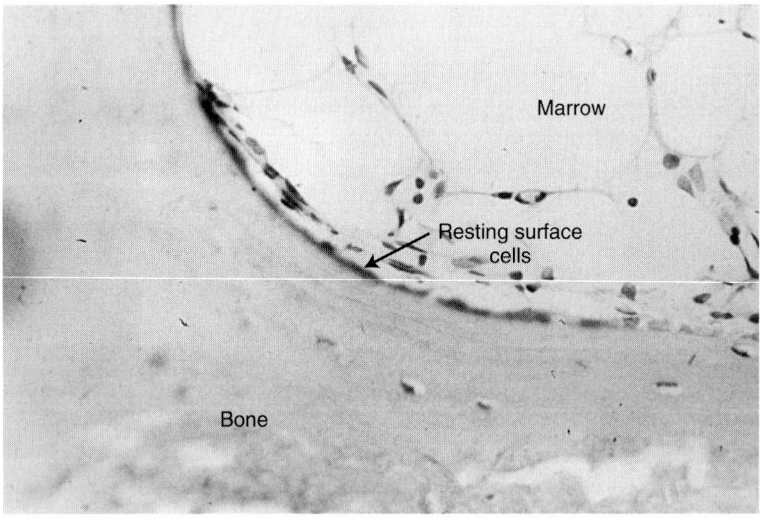

Figure 2–12. Nonradioactive in situ hybridization of resting surface cells reacted for type I collagenase mRNA.

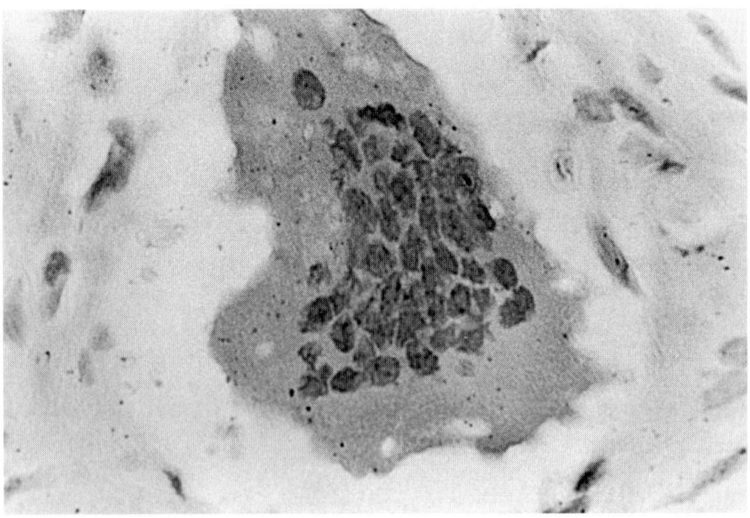

Figure 2–13. Osteoclast extracted from a giant cell tumor of bone. Although not entirely "normal," giant cells erode bone, express calcitonin receptors, and, as shown here, demonstrate the multinucleation of osteoclasts.

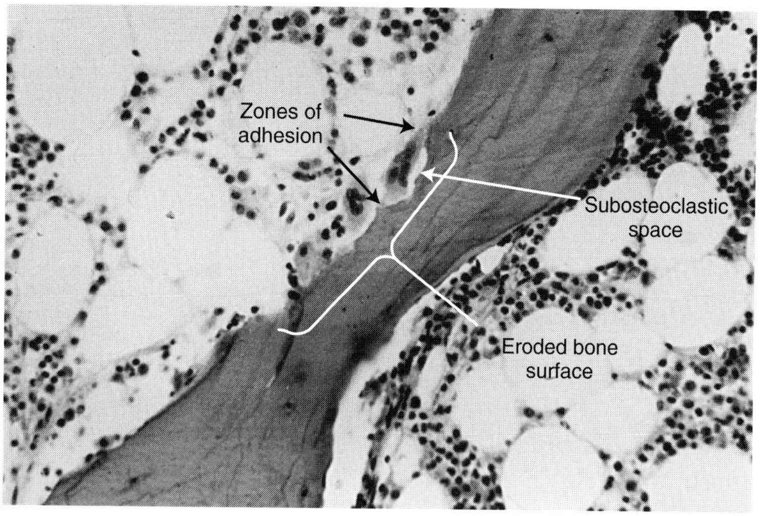

Figure 2–14. Osteoclasts on a trabecular erosive surface. Note the relationship to bone marrow.

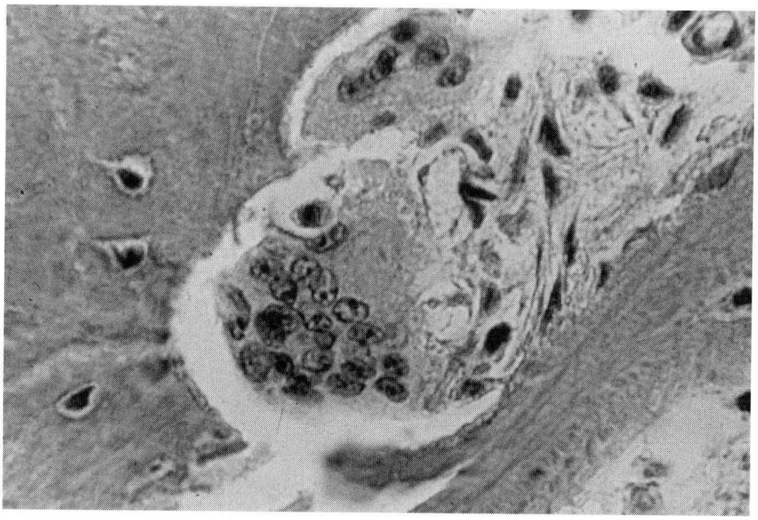

Figure 2–15. Tunneling osteoclasts are frequently seen in cortical bone, particularly as shown here in hyperparathyroidism.

osteoclasts and osteoblasts work in the same place but at different times, and the overall effect is replacement of the same amount of old bone matrix with new. This process is known as *remodeling* (Fig. 2–16).

The second case is that in which osteoclasts remove bone from one area and osteoblasts add new bone elsewhere. The two groups of bone cells can work at the same time, and the overall effect is to change the shape of the bone, either locally or more generally. This process, which is known as *modeling*, permits bone growth and allows the redistribution of bone matrix to accommodate changing load on the bone (Fig. 2–17).[28]

The Control of Bone Cell Function

Orderly modeling and remodeling necessitate an interaction between bone cells.[25, 47] The activity of bone cells is not random, and there is considerable evidence that bone cells work in concert. The most powerful example of this is the fact that although there is always osteoblastic bone deposition and osteoclastic bone resorption, between the ages of 20 and 40 years, a person's bone mass remains constant.[48] This observation has led to the concept of osteoblast and osteoclast activity being "coupled."[49]

With an increasing understanding of bone

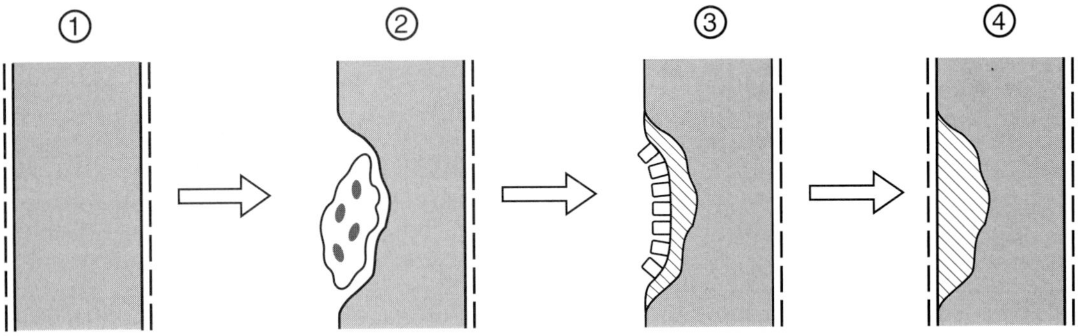

Figure 2–16. Remodeling. Osteoclasis and osteoblastic activity occur sequentially but in the same place. This leads to replacement of old bone matrix and osteocytes with new.

cells and their activity, the concepts defining the control of coupling are becoming more and more sophisticated. Indeed, it is now believed that the activity not just of the osteoblasts and osteoclasts but of all four bone cell types is linked.

This idea is best exemplified by reference to the processes of remodeling. One theory that attempts to explain how this linkage of bone cell activity is regulated in remodeling suggests that the resting surface cells, under the influence of either a local or generalized humoral factor, or following stimulation by a message sent from the osteocyte network, produce collagenase, which removes the nonmineralized fibrous tissue from the surface of bone. The exposed mineralized bone matrix, either by itself or together with an external or internal influence, initiates the formation of multinucleated osteoclasts. These cells settle on the bone and start the process of bone erosion. It is postulated that as the osteoclasts break down the matrix, they liberate latent cytokines (particularly of the TGF-β superfamily)[50] built into the matrix by previous osteoblast activity. In the microenvironment adjacent to the bone surface, active cytokine is formed that inhibits further osteoclasis and stimulates the production and localized activation of osteoblasts (Fig. 2–18).[51] These, in turn, deposit new bone matrix in the depression formed by the osteoclast. The remodeling process thus leads to the replacement of old matrix with new, and it also incorporates new osteocytes and a new complement of latent cytokines. In the interval between the cessation of osteoclastic activity and new bone deposition, a thin layer of matrix known as the *cement line* (Fig. 2–19) is laid down. The cement line demarcates the extent of the area of bone remodeling and has an important function of allowing movement of bone plates over one another under load. This, to some extent, allows energy dissipation within bone matrix that would otherwise be very brittle.

As data have accumulated over the last few years, even the mechanism just outlined has been seen to be too simplistic to explain all that is known of remodeling and is inadequate to explain modeling. It is becoming increasingly apparent that bone cells are subject to a huge number and complexity of physical and

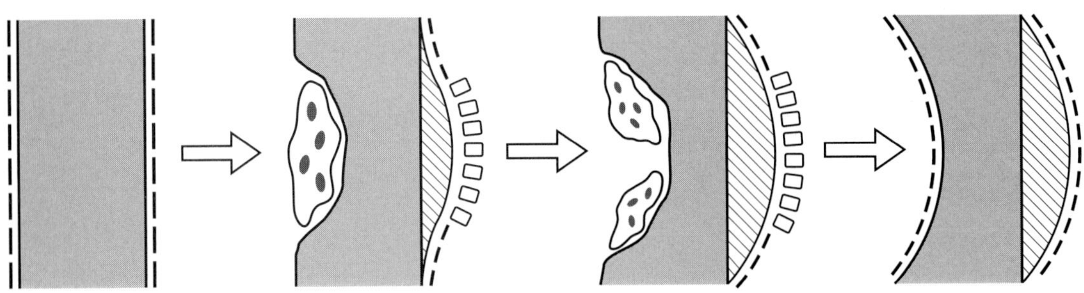

Figure 2–17. Modeling. Osteoclasis and osteoblastic activity occur at the same time but in different areas of bone. The net effect is alteration of the structure of bone.

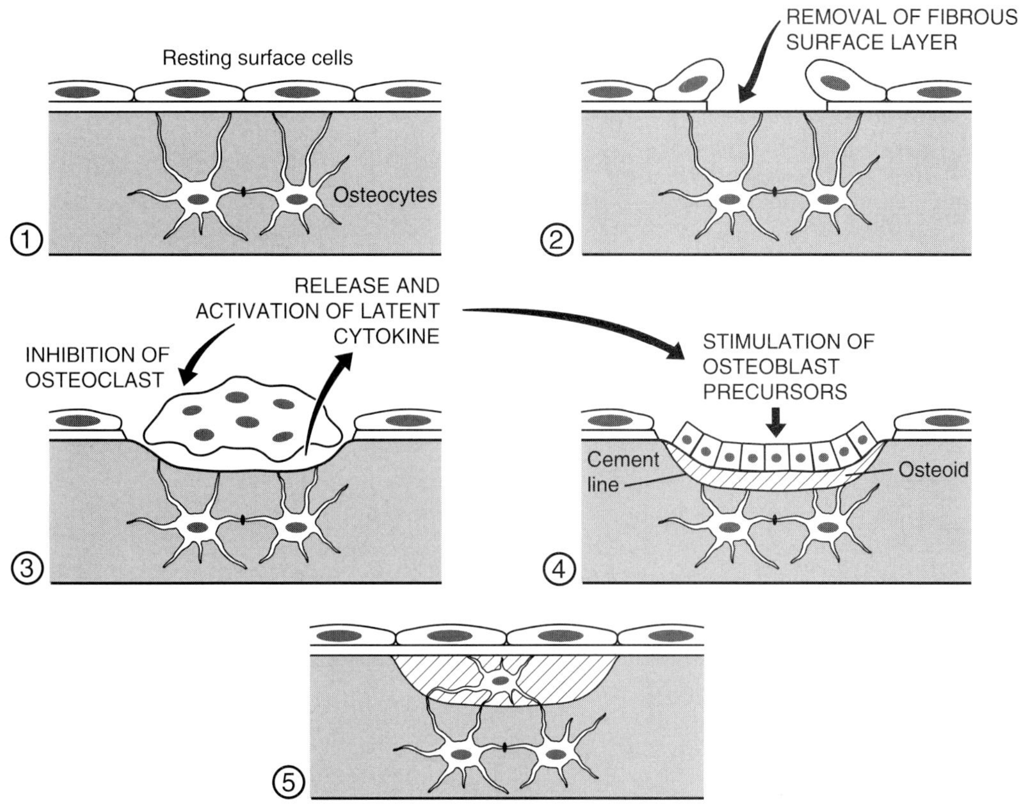

Figure 2–18. A suggested mechanism explaining cell coupling in bone remodeling in functional, cellular, and molecular terms.

Figure 2–19. Cement lines in Paget's disease. Although present in both normal and diseased bone, cement lines are more frequent and more easily visualized in Paget's disease.

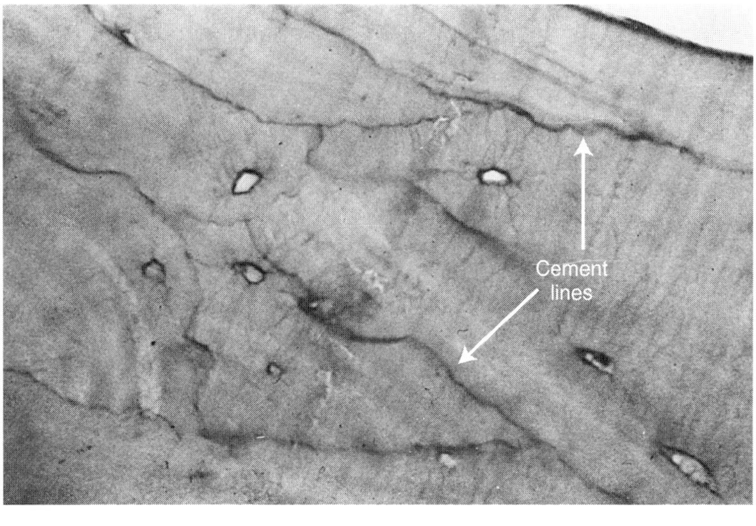

chemical environmental influences that, by affecting their function, regulate the structure, distribution, and function of bone matrix.[52, 53]

Factors Influencing Bone Cell Function

In general terms, the factors influencing bone cell function can be divided into three main groups[54, 55]:

1. Circulating hormones, such as growth hormone, parathyroid hormone (PTH), sex hormones (estrogen and androgen), and sterols, particularly $1,25(OH)_2D_3$.[40, 56, 57]
2. Locally produced chemical mediators (e.g., cytokines, growth factors, prostanoids).[58–67]
3. Mechanical load.[28, 33]

Each may act either by stimulating or by inhibiting cell function (Table 2–1), and it is probably the very complex interactions between these factors that determine the functions of individual cells. Many of the locally produced factors are manufactured by bone cells, particularly osteoblasts,[68] and act on the secretory cells by autocrine pathways as well as on other cells by paracrine mechanisms. In addition, neighboring hematopoietic and stromal cells of the marrow probably have profound effects on bone cells.[69]

The activity of the various mediators is regulated by the expression of receptors[70] on key target cells as much as, if not more than, by production of the active regulators (Fig. 2–20). Most of the cytokines, growth factors, and other locally synthesized regulators act on cell surface receptors, altering functional gene expression in target cells through cytoplasmic second messenger systems.[71] Many hormones and sterols, by contrast, enter the cell and form homodimeric or heterodimeric complexes with receptors in the nucleus. The complex cross-talk between these two receptor-regulated systems is the subject of much current investigation.

Mechanical load is believed to influence bone cell activity by conversion of mechanical distortion of osteocyte processes into chemical messages, notably prostanoids and cytokines that are transmitted to cells on the surfaces of bone. The interactions of this mechanicochemical system with the purely chemical system are unknown. It is speculated, however, that the humoral control system is more likely to have a significant influence on bone remodeling, whereas the osteocyte-mediated mechanicohumoral system is a better candidate for the regulation of modeling where bone deposition and resorption occur in parts of the bone distant from one another.

It is also becoming increasingly apparent that the chemical mediators of bone cell function act in two main ways. Many of the systemic hormones, notably the sex steroids, and some of the regulatory cytokines present in the circulation act as general stimulators or inhibitors of bone cells.[72, 73] These factors do not appear to regulate the activity of cells in spe-

Table 2–1. Stimulators and Inhibitors of Osteoblastic and Osteoclastic Functions

	Systemic	Local	Load
Osteoblasts			
Stimulators	Sex steroids	Insulin-like growth factors	Compressive (cyclical)
	Growth hormone	Transforming growth factor-β	
	Parathormone	Fibroblast growth factor	
	$1,25(OH)_2D_3$	Platelet-derived growth factor	
		Interleukin-9	
		Bone morphogenic proteins	
		Nitric oxide in low concentration	
Inhibitors	Thyroxine	Nitric oxide in high concentration	Tensile
	Retinoids		
Osteoclasts			
Stimulators	Parathormone	Interleukin-1	Tensile
	Parathormone-related peptide	Interleukin-6	
		Monocyte colony-stimulating factor	
		Blood flow	
Inhibitors	Calcitonin	Nitric oxide at low concentration	Compressive

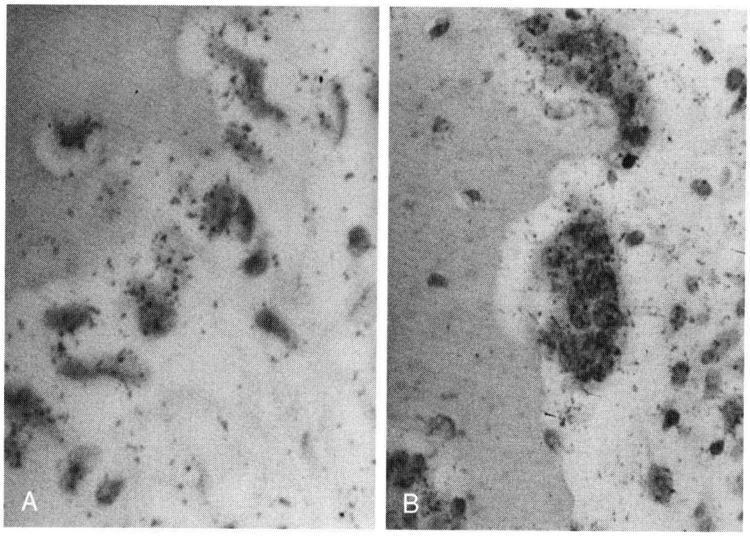

Figure 2–20. In situ hybridization studies showing osteoblast expression of interleukin 1 (IL-1) mRNA *(A)* and osteoclast expression of IL-1 receptor mRNA *(B)*.

cific localities within the bone but rather up- or down-regulate general transcription pathways,[74] thus modulating the overall activity of cells throughout the entire skeleton.[75] Changes in the production of these factors lead to generalized alterations in cell function epitomized by the metabolic bone diseases. Other humoral factors, presumably because they are produced locally or their receptors are expressed locally by target cells, control bone cell activity locally.

Osteoblasts and osteoclasts, as the cells active in bone formation and breakdown, are the ultimate targets of these regulatory systems, but they are very transient cells. One of the functions of the regulatory mechanism must therefore be recruitment of these cells from their precursors. Understanding of how this important process occurs necessitates a knowledge of the stem cells of osteoblasts and osteoclasts and the factors controlling differentiation of their precursors.

THE ORIGIN OF BONE CELLS

It is a characteristic of cells that, once they are functionally differentiated, they lose the ability to divide. From this it follows that somewhere within bone, and presumably close to their functional site, are to be found stem cells from which the two main bone cell lineages, osteoclasts and osteoblasts, derive (see Chapter 3).

Osteoclasts are related to cells of the monocyte-macrophage lineage. Their stem cells are to be found in hematopoietic bone marrow.[76–79] Osteoblast precursors also originate within marrow.[68, 80–82] In addition, cells capable of osteoblastic differentiation also populate the inner, or cambial, layer of the periosteum and are found in non–bone-associated connective tissue sites. The most primitive osteoblast precursors are undifferentiated mesenchymal stem cells with the potential to differentiate into any of the main connective tissue lines.[83, 84] These cells, known as colony forming units–fibroblastic (CFU-F), have the ability to synthesize one of the various connective tissue matrices (e.g., bone, fibrous tissue, cartilage, fat). Just as there are factors that determine the direction of differentiation of the hematopoietic stem cells, so there must be local or systemic factors that will stimulate the stromal cell precursors to form osteoblasts in preference to chondrocytes, fibroblasts, or adipocytes. When the local control mechanisms are maximally stimulated, such as in healing fractures, differentiation can occur along all or any of the main connective tissue synthetic pathways, at times simultaneously and at other times sequentially.

Fracture healing illustrates one aspect of osteoblastic activity that is generally overlooked. Lamellar bone in this situation is deposited either on calcifying cartilage or as a different type of "bone" known as *woven bone*, which forms from the primitive mesenchymal milieu. Woven bone has a disorganized collagen structure and forms around "osteoblasts" (Fig. 2–21). The matrix differs from that of lamellar bone in the apparent lack of organization of

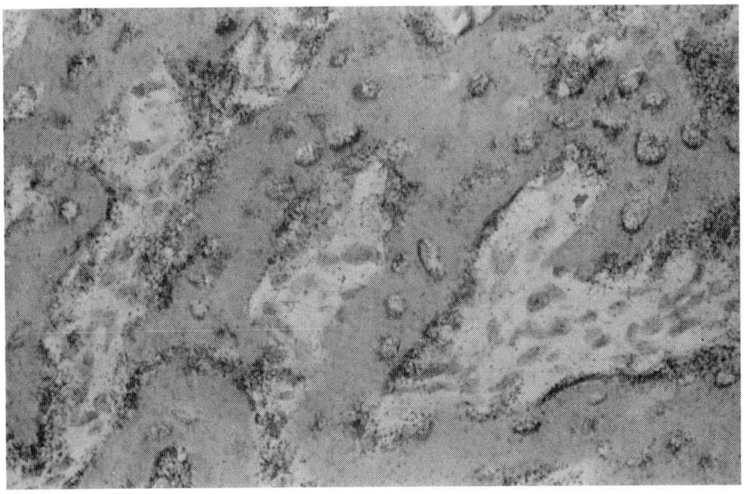

Figure 2–21. Fracture callus showing mRNA for type I collagen within surface and internalized "osteoblasts" in trabecula-like structures in newly formed woven bone.

the collagen and in the nature of the noncollagenous components of the matrix. The latter affords woven bone a distinctive and useful attribute in that the matrix is highly calcifiable and will mineralize even when lamellar bone will not. Weight for weight it is, however, weaker than lamellar bone. The "osteoblasts" do not function in the same way as bone surface osteoblasts.[85] They differentiate in situ, often expressing a mixed fibroblastic/chondrocytic/osteoblastic phenotype. They work alone, rather than in large sheets, and they induce matrix changes and bone formation in a spherical distribution about themselves rather than on one surface. Only once the primitive "skeleton" of calcified cartilage or woven bone has formed can the complex processes of cellular interactions that characterize bone remodeling be superimposed, ultimately to form normal, strong, lamellar bone.

The osteoblastic stem cell cannot be identified in vivo. It is assumed that the cell does not exhibit the usual phenotypic markers of the osteoblast, such as expression of alkaline phosphatase, osteocalcin, and type I collagen genes, an assumption supported by all the negative circumstantial data. Putative osteoblast precursors can be isolated from animal and human bone marrow.[30] When cultured with dexamethasone[86] and $1,25(OH)_2D_3$, these cells can assume an "osteoblastic" phenotype.[87]

A variety of cytokines, growth factors, and transcription factors have been implicated in the differentiation of osteoblasts. Osteoblastic differentiation is believed to be controlled by IL-6[88, 89] and the TGF-β superfamily,[90, 91] which includes most of the bone morphogenetic proteins.[92]

Because they are derived from a similar lineage to neutrophils and macrophages, it is hardly surprising that osteoclast differentiation is under the control of similar factors to those responsible for the differentiation of hematopoietic stem cells. These include M-CSF[93, 94] and GM-CSF, although cytokines such as interleukin 6 (IL-6) have also been implicated in osteoclast formation.[42, 54, 95, 96] Many of the factors that control and determine bone cell and matrix formation in adult bone and its diseases are also involved in the genesis of bones in the developing embryo.[97]

EMBRYOLOGIC DEVELOPMENT OF BONE

Of all the mechanisms described so far in this chapter, embryologic development of bone most closely mimics that occurring during fracture callus formation.[80] Embryologically bones form in two ways. The large flat bones, such as those of the calvaria, form de novo within fibrous tissue, whereas the long bones form within cartilage anlages.

The process of ossification of a flat bone starts at one or more points within the primitive fibrous connective tissue, known as *ossification centers,* The first step is a condensation of mesenchyme followed by cellular proliferation. Some of the cells enlarge in a set pattern, and between these cells a meshwork of collagen fibers forms in the shape of a crude outline of cortical and trabecular bone. This is followed by a change in the saccharide composition of the matrix and mineralization. This mineralized tissue forms the basis for remodeling and modeling to form the final shape of the bone typical of the mature skeleton.

The process of ossification in long bones is similar. The condensed mesenchyme forms a rod of hyaline cartilage (the cartilage anlage). Next, in genetically programmed fixed sites, again termed ossification centers, local chondrocytes undergo division, migrate through the matrix, and line up in columns oriented along the long axis of the developing bone. These cells undergo hypertrophy and start synthesizing a novel matrix rich in collagen type X.[98] This collagen is unique to this site and is believed to be associated with calcification of the chondroid matrix. Calcification of the matrix ensues, associated with chondrocyte apoptosis and focal transdifferentiation to cells exhibiting an "osteoblastic" phenotype and ingrowth of blood vessels into the lacunae of the now extinct chondrocytes, leaving acellular columns of calcified cartilage (Fig. 2–22).

No matter how formed, the mineralized matrix of the flat or long bone acts as a substrate for osteoclastic (chondroclastic) resorption and the initiation of the processes of remodeling. During embryologic development, to accommodate growth and development of the bone, this process of endochondral ossification is linked with bone modeling and remodeling to form the final structure of the bone.

The processes of formation of the cartilage anlage—its mineralization, remodeling, and modeling—are very intricate and highly controlled. Central to the genetic control of these processes are a group of genes that regulate intranuclear gene transcription. In humans, they are known as the homeobox, or *HOX*, genes.[99] Insects and rodents in which the animal equivalent of the *HOX* genes are overexpressed or underexpressed, following transgenic and knockout experiments, have abnormalities of skeletal development that are surprisingly focal, leading to replacement of an antenna with a limb or two full vertebrae by two hemivertebrae. Recently, a second group of morphoregulatory genes, the hedgehog genes, was described.[100]

The process of mineralization is not random either. The ossification sites in both flat and long bones form in almost constant regions of the embryo. Their occurrence and function, although the same in long and flat bones, are best illustrated by reference to a long bone. The primary center of ossification appears in the center of the rod of condensed mesenchyme and extends toward the ends, which remain cartilaginous for a length of time that varies for different bones. This part of the shaft of the bone is known as the diaphysis. Later ossification begins at one or more secondary ossification centers near the ends of the bone, and the portion of the bone formed from them constitutes the epiphysis. The cartilage between the diaphysis and the growing

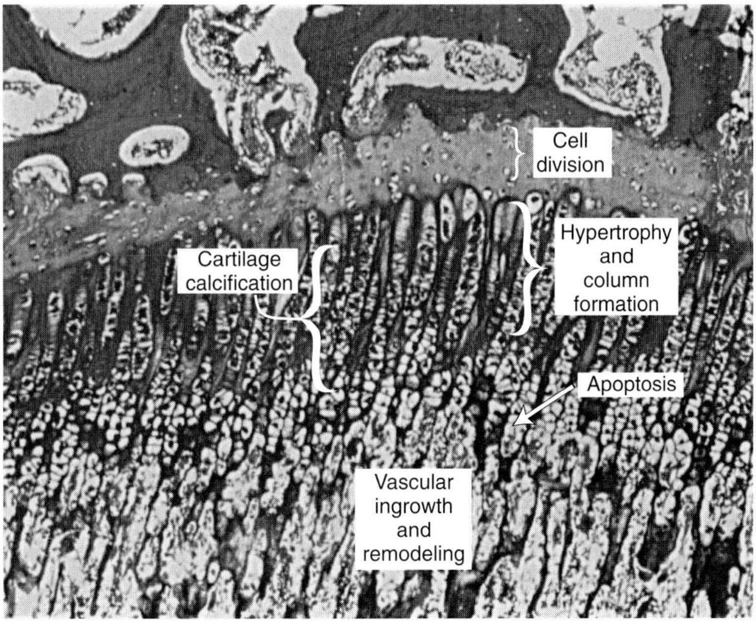

Figure 2–22. Human growth plate showing active endochondral ossification.

end is termed the *epiphyseal line*, and that part of the diaphysis adjacent to it is called the *metaphysis* (see Fig. 2–1).

VASCULAR SUPPLY OF BONE

All the processes so far described are highly energy-dependent and demand ready access to oxygen and nutrients, which come from the vasculature. The vasculature is therefore an essential part of the homeostasis of bone. Most of the bone is supplied from a small number of arteries that penetrate the cortex, supply the trabecular bone as they traverse the medullary cavity, and ramify through the cortex, having entered it from the medullary surface.[23, 101] The epiphyses are supplied in a similar way. The periosteum and adjacent bone are supplied by a different mechanism, namely by fine anastamotic vascular nets covering the surface of the bone.

This pattern of blood supply has important consequences to an understanding of pathologic processes, in particular septic and aseptic necrosis. The nature of the vasculature and particularly its endothelium also influences tumor metastasis, both into and out of bone. The veins follow the arteries and are thin-walled. The presence of lymphatics within bone marrow has never been convincingly demonstrated.

CONCLUSIONS

Bone, like all other tissues, is alive. Working through the complex interactions of the four main types of bone cell, local and systemic factors stimulate changes in the nature and distribution of bone matrix to better allow the functions of bone. As in all live tissues, perturbation of the cells, the factors controlling cell activity, or the vasculature lead to dramatic changes in the tissue; these we recognize as bone pathology. Only now are the complexities of the organization of bone coming to be appreciated. The clinical importance of this increase in knowledge is that the understanding of the processes underlying the development of neoplastic disorders of bone has improved dramatically and the route toward the development of more rational therapy is now open.

The link between bone cell activity and cytokines and growth factors[102] lies at the heart of the effects of marrow neoplasms on bone structure. As might be expected of rapidly proliferating neoplastic cells, these tumor cells are often potent synthesizers of various cytokines and growth factors. Differential overexpression of these regulatory factors causes changes as diverse as osteosclerosis (excess bone production)[103] and osteolysis (increased bone breakdown).[104, 105] The close proximity and number of hematopoietic cells to bone explain why the leukemias and lymphomas can lead to alterations in bone structure and metabolism.

The multipotential nature of the bone marrow stromal stem cells explains why such a diversity of types of tumor, as classified by the nature of their matrix, occurs in bone[106] and why such anomalies as chondroblastic osteosarcoma, in which more than one type of matrix is synthesized, exist. The small number of bone surface cells active at any one time is an indication of the relatively low turnover of bone cell precursors, which probably in turn explains the low frequency of primary neoplasms of bone. It also explains why the incidence of neoplasms is higher at times of increased skeletal growth (i.e., in childhood) and in pathologic states of high bone cell production, such as Paget's disease.

The presence of two stromal precursor cell pools, one in the marrow and one in the periosteum, explains the occurrence of medullary and periosteal neoplasms; and the vasculature and marrow microenvironment explain the relative differences in the behavior of these different neoplasms.

The most common neoplasms of bone are secondary carcinomas. Although incompletely understood, the nature of the bone vasculature and, probably, the expression of adhesion molecules on the vascular endothelium influence the process of metastasis. As metastases are not to bone, but to marrow, the influence of cytokines and growth factors synthesized during hematopoiesis on the growth of the metastasis may be significant (see Chapter 3).

REFERENCES

1. Price RA: Vitamin K–dependent bone proteins. *In* Cohn DV, Martin TJ, Meunier PJ (eds): Calcium Regulation and Bone Metabolism: Basic and Clinical Aspects. Amsterdam, Elsevier, 1987, p 419.
2. Jaworski ZFG: Haversian systems and haversian bone. *In* Hall BK (ed): Bone Metabolism and Mineralization. Boca Raton, FL, CRC Press, 1992.
3. Hoyland J, Hopkinson I, Odedra R, et al: Detection

of type I collagen mRNA in routine bone biopsies. Matrix 10:241, 1990.
4. Eyre DR, Wu JJ, Nizibizi C: The collagens of bone and cartilage: Molecular diversity and supramolecular assembly. *In* Cohn DV, Glorieux FH, Martin TJ (eds): Calcium Regulation and Bone Metabolism. Amsterdam, Elsevier, 1980, p 188.
5. Ingram RT, Clarke BL, Fisher LW, et al: Distribution on non-collagenous proteins in the matrix of adult human bone: Evidence of anatomic and functional heterogeneity. J Bone Min Res 8:1019, 1993.
6. Carlson CS, Tulli HM, Jayo M, et al: Immunolocalization of noncollagenous bone matrix proteins in lumbar vertebrae from intact and surgically menopausal cynomolgus monkeys. J Bone Min Res 8:71, 1993.
7. Termine JD, Kleinman HK, Whitson SW, et al: Osteonectin, a bone-specific protein linking mineral to collagen. Cell 26:99, 1981.
8. Fisher LW, Whitson SW, Avioli LV, et al: Matrix sialoprotein of developing bone. J Biol Chem 258:12723, 1983.
9. McKee MD, Farach-Carson MC, Butler WT, et al: Ultrastructural immunolocalization of non-collagenous (osteopontin and osteocalcin) and plasma (albumin and alpha2-HS-glycoprotein) proteins in rat bone. J Bone Min Res 8:485, 1993.
10. Chen J, McKee MD, Nanci A, et al: Bone sialoprotein mRNA expression and ultrastructural localization in fetal porcine calvarial bone: Comparison with osteopontin. Histochem J 26:67, 1994.
11. Butler WT: The nature and significance of osteopontin. Conn Tiss Res 23:123, 1989.
12. Hruska KA, Oilnick F, Huskey M: Occupancy of the osteoclast αvβ3 integrin by osteopontin stimulates a novel arc associated phosphatidylinositol 3 kinase (PI3 kinase) resulting in phosphatidylinositol triphosphate (PIP3) formation. J Bone Min Res Suppl 1:Abstract 55, 1992.
13. Romberg RW, Werness PG, Riggs BL, et al: Inhibition of hydroxapatite crystal growth by bone-specific and other calcium-binding proteins. Biochem 25:1176, 1986.
14. Ross FP, Chappel J, Alvarez JI, et al: Interactions between the bone-matrix proteins osteopontin and bone sialoprotein and the osteoclast integrin αvβ3 potentiate bone resorption. J Biol Chem 268:901, 1986.
15. Miyauchi A, Alvarez J, Greenfield E, et al: Recognition of osteopontin and related peptides by an αvβ3 integrin stimulates immediate cell signals in osteoclasts. J Biol Chem 266:369, 1993.
16. Glowacki J, Rey C, Glimcher MJ, et al: A role for osteocalcin in osteoclast differentiation. J Cell Biochem 45:292, 1991.
17. Horton MA, Davies J: Perspectives: Adhesion receptors in bone. J Bone Min Res 4:803, 1989.
18. Ali Y: Mechanism of calcification in cartilage and bone. Bone 4:18, 1987.
19. Boskey AL: Current concepts of the physiology and biochemistry of calcification. Clin Orthop Rel Res 157:225, 1981.
20. Pfeilschifter J, Bonewald L, Mundy GR: Characterization of the latent transforming growth factor β complex in bone. J Bone Min Res 5:49, 1990.
21. Glimcher MJ: The nature of the mineral component of bone and the mechanism of calcification. Instructional Course Lectures 36:49, 1987.
22. Gehron-Robey PG, Young MF, Flanders KC, et al: Osteoblasts synthesize and respond to transforming growth factor type β (TGF-β) in vitro. J Cell Biol 105:457, 1987.
23. Warwick R, Williams PL: Gray's Anatomy. 37th ed. Edinburgh, Churchill Livingstone, 1989, p 36.
24. Revell PA: Histomorphometry of bone. J Clin Pathol 36:1323, 1983.
25. Marks SC, Popoff SN: Bone cell biology: The regulation of development, structure and function in the skeleton. Am J Anat 183:1, 1988.
26. Ali SY, Ralphas JR, Stamp TCB: Matrix vesicles in human bone disorders. Bone 6:482, 1985.
27. Boyde A: Electron microscopy of the mineralizing front. *In* Jee WS, Parfitt AM (eds): Bone Histomorphometry Third International Workshop. Paris, Society Nouvelle de Publications Medicales et Dentraires, 1980, p 69.
28. Ellis HA: Metabolic bone disease. *In* Anthony PP, MacSween RNM (eds): Recent Advances in Histopathology. Edinburgh, Churchill Livingstone, 1981, p 185.
29. Fallon MD, Teitelbaum SL: The interpretation of fluorescent tetracycline markers in the diagnosis of metabolic bone diseases. Hum Pathol 13:416, 1982.
30. Udagawa N, Takahashi N, Akatsu T, et al: The bone marrow-derived stromal cell lines MC3T3-G2/PQ6 and ST2 support osteoclast-cocultures with mouse spleen cells. Endocrinology 125:1805, 1989.
31. Thomson BM, Saklavala J, Chambers TJ: Osteoblasts mediate interleukin-1 stimulation of bone resorption by rat osteoclasts. J Exp Med 164:104, 1986.
32. McSheehy PMJ, Chambers TJ: Osteoblastic cells mediate osteoclastic responsiveness to parathyroid hormone. Endocrinology 118:824, 1986.
33. Lanyon LE: The success and failure of the adaptive response to functional load-bearing in averting bone fracture. Bone 13:S17, 1992.
34. Garrett IR, Mundy GR: Relationship between interleukin-1 and prostaglandins in resorbing neonatal calvariae. J Bone Min Res 4:789, 1989.
35. Braidman AP, Davenport LK, Carter DH, et al: Preliminary in situ identification of estrogen target cells in bone. J Bone Min Res 10:74, 1995.
36. Chambers TJ: The pathophysiology of the osteoclast. J Clin Pathol 38:241, 1985.
37. Baron R, Chakraborty M, Chatterjee D, et al: The biology of the osteoclast. *In* Mundy GR, Martin TJ (eds): Physiology and Pharmacology of Bone: Handbook of Experimental Pharmacology. Berlin, Springer-Verlag, 1993, p 111.
38. Takahashi S, Goldring S, Roodman GD: Detection of calcitonin receptor (CTR) mRNA at multiple stages in the osteoclast (OCL) lineage by the polymerase chain reaction (PCR). J Bone Min Res 8(Suppl 1):1084, 1993.
39. Horton MA, Rimmer ET, Lewis D, et al: Cell surface characterization of the human osteoclast: Phenotypic relationship to other bone marrow-derived cell types. J Pathol 144:281, 1984.
40. Chambers TJ, Magnus CJ: Calcitonin alters the behaviour of isolated osteoclasts. J Pathol 136:27, 1982.
41. Blair HC, Teitelbaum SL, Ghiselli R, et al: Osteoclastic bone resorption by a polarized vacuolar proton pump. Science 245:855, 1989.
42. Mundy GR, Roodman GD: Osteoclast ontogeny and function. *In* Peck EA (ed): Bone and Mineral Research. Amsterdam, Elsevier, 1987, p 209.
43. Wright KR, Hughes DH, Guise TA, et al: Osteoclasts

undergo apoptosis at the interface between resorption and formation in bone remodelling units. J Bone Min Res 1994; 9(Suppl. 1): S174.
44. Parfitt AM: Morphometry of bone resorption: Introduction and overview. Bone 14:435, 1993.
45. Parfitt AM: Osteonatal and hemi-osteonal remodeling: The spatial and temporal framework for signal traffic in adult human bone. J Cell Biochem 55:273, 1994.
46. Revell PA: Pathology of Bone. New York, Springer-Verlag, 1986, p 102.
47. Skjodt H, Russell G: Bone cell biology and the regulation of bone turnover. *In* Gowen M (ed): Cytokines and Bone Metabolism. Boca Raton, Florida, CRC Press, 1992, p 1.
48. Rehman MTA, Hoyland JA, Denton J, et al: Age related histomorphometric changes in bone in normal British men and women. J Clin Pathol 47:529, 1994.
49. Howard GA, Bottemiller BL, Turner RT, et al: Parathyroid hormone stimulates bone formation and resorption in organ culture: Evidence for a coupling mechanism. Proc Natl Acad Sci U S A 78:3204, 1981.
50. Bonewald LF, Mundy GR: Role of transforming growth factor β on bone remodeling: A review. Conn Tiss Res 19:201, 1989.
51. Canalis E, McCarthy T, Centrella M: Growth factors and the regulation of bone remodelling. J Clin Invest 81:277, 1989.
52. Massague J: Transforming growth factor β modulates the high affinity receptors of epidermal growth factor and transforming growth factor. J Cell Biol 100:1508, 1985.
53. Massague J, Kelly B, Mottola C: Stimulation by insulin-like growth factors is required for cellular transformation by type β transforming growth factor. J Biol Chem 260:4551, 1985.
54. Smith RA: Recent advances in the metabolism and physiology of bone. *In* Baker PF (ed): Recent Advances in Physiology. Edinburgh, Churchill-Livingstone, 1984, p 317.
55. Raisz LG: Local and systemic factors in the pathogenesis of osteoporosis. N Engl J Med 318:818, 1988.
56. Hutchinson AJ, Whitehouse RW, Boulton HF, et al: Correlation of bone histology with parathyroid hormone, vitamin D_3 and radiology in end-stage renal disease. Kidney Int 44:1071, 1993.
57. Teti A, Rizzoli R, Zambonin-Zallone A: Parathyroid hormone binding to cultured avian osteoclasts. Biochem Biophys Res Comm 174:1217, 1991.
58. Smith D, Gowen M, Mundy GR: Effects of interferon gamma and other cytokines on collagen synthesis in fetal rat bone cultures. Endocrinology 120:2494, 1987.
59. Noda M, Camilliere JJ: In vivo stimulation of bone formation by transforming growth factor beta. Endocrinology 124:2991, 1989.
60. Marcelli C, Yates AJP, Mundy GR: In vivo effects of human recombinant transforming growth factor β turnover in normal mice. J Bone Min Res 5:1087, 1990.
61. Lowik CWGM, van der Pluijm G, Bloys H, et al: Parathyroid hormone (PTH) and PTH-like protein (Plp) stimulate interleukin-6 production by osteogenic cells: A possible role of interleukin-6 in osteoclastogenesis. Biochem Biophys Res Comm 162:1546, 1989.
62. Gowen M, Wood DD, Ihrie EJ, et al: An interleukin-1 like factor stimulates bone resorption in vitro. Nature 306:378, 1993.
63. Garrett IR, Boyce BF, Oreffo ROC, et al: Oxygen derived free radicals stimulate osteoclastic bone resorption in rodent bone in vitro and in vivo. J Clin Invest 85:632, 1990.
64. Gallwitz WE, Mundy GR, Lee C, et al: 5-Lipoxygenase metabolites of arachidonic acid stimulate isolated osteoclasts to resorb calcified matrix. J Biol Chem 368:10087, 1993.
65. Chambers TJ, Ali HN: Inhibition of osteoclastic motility by prostaglandins I_2, E_1, E_2, and 6-oxoE_1. J Pathol 139:383, 1983.
66. Boyce BF, Aufdemorte TB, Garrett IR, et al: Effects of interleukin-1 on bone turnover in normal mice. Endocrinology 125:1142, 1989.
67. Evans DM, Ralston SH: Nitric oxide and bone. J Bone Min Res 11:300, 1996.
68. Owen TA, Aronow M, Shalhoub V, et al: Progressive development of the rat osteoblast phenotype in vitro: Reciprocal relationships in expression of genes associated with osteoblast proliferation and differentiation during formation of the bone extracellular matrix. J Cell Physiol 143:420, 1990.
69. Manolagas SC, Jilka RL: Bone marrow, cytokines, and bone remodeling: Emerging insights into the pathophysiology of osteoporosis. N Engl J Med 332:305, 1995.
70. Garett IR, Guise TA, Bonewald LF, et al: Evidence that interleukin-1 mediates its effects on bone resorption via the 80 kilodalton interleukin-1 receptor. Calcif Tiss Int 52:438, 1993.
71. Martin TJ, Ingleton PM, Underwood JC, et al: Parathyroid hormone-responsive adenylate cyclase in induced transplantable osteogenic rat sarcoma. Nature 260:436, 1975.
72. Canalis E, McCarthy T, Centrella M: The role of growth factors in skeletal remodeling. Endocrin Metab Clin North Am 18:903, 1989.
73. Canalis E, Centrella M, Burch W, et al: Insulin-like growth factor 1 mediates selective effects of parathyroid hormone in bone cultures. J Clin Invest 83:60, 1989.
74. Canalis E: Effect of insulin-like growth factor 1 on DNA and protein synthesis in cultured rat calvaria. J Clin Invest 66:709, 1980.
75. Farley JR, Tarbaux NM, Hall SL, et al: The anti-bone resorptive agent calcitonin also acts in vitro to directly increase bone formation and bone cell proliferation. Endocrinology 123:159, 1988.
76. Kurihara N, Chenu C, Civin CL, et al: Identification of committed mononuclear precursors for osteoclast-like cells formed in long-term narrow cultures. Endocrinology 126:2733, 1990.
77. Kurihara N, Gluck S, Roodman GD: Sequential expression of phenotype markers for osteoclasts during differentiation of precursors for multinucleated cells formed in long-term human marrow cultures. Endocrinology 127:3215, 1990.
78. Coccia PF, Krivit W, Cervenka J, et al: Successful bone marrow transplantation for infantile malignant osteoporosis. N Engl J Med 302:701, 1980.
79. Baron R, Neff F, Van PT, et al: Kinetic and cytochemical identification of osteoclast precursors and their differentiation into multinucleated osteoclasts. Am J Pathol 121:323, 1986.
80. Caplan AL, Pechak DG: The cellular and molecular embryology of bone formation. In Peck WA (ed):

Bone and Mineral Research. Amsterdam, Elsevier, 1987, p 209.
81. Owen M: Lineage of osteogenic cells and their relationship to the stromal system. *In* Peck WA (ed): Bone and Mineral Research. Amsterdam, Elsevier, 1985, p 1.
82. Khan AJ, Simmons DJ: Investigation of the cell lineage in bone using a chimera of chick and quail embryonic tissue. Nature 258:325, 1975.
83. Ham AW: A histologic study of the early phases of bone repair. J Bone Joint Surg 12:827, 1930.
84. Mindell ER, Rodbard S, Kwasman BG: Chondrogenesis in bone repair. A study of the healing fracture callus in the rat. Clin Orthop Rel Res 79:187, 1971.
85. Mackie EJ, Trechsel U: Stimulation of bone formation in vivo by transforming growth factor beta remodeling of woven bone and lack of inhibition by indomethacin. Bone 11:295, 1990.
86. Kasugi S, Todescau R, Nagata T, et al: Expression of bone matrix proteins associated by adult rat bone marrow cells in vitro: Inductive effects of dexamethasone on the osteoblastic phenotype. J Cell Physiol 147:111, 1991.
87. Ishida H, Bellows CG, Aubin JE, et al: Characterization of the 1,25-$(OH)_2D_3$ induced inhibition of bone nodule formation in long-term cultures of fetal rat calvaria cells. Endocrinology 132:61, 1993.
88. Hoyland JA, Freemont AJ, Sharpe P: Interleukin 6 (IL-6), IL-6 receptor and IL-6 nuclear factor gene expression in Paget's disease. J Bone Min Res 9:75, 1994.
89. Andrew JG, Hoyland JA, Freemont AJ, et al: Platelet derived growth factor expression in normally healing human fractures. Bone 16:455, 1995.
90. Andrew JG, Hoyland JA, Andrew SM, et al: Demonstration of TGF-β_1 in normally healing fracture callus by in-situ hybridisation. Calcif Tiss Int 52:74, 1993.
91. Andrew JG, Hoyland JA, Freemont AJ, et al: Insulin like growth factor gene expression in human fracture callus. Calcif Tiss Int 53:97, 1993.
92. Wozney JM, Rozen V: Bone morphogenetic proteins. *In* Mundy GR, Martin TJ (eds): Physiology and Pharmacology of Bone. Berlin, Springer-Verlag, 1993, p 725.
93. MacDonald BR, Mundy GR, Clark S, et al: Effects of human recombinant CSF-GM and highly purified CSF-1 on the formation of multinucleated cells with osteoclast characteristics in long-term bone marrow cultures. J Bone Min Res 1:227, 1986.
94. Felix R, Cecchini MG, Fleisch H: Macrophage colony stimulating factor restores in vivo bone resorption in the op/op osteopetrotic mouse. Endocrinology 127:2592, 1990.
95. Frost HM: Bone mass and the mechanostat: A proposal. Anat Rec 219:1, 1987.
96. Vaughan J: The Physiology of Bone. 3rd ed. Oxford, Oxford University Press, 1981.
97. Harris SE, Harris MA, Feng JW, et al: Expression of bone morphogenetic proteins (BMPs) during differentiation of fetal rat calvarial osteoblasts in vitro. J Bone Min Res 7(Suppl 1):112, 1992.
98. Kwan APL, Freemont AJ, Grant ME: Immunoperoxidase localisation of Type X collagen in chicken tibiae. Bioscience Reports 6:155, 1986.
99. Roberts DJ, Tabin C: The genetics of human limb development. Am J Hum Genet 55:106, 1994.
100. Duprez DM, Kostakopolou K, Francis-West PH, et al: Activation of Fgf-4 and HOXD gene expression by BMP-2 expressing cells in the developing chick limb. Development 122:1821, 1996.
101. Bullough PG, Vigorita VJ: Atlas of orthopaedic pathology with clinical and radiologic correlations. London, Gower Medical Publishing, 1983.
102. Klein B, Battaille R: Recent advances in the biology of IL-6 in multiple myeloma. Cancer J 4:81, 1991.
103. McCullum P, Freemont AJ, Geary C, et al: A case of IgD myeloma presenting as diffuse osteosclerosis. J Clin Pathol 41:486, 1988.
104. Stewart AF, Vignery A, Silvergate A, et al: Quantitive bone histomorphometry in humoral hypercalcaemia of malignancy: Uncoupling of bone cell activity. J Clin Endocr Metab 55:219, 1988.
105. Mundy GR, Luben RA, Raisz LG, et al: Evidence for the secretion of an osteoclast stimulating factor in myeloma. N Engl J Med 291:1041, 1974.
106. Young M, Freemont AJ: Primary leiomyosarcoma of bone. Histopathology 19:257, 1991.

Chapter

3

CELL AND ORGAN CULTURE IN THE UNDERSTANDING OF BONE AND ITS NEOPLASMS

NICHOLAS A. ATHANASOU

Cell and organ (or tissue) culture refers to the growth and maintenance of isolated cells or whole tissue components outside the body under suitable conditions in which a number of their characteristics can be studied. Cell and organ culture is a commonly used technique in the study of bone biology but, with the exception of the cytogenetic analysis (see Chapter 4), is not commonly employed in the diagnosis of bone tumors. Nevertheless, isolation and culture of cells from bone and other osteoarticular tissues does provide a unique means of studying these cells, permitting analysis of their various structural, cytochemical, biochemical, functional, and other characteristics. Definition of these characteristics is clearly important in this study of bone tumors, which are classified according to the structural and functional features of the neoplastic cells. Organ and cell culture studies have greatly increased our understanding of the pathogenesis of skeletal neoplasms and have provided a basis for the development of new methods of diagnosis and treatment of these tumors. The studies on primary malignant bone tumors are considered here in detail, and the pathobiology of malignant bone resorption associated with skeletal metastases is discussed.

BONE ORGAN AND CELL CULTURE SYSTEMS

Organ Culture Systems

In bone organ culture systems, explants of bone are maintained in a chemically defined medium, supplemented with low levels of serum for a relatively short incubation time. These systems have the advantage of preserving the skeletal microenvironment, particularly the anatomic status between bone cells and the extracellular matrix; the response of explanted bone to particular stimuli can then be analyzed in vitro to determine changes in these components. In fetal long bone and neonatal calvarial bone organ culture systems, bone that is newly formed is labeled by injection of radio-isotopes in vivo; the prelabeled isotope (e.g., ^{45}Ca) in the bone explants is released under experimental conditions and this is then measured over a defined period of organ culture, being expressed as a percentage of the total bone isotope originally present.[1, 2] Such systems are essentially limited to studying bone resorption because under most organ culture conditions the net effect is one of bone resorption. It is through organ culture that the stimulatory effect on bone resorption of major systemic osteotropic hormones, such as 1,25 dihydroxyvitamin D_3 ($1,25(OH)_2D_3$) and parathyroid hormone (PTH), was first demonstrated; the stimulatory effect of local factors, such as various prostaglandins, cytokines, and growth factors on bone resorption can also be measured by this method.[3] An inhibitory effect on bone resorption by systemic and local hormonal factors (e.g., calcitonin, interferon-γ) can be detected in organ culture systems,[4] and the effect of combinations of hormones on bone resorption (i.e., whether one factor can overcome the stimulatory or inhibitory effect of another) can be examined.[5]

Organ culture systems can also be used to study bone formation. Cultured explants are allowed to incorporate an isotope (e.g., ^{3}H proline) from the culture medium so that the bone matrix becomes labeled. Agents such as insulin-like growth factor (IGF) specifically increase collagen synthesis,[6] whereas agents known to stimulate bone resorption specifically switch off collagen synthesis.[7, 8] Mineralization does not ordinarily take place in organ culture, and there is still some doubt over how closely organ culture studies of bone formation relate to matrix synthesis and mineralization in vivo.

Organ culture techniques are of limited use in determining the ontogeny of bone cells, owing to the heterogeneous nature of the cell population found in skeletal explants. However, an organ culture technique developed by Burger et al.[9] that employs fetal mouse metatarsal bones from which the periosteum has been removed has been used extensively to study the ontogeny of the osteoclast. These bone rudiments do not contain osteoclasts or their progenitors but do contain chondrocytes and osteoblasts. Osteoclast formation is seen when these bone rudiments are cocultured with immature marrow mononuclear cells containing osteoclast progenitors (derived from the pluripotential hematopoietic stem cell), but not with mature adherent bone marrow cells or mature monocytes or tissue macrophages.[10, 11]

Cell Culture Systems

The primary objective of developing methods to isolate and culture bone cells is to obtain a homogeneous cell population on which experiments can be reproducibly performed. Bone organ culture systems have proved too complex to ascribe a particular hormonal response or observed function to a specific bone cell type. To analyze the functional activity of bone cells and, in particular, to characterize the origin and developmental pathway of specific cell populations in bone (Fig. 3–1), it is necessary to isolate and establish cultures of purified bone cells. It is not possible, however, to isolate from bone a wholly pure population of one bone cell type, and more realistically the aim is to isolate cell populations that contain predominantly a single bone cell type.

Osteoblast Culture

Osteoblast populations that are relatively pure and suitable for cell culture studies have proved particularly difficult to isolate satisfactorily, as the criteria for their definition are not precise, certainly less so than for osteoclasts. Primary cultures of osteoblasts derived by sequential enzymatic digestion of neonatal rodent calvaria have been used for a number of studies. These mononuclear osteoblast-like cell preparations are defined primarily by biochemical criteria, including PTH stimulation of adenyl cyclase activity, elevated levels of alkaline phosphatase, and secretion of type I collagen and osteocalcin[12, 13]; they maintain certain differentiated characteristics if they are subcultured at high density and also proliferate in culture. However, cells within this osteoblast-like population are by no means homogeneous by histochemical or morphologic criteria.[14, 15] The developmental or metabolic status of these isolated cells is particularly important because many of the effects caused by a particular agent depend greatly on whether these cells are proliferating or stable. Receptor studies have indicated that osteoblast function may be related to the number of surface receptors, and that after the second or third passage, cell cultures contain a majority of cells exhibiting the osteoblastic phenotype.[16]

Pluripotential haematopoietic stem cell → Marrow CFU-GM → Circulating Monocytes/Osteoclast precursors → Osteoclast precursors in bone → (M-CSF, $1,25(OH)_2D_3$) → Osteoclasts (→ Bone resorption)

Pluripotential bone stromal cell → Committed osteoprogenitor cell → Preosteoblast → Osteoblast (→ Osteoid/bone formation)

↘ Committed progenitors for other mesenchymal cells in bone [e.g., chondrocytes, fibroblasts, adipocytes]

Figure 3–1. Schematic outline of the cell lineage of osteoclasts and osteoblasts favored by current cell culture studies. Osteoblasts are necessary for the proliferation and differentiation of osteoclast precursors, and they control osteoclastic bone-resorbing activity.

It has also been possible to study bone formation using osteoblast-rich populations from various animal and human sources.[17] In culture, these osteoblasts synthesize type I collagen and numerous non-collagen proteins.[17, 18] A number of cytokines such as transforming growth factor-β (TGF-β) appear to be involved in osteoblast differentiation.[19] The matrix produced by stromal cell populations can be altered when culture conditions are manipulated, so that the matrix produced by osteoblasts can be induced to mineralize in culture when an exogenous source of phosphate (usually β-glycerolphosphate) is supplied.[20, 21] It is assumed that alkaline phosphatase produced by osteoblasts releases phosphate from the substrate and that once a critical concentration is reached, crystals of calcium phosphate are deposited. Whether this process of mineralization in vitro truly reflects bone formation in vivo remains uncertain.

To provide a relatively homogeneous cell population uncontaminated by other bone cell types, cloned or transformed stromal cell lines of osteoblasts or chondrocytes are commonly employed. Many of these cell lines were originally derived from animal and human bone neoplasms. Clonal variants of primary rat osteosarcoma cell lines such as UMR and ROS cells are commonly used in bone cell biology,[22] and it is important to ensure that such cells continue to express the differentiated phenotype of interest. In general, these cells express a highly characteristic osteoblast-like phenotype, although mineralization and bone formation are not generally seen. The practical value of such cell lines is that they permit large-scale studies to be carried out for investigation of the bone cell response to particular agents.

Osteoclast Culture

In contrast to osteoblasts, osteoclasts can be isolated directly from bone and identified with some certainty. Osteoclasts are generally isolated by curettage of the endosteal surface of neonatal avian or rodent/murine bone after the marrow has been removed.[23] Human osteoclasts have proved more difficult to isolate, and the most fruitful source of osteoclast-like cells has proved to be giant cells isolated from giant cell tumor of bone.[24] Although curettage of bone generates a mixed population of cells, it does provide a relatively pure population of osteoclasts that are suitable for functional, morphologic, and cytochemical characterization. Osteoclasts isolated in this way adhere strongly to a plastic, glass, or bone substrate after settling; they rapidly expand their cytoplasm and are highly motile (Fig. 3–2). This activity is directly inhibited by calcitonin (Fig. 3–3) and, to a lesser extent, prostaglandin.[23, 25] When cultured on a smooth-surfaced bone or other mineralized (e.g., dentine) substrate, osteoclasts produce highly characteristic resorption lacunae (Fig. 3–4). These are single or multiple well-defined oval or circular areas of excavation of the bone surface.[26, 27] An assessment of the amount of bone resorbed by these

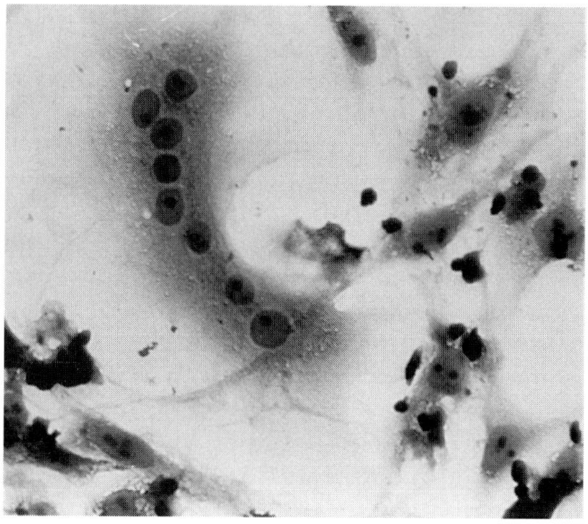

Figure 3–2. Rat osteoclast in coculture with osteoblasts. Osteoclast cytoplasm is extensive where it is in contact with osteoblasts, indicating an increase in osteoclastic activity. (Giemsa.)

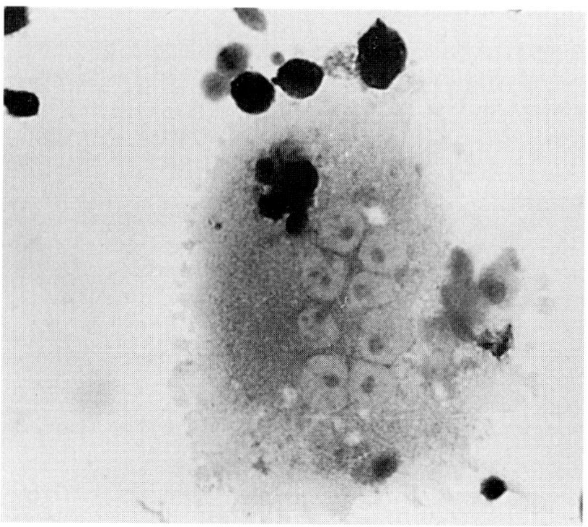

Figure 3–3. Isolated rat osteoclast after administration of salmon calcitonin (1 ng/mL), showing retraction and blunting of cytoplasmic processes. (Giemsa.)

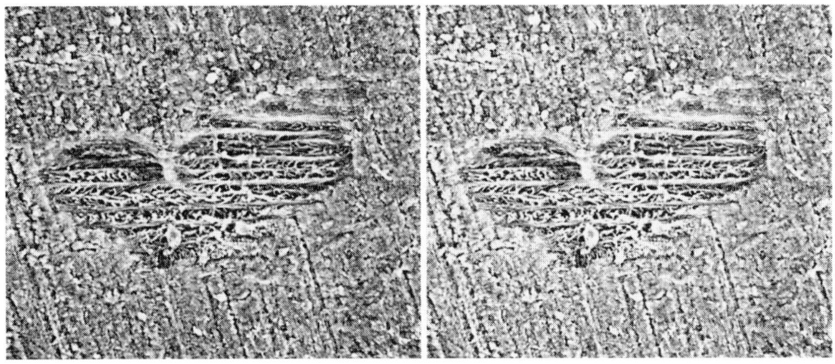

Figure 3–4. Scanning electron microscopic stereopair photomicrographs of lacunar resorption pits formed by isolated rat osteoclasts after 24 hours in culture on a smooth-surfaced cortical bone slice. (Field width = 150 μm.)

cells can be made by measuring the surface area (or volume) of resorption pits produced on the bone slice. The addition of hormones or other agents to this culture system thus provides a means of directly determining the influence of these factors on osteoclast activity. This system can be modified by the addition of other cell types (e.g., osteoblasts, other stromal cells, or tumor cells) that are thought to influence osteoclast activity. It has been shown that hormones that stimulate osteoclast resorptive activity, such as PTH, 1,25$(OH)_2D_3$, interleukin-1 (IL-1), tumor necrosis factor (TNF), and prostaglandins achieve their effects by acting primarily via the osteoblast, which then stimulates osteoclast activity.[28–31]

One of the disadvantages of the isolated osteoclast bone resorption assay is that insufficient cells are isolated for biochemical studies to be performed. Sequential enzyme digestion techniques isolate larger numbers of "osteoclast-like" cells. This cell population, however, is heterogeneous, and the ability of these cells to resorb bone is questionable.[12, 14, 32] For the same reason, various mononuclear phagocyte populations (monocytes, tissue macrophages) were used as osteoclast surrogates in cell culture studies; these cells are capable of releasing both mineral and organic matrix components from devitalized bone fragments,[33–35] but they are not capable of lacunar bone resorption when cultured alone on bone slices.[36] Mononuclear phagocytes also lack several specific osteoclastic characteristics, such as the presence of membrane ruffled borders and calcitonin receptors.[33, 37]

Culture of Bone Cell Precursors

Cell culture studies have added to evidence from experimental animal and hormone culture work that showed that osteoblasts and osteoclasts have separate cell lineages (see Fig. 3–1).[9, 10, 38–40]

Osteoclasts

Cell culture studies on the osteoclast cell lineage have often provided conflicting results, and the nature of osteoclast precursor cells and the precise osteoclast lineage pathway remains controversial. Although a number of studies appear to show that the osteoclast has an entirely separate lineage from that of mononuclear phagocytes (with even its own unique primordial stem cell), it is now known that the osteoclast is derived from the pluripotential hematopoietic stem cell and that it shares its more committed progenitors (e.g., colony forming unit–GM) with monocytes and macrophages.[41–43] Recent studies of long-term mammalian, avian, spleen, and bone marrow cell culture systems have shown that a number of cellular and hormonal factors are required for the generation of osteoclasts from hematopoietic precursors. These include the presence of osteoblasts or specific bone-derived stromal cells and incubation with 1,25$(OH)_2D_3$ and macrophage colony-stimulating factor (M-CSF).[44–48] It has recently been shown that monocytes and tissue macrophages are also capable of osteoclastic differentiation under the same cellular and hormonal conditions (Fig. 3–5).[49, 50] These findings are of considerable significance in the pathologic bone resorption associated with inflammatory and neoplastic lesions of bone, in which a significant macrophage infiltrate is generally present. Macrophages isolated from these lesions are capable of osteoclastic differentiation.[51–53] Cell culture studies have also shown that extraskeletal tumors and inflammatory lesions containing numerous macrophages and macrophage polykaryons include a subset of mononuclear phagocytes that exhibit osteoclastic

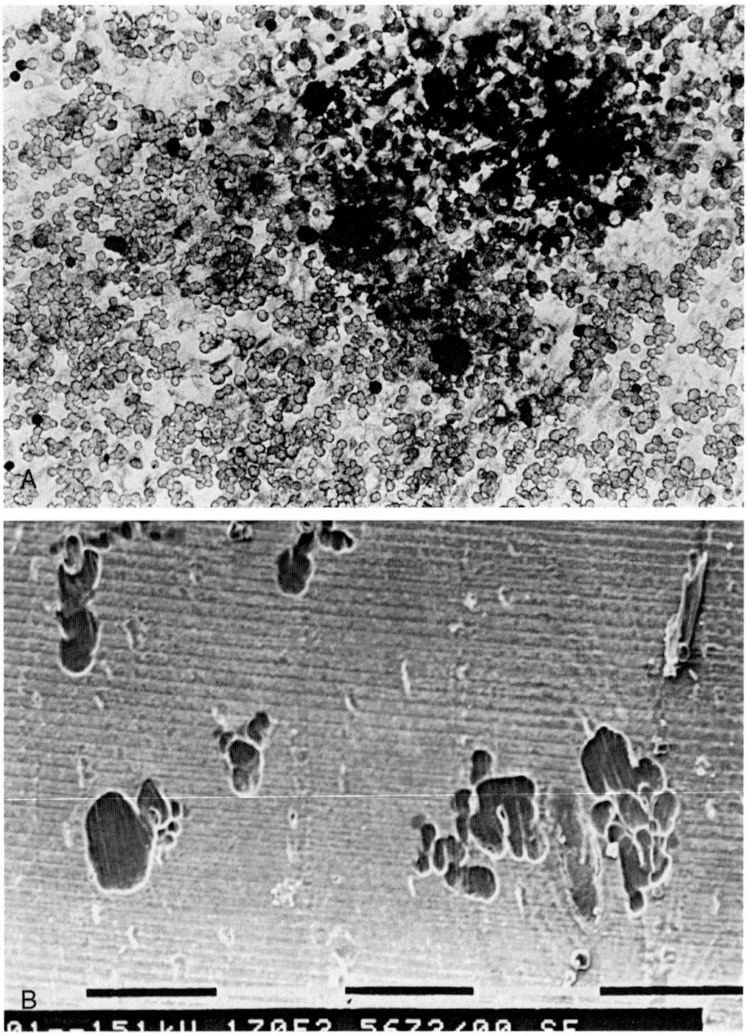

Figure 3–5. Osteoclastic differentiation of monocytes and tissue macrophages. *A*, A cluster of TRAP positive cells formed after coculture of mouse monocytes with UMR 106 rat osteosarcoma cells. *B*, Scanning electron microscopic photomicrograph of corresponding coculture on bone slice where cells have been removed; numerous resorption lacunae are present. (Black bar = 0.1 mm.)

properties, including that of bone resorption.[54–57] These findings argue strongly in favor of the osteoclast being considered a member of the mononuclear phagocyte system; osteoclasts have a common hematopoietic origin with that of monocytes and macrophages, and their mononuclear precursor clearly circulates in the monocyte fraction. More recent cell culture studies have demonstrated the importance of the role of osteoblasts not only in the regulation of osteoclast activity but also in osteoclast formation.[47, 48]

Osteoblasts

The origin of osteoblasts, chondrocytes, and other bone stromal cells has proved more difficult to determine than that of osteoclasts. This is on account of the numerous similar morphologic and other features exhibited by the precursors of each of these specific stromal cell types, and the relative lack of specific defining features to distinguish immature from differentiated stromal cell types. Friedenstein[58, 59] used a combination of in vitro and in vivo techniques, including diffusion chambers, to study the differentiation of bone marrow stromal cells and showed that single bone marrow cells could give rise to a variety of stromal cell lines. Single cells were cloned after up to 20 days in culture, and then single colonies were transferred to live animals, where they subsequently formed plaques, some of which contained a mixture of connective tissues, including bone. Using the same methodology, fibroblasts cultured from lymphoreticular tissue, including spleen, thymus, and lymph nodes, were shown to be incapable of bone formation. When an osteogenic inducing factor, such as transitional epithelium of the urinary tract, decalcified bone matrix, or bone morphogenetic protein (BMP) was added to diffusion chambers containing fibroblasts, a calcified tissue was formed.[60, 61] Thus, bone marrow appears to contain undifferentiated mesenchymal stromal cells that are capable of differentiating into committed progenitors of osteoblasts (determined osteogenic precursor cells) and that extraskeletal tissue contains cells that, when appropriately stimulated, are capable of osteogenic differentiation (inducible osteogenic precursor cells).[61]

It has been proposed that, analogous to the hematopoietic system, pluripotential primordial stromal stem cells are present within bone and marrow, and that from these cells are derived more committed progenitors, each of which gives rise to a different specific stromal cell line (see Fig. 3–1).[61, 62] This process occurs in a number of steps each of which leads to commitment or restriction to a particular stromal cell phenotype.[63] The factors controlling this differentiation process are not fully characterized, but it is known that glucocorticoids, fibroblast growth factor (FGF), platelet-derived growth factor (PDGF), TGF-β, and BMPs are involved in the regulation of some of these steps.[63, 64] Cell lines and primary cultures have been used to investigate the transitional steps in osteoblast and chondroblast differentiation. Osteoblasts and chondroblasts share expression of some molecules, and hypertrophic chondrocytes down-regulate expression of some cartilage markers and up-regulate osteoblast marker expression.[64, 65]

CELL AND ORGAN CULTURE STUDIES ON BONE NEOPLASMS

The mechanisms underlying the induction of neoplastic change in the cellular components of bone are unknown. It is widely accepted that neoplastic transformation occurs in a number of steps. The net effect of the changes associated with each of these steps is production of a malignant tumor cell with unlimited growth potential. The characterization of genes and proteins expressed in malignant cells is an important area of study in bone tumor biology because it identifies those crucial areas of the genome and their protein products that are associated with the chaotic state of cellular malignancy. There is evidence that inherited chromosomal abnormalities related to the loss of a tumor suppressor gene or expression of an oncogene are involved (e.g., deletion of the same locus in chromosome 13 in patients with hereditary retinoblastoma who also have a higher incidence of osteosarcoma).[66] Such changes can be identified by cytogenetic analysis, which employs short-term in vitro culture. Cytokines and growth factors play an important role in inducing expression of particular oncogenes, which can be identified in cultured neoplastic cells.

Osteosarcoma

Osteosarcomas are malignant tumors that may have variable histologic features but are characterized by the presence of malignant cells that directly form osteoid or bone. In vitro studies on isolated osteosarcoma cells have been employed to explain the great variation in histologic patterns of osteosarcoma, to determine the factors governing their oncogenesis and growth, and to provide a theoretical basis for the selection of anticancer therapy. As mentioned earlier, a number of animal and human osteosarcoma cell lines are also commonly used as surrogates for osteoblast-like cells in the study of osteoblast biology and bone formation.

Culture of Murine Osteosarcomas

Several transplantable osteosarcomas have been studied in mice or rats, including spontaneous osteosarcomas and osteosarcomas induced by radiation or viral or chemical agents. One of the characteristics of a number of murine osteosarcomas is their strong bone-inducing ability. This was first shown using diffusion chamber techniques[67] and pointed to the existence of an osteogenic factor in all osteosarcomas. Amitani and Nakata[68] showed that an established rat clonal osteosarcoma cell line, BFO, exhibits rapid growth in culture with a serum requirement and no contact inhibition. In vitro, BFO cells show a decrease in the synthesis of an osteo-inductive factor, which is regained when the tumor is reimplanted into an isologous host. Tumor cell culture transplants of Dunn and Ridgway mouse osteosarcomas—standard experimental tools of tumor immunology, chemotherapy, and bone cell differentiation—are capable of osteogenesis and chondrogenesis.[69] Of relevance to the known variation in histologic appearances of osteosarcoma is the finding that distinct osteogenic neoplastic subclones can be obtained from a primary mouse osteosarcoma.[70] These clones exhibit significant morphologic, functional, and molecular diversity but retain the basic pathogenic properties of the tumor from which they were derived.

Culture of Human Osteosarcomas

Relatively few human osteosarcoma cell lines have been established, not only because of the relative infrequency of this tumor but also because of the difficulty in isolating osteosarcoma cells from the abundant calcified matrix that surrounds them. In addition, maintaining these cells in culture is problematic, as they are commonly overgrown by fibroblast-like cells. A number of early studies succeeded in establishing human osteosarcoma cell lines (Fig. 3–6), which exhibit many of the criteria commonly used to define malignant transformation.[71–74] Yamane et al.[75] established continuously growing osteosarcoma cell lines in vitro after transplantation of a human osteosarcoma into athymic nude mice. These cells showed alkaline phosphatase activity (increased by $1,25(OH)_2D_3$), and cytogenetic studies showed that they were aneuploid. Kawai[76] established a human osteosarcoma cell line HuO9 from a tumor that was transplanted into athymic nude mice. This cell line expresses a well-differentiated osteoblastic phenotype and provides a useful model for the study of osteoblasts. Tumor cells have alkaline phosphatase activity and secrete osteocalcin, both of which are stimulated by the addition of $1,25(OH)_2D_3$. HuO9 cells respond to human PTH with an increase in production of intracellular cyclic adenosine monophosphate (cAMP). Addition of antiserum against nude mouse spleen cells was found to facilitate the elimination of the fibroblastic cells derived from host tissue.

The production of organic matrix (osteoid) components and their mineralization is considered the most characteristic feature of both normal and malignant osteoblasts. Rodan et al.[77] isolated and maintained a human osteosarcoma cell line (SAOS-2) that showed several osteoblastic properties, including a cAMP response to PTH and the ability to bind $1,25(OH)_2D_3$. It is often used as a source of human osteoblast-like cells and osteoblast-related molecules such as alkaline phosphatase and noncollagen matrix proteins such as osteonectin. These cells form a calcified matrix in diffusion chambers implanted into nude mice, although the cells do not produce tumors when injected subcutaneously into nude mice. Other human osteosarcoma cell lines, such as MG-63 and SAOS-1 cells, have very low levels of alkaline phosphatase activity compared to SAOS-2 cells. A bone-inducing agent has been isolated from cultured SAOS-2 cells that can induce heterotopic bone formation in the muscle of Nu/Nu mice.[78] It has been suggested that these cells contain an optimal admixture of known bone growth factors, BMP-1,2,3,4,6, and other unknown components that, acting alone or in combination with BMP or TGF-β, or both, can induce bone formation. Phorbol esters are also known to induce secretion of alkaline phosphatase by

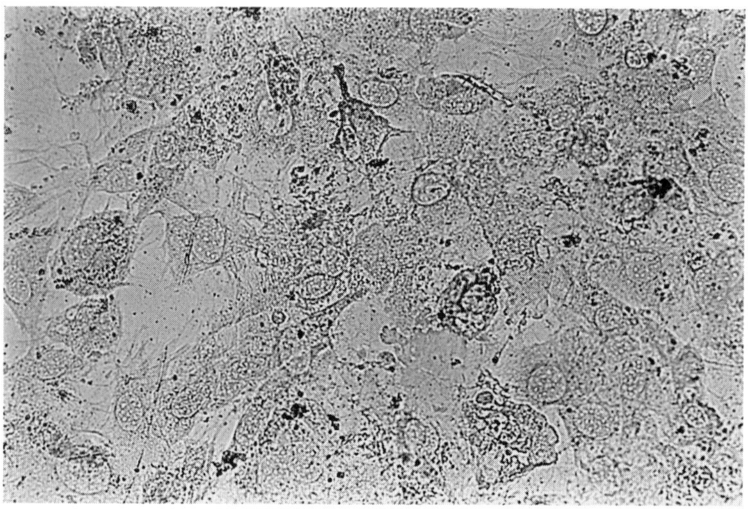

Figure 3–6. Human osteosarcoma cells in confluent culture. (Phase contrast.)

tumor cells of another established human osteosarcoma line, U-2 OS.[79] It is thought that phorbol esters trigger changes in the plasma membrane of human osteosarcoma cells and that this leads to the release of native alkaline phosphatase–enriched matrix vesicles. Both these human osteosarcoma cell lines provide models for the study of cell differentiation and mineralization in vitro.

Sonobe et al.[80] established a new human osteosarcoma cell line, HS-Os-1, that was strongly positive for specific markers of osteoblasts such as alkaline phosphatase and osteocalcin; following inoculation into nude mice, typical osteoblastic osteosarcomas were induced. Both in vitro and in vivo, HS-Os-1 cells showed numerous ultrastructural features characteristic of osteoblasts. Anaplastic fibroblastic and osteoblastic cells with various transitional forms were also noted, suggesting that some of the tumor cells may arise from multipotential mesenchymal cells rather than osteoblasts or their immediate precursors. Oshima et al.[81] have also highlighted this feature of divergent differentiation in osteosarcoma. They succeeded in transplanting human osteosarcomas into nude mice and found that morphologically, the transplanted tumor was a chondrosarcoma that manifested calcification but not ossification. Collagen types I and II mRNA were produced by cells of the transplanted tumor. Collagen type III mRNA was not expressed by the transplanted tumor. These results suggest that the character of progenitor chondrogenic cells might be transferred with the transplanted tumor, and that the tumor cells change expression of collagen genes with differentiation or maturation.

Hormonal Control of Osteosarcoma Cells

A number of osteosarcomas have been established in culture under conditions that allow the effects of hormones on cell replication and function to be studied. Hormonal control of human osteosarcoma cell growth is suggested by the specific regulatory effect of $1,25(OH)_2D_3$ on the growth, morphology, and fibronectin production of the MG-63 human osteosarcoma cells[82]; there is also evidence that both estrogens and androgens directly influence the response of SAOS-2 osteosarcoma cells to human PTH and PTH-related peptide (PTH-rP).[83] McMaster et al.[84] studied the effects of human serum, estradiol, and growth hormone on the incorporation of ^{3}H-thymidine into cultured human articular chondrocytes and osteosarcoma cells. In this system, serum from osteosarcoma patients stimulated tumor cell replication many times more effectively than did control serum; this stimulation could be partially inhibited by estradiol. Estrogens are known to be growth inhibitory, and most human osteosarcomas occur in males. It is therefore possible that estrogens or androgens, or both, may influence tumor growth. Glucocorticoids have also been shown to affect the metabolism of osteosarcoma cells[85]; hydrocortisone produces marked ultrastructural changes in human osteosarcoma cell lines, including an increase in cell size and nuclear and mitochondrial enlargement. In a tumor as hormone-responsive as osteosarcoma appears to be, there is clearly a need to define precisely the effects of hormones on osteosarcoma cells.

Growth Factors and Osteosarcomas

Both protein growth factors and growth inhibitory factors significantly influence the growth of normal and neoplastic cells of the stromal cell system. Abnormal growth factor production or an abnormality in the cellular response to a particular growth factor that stimulates or inhibits mitotic activity may result in uncontrolled cell proliferation and malignant transformation. The bone matrix itself is a rich source of growth factors, which are known to influence bone cell growth and behavior; growth factors are also present in the circulation.

A number of studies have focused on the role of PDGF, a major growth factor for connective tissue cells. The amino acid sequence of PDGF is homologous to that of $p28^{sis}$, the transforming protein of simian sarcoma virus. A PDGF-like growth factor has been isolated from the U-2 OS cell line and shown to have a structure similar to a homodimer of the PDGF A-chains[86, 87]; this PDGF-like growth factor induces tyrosine-specific phosphorylation and early actin reorganization in U-2 OS cells. Disorders in the PDGF-related pathways have since been described in a number of osteosarcoma cell lines, and its RNA has been isolated from some primary osteosarcomas.[88] It is known that some osteosarcoma cell lines can be maintained in the absence of PDGF,[89] and one means whereby osteosarcoma cell growth may become independent of PDGF is by autologous production of PDGF chains, as shown for U-2 OS cells.[86, 87] Amplification of the PDGF A-chain gene and reduplication of the portion of chromosome 22 containing the c-*sis* proto-oncogene has also been found in the DNA extracted from osteosarcomas.[90]

Mioh and Chen[91] showed that a number of growth factors, including PDGF, epidermal growth factor (EGF), heparin-binding growth factor, and TGF-β influence the growth of MG63 human osteosarcoma cells. TGF-β inhibited the mitogenic effects of EGF and PDGF. TGF-β is also known to influence phenotypic expression of the osteoblast and chondroblast phenotypes in vitro, and this activity may be mediated through cell-matrix interactions.[92] Tumor necrosis factor may be a growth factor for human osteosarcoma cells, stimulating cell proliferation and the accumulation of c-*myc* mRNA.[93] Other growth factors such as IGF may also play a role, U-2 OS cells being dependent on IGF-1 for in vitro growth, having receptors for IGF-1 and synthesizing IGF-2.[94, 95] The significance of the effects of many of these growth factors in vitro is often difficult to interpret, as they may differ depending on the type of human osteosarcoma cell line employed.[96]

Oncogene Expression in Osteosarcoma Cells

Analysis of oncogene expression in human osteosarcoma cells has been studied in relation to the known proliferative response to various growth factors. In addition to c-*sis* proto-oncogene expression mentioned above, the c-*myc* proto-oncogene has also been identified. This codes for a nuclear protein that is known to influence cell growth, transformation, and differentiation. The amplification and expression of c-*myc* has been demonstrated in vitro in cell lines isolated from a patient with osteosarcoma of the femur, and this was found to correlate with c-*myc* expression in vivo.[97] Womer[88] noted that PDGF induced c-*myc* mRNA expression in MG-63 human osteosarcoma cells but found that this did not stimulate cell replication. Chan and Song[98] showed that, following transformation with the K-*ras* oncogene, human HDS osteosarcoma cells can be induced to produce matrix metalloproteinases.

Other genes have also been reported to affect bone tumor formation, including the retinoblastoma gene, rearrangement of which is found in several osteosarcomas.[66, 99] The reintroduction of the intact retinoblastoma gene in cell lines derived from bone tumors strongly reduces tumor growth. Huang et al.[100] transfected cultured osteosarcoma cells that did not express the retinoblastoma (*RB*) mRNA with a genetically engineered *RB* gene. The transfected cells were found to express *RB* mRNA and to revert to a nontransformed phenotype in culture. In another osteosarcoma cell line that expressed the *RB* gene normally, transfection with the *RB* gene had no effect. Thus, the loss of *RB* gene function may be a primary event in the genesis of some osteosarcomas, and the restoration of *RB* gene function by genetic replacement may represent a possible treatment in these cases. Changes in tumor suppressor or growth suppressor genes such as p53 have also been reported. Overexpression of wild-type p53 in the SAOS-2 osteosarcoma-derived cell line blocks growth of tumor cells.[101]

Viruses and c-fos *in the Genesis of Osteosarcoma*

Cell culture has proved useful in studying the role that viruses and other factors play in the induction of bone tumors in experimental animals. Early reports showing cell-free passage of avian osteosarcoma suggested that viruses may play a role in the induction of bone sarcomas.[102] This was supported by the appearance of bone tumors in 22% of mice inoculated at birth with SE polyoma virus, a DNA virus.[103] The SV40 virus, also a DNA virus, when injected into hamsters, can result in the formation of osteogenic sarcomas.[104, 105] Many other types of DNA and RNA viruses have similarly been shown to induce bone tumors in different species.[104, 105] A number of murine sarcoma viruses that have a C-type virus particle morphology have been associated with osteosarcoma induction. These type C retroviruses include the FBJ and FBR osteosarcoma viruses derived respectively from a spontaneous osteosarcoma arising in a CF-1 mouse[106] and a radiation-induced osteosarcoma arising in a X/Gf mouse.[107] Neonatal mice of several strains develop osteosarcomas following injections of the FBJ and FBR viruses. Horizontal and vertical transmission from tumor-bearing animals to cage mates and offspring has not been successful.

DNA and RNA tumor viruses induce neoplastic transformation through host cellular genes, which are important for the processes of cell growth regulation. These genes have been shown to be potentially oncogenic themselves. Both FBJ and the FBR viruses contain sequences derived from the mouse *c-fos* gene.[108] The *c-fos* gene has numerous upstream regulatory sequences including response elements to factors such as calcium, cAMP, PDGF, estrogen, and TNF, which influence both the basal and inducible expression of *c-fos* mRNA. The *c-fos* protein is a nuclear phosphoprotein associated with members of the Jun family in the AP-1 transcription complex. Alterations in the regulation of the *c-fos* gene in mRNA translation or protein transcription can result in the *c-fos* protein becoming an active oncogene.[109] In itself, *c-fos* does not transform primary cultures of fibroblasts in vitro, but elimination of the carboxy terminal part of the coding sequence and of a short noncoding domain of the *c-fos* gene converts it into an oncogene in vitro.[110] Activation of *c-fos* is achieved in different ways by FBJ and FBR viruses, but both are essentially associated with identifiable gene mutations or a sequence substitution.[108]

Abnormal *c-fos* expression affects bone growth and differentiation. Overexpression of *c-fos* in transgenic mice interferes with bone development, resulting in excessive new bone formation and the development of osteosarcomas in some animals. Chondrogenic cells and earlier progenitors are also specifically transformed by Fos/Jun, and *c-fos* overexpression appears to favor transformation of the mesenchymal cells.[111] Using an in vitro organ culture model of differentiation of bone-forming cells, in which distinct layers of phenotypically different cells are formed, mesenchymal-like stem cells have been shown to differentiate into osteogenic cells and to form chondroid bone[112]; it was shown that *c-fos* expression in these stem cells precedes osteogenic differentiation.[113] Infection of this organ culture with the FBR virus complex results in the transformation of mesenchymal progenitor cells and formation of a transplantable osteosarcoma-like lesion.[114] The relevance of these studies to human osteosarcoma is not certain, but it has been shown that in 61% of human osteosarcomas, *c-fos* expression is elevated.[115]

Cell Culture and the Treatment of Osteosarcomas

A number of assay systems have been developed to determine the effect of various chemotherapeutic agents and regimes on the growth of osteosarcomas. The application of human tumor clonogenic assay systems, which have been widely used to assess the sensitivity of different carcinoma cells to various antineoplastic drugs, is limited by the low colony-forming activity of sarcoma cells. However, Tomita et al.[116] used a modified form of human tumor clonogenic assay to assess the response of individual tumors to various cytotoxic drugs including methotrexate, doxorubicin (Adriamycin), cisplatin, and vincristine. They found that chemotherapeutic agents that reduced or stimulated colony growth in vitro were correspondingly effective or ineffective clinically.

Gebhardt et al.[117] described an in vitro assay system to measure Adriamycin binding in osteosarcoma cells. Cells were incubated with Adriamycin, and cell viability and the intensity of Adriamycin fluorescence in the nuclei was measured. Adriamycin acts by intercalating to DNA, and its absence from the nucleus probably indicates a resistant cell, thus permitting prediction of Adriamycin sensitivity at the time of diagnosis or relapse. Another in vitro chemosensitivity assay for human osteosarcoma used the large number of viable tumor cells obtained from xenografts of osteosarcoma in athymic nude mice.[118] Ishii et al.[119] described a similar in vitro method for determining sensitivity of drugs used to treat human osteosarcomas. They found that cells that had been grafted onto nude mice were highly sensitive to Adriamycin and mitomycin C and less sensitive to bleomycin and methotrexate in all the tumors tested; similar results were obtained with cells cultured directly from the original tumor. Hall and Wong[120] also showed that certain types of hypolipidemic agents may function as cytotoxic agents that inhibit osteosarcoma cell culture growth.

Other Uses of Osteosarcoma Cell Cultures

Another use of culturing of human osteosarcoma cells is the production of a bone-inducing agent by which bone healing can be enhanced.[121] Further uses include development of monoclonal antibodies, which can be formed following immunization of mice with a human osteosarcoma cell line. Some of these antibodies have been reported to react strongly with osteosarcomas but not with other bone and soft tissue tumors.[122] A different approach to tumor diagnosis using tumor cell culture was employed by Stern et al.,[123] who showed that different sarcoma cell lines (including those of osteosarcoma and Ewing's sarcoma) elaborate different procollagen types. The authors proposed that examination of the matrix proteins produced by sarcoma cell lines may provide a general classification scheme for human sarcomas and permit distinction of one malignant tumor from another.

Chondrosarcoma

General Aspects

When removed from their matrix, normal chondrocytes are difficult to study in long-term culture because they have an extremely limited proliferative potential, generally ceasing cell division after several generations. Cartilage cell cultures also have a marked tendency to revert phenotypically to a more fibroblastic phenotype, a process that involves down-regulation in the biosynthesis of cartilage-specific molecules and a shift in the synthesis of proteoglycans to that of more immature cells. Cell culture studies employing freshly isolated chondrocytes are also limited by the extensive morphologic variability that exists among chondrocytes derived from different animals or from different joints of the same animal, or even different sites within a single joint.[124, 125] These cells also have the ability to switch collagen synthesis from type II to type I collagen and vice versa under a variety of experimental conditions.[124]

Chondrocytes from human fetal and adult articular tissues have been successfully isolated and cultured[126] and used to show the effects of various growth factors, including IGF-1, IGF-2, and growth hormone, on chondrocyte proliferation and clonal growth. Clonal analysis studies of human chondrosarcomas have shown that clones of phenotypically distinct chondrocytes may be derived from a single human chondrosarcoma and can be maintained in long-term culture. The range of proteoglycans produced shows some variation from clone to clone.[127, 128] This is in keeping with previous studies, which have shown that there is marked variability in the proteoglycan composition of human chondrosarcomas.[129, 130] A major problem with culturing cartilage cells from human chondrosarcomas is a tendency for the cultures to be overgrown by contaminating fibroblasts.

One approach to minimizing the problems of variability in cartilage cell cultures and fibroblast overgrowth is the use of cultures of transformed chondrocytes derived from a transmissible malignant cartilage tumor of rats, the Swarm-rat chondrosarcoma (SRC). This tumor originally arose spontaneously in a female Sprague-Dawley rat and has been maintained for several years by serial subcutaneous transplantation.[131] The tumor was originally composed of bone and cartilage elements but, with successive transplantations, the osseous elements disappeared and only the cartilaginous elements remained.[132] The composition of the SRC has remained stable for many years and has proved a useful chondrosarcoma model for morphologic and biochemical studies.[132–135] When the SRC is experimentally implanted into bone it shows an essentially similar morphology and growth pattern to that of a well-differentiated (Grade I) human chondrosarcoma[136]; there is invasion of cortical and cancellous bone and extension into the soft tissues with metastases occurring only rarely. S100 protein is positive in SRC, although the reaction is weaker than that in human chondrosarcoma.[136, 137] The matrix of SRC reacts positively with alcian blue in the same fashion as hyaline cartilage and human chondrosarcoma, indicating the presence of sulfated glycosaminoglycans[136, 138, 139]; SRC proteoglycans differ from those in mature hyaline cartilage and human chondrosarcoma, which contain mostly chondroitin-4 sulfate and hyaluronic acid.[129, 130] SRC cells, however, do synthesize major cartilage matrix molecules including type II and type IX collagen and chondroitin sulfate.

Growth Factors and Oncogenes and Chondrosarcoma Cells

Guerne and Lotz[140] identified TGF-β as the most potent growth factor for SRC chondrocyte proliferation in vitro and noted a serum-dependent effect of IL-6 on SRC growth; the effect of TGF-β and IL-6 on SRC growth was synergistic. Seong et al.[141] analyzed the response of cultured SRC chondrocytes to IGF-1 with respect to DNA and glycosaminoglycan synthesis and found that both were increased in the presence of IGF-1. Their results suggested that chondrosarcoma may be a somatomedin-responsive tumor and that it may be susceptible to interventions directed toward mechanisms that block IGF action. Cultured SRC cells produce a heat-labile collagenase and a heat-stable collagenase inhibitor and show differences in enzyme profile and activity from normal cartilage[142]; these differences may indicate that chondrosarcoma develops in vivo because the inherent proteolytic balance between the production of proteases and their endogenous inhibitors is shifted in favor of enzyme activity.

A number of immortalized human chondrosarcoma cell lines have been established, allowing the evaluation of cartilage tumor cell responses to specific factors. The HL52A human chondrosarcoma cell line shows high tumorigenicity in vivo and is able to form proteoglycan-rich cartilage-like nodules and type II collagen[143]; this proteoglycan production was found to be responsive to insulin in vitro. Zhu et al.[144] analyzed the proto-oncogene expression of the human chondrosarcoma cell line HCS02/8 and detected transcripts of several proto-oncogenes in these tumor cells including c-*fos*, c-*raf*-I, *int*-2, c-*mos*, and K-*ras*, which showed variable expression depending on the growth phase of the tumor cells. Some studies have shown that when a human osteogenic sarcoma is transplanted into nude mice, a chondrosarcoma showing calcification but not ossification may develop.[111, 145] This would indicate that the character of progenitors of chondrogenic tumor cells can be transferred to the transplanted tumor and that the tumor cells can change expression of collagen species upon differentiation and maturation. A different approach has been adopted by Wang et al.,[111] who used different embryonic stem cell clones to generate chimeric mice selected for high exogenous c-*fos* expression; these mice did not develop cartilage tumors during embryonic development but commonly developed these tumors as early as 3 to 4 weeks of age. This was apparently independent of the extent of chimerism. Expression of exogenous c-*fos* RNA and c-*fos* protein was observed during development and was highest in the tumor tissue, predominantly in differentiating chondrocytes. A number of primary and clonal tumor-derived cell lines established from this chimeric tissue also expressed high levels of c-*fos* and c-*jun*, as well as the type II collagen gene. These cells also gave rise to cartilage tumors in vivo. Thus, chondrogenic cells and early progenitors may represent a novel mesenchymal cell target for c-*fos* overexpression.

Human chondrosarcoma cell lines that synthesize chondrocytic keratin sulphate–containing proteoglycans have been established and are of use in studying the structure and regulation of matrix proteoglycans produced by cartilage cells as well as in providing an in vitro model of human chondrosarcoma.[128] Other uses of human chondrosarcoma cell cultures include the production of monoclonal antibodies that react with cartilaginous tumours[146]; none thus far appears to be specific for tumors of this type.

Ewing's Sarcoma

Cell Culture and the Histogenesis of Ewing's Sarcoma

Ewing's sarcoma is a malignant round cell neoplasm most often diagnosed in the second decade of life. The histogenesis of Ewing's sarcoma has long been disputed, and, largely on the basis of morphologic studies, the cell of origin has variously been postulated to be an endothelial cell, a plasma cell, a mesenchymal cell, a neuroblast, a myeloblast, a pericyte, or a smooth muscle cell. Culture of cells from Ewing's sarcomas has played an important role in the elucidation of the nature of this tumor. Ewing's sarcoma cells take on a variety of shapes when grown in tissue culture, ranging from floating cells to cells that grow as a monolayer of small, plump, refractile cells that may become more fibroblastic at or near confluence.[147–149] Cell types vary from slender, spindle-shaped to more blunted, rounded forms showing nuclear angulation and convolutions with atypical nucleoli. Ultrastructurally, tumor cells grown in vitro resemble those of the original tumor.[148, 149] Glycogen is also present but is not as prominent as in tumor cells in vivo.

On the basis of the morphology of the tumor cells in culture, and analysis of the type of collagen produced by the tumor cells, a myelogenous or vascular smooth muscle origin was originally proposed for Ewing's sarcoma.[123, 147] Dickman et al.,[148] however, found production of collagen types I, III, and IV in vitro; this collagen profile, coupled with the morphologic and ultrastructural features of the sarcoma cell lines, suggested that Ewing's sarcoma cells were derived from a multipotential primitive mesenchymal cell that was uncommitted to osteoblastic, fibroblastic, or epithelial differentiation. Scarpa et al.[150] showed that Ewing's sarcoma cell lines synthesized laminin and fibronectin in addition to various collagen proteins, indicating that histogenetic classification of Ewing's tumor was not possible on the basis of the extracellular matrix proteins synthesized by the tumor cells in vitro.

Cell culture of three malignant small round cell tumors of bone arising in children was carried out by Jaffe et al.[151] Neuron-specific enolase was present in all cultured cells, but other features of neuroblastoma, including catecholamine fluorescence, were absent. The addition of dibutyryl cAMP failed to induce neural differentiation; however, neurite outgrowth was noted when cells were grown on glass in a serum-free medium. Cavazzana et al.[152] found that under normal culture conditions and following treatment with retinoic acid (an agent that induces neural differentiation in neuroblastoma), evidence of neural differentiation could not be detected in cultures of Ewing's sarcoma cells. However, treatment with cAMP and phorbol-12-myristate-13-acetate (TPA) induced pronounced neural differentiation, the cells developing elongate processes with varicosities, accompanied by the ultrastructural demonstration of filaments, microtubules, and dense core granules. Three neural markers (neuron-specific enolase, neural filament triplet protein, and cholinesterase) were absent or barely detectable in untreated cells but became abundant after treatment. These studies provided strong evidence for a neural histogenesis of Ewing's sarcoma.

The now well-recognized reciprocal translocation t(11:22)(q24:12) was originally reported in primary cultures of tumor cells and in cell lines derived from Ewing's sarcoma.[149, 153] Lipinski et al.[154] also showed the presence of neural ectodermal antigens on several Ewing's sarcoma cell lines having the t(11:22) translocation. Kodama et al.[155] established and characterized a Ewing's sarcoma cell line (CADO-ES1), which showed the t(11:22) translocation, no morphologic evidence of neural differentiation under normal culture conditions, and cells strongly positive for vimentin and weakly positive for neurofilament and neuron-specific enolase. Treatment with cAMP induced neural differentiation and strong expression of neurofilaments in cultured cells. S100 protein, glial fibrillary acidic protein, desmin, cytokeratin, and epithelial membrane antigen were not detected. The authors concluded that this cell line was derived from an undifferentiated neural cell with high chromosomal clonality and that under certain conditions neural differentiation occurred. Although the majority of CADO-ES1 cells express a neural phenotype, a minor proportion of cells appear flattened and have short processes. When transplanted to nude mice, cartilage was formed by these cells, indicating that CADO-ES1 cells differentiate not only toward neural but also toward mesenchymal cells.[156] Scanning electron microscopy studies have also shown evidence for neural differentiation in Ewing's cell lines, providing further evidence for the neural character of Ewing's sarcoma and its close relationship to peripheral neuroectodermal tumor (PNET).[157] Ohta et al.[158] showed neural differentiation in a Ewing's sarcoma cell line established from a metastatic lesion in the marrow of a patient with advanced disease. The cells expressed neurofilaments and Leu 7 but there was absence of the S100 protein and no evidence of glial differentiation. They concluded that Ewing's sarcoma is of more primitive neural origin than neuroblastoma, PNET, and other related neural tumors. Hara et al.[159] studied cell lines established from extraosseous Ewing's sarcomas and found cellular heterogeneity in the ability to undergo neuronal differentiation following stimulation with cAMP. Noguera et al.[160] found that Ewing's sarcoma cells in vitro display a variable neural phenotype, there being a variety of biologic responses to diverse culture media, with no consistent effect on N-*myc*, c-*myc*, and *dbl* oncogene expression. These and other studies highlight the strong relationship between Ewing's sarcoma and other primitive round cell sarcomas of bone and soft tissue, including PNET. Peripheral neuroectodermal tumors show a consistent pattern of proto-oncogene expression with high levels of RNA for c-*myc*, c-*myb*, c-*mil*, and c-*rap*, a lack of N-*myc* amplification or overproduction, and production of acetylcholinesterase,[161] consistent with their presumed origin from neural cells of parasympathetic lineage. Histologic differences between PNET and Ewing's sarcoma reflect differences in their degree of neural differentiation.

Growth Factors, Cytokines, and the Treatment of Ewing's Sarcoma

Insulin-like growth factor-1 is thought to play an important role in the growth of Ewing's sarcoma and PNET cells. Hamilton et al.[162] showed that the monoclonal antibody HBA-71 recognizes a Ewing's sarcoma–associated antigen (MIC2, CD99) that is also highly expressed on the cell surface of human cortical thymocytes and cells of the islets of Langerhans (see Chapters 5 and 14). This antibody partially inhibits the growth of Ewing's sarcoma cell lines and triggers proliferation in thymocyte cultures. Ewing's sarcoma cell growth also depends on the presence of IGF-2 or insulin. The HBA-71 antibody enhances the growth stimulatory effect of IGF-1 under serum-free conditions. Van Valen et al.,[163] using recombinant human ^{125}I labeled IGF-1, showed the presence of IGF-1 receptors in three Ewing's sarcoma cell lines. They showed that IGF-1 and IGF-2 induce rapid and long-term biologic responses in Ewing's sarcoma cells exclusively through interaction with IGF type 1 receptors. Yee et al.[164] showed that IGF-1 expression is a property of neuroectodermal tumors with a t(11;22) translocation and that interruption of an IGF-1 autocrine loop inhibits the growth of these tumor cells.

Cell culture has also provided information regarding possible treatment strategies for Ewing's sarcoma. Van Valen et al.,[165] using three Ewing's sarcoma cell lines, showed that among various cytokines tested, only interferon-γ and TNF-α were capable of reducing Ewing's sarcoma cell growth in vitro, which suggested that these cytokines might be useful in the design of novel therapeutic strategies for Ewing's sarcoma. Ewing's sarcoma and PNET are both sensitive to doxorubicin but may escape treatment by expression of a multi-drug-resistant phenotype. Doxorubicin coupled to albumin (a growth-supporting factor for Ewing's and PNET tumor cells in IGF-1 supplemented tissue cultures) inhibits the growth Ewing's sarcoma and PNET tumor cell lines selectively.[166]

Giant Cell Tumor of Bone

Giant cell tumors (GCTs) are uncommon primary tumors of bone (see Chapter 15), characterized by the presence of abundant multinucleated, osteoclast-like giant cells that are interspersed among mononuclear cells. The nature of these two components and the relationship between the giant cells of GCT, normal osteoclasts, and giant cells in other giant cell–rich lesions of bone and soft tissue have been studied in cell cultures.

Histogenesis of Giant Cells in Giant Cell Tumor of Bone

The osteoclastic nature of the giant cells in GCTs has long been suspected from their close morphologic and cytochemical resemblance to osteoclasts.[167] The criteria for osteoclast definition were alluded to earlier, and the giant cells of GCTs fulfill all the essential criteria for osteoclast definition. The presence of calcitonin receptors on giant cells and a minor population of mononuclear cells was confirmed by autoradiography using ^{125}I salmon calcitonin.[168] The giant cells possess a great number of calcitonin receptors (approximately 1,000,000 sites per cell) and, like osteoclasts, respond to calcitonin with a rise in cAMP.[168–170] Functional studies provided definitive evidence of the osteoclastic nature of giant cells in GCT, by showing that these cells, when directly isolated from tumors, formed resorption pits on bone slices in a manner identical to that of osteoclasts (Fig. 3–7).[171] Factors that inhibit the cytoplasmic motility and bone-resorbing activity of mammalian osteoclasts, such as calcitonin, prostaglandins, and dibutyryl cAMP, also inhibit these activities in giant cells, but PTH does not significantly influence the bone resorbing activity of these cells.[24] Kanehisa et al.[172] provided ultrastructural support for the osteoclastic nature of the giant cells forming these resorption lacunae by demonstrating the presence of ruffled borders and clear zones on these cells, even though these features are poorly developed in giant cells in vivo.[167] Giant cell degradation of the bone matrix is associated with the release of an osteoclast cathepsin as well as a 92kd type IV collagenase/gelatinase.[173, 174]

Histochemical and immunohistochemical studies also point to giant cells of GCT having an osteoclastic phenotype. The giant cells are positive for tartrate-resistant acid phosphatase (TRAP),[175] and biochemical studies have confirmed that this phosphatase, like that of osteoclasts, differs from that of other cells.[176, 177] The giant cells of GCT also express a similar, restricted range of macrophage-associated antigens to osteoclasts.[170, 178–180] The giant cells lack surface markers for Fc and C_3 receptors, HLA-DR, and a number of mononuclear phagocyte antigens,[179–181] but they strongly express CD45 (leucocyte common antigen) and CD68 (a macrophage-associated antigen).[180–183] Monoclonal antibodies to CD45 and CD68, which work on routinely processed sections

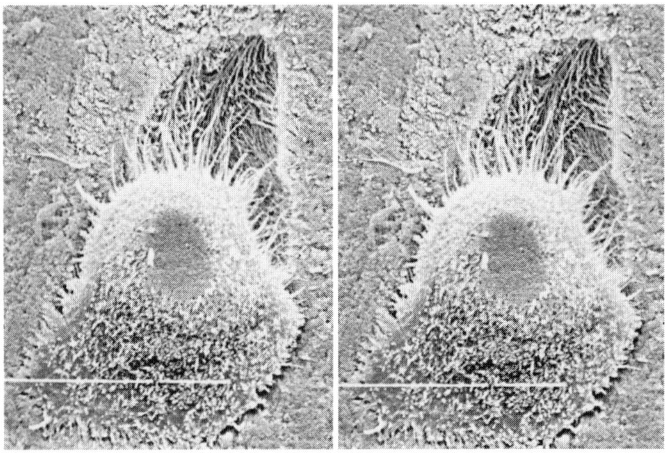

Figure 3–7. Scanning electron microscopic stereopair photomicrographs of a giant cell from a giant cell tumor forming resorption pit on cortical bone slice. (Field width = 105 μm.)

from decalcified tissues, are particularly useful in bone tumor diagnosis in distinguishing osteoclasts (and macrophage polykaryons) from tumor giant cells of nonhematopoietic origin.[184, 185] The only other tumor in which the giant cells have been reported to show an identical phenotype to those of GCT is the giant cell granuloma of the jaw, as the giant cells in both conditions do not express HLA-DR.[186] Rathod et al.[187] identified an uncommon subtype of "aggressive" GCT in which the giant cells are HLA-DR positive. These cells exhibit avid bone resorbing activity that is insensitive to calcitonin, despite the fact that the giant cells appear to possess calcitonin receptors.

Antigenic phenotype, however, does not strictly conform to the functional ability to form resorption lacunae. In other extraskeletal giant cell–rich lesions, including breast carcinomas containing numerous giant cells, giant cell tumor of tendon sheath, and pilar tumor of scalp, the giant cells strongly express only macrophage markers yet are capable of extensive lacunar resorption of bone.[54–56]

Cell Surface Receptors on Giant Cells

A number of monoclonal antibodies have been raised against cell preparations isolated from GCT that react strongly with osteoclasts.[188, 189] An antigen highly expressed by osteoclasts and their precursors is the α-chain of the vitronectin receptor (CD51).[188] This antigen was originally thought to be osteoclast-specific but is now known to be expressed by macrophages and macrophage polykaryons.[190] It has been identified on giant cells in the giant cell–rich variant of malignant fibrous histiocytoma of soft tissue.[191] Nevertheless, CD51 is a highly osteoclast-associated antigen, and its presence on giant cells of GCT has led to studies of osteoclast/giant cell adhesion molecules and matrix receptors. Zambonin-Zallone et al.[192, 193] showed that GCT-derived osteoclasts elaborate the β_3 subunit of the vitronectin receptor in osteoclast adhesion structures; this was not found on monocytes or macrophages. Cell preparations from GCT have led to the characterization of cell surface receptors to extracellular matrix molecules, which contain the tripeptide Arg-Gly-Asp (RGD) sequence.[194, 195] RGD peptides and anti-vitronectin receptor antibodies also inhibit osteoclastic bone resorption.[196, 197] These agents may potentially be useful in treating GCT and other giant cell lesions of bone in a manner analogous to that reported for calcitonin, which has been shown to cause regression of giant cell granulomas of the jaw.[198]

Relationship Between Mononuclear Cells and Giant Cells

Grano et al.[175] studied the cell culture characteristics of twelve GCTs over several passages in which cells maintained their multinuclearity. The giant cells expressed a number of osteoclast phenotypic features including TRAP and a calcitonin-induced increase in intracellular cAMP, with induction of cytoplasmic quiescence and inhibition of bone resorption. Cell proliferation, as assessed by incorporation of ^{3}H thymidine, showed that the number of labeled multinucleated cells in culture increased constantly over the incubation period, strongly supporting the hypothesis of giant cell formation mainly through fusion of mononuclear elements. Goldring et al.[199, 200] identified two populations of cells in GCT; one population expressed monocyte-macrophage markers but lacked receptors for PTH, calcitonin, and prostaglandins, and the other population, which proliferated in culture, resembled connective tissue stromal cells, possessed receptors for PTH, produced collagen type I and III, and did not express macrophage antigens. This population was thought most likely to represent the neoplastic cellular component of GCT.

The cell culture studies of Joyner et al.[201] also found that the mononuclear cell component was heterogeneous with both macrophage-like cells, which persisted for a short time in culture, and fibroblast-like cells, which actively proliferated. Subcutaneous implantation of the fibroblast-like cells in nude mice resulted in bone formation in those areas in which the cells showed strong alkaline-phosphatase activity. These observations were interpreted as being consistent with the concept that osteoblastic differentiation is exhibited by the proliferating neoplastic stromal cell component of GCT and that it is likely that these cells actively recruit osteoclast precursors from the circulation. Alkaline phosphatase-positive mononuclear cells were also found in a giant cell–rich malignant fibrous histiocytoma from which bone resorbing giant cells were isolated.[191]

In other cell culture studies in which giant cells have been isolated by either chemical or enzymatic dispersion from tumors or have been obtained from outgrowth cultures of GCT, giant cells were found not to persist in culture, although this depends on the culture conditions.[202, 203] Zheng et al.[204] showed that TGF-β_1 may play a role in the interaction between tumor cells and giant cells. They showed that the TGF-β_1 mRNA transcript is consistently detected in both mononuclear cells and giant cells, whereas the TGF-β_1 type II receptor gene transcript is only present in osteoclast-like cells. They concluded that TGF-β_1, possibly in concert with other cytokines, may be involved in the chemotactic recruitment of osteoclast-like cells in GCT through autocrine or paracrine mechanisms.

CELL AND ORGAN CULTURE STUDIES OF TUMOR-ASSOCIATED BONE RESORPTION

The most common malignant tumor to affect bone is metastatic cancer, and bone is the third most common site of metastasis after the lung and the liver.[205] Bone resorption is associated with the establishment of a tumor metastasis. The cellular and hormonal mechanisms accounting for tumor-associated osteolysis are poorly understood, partly because few tumors in experimental animals metastasize consistently to bone. For this reason in vitro models of tumor-associated osteolysis have been developed.

Cell Types Associated with Tumor-Associated Bone Resorption

One of the principal questions concerning malignant bone resorption is whether tumor cells are capable of directly resorbing bone or whether they act indirectly by stimulating host osteoclasts to resorb bone. Histologic studies in humans and animals have suggested that both cellular mechanisms may operate and have defined two distinct phases of osteolysis connected with bone metastases.[206, 207] Osteoclasts and osteoclastic bone resorption are prominent in the early phase when the metastasis is becoming established and bone resorption proceeds rapidly; but later, when the metastasis grows more slowly, there is little or no osteoclastic resorption, and tumor cells and cells in the host inflammatory response to the tumor are the most prominent feature. Tumor cells lack specialized cell surface structures (such as the ruffled border of osteoclasts), which are thought to be necessary for the optimal dissolution of mineralized bone matrix. Nevertheless, tumor cells do possess the intracellular machinery to degrade bone; they produce several acid proteases and release a type I collagenase that may be of importance both in the direct resorption of bone[208] and in the initiation and promotion of osteoclastic bone resorption.[209] Cultured human breast cancer cells (MCF-7) are capable of releasing radiolabeled calcium and proline from devitalized bone particles,[210] but lacunar resorption by tumor cells has not been reported; at best, it is considered that these cells exhibit only a low-grade form of bone resorption that is quite unlike the high-grade, lacunar resorption of osteoclasts.[211–213]

Quinn et al.[214] developed an in vitro model of tumor osteolysis that proved definitively that tumor cells did not effect lacunar bone resorption. They isolated tumor cells and tumor-infiltrating macrophages (TIMs) from carcinomas that had developed in nude mice following subcutaneous implantation of human breast, colon, and cervical carcinoma cell lines. Isolated carcinoma cells and TIMs were cultured separately with osteoblast-like cells on bone slices; evidence of osteoclast differentiation and lacunar resorption was found only in those cultures that contained TIMs. Both $1,25(OH)_2D_3$ and osteoblast-like cells were absolute requirements for osteoclast differentiation to occur from the TIMs. This process is analogous to osteoclast differentiation exhibited by mouse monocytes and various tissue macrophages, including those isolated from inflammatory and neoplastic lesions.[49–53, 215] Osteoclast differentiation from mononuclear phagocyte precursors may thus represent a mechanism whereby osteolysis is generally effected by pathologic lesions in bone.

A number of humoral factors produced by tumor cells may influence macrophage-osteoclast differentiation. Bottazzi et al.[216] showed that TIMs isolated from two murine sarcomas had high levels of proliferative activity compared with peritoneal macrophages. TIMs had high levels of mRNA transcripts of the c-*fms* proto-oncogene, the M-CSF receptor, but did not express M-CSF transcripts; sarcoma cells, however, had high levels of M-CSF mRNA. The proliferative activity of sarcoma cells on macrophages was also blocked by anti–M-CSF antibodies. These findings point to possible paracrine regulation of TIM proliferation by a mechanism involving M-CSF, the latter being secreted by sarcoma cells and acting on TIMs that express c-*fms*. Given the known importance of M-CSF in the proliferation and differentiation of osteoclast precursors,[45] this could represent one means whereby an immature subpopulation of TIMs could be stimulated to proliferate and differentiate into osteoclastic bone-resorbing cells. A small proportion of proliferating mononuclear phagocytes are present in the macrophage pool in various body cavities and organs,[217] as well as in inflammatory and neoplastic lesions.[218, 219] These DNA-synthesizing mononuclear phagocytes are morphologically and histochemically indistinguishable from resident macrophages and may represent the subpopulation of TIMs from which osteoclastic cells are formed. Low-grade bone resorption by TIMs has also been reported in both murine and human TIM cell cultures on bone slices, in the absence of bone stromal cells and $1,25(OH)_2D_3$.[51, 52] In the context of a bone metastasis, the net effect of a large number of TIMs (or tumor cells) carrying out low-grade resorption may be quite significant. This mechanism could partly account for the continuing osteolysis, which occurs in the apparent absence of osteoclasts.

Chemical Mediators of Tumor-Associated Bone Resorption

Stimulation of bone-resorbing activity by host osteoclasts is undoubtedly important in the bone destruction associated with both metastatic and primary malignant tumors. Both tumor cells and inflammatory cells produce numerous local factors that stimulate osteoclastic bone resorption. Many of these have been identified by cell and organ culture studies including prostaglandins of the E series, TNF, IL-1, TGF-α and TGF-β, interleukin-6 (IL-6), and procathepsin D.[220] With the exception of procathepsin D, most of these factors act primarily on osteoblasts to stimulate osteoclastic bone resorption.

Prostaglandins

Prostaglandins, particularly of the E series, are believed to be implicated in the osteolysis associated with inflammation and neoplasia. PGE_2 is synthesized by human primary and metastatic bone tumors in culture, and significantly higher levels of PGE_2 are found in organ cultures derived from highly osteolytic tumors.[221] Prostaglandins strongly stimulate bone resorption in organ cultures and, in some tumors, humoral factors such as TGF and IL-1 stimulate prostaglandin production and bone resorption. Prostaglandins stimulate osteoclastic bone resorption indirectly via osteoblasts. When indomethacin is added to organ cultures of tumors, a significant reduction in PGE_2-induced osteolysis (as assessed by the release of calcium from neonatal calvariae) occurs.[222] However, other studies have found no correlation between tumor prostaglandin production and osteolysis or the development of malignant hypercalcemia.[223]

Cytokines and Growth Factors

Tumors that metastasize to bone, and hematologic malignancies such as myeloma and lymphoma, produce a variety of osteoclast-stimulating factors. Tumor cells also secrete factors that stimulate reactive inflammatory cells, such as TIMs and lymphocytes, to release cytokines and growth factors, which stimulate osteoclast activity and influence osteoclast formation.[224–228] Both IL-1 and TNF are potent stimulators of osteoclastic bone resorption and inhibit bone formation, and both are produced by macrophages and osteoblasts. Some human tumors associated with the humoral hypercalcemia of malignancy, particularly squamous cell carcinomas, have been shown to produce IL-1. It is also likely that tumor cells produce TNF or that the tumor cells stimulate host immune cells (possibly through the secretion of GM-CSF and other factors) to produce TNF and IL-1.[229]

Transforming growth factor-α and TGF-β are produced by human breast cancer cells in vitro, and TGF-α is present in high concentration in patients with breast tumors.[230] Breast cancer cells with estrogen receptors show increased production of TGF-α, which stimulates osteoclast formation and bone resorption in vitro[231, 232] and enhances the effects of PTH, PTHrP, and IL-1 on osteoclastic bone resorption in vitro.[233–235] TGF-α is probably a mediator of the osteoclastic bone resorption occurring in metastatic breast cancer. TGF-β has complex and multiple effects on bone cell function; it is found in most normal tissues and is produced by tumor cells, and it is present in particularly high concentrations in bone matrix, where it may act as a coupling factor between the processes of bone formation and resorption (see Chapter 2). The stimulatory effects of TGF-β on osteoclast activity appear to be mediated by prostaglandins, and the role of TGF-β in malignant bone resorption is uncertain. Carcinomas, particularly squamous cell carcinomas, have been reported to produce colony-stimulating factors such as GM-CSF, which influence osteoclast formation and activity in vitro, and may have complex interactions with other local humoral factors.[227, 228]

Interleukin-6, a cytokine produced by fibroblasts, osteoblasts, keratinocytes, and other cells, stimulates bone resorption in vitro and may be an important factor in osteoclast formation in long-term human and other mammalian bone marrow culture systems.[47, 236] IL-6 has complex interactions with other humoral factors. PTH-related peptide (PTH-rP), IL-1, and TNF-α each increase production of IL-6 by bone-forming cells. Endogenous IL-6 production also increases when mouse calvarial cultures are treated with IL-1 or TNF, and neutralizing antibodies to IL-6 abolish the bone resorbing activity of exogenously administered IL-1 or TNF. IL-6 is a growth factor for myeloma and has been strongly implicated in the osteolytic bone destruction associated with myeloma.[237, 238] IL-6 may mainly stimulate the generation of new osteoclasts rather than increase the activity of mature osteoclasts. Treating patients with anti–IL-6 decreases the tumor burden in some patients. Multiple myeloma cells also produce numerous locally acting cytokines and growth factors, including IL-1, TNF-α, and TNF-β, that can stimulate osteoclast formation and activity. IL-6 may be a pathogenic factor in the bone resorption associated with Gorman's disease.[239]

Purification of PTH-like biologic activity from neoplasms associated with humoral hypercalcemia of malignancy resulted in the discovery of a PTH-rP that may play a central role in the pathogenesis of this condition. PTH-rP is secreted by both normal and neoplastic cells in vitro.[240, 241] Numerous factors influence the transcription, translation, post-translational modification, and secretion of PTH-rP, including $1,25(OH)_2D_3$, TGF-β, and other cytokines and growth factors. Stromal cells may regulate PTH-rP production by some carcinomas, and this is important in both the production and the secretion of PTH-rP by malignant cells. Breast carcinoma cells produce PTH-rP in sufficient amounts to stimulate osteoclastic bone resorption, and local PTH-rP production by metastatic breast carcinoma could be involved in osteoclast activation at sites of skeletal metastasis.[241–243]

Cell culture studies have shown that bone undergoing resorption is stimulatory for tumor cell growth, suggesting that the microenvironment of host bone can promote enlargement of skeletal metastases.[244] This is presumably caused by the release by osteoclastic bone resorption of growth factors from the bone matrix, which stimulate tumor cell growth and reactive bone formation. Some tumors that metastasize to bone, notably prostatic carcinoma, are often associated with increased localized bone formation (osteoblastic metastases). Both hyperplastic and adenocarcinomatous prostate tissue can release substances that stimulate osteoblast activity and bone formation.[245–247] These cells have also been shown to contain other factors such as BMP types III and IV, basic fibroblast growth factor, and tissue plasminogen activator, all of which are known to be mitogenic for osteoblasts.[245–252]

CONCLUSION

Cell and organ culture techniques developed to study bone biology and physiology have greatly increased our understanding of the origin, nature, and function of bone cells. These techniques have also been used to study several aspects of bone tumors, including their origin and pathogenesis, and to develop treatments to control their growth and spread. Cell and organ culture studies have also led to the identification of the defining characteristics of a number of bone cells; these have proved useful in the diagnosis of bone tumors by immunohistology and other means. An understanding of the cellular mechanisms by which tumor cells influence bone cell function and vice versa is essential for rational development of treatments to control the growth, spread, and destruction of bone tumors.

REFERENCES

1. Reynolds JJ, Dingle JT: A sensitive in vitro method for studying the induction and inhibition of bone resorption. Calcif Tissue Res 4:339, 1970.
2. Reynolds JJ, Holick MF, DeLuca HF: The role of vitamin D metabolites in bone resorption. Calcif Tissue Res 12:295, 1973.
3. Heath JK, Saklatvala J, Meikle MC, et al: Pig interleukin 1 (catabolin) is a potent stimulator of bone resorption in vitro. Calcif Tissue Int 37:95, 1985.
4. Gowen M, Nedwin GE, Mundy GR: Preferential inhibition of cytokine stimulated bone resorption by recombinant interferon gamma. J Bone Miner Res 1:469, 1986.
5. Tashjian AH, Voelkel EF, Lazzaro M: Alpha and beta human transforming growth factors stimulate prostaglandin production and bone resorption in cultured mouse calvaria. Proc Natl Acad Sci 82:4535, 1985.
6. Kream BE, Rowe DW, Gworek SC, et al: Parathyroid hormone alters collagen synthesis and procollagen mRNA levels in fetal rat calvaria. Proc Natl Acad Sci 77:5654, 1980.
7. Hock JM, Centrella M, Canalis E: Insulin-like growth factor I has independent effects on bone matrix formation and cell replication. Endocrinology 122:254, 1988.
8. Bertolini DR, Nedwin GE, Bringman TS: Stimulation of bone resorption and inhibition of bone formation in vitro by human tumor necrosis factor. Nature 319:516, 1986.
9. Burger EH, van der Meer JWM, van de Gevel JS, et al: In vitro formation of osteoclasts from long-term cultures of bone marrow mononuclear phagocytes. J Exp Med 156:1604, 1982.
10. Thesingh CW: Formation sites and distribution of osteoclast progenitor cells during the ontogeny of the mouse. Dev Biol 117:127, 1986.
11. Scheven BAA, Visser JWM, Nijweide PJ: In vitro osteoclast generation from different bone marrow fractions, including a highly enriched haematopoietic stem cell population. Nature 321:79, 1986.
12. Luben RA, Wong GL, Cohn DV: Biochemical characterisation with parathormone and calcitonin of isolated bone cells: Provisional identification of osteoclasts and osteoblasts. Endocrinology 99:526, 1976.
13. Wong GL, Cohn DV: Separation of parathyroid hormone and calcitonin-sensitive cells from non-responsive bone cells. Nature 252:713, 1974.
14. Wong GL: Characterisation of subpopulations of OC and OB bone cells obtained by sedimentation of unit gravity. Calcif Tissue Int 34:67, 1982.
15. Burger EH, Boonekamp PM, Nijweide PJ: Osteoblast and osteoclast precursors in primary cultures of calvarial bone cells. Anat Rec 214:32, 1986.
16. Chen TL, Hauschka PV, Cabrales S, et al: The effects of 1,25 dihydroxyvitamin D3 and dexamethasone on rat osteoblast-like primary cell cultures: Receptor occupancy and functional expression patterns for three different bioresponses. Endocrinology 118:250, 1986.
17. Gehron Robey P, Termine JD: Human bone cells in vitro. Calcif Tissue Int 37:453, 1985.
18. Heath JK, Atkinson SJ, Meikle MC, et al: Mouse osteoblasts synthesise collagenase in response to bone resorbing agents. Biochem Biophys Acta 802:151, 1984.
19. Robey PG, Young MF, Flanders KC, et al: Osteoblasts synthesise and respond to transforming growth factor-type-beta in vitro. J Cell Biol 105:457, 1987.
20. Williams DC, Boder GB, Toomey RE, et al: Mineralisation and metabolic response in serially passaged adult rat bone cells. Calcif Tissue Int 30:233, 1980.
21. Nijweide PJ, van Iperen-van Gent AS, Kawilarang-de Hass EWM, et al: Bone formation and calcification by isolated osteoblast-like cells. J Cell Biol 93:318, 1982.
22. Rodan GA, Rodan SB: Expression of the osteoblastic phenotype. *In* Peck WA (ed): Bone and Mineral Research. Amsterdam, Elsevier, 1984, p 244.
23. Chambers TJ, Magnus CJ: Calcitonin alters behaviour of isolated osteoclasts. J Pathol 136:27, 1982.
24. Chambers TJ, Fuller K, McSheehy PMJ: The effects of calcium regulating hormones on bone resorption by isolated human osteoclastoma cells. J Pathol 145:297, 1985.
25. Chambers TJ, Ali NN: Inhibition of osteoclastic motility by prostaglandins I_2, E_1, E_2 and 6-oxo-E_1. J Pathol 139:383, 1983.
26. Chambers TJ, Revell PA, Fuller K, et al: Resorption of bone by isolated rabbit osteoclasts. J Cell Sci 66:383, 1984.
27. Boyde A, Ali NN, Jones SJ: Resorption of dentine by isolated osteoclasts in vitro. Br Dent J 156:216, 1984.
28. McSheehy PMJ, Chambers TJ: Osteoblastic cells mediate osteoclastic responsiveness to parathyroid hormone. Endocrinology 118:824, 1986.
29. Chambers TJ, McSheehy PMJ, Thomson BM, et al: The effect of calcium-regulating hormones and prostaglandins on bone resorption by osteoclasts disaggregated from neonatal rabbit bones. Endocrinology 116:234, 1985.
30. Thomson BM, Saklatvala J, Chambers TJ: Osteoblasts mediate interleukin 1 stimulation of bone resorption by rat osteoclasts. J Exp Med 164:104, 1986.
31. Thomson BM, Mundy GR, Chambers TJ: Tumor necrosis factors alpha and beta induce osteoblastic cells to stimulate osteoclastic bone resorption. J Immunol 138:775, 1987.
32. Braidman IP, Anderson DC, Jones CJP, et al: Separa-

tion of two bone populations from fetal rat calvaria and a study of their responses to parathyroid hormone and calcitonin. J Endocrinol 99:387, 1983.
33. Kahn AJ, Stewart CC, Teitelbaum SL: Contact-mediated bone resorption by human monocytes in vitro. Science 199:988, 1978.
34. Teitelbaum SL, Stewart CC, Kahn AH: Rodent peritoneal macrophages as bone resorbing cells. Calcif Tissue Int 27:255, 1979.
35. Mundy GR, Altman AJ, Gondek MD: Direct resorption of bone by human monocytes. Science 196:1109, 1977.
36. Chambers TJ, Horton MA: Failure of cells of the mononuclear phagocyte series to resorb bone. Calcif Tissue Int 36:556, 1984.
37. Nicholson GC, Moseley JM, Sexton PM, et al: Abundant calcitonin receptors in isolated rat osteoclasts. J Clin Invest 78:355, 1986.
38. Jotereau FV, LeDouarin NM: The developmental relationship between osteocytes and osteoclasts: A study using the quail-chick nuclear marker in endochondral ossification. Dev Biol 63:253, 1978.
39. Walker DG: Osteopetrosis cured by temporary parabiosis. Science 180:875, 1973.
40. Ash P, Loutit KM, Townsend MS: Osteoclasts derived from haematopoietic stem cells. Nature 283:669, 1980.
41. Hattersley G, Chambers TJ: Generation of osteoclasts from haemopoietic cells and a multipotential cell line in vitro. J Cell Physiol 140:478, 1989.
42. Alvarez JI, Teitelbaum SL, Blair HC: Generation of avian cells resembling osteoclasts from mononuclear phagocytes. Endocrinology 128:2324, 1990.
43. Kurihara N, Chenu C, Civin C, et al: Identification of committed mononuclear precursors for osteoclast-like cells formed in long term human marrow cultures. Endocrinology 126:2733, 1990.
44. Takahashi N, Akatsu T, Udagawa N: Osteoblastic cells are involved in osteoclast formation. Endocrinology 123:2600, 1988.
45. Tanaka S, Takahashi N, Udagawa N: Macrophage colony stimulating factor is indispensable for both proliferation and differentiation of osteoclast progenitors. J Clin Invest 91:257, 1993.
46. Felix R, Cecchini MG, Fleisch H: Macrophage colony stimulating factor restores in vivo bone resorption in the op/op osteopetrotic mouse. Endocrinology 127:2592, 1990.
47. Suda T, Udagawa N, Nakamura I: Modulation of osteoclast differentiation by local factors. Bone 17:87S, 1995.
48. Suda T, Takahashi N, Martin TJ: Modulation of osteoclast formation. Endocrine Rev 13:66, 1992.
49. Udagawa N, Takahashi N, Akatsu T, et al: Origin of osteoclasts: Mature monocytes and macrophages are capable of differentiating into osteoclasts under a suitable microenvironment prepared by bone marrow-derived stromal cells. Proc Natl Acad Sci 87:7260, 1990.
50. Quinn J, McGee JOD, Athanasou NA: Cellular and hormonal factors influencing monocyte differentiation to osteoclast-like bone resorbing cells. Endocrinology 134:2416, 1994.
51. Athanasou NA, Quinn J: Human tumour-associated macrophages are capable of bone resorption. Br J Cancer 65:523, 1992.
52. Quinn J, Athanasou NA: Tumour infiltrating macrophages are capable of bone resorption. J Cell Sci 101:681, 1992.
53. Quinn JM, Joyner C, Triffitt JT, et al: Polymethyl methacrylate-induced inflammatory macrophages resorb bone. J Bone Joint Surg 74B:652, 1992.
54. Athanasou NA, Wells CA, Quinn J: The origin and nature of stromal osteoclast-like multinucleated giant cells in breast carcinoma: Implications for tumour and macrophage biology. Br J Cancer 59:491, 1989.
55. Athanasou NA, Quinn J, Bulstrode CJK: Resorption of bone by inflammatory cells derived from the capsule of hip arthroplasties. J Bone Joint Surg 74B:57, 1992.
56. Athanasou NA, Quinn J, Ferguson D, et al: Bone resorption by macrophage polykaryons of a giant cell tumour of tendon sheath. Br J Cancer 63:527, 1991.
57. Athanasou NA, Quinn J: Bone resorption by macrophage polykaryons of a pilar tumour of scalp. Cancer 70:469, 1992.
58. Freidenstein AJ: Precursor cells of mechanocytes. Int Rev Cytol 47:327, 1976.
59. Freidenstein AJ: Stromal mechanism of bone marrow: Cloning in vitro and retransplantation in vivo. *In* Thientelder S (ed): Immunobiology of Bone Marrow Transplantation. Berlin, Springer-Verlag, 1980, p 19.
60. Urist MR, Nakagawa M, Nakata N, et al: Experimental myositis ossificans: Cartilage and bone formation in muscle in response to a diffusible bone matrix-derived morphogen. Arch Pathol Lab Med 102:312, 1978.
61. Owen M: Lineage of osteogenic cells and their relationship to the stromal system. *In* Peck WA (ed): Bone and Mineral Research. Amsterdam, Elsevier, 1985, p 1.
62. Owen MR, Cave J, Joyner CG: Clonal analysis in vitro of osteogenic differentiation of marrow CFU-F. J Cell Sci 87:731, 1987.
63. McCulloch CAG, Tenenbaum HC: Dexamethasone induces proliferation and terminal differentiation of osteogenic cells in tissue culture. Anat Rec 215:397, 1986.
64. Aubin JE, Liv L, Malaval L, et al: Osteoblast and chondroblast differentiation. Bone 17:77S, 1995.
65. Mundy GR, Boyce B, Hughes D, et al: The effect of cytokines and growth factors on osteoblastic cells. Bone 175:71S, 1995.
66. Benedict WF, Hong-Ji X, Hu S-X, et al: Role of the retinoblastoma gene in the initiation and progression of human cancer. J Clin Invest 85:988, 1990.
67. Heiple KG, Herndon CH, Chase WS, et al: Osteogenic induction by osteosarcoma and normal bone in mice. J Bone Joint Surg 58A:311, 1968.
68. Amitani K, Nakata Y: Characteristics of osteosarcoma cells in culture. Clin Orthop 122:315, 1977.
69. Hanamura H, Urist MR: Osteogenesis and chondrogenesis in transplants of Dunn and Ridgway osteosarcoma cell cultures. Am J Pathol 91:277, 1978.
70. Schmidt J, Strauss GP, Schon A, et al: Establishment and characterisation of osteogenic cell lines from a spontaneous murine osteosarcoma. Differentiation 39:151, 1985.
71. McAllister RM, Gardner MB, Greene AE, et al: Cultivation in vitro of cells derived from a human osteosarcoma. Cancer 27:397, 1971.
72. Smith HS, Owens RB, Hiller AJ, et al: The biology of human cells in tissue culture. I Characterisation of cells derived from osteogenic sarcomas. Int J Cancer 17:219, 1976.
73. Weichselbaum R, Epstein J, Little JB: A technique

for developing established cell lines from human osteosarcomas. In Vitro 12:833, 1976.
74. Tsang K-Y, Pai GS, Fudenberg HH: Characterisation of newly established human osteosarcoma cell line, LM-1. In Vitro 17:308, 1981.
75. Yamane I: Establishment and characterisation of cell lines derived from human osteosarcoma. Clin Orthop 199:261, 1985.
76. Kawai A: A newly established human osteosarcoma cell line with osteoblastic properties. Clin Orthop 259:256, 1990.
77. Rodan SB, Imai Y, Thiede MA, et al: Characterisation of a human osteosarcoma cell line (SAOS-2) with osteoblastic properties. Cancer Res 47:4961, 1987.
78. Clarke Anderson H, Sugamoto K, Morris DC, et al: Bone inducing agent (BIA) from cultured human SAOS-2 osteosarcoma cells. Bone Miner 16:42, 1992.
79. Ringbom-Anderson T, Akerman KEO: A phorbol ester secretion of alkaline phosphatase activity in human osteosarcoma cells. Calcif Tissue Int 50:533, 1992.
80. Sonobe H, Mizobuchi H, Manabe Y, et al: Morphological characterisation of a newly established human osteosarcoma cell line, HS-Os-1, revealing its distinct osteoblastic nature. Virchows Arch 60:181, 1991.
81. Oshima O, Haraki T, Kakuta S, et al: Expression of collagen species in a cartilaginous tumour derived from a human osteogenic sarcoma. Calcif Tissue Int 54:516, 1994.
82. Franceschi RT, James WM, Zerlauth G: 1α, 25-dihydroxyvitamin D_3 specific regulation of growth, morphology, and fibronectin in a human osteosarcoma cell line. J Cell Physiol 123:401, 1985.
83. Fukuyama S, Tashjian AH: Direct modulation by androgens of the response of human bone cells (SAOS-2) to human parathyroid hormone (PTH) and PTH-related protein. Endocrinology 125:1789, 1989.
84. McMaster JH, Suorton PE, Drash AL: Growth and hormone control mechanisms in osteosarcoma. Clin Orthop 106:366, 1975.
85. Singh I, Tsang KY, Ludwig GD: Alterations in the mitochondria of human osteosarcoma cells with glucocorticoids. Cancer Res 34:2946, 1974.
86. Betsholtz C, Westermark B, Ek B, et al: Coexpression of a PDGF-like growth factor and PDGF receptors in a human osteosarcoma cell line: Implications for autocrine receptor activation. Cell 39:447, 1984.
87. Heldin C-H, Johnsson A, Weinergren S, et al: A human osteosarcoma cell line secretes a growth factor structurally related to a homodimer of PDGF A-chain. Nature 319:511, 1986.
88. Womer RB: The cellular biology of bone tumors. Clin Orthop 262:12, 1991.
89. Womer RB, Frick K, Mitchell CD: PDGF induces c-myc mRNA expression in MG-63 human osteosarcoma cells but does not stimulate cell replication. J Cell Physiol 132:65, 1987.
90. Masuda H, Yokota J, Battifora H, et al: Events on different chromosomes alter the genes for the two peptides of platelet-derived growth factor in an osteogenic sarcoma. Cancer 29:303, 1987.
91. Mioh H, Chen J-K: Differential inhibitory effects of TGF-β on EGF-, PDGF-, and HBGF-1-stimulated MG63 human osteosarcoma cell growth: Possible involvement of growth factor interactions at the receptor and post receptor levels. J Cell Physiol 139:509, 1989.
92. Rosen DM, Stempien SA, Thompson AY, et al: Transforming growth factor-beta modulates the expression of osteoblast and chondroblast phenotypes in vitro. J Cell Physiol 134:337, 1988.
93. Kirstein M, Baglioni C: Tumour necrosis factor stimulates proliferation of human osteosarcoma cells and accumulation of c-myc messenger RNA. J Cell Physiol 134:479, 1988.
94. Raile K, Hoflich A, Kessler U, et al: Human osteosarcoma (U-2 OS) cells empress both insulin-like growth factor 1 (IGF-I) receptors and synthesise IGF-II: autocrine stimulation by IGF-II via the IGF-I receptor. J Cell Physiol 159:531, 1994.
95. Kappel CC, Velez Yanguras MC, Hirschfield S, et al: Human osteosarcoma cell lines are dependent on insulin-like growth factor I for in vitro growth. Cancer Res 54:2803, 1994.
96. Harju VT, Alitalo R, Andersson LC: Divergent in vitro effects of recombinant interferons on human osteosarcoma cells. Bone 11:247, 1990.
97. Bogenmann E, Moghadam H, DeClerck YA, et al: c-myc amplification and expression in newly established human osteosarcoma cell lines. Cancer Res 47:2808, 1987.
98. Chan JC, Song WT: Activated production of metalloproteinases in Ki-ras transformed human osteosarcoma cells. Leukaemia 1994; 8(Suppl. 1): S30.
99. Cowell JK: The genetics of retinoblastoma. Br J Cancer 63:333, 1991.
100. Huang H-J, Yee J-K, Sheu J-Y, et al: Suppression of the neoplastic phenotype by explacement of the RB gene in human cancer cells. Science 242:1563, 1989.
101. Diller L, Kassel J, Nelson CE, et al: p53 functions as a cell cycle control protein in osteosarcomas. Mol Cell Biol 10:5772, 1990.
102. Rous P, Murphy JB, Tytler WH: A filterable agent the cause of a second chicken-tumour, an osteochondrosarcoma. JAMA 59:1793, 1912.
103. Stewart SE: The polyoma virus. *In* Smith KM, Lavffer MA (eds): Advances in Virus Research. New York, Academic Press, 1960, p 61.
104. Laterjet R: On the viral aetiology of certain osteogenic sarcomas: A critical review. Bull Cancer 58:277, 1971.
105. Shenein R, Mak TW, Clark SP: Viruses and cancer. *In* Tannock IA, Hill RP (eds): The Basic Science of Oncology. New York, Pergamon Press, 1987, p 52.
106. Finkel MP, Biskis BO, Jinkins PB: Virus induction of osteosarcomas in mice. Science 155:698, 1966.
107. Finkel MP, Reilly CA, Biskis BO: Pathogenesis of radiation and virus induced bone tumour. *In* Grundmann E (ed): Malignant Bone Tumors. Heidelberg, Springer-Verlag, 1976, p 92.
108. Michiels L, Merregaart J: Retroviruses and oncogenes associated with osteosarcoma. *In* Humphrey GB (ed): Osteosarcoma in adolescents and young adults. Boston, Kluwer, 1993, p 62.
109. Jenuwein T, Müller R: Structure-function analysis of fos protein: A single amino acid changes the immortalising potential of v-fos. Cell 48:647, 1987.
110. Shyu AB, Belasco JG, Greenberg ME: Two distinct destabilising elements in the c-fos message trigger deadenylation as a first step in rapid mRNA decay. Genes Dev 5:221, 1991.
111. Wang ZQ, Grigoriadis AE, Möhle-Steinlein U, et al: A novel target cell for c-fos induced oncogenesis: Development of chondrogenic tumors in embryonic stem cell chimeras. EMBO J 10:2437, 1991.
112. Sibermann M, Reddi AH, Hand A, et al: Chondroid

bone arises from mesenchymal stem cells in organ culture of mandibular condyles. J Cranial Genet Dev Biol 7:39, 1987.
113. Closs EI, Murray AB, Schmidt J, et al: c-fos expression precedes osteogenic differentiation of cartilage cells in vitro. J Cell Biol 111:1313, 1990.
114. Schmidt J, Closs EI, Livne E, et al: Biochemical characterisation of virus-induced osteosarcoma-like osseous lesion in vitro. Calcif Tissue Int 45:232, 1989.
115. Wu JX, Carpenter JK, Gresens C, et al: The proto oncogene c-fos is overexpressed in the majority of human osteosarcomas. Oncogene 5:989, 1990.
116. Tomita K, Yokogawa A, Nomura S: Human tumour clonogenic assay in osteosarcoma for evaluation of clinical efficacy of anticancer drugs. Cancer Chemother Pharmacol 18:133, 1986.
117. Gebhardt MC, Kusuzaki K, Mankin HJ, et al: An assay to measure Adriamycin binding in osteosarcoma cells. J Orthop Res 12:621, 1994.
118. Fujisaki T, Wada T, Takahashi M, et al: In vitro chemosensitivity assay for human osteosarcoma using tumour xenografts. Clin Orthop 313:279, 1995.
119. Ishii S, Yamawaki S, Sasaki T, et al: An in vitro method for testing the sensitivities to drugs of human osteosarcomas grafted onto nude mice. Clin Orthop 172:281, 1983.
120. Hall IH, Wong OT: The cytotoxicity of 3-imino-1-oxoisoindolines in murine and human tissue culture cells. Anticancer Drugs 5:207, 1994.
121. Clarke Anderson H, Hsu HHT, Raval P, et al: The mechanism of bone induction and bone healing by human osteosarcoma cell extracts. Clin Orthop 313:129, 1995.
122. Wada T, Uede T, Ishii S, et al: Monoclonal antibodies that detect different antigenic determinants of the same human osteosarcoma-associated antigen. Cancer Res 48:2273, 1988.
123. Stern R, Wilczek J, Thorpe WP, et al: Procollagens as markers for the cell of origin of human bone tumors. Cancer Res 40:325, 1980.
124. Webber RJ, Malemud CJ, Sokoloff L: Species differences in cell culture of mammalian articular chondrocytes. Calcif Tissue Res 23:61, 1977.
125. Kuettner KE, Pauli BU, Gall G, et al: Synthesis of cartilage matrix by mammalian chondrocytes in vitro I isolation, culture characteristics, and morphology. J Cell Biol 93:743, 1982.
126. Vetter U, Zapf J, Heit W, et al: Human fetal and adult chondrocytes. J Clin Invest 77:1903, 1986.
127. Gitelis S, Kimura J, Block J, et al: Clonal analysis of human chondrosarcoma. Chir Orgagni Mov LXXV(suppl N1):11, 1990.
128. Block JA, Inerot SE, Gitelis S, et al: Synthesis of chondrocytic keratan sulphate-containing proteoglycans by human chondrosarcoma cells in long-term cell culture. J Bone Joint Surg 73A:647, 1991.
129. Mankin HJ, Cantley KP, Lippiello L, et al: The biology of human chondrosarcoma. J Bone Joint Surg 62A:160, 1980.
130. Buckwalter JA: The structure of human chondrosarcoma proteoglycans. J Bone Joint Surg 65A:958, 1983.
131. Marbenco HC, Krehbiel RH, Nelson D: Transplantable osteogenic tumour in the rat. Cancer Res 27:362, 1967.
132. Breitkreutz D, Diaz deLeon L, Paglia L, et al: Histological and biochemical studies of transplantable rat chondrosarcoma. Cancer Res 39:5093, 1979.
133. DegingSun MB, Maldonado AB, Kuettner KE, et al: Clonal analysis of the population of chondrocytes from the Swarm rat chondrosarcoma in agarose cultures. J Orthop Res 4:427, 1986.
134. Kimura JH, Lohmander LS, Hascall VC: Studies on the biosynthesis of cartilage proteoglycans in a model system of cultured chondrocytes from the Swarm rat chondrosarcoma. J Cell Biochem 26:261, 1984.
135. Steven JW, Oike Y, Mandley C, et al: Characteristics of the core protein of the aggregation proteoglycans from the Swarm rat chondrosarcoma. J Cell Biochem 26:247, 1984.
136. Kennan S, Steiner GC: Experimental transplantation of the Swarm rat chondrosarcoma into bone: Radiological and pathological studies. J Orthop Res 9:445, 1991.
137. Weiss APC, Dorfman HD: S100 protein in human cartilage lesions. J Bone Joint Surg 68A:521, 1986.
138. Choi HU, Meyer K, Swarm RL: Mucopolysaccharide and protein-polysaccharide of a transplantable rat chondrosarcoma. Proc Natl Acad Sci 68:877, 1971.
139. Oegama TR, Hascall VC, Dziewiatkowski DD: Isolation and characterisation of proteoglycans from Swarm rat chondrosarcoma. J Biol Chem 250:6151, 1975.
140. Guerne PA, Lotz M: Interleukin-6 and transforming growth factor-beta synergistically stimulate chondrosarcoma cell proliferation. J Cell Physiol 149:117, 1991.
141. Seong SC, Matsumura T, Lee FY, et al: Insulin-like growth factor I regulation of Swarm rat chondrosarcoma. Exp Cell Res 211:238, 1994.
142. Moses MA, Shing Y: Production of matrix metalloproteinases and a metalloproteinase inhibitor by Swarm rat chondrosarcoma. Biochem Biophys Res Comm 199:418, 1994.
143. Takigawa M, Pan HO, Kinoshita A, et al: Establishment from a human chondrosarcoma of a new immortal cell line with high tumorigenicity in vivo, which is able to form proteoglycan-rich cartilage-like nodules and to respond to insulin in vitro. Int J Cancer 48:717, 1991.
144. Zhu JD, Pan HO, Suzuki F, et al: Proto oncogene expression in a human chondrosarcoma cell line: HCS02/8. Jpn J Cancer Res 85:364, 1994.
145. Haraki T, Oshima O, Kakuta S, et al: Localisation of Types I, II and X collagen in the transplanted tumour derived from human osteogenic sarcoma. Bone 13:121, 1992.
146. Eisenbrey AB, Chen JC, Dyer CA, et al: Monoclonal antibody to human cartilage cells and its reactivities to chondrocytic tumors. J Clin Lab Anal 5:180, 1991.
147. Kadin ME, Bensch KG: On the origin of Ewing's tumour. Cancer 27:257, 1971.
148. Dickman PS, Liotta LA, Triche TJ: Characterisation in established cultures and evidence of its histogenesis. Lab Invest 47:375, 1982.
149. Maletz N, McMorrow L, Greco A, et al: Ewing's sarcoma. Pathology, tissue culture, and cytogenetics. Cancer 58:252, 1986.
150. Scarpa S, D'Orazie G, Modesti M, et al: Ewing's sarcoma lines synthesise laminin and fibronectin. Virchows Arch 410:375, 1987.
151. Jaffe R, Santamaria M, Yunis EJ, et al: The neuroectodermal tumour of bone. Am J Surg Pathol 8:885, 1984.
152. Cavazzana AO, Miser JS, Jefferson J, et al: Experimental evidence for a neural origin of Ewing's sarcoma of bone. Am J Pathol 127:507, 1987.

153. Turc-Carel D, Philip I, Berger M, et al: Chromosome study of Ewing's sarcoma (ES) cell lines: Consistency of a reciprocal translocation t(11;22)(q24;q12). Cancer Genet Cytogenet 12:1, 1984.
154. Lipinski M, Braham K, Tursz T: Neuroectodermal traits in Ewing's sarcoma. Fed Proc 43:1510, 1984.
155. Kodama K, Doi O, Higashiyama M, et al: Establishment and characterisation of a new Ewing's sarcoma cell line. Cancer Genet Cytogenet 57:19, 1991.
156. Kodama K, Doi O, Higashiyama M, et al: Differentiation of a Ewing's sarcoma cell line towards neural and mesenchymal cell lineages. Jpn J Cancer Res 85:335, 1994.
157. Navarro S, Ganzalez-Devesa M, Ferrandez-Izquierdo A, et al: Scanning electron microscopic evidence for neural differentiation in Ewing's sarcoma cell lines. Virchows Arch 416:383, 1990.
158. Ohta S, Suzuki A, Shimada M, et al: Neuronal differentiation of Ewing's sarcoma induced by cholera toxin B and bromodeoxyuridine establishment of Ewing's sarcoma cell line and histochemical study. Acta Ped Jpn 33:428, 1991.
159. Hara S, Adachi Y, Kaneko Y, et al: Evidence for heterogeneous groups of neuronal differentiation of Ewing's sarcoma. Br J Cancer 64:1025, 1991.
160. Noguera R, Triche TJ, Navarro S, et al: Dynamic model of differentiation in Ewing's sarcoma cells. Comparative analysis of morphologic, immunocytochemical, and oncogene expression parameters. Lab Invest 66:143, 1992.
161. McKeon C, Thiele CJ, Ross RA, et al: Indistinguishable patterns of protooncogene expression in two distinct but closely related tumours: Ewing's sarcoma and neuroepithelioma. Cancer Res 48:4307, 1988.
162. Hamilton G, Mallinger R, Hofbauer S, et al: The monoclonal antibody HBA-71 antibody modulates proliferation of thymocytes and Ewing's sarcoma cells by interfering with the action of insulin like growth factor 1. Thymus 18:33, 1991.
163. van Valen F, Winkelmann W, Jurgens J: Type I and type II insulin-like growth factor receptors and their function in human Ewing's sarcoma cells. J Cancer Res Clin Oncol 118:269, 1992.
164. Yee D, Favoni RE, Lebovic GS, et al: Insulin like growth factor 1 expression by tumors of neuroectodermal origin with the t(11;22) chromosomal translocation: A potential autocrine growth factor. J Clin Invest 86:1806, 1990.
165. van Valen F, Winkelmann W, Burdach S, et al: Interferon gamma and tumour necrosis factor alpha induce a synergistic antiproliferative response in human Ewing's sarcoma cells in vitro. J Cancer Res Clin Oncol 119:615, 1993.
166. Gabor F, Wollmann K, Theyer G, et al: In vitro antiproliferative effects of albumin doxorubicin conjugates against Ewing's sarcoma and peripheral neuroectodermal tumour cells. Anticancer Res 14:1943, 1994.
167. Gothlin G, Ericsson JLE: The osteoclast. Clin Orthop 120:201, 1976.
168. Nicholson GC, Horton MA, Sexton PM, et al: Calcitonin receptors of human osteoclastoma. Hormon Metab Res 19:585, 1987.
169. Goldring S, Dayer J-M, Russell RGG, et al: Response to hormones of cells cultured from human giant cell tumors of bone. J Clin Endocrinol Metab 46:425, 1978.
170. Komiya S, Sasaguri Y, Inoue A, et al: Characterisation of cells cultured from human giant cell tumors of bone. Clin Orthop 258:304, 1990.
171. Athanasou NA, Pringle JAS, Revell PA, et al: Resorption of bone by human osteoclastoma cells. J Pathol 141:508, 1983.
172. Kanehisa J, Izumo T, Takaeuchi M, et al: In vitro bone resorption by isolated multinucleated giant cells from giant cell tumour of bone: Light and electron microscopy study. Virchows Arch 499:327, 1981.
173. Page AE, Hayman AR, Andersson LM: Degradation of bone matrix proteins by osteoclast cathepsins. Int J Biochem 25:545, 1993.
174. Wuchepfennig AL, Li TP, Stetler Stevenson WG: Expression of 92 kD type IV collagenase/gelatinase B in human osteoclasts. J Bone Miner Res 9:549, 1994.
175. Grano M, Colucci S, De Bellis M, et al: New model for bone resorption study in vitro: Human osteoclast-like cells from giant cell tumors of bone. J Bone Miner Res 9:1013, 1994.
176. Hoyman AR, Warburton MJ, Pringle JA: Purification and characterisation of a tartrate-resistant acid phosphatase from human osteoclastomas. Biochem J 15:601, 1989.
177. Hoyman AR, Dryden AJ, Chambers TJ, et al: Tartrate resistant acid phosphatase from human osteoclastomas is translated as a single polypeptide. Biochem J 277:631, 1991.
178. Burmester GR, Winchester RJ, Dimitiu Bona A: Delineation of four cell types comprising the giant cell tumour of bone. Expression of Ia and monocyte-macrophage lineage antigens. J Clin Invest 71:1633, 1983.
179. Horton MA, Rimmer EF, Lewis D: Cell surface characterisation of the human osteoclast: Phenotypic relationship to other bone marrow-derived cell types. J Pathol 144:281, 1984.
180. Athanasou NA, Quinn J, McGee JDO: Immunocytochemical analysis of the human osteoclast: Phenotypic relationship to other marrow-derived cells. Bone Mineral 3:317, 1988.
181. Athanasou NA, Bliss E, Gatter KC, et al: An immunohistological study of giant-cell tumour of bone: Evidence for an osteoclast origin of the giant cells. J Pathol 147:153, 1985.
182. Athanasou NA, Quinn J: The antigenic phenotype of osteoclasts and macrophage polykaryons: Immunohistological distinction and implication for osteoclast ontogeny and function. J Clin Pathol 43:997, 1990.
183. Roessner A, Vollmer E, Zwadlo G, et al: The cytogenesis of macrophages and osteoclast-like giant cells in bone tumors with special emphasis on the so-called fibrohistiocytic tumors. Curr Top Pathol 79:205, 1981.
184. Doussis I, Puddle B, Athanasou NA: The immunophenotype of mononuclear and multinucleated cells in giant cell lesion of bone and soft tissue. J Clin Pathol 45:398, 1992.
185. Athanasou NA, Puddle B, Woods CG: Use of monoclonal antibodies to recognise osteoclasts in routinely processed bone biopsies. J Clin Pathol 44:664, 1991.
186. Flanagan A, Tinkler SMB, Horton MA, et al: The multinucleate cells in giant cell granuloma of the jaw are osteoclasts. Cancer 62:1139, 1988.
187. Rathod H, Malcolm AJ, Gillespie JI, et al: Characterisation of a subtype of primary osteoclastoma: Extracellular calcium but not calcitonin inhibits aggressive HLA-DR-positive osteoclastoma possessing

"functional" calcitonin receptors. J Pathol 175:293, 1994.
188. Horton MA, Lewis D, McNulty, et al: Monoclonal antibodies to osteoclastomas (giant cell bone tumors): Definition of osteoclast-specific cellular antigens. Cancer Res 45:5663, 1985.
189. James IE, Walsh S, Dodds RA, et al: Production and characterisation of osteoclast-selective monoclonal antibodies that distinguish between multinucleated cells derived from different human tissues. J Histochem Cytochem 39:905, 1991.
190. Athanasou NA, Quinn J, Horton MA, et al: New sites of cellular vitronectin receptor immunoreactivity detected with osteoclast-reacting monoclonal antibodies 13C2 and 23C6. Bone Miner 8:7, 1990.
191. Flanagan AM, Chambers TJ: Osteoclasts are present in the giant cell variant of malignant fibrous histiocytoma. J Pathol 159:53, 1989.
192. Zambonin-Zallone A, Teti A, Gaboli M, et al: β3 subunit of vitronectin receptor is present in osteoclast adhesion structures and not in other monocyte-macrophage derived cells. Conn Tissue Res 20:143, 1989.
193. Zambonin-Zallone A, Teti A, Grano M, et al: Immunocytochemical distribution of extra cellular matrix receptors in human osteoclasts: A β3 integrin is colocalised with vinculin and talin in the polysomes of osteoclastoma giant cells. Exp Cell Res 182:645, 1989.
194. Nesbitt S, Nesbit A, Helfrich M, et al: Biochemical characterisation of human osteoclast integrins. Osteoclasts express αvβ3, α2β1 and αvβ1 integrins. J Biol Chem 287:16737, 1993.
195. Glover J, Dodds RA, Gowen MA: Integrin subunit expression by human osteoblasts and osteoclasts in situ and in culture. J Cell Sci 103:267, 1992.
196. Chambers TJ, Fuller K, Darby JA, et al: Monoclonal antibodies against osteoclast inhibit bone resorption in vitro. Bone Miner 1:127, 1986.
197. Horton MA, Taylor ML, Arnett TR, et al: Arg-Gly-Asp (RGD) peptides and the antivitronectin receptor antibody 23C6 inhibit dentine resorption and cell spreading by osteoclasts. Exp Cell Res 195:368, 1991.
198. Harris M: Central giant cell granulomas of the jaw regress with calcitonin therapy. Br J Oral Maxil Surg 31:89, 1993.
199. Goldring SR, Roelke MS, Petrison KK, et al: Human giant cell tumors of bone: Identification and characterisation of cell types. J Clin Invest 79:482, 1987.
200. Goldring S, Schiller AL, Mankin JH, et al: Characterisation of cells from human giant cell tumors of bone. Clin Orthop 204:59, 1978.
201. Joyner CJ, Quinn JM, Triffitt JT, et al: Phenotypic characterisation of mononuclear and multinucleated cells of giant cell tumour of bone. Bone Mineral 16:37, 1992.
202. Gallardo H, DeLustig ES, Schajowicz F: Growth and maintenance of human giant cell tumors (osteoclastomas) in continuous culture. Oncology 24:146, 1970.
203. Wientroub S, Binderman I, Somjen D, et al: Response to parathyroid and calcitonin of human giant cell tumour of bone cultured in patients' serum. Clin Orthop 167:277, 1992.
204. Zheng MH, Fan Y, Wysocki SJ, et al: Gene expression of transforming growth factor beta 1 and its type II receptor in giant cell tumors of bone. Possible involvement in osteoclast like cell migration. Am J Pathol 145:1095, 1994.
205. Stoll BA: Natural history, prognosis and staging of bone metastases. *In* Stoll BA, Parbhoo S (eds): Bone Metastases: Monitoring and Treatment. New York, Raven Press, 1983, p 1.
206. Galasko CSB: Mechanisms of bone destruction in the development of skeletal metastases. Nature 263:507, 1986.
207. Galasko CSB, Bennett A: Relationship of bone destruction in skeletal metastases to osteoclast activation and prostaglandin. Nature 263:508, 1976.
208. Eilon G, Mundy GR: Effects of inhibition of microtubule assembly on bone mineral release and enzyme release by human breast cancer cells. J Clin Invest 87:69, 1981.
209. Chambers TJ, Darby JA, Fuller K: Mammalian collagenase predisposes bone surfaces to osteoclastic resorption. Cell Tissue Res 241:671, 1985.
210. Eilon G, Mundy GR: Direct resorption of bone by human breast cancer cells in vitro. Nature 276:726, 1978.
211. Boyde A, Maconnachie E, Reid SA, et al: Scanning electron microscopy in bone pathology: Review of methods. potential and applications. Scan Electron Microsc 4:1537, 1986.
212. Carter RL: Patterns and mechanisms of bone metastases. J Royal Soc Med 78(suppl):2, 1985.
213. Athanasou NA, Quinn J, McGee JOD: Mechanism of osteolysis by U937 and M5076 tumour cells. Calcif Tissue Int 42(suppl):A39, 1988.
214. Quinn JMW, Matsumura Y, Tarin D, et al: Cellular and hormonal mechanisms associated with malignant bone resorption. Lab Invest 71:465, 1994.
215. Quinn JMW, Sabokbar A, Athanasou NA: Cells of the mononuclear phagocyte series differentiate into osteoclastic lacunar bone resorbing cells. J Pathol 179:106, 1996.
216. Bottazzi B, Erba E, Nobili N: A paracrine circuit in the regulation of the proliferation of macrophages infiltrating murine sarcomas. J Immunol 144:2409, 1990.
217. Van Furth R: Origin and turnover of monocytes and macrophages. Curr Top Pathol 79:125, 1989.
218. Spector W, Lykke AWJ: The cellular evolution of inflammatory granulomata. J Pathol 92:163, 1966.
219. Whitworth W, Pak CC, Esgro J, et al: Macrophages and cancer. Cancer Metast Rev 8:319, 1989.
220. Mundy GR: Mechanisms of osteolytic bone destruction. Bone 2:S1, 1991.
221. Gebhardt MC, Lippsello L, Bringhurst FR, et al: Prostaglandin E2 synthesis by human primary and metastatic bone tumors in culture. Clin Orthop 196:300, 1985.
222. Galasko CSB, Samuel AW, Rushton S, et al: The effect of prostaglandin synthesis inhibition and diphosphonates on tumour-mediated osteolysis. Br J Surg 67:453, 1980.
223. Bennett A, Stamford IF, Berstock DA, et al: Breast cancer, prostaglandins and patient survival. Br J Cancer 59:268, 1989.
224. Sabatini M, Chavez J, Mundy G, et al: Stimulation of tumour necrosis factor release by monocytic cells by the A375 human melanoma via granulocyte-macrophage colony stimulating factor. Cancer Res 50:2673, 1990.
225. Sabatini M, Yates AJ, Garrett R, et al: Increased production of tumour necrosis factor by immune cells in a model of the humoral hypercalcaemia of malignancy. Lab Invest 63:678, 1990.

226. Lee MY, Lui CC, Lottsfeldt JL, et al: Production of granulocyte-stimulating and bone cell-modulating activities from a neutrophilia hypercalcaemia-inducing murine mammary cancer cell line. Cancer Res 47:4059, 1987.
227. Sato K, Fujii Y, Ono M, et al: Production of interleukin 1 alpha-like factor and colony-stimulating factor by a squamous cell carcinoma of the thyroid (T3M-5) derived from a patient with hypercalcaemia and leucocytosis. Cancer Res 47:6474, 1976.
228. Sato K, Mimura H, Han DC, et al: Production of bone resorbing activity and colony stimulating activity in vivo and in vitro by a human squamous cell carcinoma associated with hypercalcaemia and leucocytosis. J Clin Invest 78:145, 1986.
229. Mundy GR: Ectopic production of calciotropic peptides. Endocrinol Metab Clin North Am 20:473, 1991.
230. Derynck R, Goeddel DV, Ullrich A: Synthesis of messenger RNAs for transforming growth factor alpha and beta and the epidermal growth factor receptor by human tumors. Cancer Res 47:707, 1987.
231. Gregory J, Thomas CE, Willshire IR, et al: Epidermal and transforming growth factor alpha in patients with breast tumors. Br J Cancer 59:605, 1989.
232. Salomon DS, Kidwell WR, Liu S: Presence of alpha TGF mRNA in human breast cancer cell lines and in human breast carcinomas. Breast Cancer Res Treat 8:106a, 1986.
233. Rosol TJ, Merryman JI, Nohuteu RM, et al: Effects of transforming growth factor beta on parathyroid hormone and parathyroid hormone related protein mediated bone resorption and adenylate cyclase stimulation in vitro. Dom Anim Endocrinol 8:501, 1991.
234. Lorenzo JA, Sousa SL, Centrella M: Interleukin-1 in combination with transforming growth factor beta produces enhanced bone resorption in vitro. Endocrinology 123:2194, 1988.
235. Yates AJ, Marcelli C, Bonewald L, et al: Human transforming growth factor (TGF-beta) causes marked hypercalcaemia in mice and is synergistic with low-dose parathyroid hormone related protein. J Bone Miner Res 5:741, 1990.
236. Manolagas SC: Role of cytokines in bone resorption. Bone 17:63S, 1995.
237. Klein B, Bataille R: Cytokine network in human multiple myeloma. Hematol Oncol Clin North Am 6:273, 1992.
238. Roodman GD: Osteoclast function in Paget's disease and multiple myeloma. Bone 17:57S, 1995.
239. Devlin RD, Bone JG, III, Roodman GD: Stimulation of osteoclast-like multinucleated cell (MNC) formation in long-term human bone marrow culture by the serum of patients with Gorham-Stout or disappearing bone disease [abstract]. J Bone Miner Res 9:S140, 1994.
240. Moseley JM, Kubota M, Diefenback-Jagger H: Parathyroid hormone related protein purified from a human lung cancer cell line. Proc Natl Acad Sci 84:5048, 1987.
241. Docherty HM, Dixon-Lewis MJ, Milton PG, et al: Parathyroid hormone related proteins in cultured epithelial cells. J Endocrinol 123:487, 1989.
242. Powell GJ, Southby J, Danks JA, et al: Localisation of parathyroid hormone related protein in breast cancer metastases: Increased incidence in bone compared to other sites. Cancer Res 51:3059, 1991.
243. Bundred NJ, Walker RA, Ratcliffe WA, et al: Parathyroid hormone related protein and skeletal morbidity in breast cancer. Eur J Cancer 28:690, 1992.
244. Manisken WJ, Sivanathan K, Orr FW: Resorbing bone stimulates tumour cell growth: A role for the host microenvironment in bone metastasis. Am J Pathol 123:39, 1986.
245. Jacobs SC, Pikna D, Lawson RK: Prostatic osteoblastic factor. Invest Urol 17:195, 1979.
246. Simpson EL, Harrod J, Eilon G, et al: Identification of a mRNA fraction in human prostatic cancer cells coding for a novel osteoblast stimulating factor. Endocrinology 117:1615, 1985.
247. Koutsilieris M, Rabbani SA, Bennett HP, et al: Characteristics of prostate derived growth factors for cells of the osteoblast phenotype. J Clin Invest 80:941, 1989.
248. Harris SE, Harris MA, Mahy P, et al: Expression of BMP and BMP-like mRNA by human prostate carcinoma cells. J Bone Miner Res 6:S193, 1991.
249. Hart KA, Bentley H, Seid J, et al: Detection of bone morphogenetic protein (BMP) expression in human prostatic tissue and cell lines. J Bone Miner Res 6:S260, 1991.
250. Rabbani SA, Desjardins J, Bell AW, et al: Identification of a new osteoblast mitogen from a human prostate cancer cell line PC-3. J Bone Miner Res 5:S211, 1990.
251. Kaplan RL, Mickey DD, Gray TK: Rat prostate tumour cells secrete a mitogen for osteosarcoma cells that is similar to basic fibroblast growth factor. J Bone Miner Res 6:S143, 1991.
252. Gottzman D, Bolivar I, Moroz LA, et al: Urokinase and the mechanism of osteoblastic metastases by prostate cancer. Fibrinolysis 6:63, 1992.

Chapter

4

CYTOGENETIC ANALYSIS OF BONE AND JOINT NEOPLASMS

JULIA A. BRIDGE and CHARLOTTE ORNDAL

BASIC PRINCIPLES OF CYTOGENETIC ANALYSIS

Cytogenetic analysis of solid tumors (including bone tumors) or other types of tissue, such as bone marrow and peripheral blood, requires dividing cells. Mitotically active cells are arrested in prometaphase or metaphase by the addition of a microtubule inhibitor. Individual chromosomes are examined by special staining techniques that produce a pattern of alternating light and dark bands. These bands, which are most commonly obtained with Giemsa staining and thus referred to as *G-bands*, are unique for each of the sex chromosomes and the 22 pairs of autosomal chromosomes present in a normal human somatic cell.

Cytogenetic analyses of both benign and malignant tumors have revealed abnormalities in the number or structure, or both, of the chromosomes. Many of these changes are specific for a particular tumor type and thus play a direct, potentially decisive role in the examination of these neoplasms.[1] In addition to adding a new dimension to the formulation of a diagnosis, the cytogenetic findings in bone and joint neoplasms have provided resolution of cellular origin.[2] Identification of the aberrant chromosomal bands has served as a basis for molecular approaches in establishing the definitive genes affected and the associated consequences of these gene alterations.[3] In some instances, recognition of the cytogenetic abnormality is the first clue that a mutated gene resides at a particular locus. For example, the autosomal dominant disorder, Langer-Giedion syndrome (characterized by multiple exostoses, mental retardation, and abnormal facial features) has been mapped to the long arm of chromosome 8 following observation of constitutional deletions of 8q24 cytogenetically in affected patients.[4, 5]

USES AND LIMITATIONS OF CYTOGENETICS IN THE DIAGNOSIS OF BONE TUMORS

The cytogenetic examination of benign and malignant primary bone tumors has revealed tumor-specific chromosomal abnormalities that are of diagnostic importance and potential prognostic value. The histologic classification of mesenchymal neoplasms, especially the so-called high-grade lesions, often presents a challenge to the surgical pathologist. Electron microscopy can be helpful, but sampling errors can occur with this technique. Many lesions defy histologic classification, even with the aid of immunohistochemistry.

An accurate diagnosis is essential for determination of appropriate therapy. Chromosomal analysis is not only used to supplement conventional pathologic examination in the classification of bone and joint neoplasms, but also serves as a vital diagnostic tool when other investigations have failed.[1] For example, demonstration of characteristic chromosomal abnormalities can be especially useful in the differential diagnosis of "small round cell neoplasms" such as Ewing's sarcoma and peripheral primitive neuroectodermal tumors (PNETs), neuroblastoma, rhabdomyosarcoma, lymphoma, and small cell osteosarcoma.[6] A distinct advantage of cytogenetic analysis as a diagnostic tool is that chromosomal aberrations are not lost as a neoplasm becomes less differentiated. This is in contrast to some immunohistochemical and ultrastructural features.

Cytogenetic analysis has also provided insight into the histopathogenesis of certain types of primary bone tumors for which the derivation was previously unknown.[1] For example, Ewing's sarcoma (a tumor of unknown histopathogenesis) has been shown to share a functionally identical chromosomal rearrangement involving chromosomes 11 and 22, with peripheral neuroepithelioma, esthesioneuroblastoma, and Askin's tumor (tumors with evidence of a neural origin), indicating a common mechanism of oncogenesis and a similar tissue of origin for these distinct clinicopathologic entities.[6] Recognition of the chimeric gene produced with this translocation has also been valuable diagnostically.[3] Ultimately, specific gene therapies may be developed based on the biologic functions of these chromosomal rearrangements.

Despite the significant diagnostic and etiologic information cytogenetics has provided in the evaluation of bone and joint neoplasms, there are some limitations to the findings. (1) Several histologic subtypes of the various benign and malignant primary bone tumors are rare and have not yet been subjected to cytogenetic analysis. (2) Successful cytogenetic analysis is dependent on the ability of the cytogeneticist to culture the tumor cells in question, which can be a formidable task for many of the bone tumors; with the exception of a few high-grade malignancies, most neoplasms do not have a sufficient number of endemic mitoses and must undergo tissue culture for satisfactory analysis. (3) The cytogenetic findings in bone sarcomas are often complex, and thus distinguishing primary from secondary chromosomal abnormalities is difficult. Secondary changes may be consistent in a particular neoplasm, but are also observed in other histologic tumor types, thereby lacking the specificity of the primary change. Secondary changes appear to contribute to tumor progression.

METHODS FOR TRADITIONAL CYTOGENETIC ANALYSIS

Specimen Requirements

Tissue submitted for cytogenetic analysis must be fresh, not frozen or fixed in formalin, because living, dividing cells are required. Samples should be sterile, and transportation time to the laboratory should be kept to a minimum. Specimens can be transported at room temperature or refrigerated (not frozen) in sterile isotonic saline or culture media containing serum. For specimens requiring longer transport times (5–48 hours), the latter solution is preferable.

Cytogenetic analysis can be performed on both benign and malignant tumors. An optimal sample submission size is 1 cm^3 or greater. Depending on the cellularity of the specimen, however, samples smaller than 1 cm^3 can yield enough cells to initiate cultures and even to attempt direct harvest of spontaneously dividing cells in cases in which a rapid result is desired. Curettaged material and, in some cases, fine needle aspiration biopsy samples, are suitable for analysis.[7, 8] Efforts to perform cytogenetic analysis are worthwhile even when material is limited, as the presence of a single cell exhibiting a tumor-specific chromosomal abnormality provides strong diagnostic support.

In general, successful cytogenetic analysis of primary bone tumors is more difficult to achieve than analysis of soft tissue tumors. Difficulties encountered with bone tumors include low cell density and release of cells from the bone matrix. Tissue selected for analysis should appear viable without evidence of necrosis. Ideally, all normal tissue should be trimmed from the submitted sample as its presence interferes with processing and analysis.[9] For some tumors, sampling of separate or distinct areas of a particular lesion will reveal different but related or overlapping cytogenetic clones, that is, intratumor heterogeneity. Importantly, tumors that are characterized by a specific aberration appear to exhibit that abnormality in all analyzed areas from the tumor.[10]

Cell Culture and Chromosome Banding

The basic process of cell culturing for all mesenchymal lesions is the same. Briefly, sterile tumor tissue is mechanically minced with scissors or a scalpel and enzymatically disaggregated by being incubated in collagenase (usually type II collagenase).[11] The resulting cell suspension is washed, diluted in culture media, and allocated to tissue culture flasks, chamber slides, or coverslips. Standard culture media preparations such as RPMI 1640 with fetal bovine serum are most commonly used. To minimize contamination, a low concentration of antibiotics and antimycotics is added to the media. (For more detailed information on culture media composition and processing protocols, the reader is referred to Sandberg and Bridge[2] and Mandahl[12]).

The cells suspended in culture media are incubated at 37°C, 5% CO_2 and are inspected for growth under an inverted microscope. A short-term culture usually results in a satisfactory number of mitoses in 10 days or less. Lengthy culture times should be avoided because undesired overgrowth by normal fibroblasts is more likely to occur.

When an optimal number of mitoses is observed, the dividing cells are arrested in metaphase with the addition of colchicine, to block the assembly of the mitotic spindle. The cells are then subjected to a hypotonic salt solution to induce swelling and subsequently fixed in multiple changes of glacial acetic acid and methanol (3:1).

A method referred to as *direct harvest* is an alternative to tissue culture. With this technique, endemic dividing cells are arrested following a 1- to 12-hour incubation in colchicine and culture media. This method is useful for obtaining fast or preliminary results but is limited by the in vivo mitotic index.[8]

G-banding is the most commonly utilized form of banding. G-bands can be obtained with Giemsa or Wright stains pretreated with trypsin or phosphate buffer respectively. The number of alternating light and dark bands detectable with G-banding in the haploid genome varies with the level of chromosomal contraction in each metaphase cell. The number of bands provided in the ideogram is 400 (Fig. 4–1). A special approach designated *high-resolution analysis* provides additional bands (greater than 850 per haploid set) by synchronizing the dividing cells and arresting their division earlier in the mitotic cycle (prophase or prometaphase). This form of analysis is difficult to perform with solid tumors and is, therefore, infrequently used.

The banded chromosome preparations are visualized with standard light microscopy and karyotypes are produced by photographing a metaphase spread, manually cutting out the chromosomes from the photograph, and arranging and pasting them in order. Automated or computerized systems have been developed in recent years that facilitate analysis by eliminating the need for photography and other darkroom activities as well as the manual preparation of the karyotype.[13]

Cytogenetic Nomenclature

A normal chromosomal complement is composed of 22 pairs of autosomal chromosomes, numbered 1 through 22, and two sex chromosomes, XX and XY. The primary constriction of a chromosome, the centromere, divides the chromosome into an upper (short) arm and lower (long) arm designated p (petite) and q, respectively. The distal ends of each chromosome are termed *telomeres*. Banded chromosomal arms are divided into regions, bands, and sometimes sub-bands. Regions are numbered consecutively from the centromere to the telomere on each arm; within each region, the individual bands are numbered in the same direction. Thus, the complete designation for a band would consist of the chromosome number, a letter to indicate the short or long arm, a number for the region, and a number for the band. For example, 1p36 refers to the long arm of chromosome 1, region 3, band 6. This numbering system is necessary for specifying breakpoints in structurally aberrant, rearranged, or deleted chromosomes and for defining the location of genes on chromosomes.

A uniform system for defining abnormalities in human chromosomes, the International System for Cytogenetic Nomenclature, was introduced and subsequently implemented at a conference in Paris in 1971.[14] One example of the abbreviations provided in this system is the use of a minus sign to signify loss of a chromosome or chromosomal arm; −12 is interpreted as loss of one copy of chromosome 12. A translocation is designated by t and is defined as the exchange of chromosomal material between two or more nonhomologous chromosomes. An abnormal clone is defined as the presence of two or more cells exhibiting

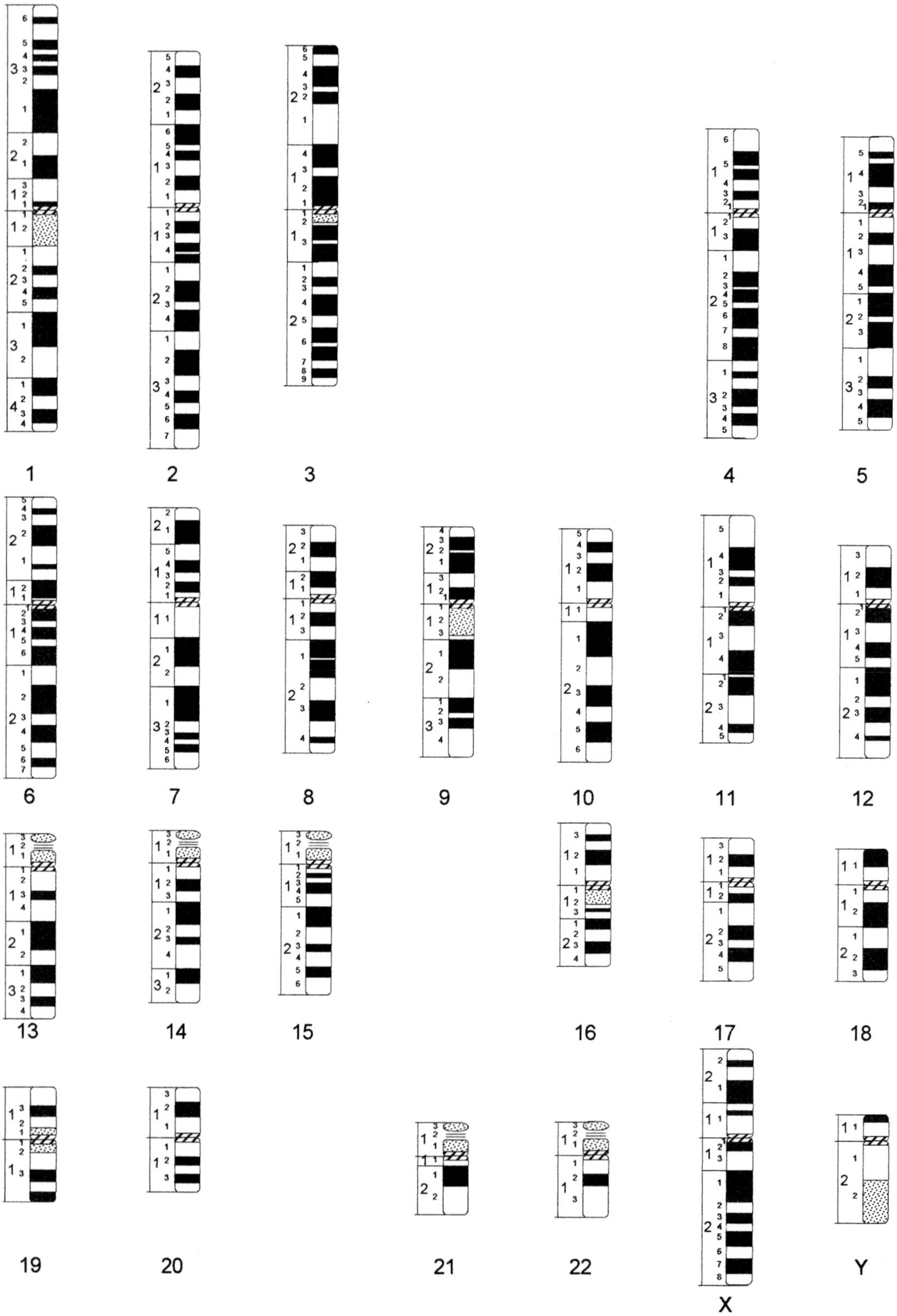

Figure 4–1. G-banding pattern for human chromosomes at the metaphase stage of condensation, with about 400 bands per haploid karyotype. The chromosomes are represented as single-chromatid structures rather than as the two-chromatid structures seen in mitotic chromosomes under the microscope.

Table 4–1. Summary of Cytogenetic Nomenclature*

Shorthand Symbol	Term	Explanation
add	Addition	Addition of chromosome material of unknown origin to denoted band
del	Deletion	Loss of material distal to, or between, breakpoint(s)
der	Derivative chromosome	Rearranged chromosome, containing material from more than one chromosome, defined by the centromeric region
ins	Insertion	Insertion of chromosome material between breakpoints
inv	Inversion	Rotation of segment 180 degrees
mar	Marker	Structurally abnormal chromosome in which no part can be identified
r	Ring	Ring chromosome; may contain identified or unidentified material
t	Translocation	Exchange of material between chromosomes; may be reciprocal
[cp]	Composite	Denotes clone to be composed from a number of cells; where all changes are not present in all cells
inc	Incomplete	Karyotype contains additional aberrations, which are unidentifiable
[n]	Number of cells	Number of cells in the clone

*For details, see ISCN: An International System for Human Nomenclature. Basel, S. Karger, 1995.

the same structural abnormality or supernumerary chromosome, or three or more cells exhibiting loss of the same chromosome. A list of some of the most commonly utilized terms is provided in Table 4–1.

MOLECULAR CYTOGENETIC ANALYSIS

Technical advances in the study of the organization and function of nucleic acid sequences have made it possible to gain information about the chromosomes in an interphase or terminally differentiated cell by means of specially developed chromosome-specific probes and in situ hybridization.[15] Hybridization refers to the binding or annealing of complementary DNA or RNA sequences.

A major limitation of traditional cytogenetic analysis is the dependency on tumor growth in culture and production of high-quality metaphase preparations. With *in situ hybridization,* specific DNA or RNA target sequences can be detected in individual cells from fresh or aged samples (such as blood smears or touch and cytospin preparations), paraffin-embedded tissue sections, and disaggregated cells retrieved from fresh, frozen, or paraffin embedded material in addition to chromosome preparations. Importantly, analysis with in situ hybridization is not contingent on dividing or mitosing cells and is the only form of analysis that provides cellular localization of DNA and RNA sequences in a heterogeneous cell population.[1, 2]

Chromosome-specific probes are most commonly labeled with fluorescent dyes (directly or indirectly) and are used to visualize the chromosome or chromosomal sequence of interest. This technique is called *fluorescence in situ hybridization* (FISH). Different combinations of haptenated probes (e.g., labeled with biotin, digoxigenin, or dinitrophenol) and different fluorophores (green [fluorescein], red [rhodamine or Texas Red], and blue [AMCA or Cascade Blue]) allow visualization of three or more separate chromosomal DNA sequences concurrently.[16, 17] The results are evaluated under a fluorescence microscope.

Several different types of chromosomal probes are available. Those most commonly used in the examination of bone tumors include probes specific for the centromeric region of different chromosomes (Fig. 4–2*A* [see also color figure]), sequence- or loci-specific probes such as breakpoint flanking or breakpoint spanning cosmid and yeast artificial chromosome (YAC) probes (see Fig. 4–2*B* [see also color figure]), and whole chromosome "painting" probes (Fig. 4–3 [see also color figure]). Whole chromosome painting probes are composed of a mixture of sequences that will bind to the entire length of a particular chromosome.

Fluorescence in situ hybridization has revolutionized the field of cytogenetics. With this approach, an investigator can (1) map DNA sequences on specific chromosomes, (2) directly detect repositioning of sequences between chromosomes or within a particular chromosome as a result of a chromosomal rearrangement, (3) uncover small rearrangements that are not detectable with stan-

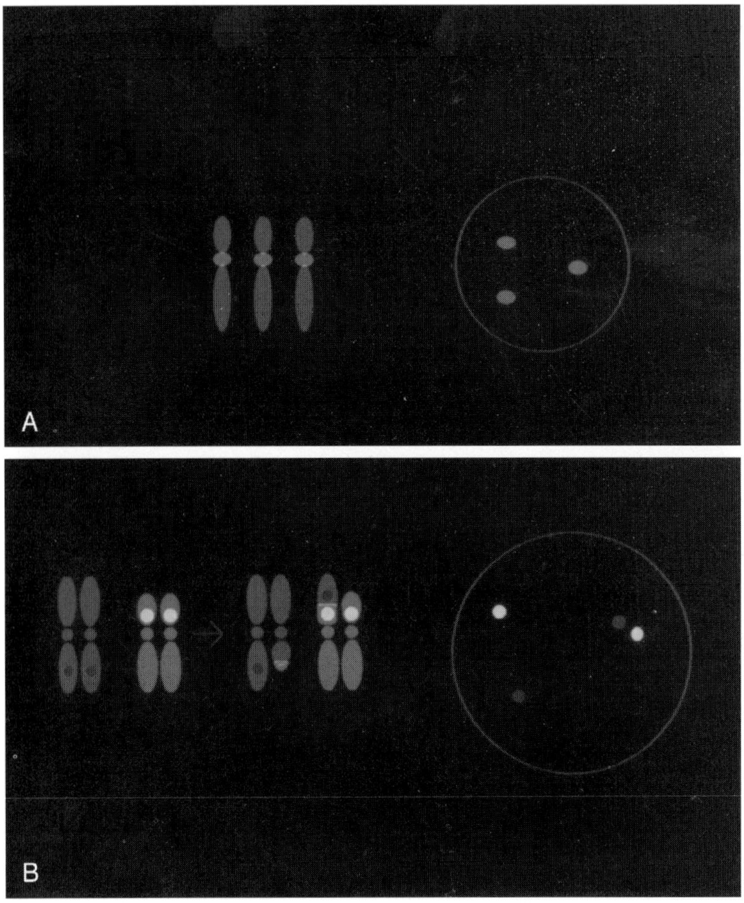

Figure 4–2. Fluorescence in situ hybridization (FISH). *A*, Schematic representation of FISH with a centromere specific probe (labeled in green). Three green signals are seen in an interphase cell demonstrating trisomy (*right*). *B*, Schematic representation of the detection of a reciprocal translocation utilizing FISH with breakpoint flanking probes (yellow and blue signals). In the interphase cell, the two different colored probes will lie in close proximity (*right*) to each other if a rearrangement has occurred, and may be visualized as a third color; for example, a green and red probe may create a yellow signal. (See also color figure.)

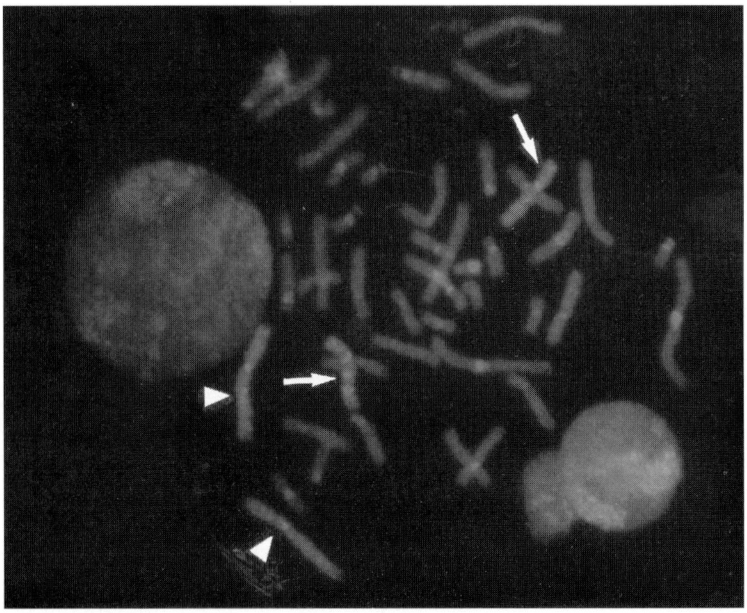

Figure 4–3. Multicolor FISH with chromosomal paint probes for specific identification of chromosomes 2 (spectrum orange, *arrowheads*) and 7 (spectrum green, *arrows*), performed on karyotypically normal male peripheral blood lymphocytes. The remaining nonprobed chromosomes are counterstained with DAPI (4,6-diamino-2-phenylindolhydrochloride, blue). These probes can be used to define or uncover various structural abnormalities. (See also color figure.)

dard karyotypic analysis, and (4) detect aneuploidy in interphase cells from both fresh and fixed tissue preparations. Limitations of FISH include the availability of probes and technical adjustments required for individual tumors. Additionally, unless the anomaly of interest is known, the number of hybridization reactions needed to resolve the question may be quite large.[18]

Another powerful method in the armament of molecular cytogenetic analysis of cancer is *comparative genomic hybridization* (CGH).[19–21] In a single hybridization, CGH provides an overview of DNA sequence copy number changes (including losses or deletions and gains or amplifications) in a tumor specimen and maps these changes on normal chromosomes. With this assay, normal human metaphase chromosomes are competitively hybridized with two differentially labeled genomic DNAs (test and reference). Analysis with fluorescence microscopy reveals the chromosomal locations of copy number changes in DNA sequences between two complements. Following hybridization and fluorescent staining of the bound DNAs, copy number variations among the different sequences in the tumor DNA are detected by measuring the tumor-to-normal fluorescence intensity ratio for each locus in the target metaphase chromosomes. CGH is particularly useful for analysis of DNA sequence copy number changes in bone tumors where high quality metaphase preparations are often difficult to make and where complex karyotypes with numerous markers, double minutes, and homogeneously stained chromosomal regions are common. CGH can be performed using total genomic tumor DNA from fresh, frozen, or paraffin-embedded tissue.

CYTOGENETIC ANALYSIS OF BENIGN BONE TUMORS

Osteochondroma

Osteochondroma, also referred to as osteocartilaginous exostosis, is the most common benign tumor of bone (see Chapter 11). Osteochondroma may arise as a sporadic solitary lesion or as multiple lesions characterizing the autosomal dominant disorders, hereditary multiple exostoses (osteochondromatosis), and Langer-Giedion syndrome (trichorhinophalangeal syndrome type II). In addition to multiple osteochondromas, patients with hereditary multiple exostoses exhibit short stature and patients with Langer-Giedion syndrome exhibit abnormal scalp hair and facial features and mental retardation. Constitutional deletions of 8q24.1 are seen in Langer-Giedion syndrome, a contiguous gene syndrome.[4] Genetic linkage studies have shown that the locus for hereditary multiple exostosis (EXT1) is also within 8q24.1, but that this disease is genetically heterogeneous.[22] Recently, EXT1 has been cloned, but its function remains elusive.[5]

Six osteochondromas with acquired clonal cytogenetic aberrations have been described; four sporadic tumors and two from patients with hereditary multiple exostoses.[23, 24] Importantly, an abnormality of the long arm of chromosome 8 was detected in five of these six tumors (Fig. 4–4). Thus, abnormalities of 8q appear to play a role in the development of both sporadic and hereditary osteochondromas.

The chromosomal association of a sporadically occurring neoplasm and a specific genetic syndrome featuring that neoplasm is not a novel one. One well-documented example is the involvement of 5q in sporadically occurring colonic polyps and desmoid tumors and the localization of the gene for familial polyposis coli and Gardner's syndrome to that same chromosomal segment.[2] Analogous to the homozygous inactivation of 5q in sporadic and hereditary colonic polyps, homozygous inactivation of 8q may be responsible for the expression of either sporadic or hereditary exostoses. Recent studies have demonstrated loss of heterozygosity for markers in 8q24.1 and chromosome 11 in chondrosarcoma, the malignant counterpart of osteochondroma, suggesting that the genes responsible for multiple exostoses may be tumor suppressor genes.[25, 26] Further molecular genetic studies will be important in testing this hypothesis.

Fibro-osseous Lesions of Bone

Osteofibrous Dysplasia

Osteofibrous dysplasia, also referred to as extragnathic ossifying fibroma, classically arises as a painless lesion in the tibia during the first decade of life (see Chapter 13). Anterior or anterolateral bowing of the tibia may be prominent. The most controversial aspect of osteofibrous dysplasia is its possible histogenetic relationship to adamantinoma of long bone. It

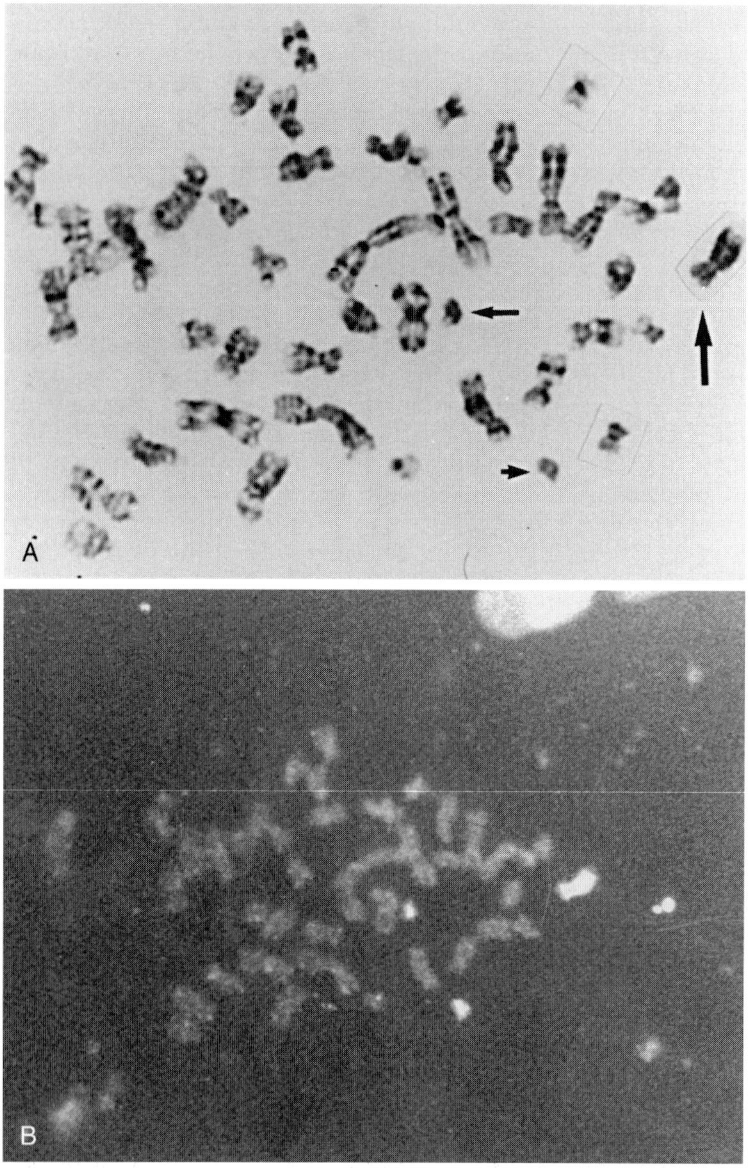

Figure 4–4. Acquired clonal cytogenetic aberration in osteochondroma. *A*, GTG-banded metaphase cell from a solitary osteochondroma of the hip demonstrating the normal chromosome 8 homologue (*large arrow*), the del(8)(q11) (*small arrow*), and der(?)t(?;8)(?;?q) (*arrowhead*). *B*, Fluorescence in situ hybridization of the same metaphase cell utilized to construct the karyotype showing positive hybridization of the deleted and derivative chromosomes (and the normal chromosome 8 homologue), with a chromosome 8 specific painting probe. (From Bridge JA, Bhatia PS, Anderson JR, et al: Biologic and clinical significance of cytogenetic and molecular cytogenetic abnormalities in benign and malignant cartilaginous lesions. Cancer Genet Cytogenet 69:79, 1993.)

has been proposed that osteofibrous dysplasia is the benign counterpart of a neoplastic process that produces an adamantinoma, that osteofibrous dysplasia is a precursor lesion to adamantinoma, or that osteofibrous dysplasia is the residual of a spontaneously regressing adamantinoma.[27]

Cytogenetic studies of osteofibrous dysplasia are few but have revealed clonal karyotypic abnormalities. Specifically, extra copies of chromosome 12 (Fig. 4–5) or chromosomes 7, 8, and 22 have been observed.[28] Trisomy 7 and 12 are abnormalities that have been described as part of an abnormal complement in one of two reportedly analyzed adamantinomas.[29] These shared cytogenetic abnormalities provide additional evidence for a histogenetic relationship between osteofibrous dysplasia and adamantinoma.

Fibrous Dysplasia and Cemento-Ossifying Fibroma

Cemento-ossifying fibroma involves the craniofacial bones and is thought to arise from the periodontal membrane.[30] The differential diagnosis of fibrous dysplasia versus ossifying fibroma may be problematic; however, radio-

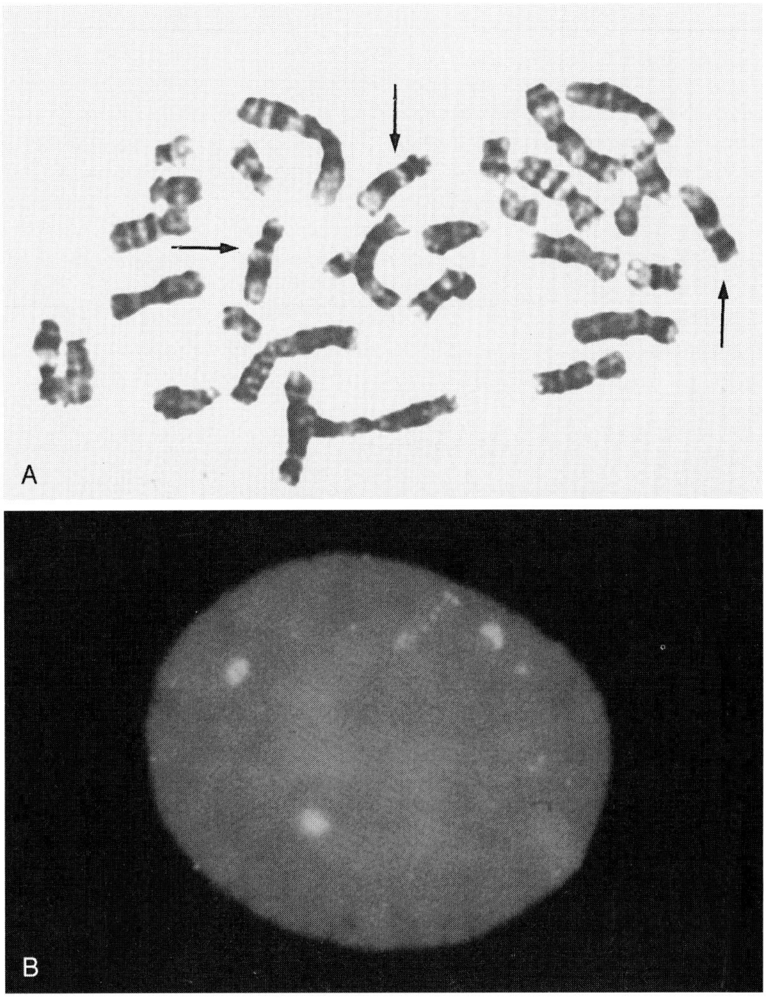

Figure 4–5. Clonal karyotypic abnormalities in osteofibrous dysplasia. *A*, GTG-banded partial metaphase cell showing trisomy 12 in osteofibrous dysplasia (*arrows*). *B*, Three copies of chromosome 12 were also detected in the interphase cells of this lesion utilizing a chromosome 12 specific alpha-satellite probe (ONCOR, Gaithersburg, MD). (From Bridge JA, Dembinski A, DeBoer J, et al: Clonal chromosomal abnormalities in osteofibrous dysplasia of the tibia: Implications for histopathogenesis and its relationship with adamantinoma. Cancer 73(6):1746, 1994. Copyright 1994, American Cancer Society. Reprinted by permission of Wiley-Liss, Inc., a subsidiary of John Wiley & Sons, Inc.)

graphic evidence of spherical calcifications supports a diagnosis of cemento-ossifying fibroma (see Chapter 13).

Cytogenetic analyses of fibrous dysplasia and nonossifying fibroma have not yet produced a consistent or characteristic chromosomal abnormality.[31–33] Recent reports of cemento-ossifying fibroma, however, have revealed consistent chromosomal breakpoints involving chromosomes X and 2. For example, two lesions of the orbit have shown an identical (X;2)(q26;q33) translocation as the sole abnormality.[34] These recurring breakpoints provide a new cytogenetic tumor marker for the identification of this tumor subtype. Overall, five fibro-osseous lesions of the jaw and frontal bones have shown clonal chromosomal abnormalities involving 2q31-35.[34, 35] Molecular examination of this region should provide important information regarding the underlying histogenetic events.

CYTOGENETIC ANALYSIS OF MALIGNANT BONE TUMORS

Giant Cell Tumor

Giant cell tumor of bone is a tumor of borderline malignancy with a distinct tendency for local recurrence (see Chapter 15). Cytogenetic investigations of giant cell tumor of bone have revealed prominence of an unusual cytogenetic phenomenon entitled *telomeric association* (tas).[36] The telomeres represent the distal ends of a chromosome and contain variable quantities of a repeat sequence TTAGGG. Telomeric association is the end-to-end fusion of cytogenetically appearing "whole" or "intact" chromosomes. There appears to be no loss of chromosomal material with tas by light microscopy. At the molecular level, however, a reduction in telomere length (average loss of 500 base pairs) has been demonstrated,[37] both in giant cell tumors cytogenetically demonstrating tas and also in tumors not demonstrating tas, although reduction appears to be greatest in giant cell tumors exhibiting tas.

Telomeric associations have been detected in approximately 75% of giant cell tumors of bone evaluated. In addition to tas, structural rearrangements involving the same chromosomal arms are common (Fig. 4–6*A–D*).[38] A histogram summarizing chromosomal short and long arm involvement in tas and/or structural rearrangements in all reported cases in which the number of normal and abnormal cells was defined, as well as a description of the specific abnormalities, is provided in Figure 4–7.[2] The telomeres most commonly affected include 19p, 11p, 15p, 21p, 20q, and 18p (in decreasing order of frequency).

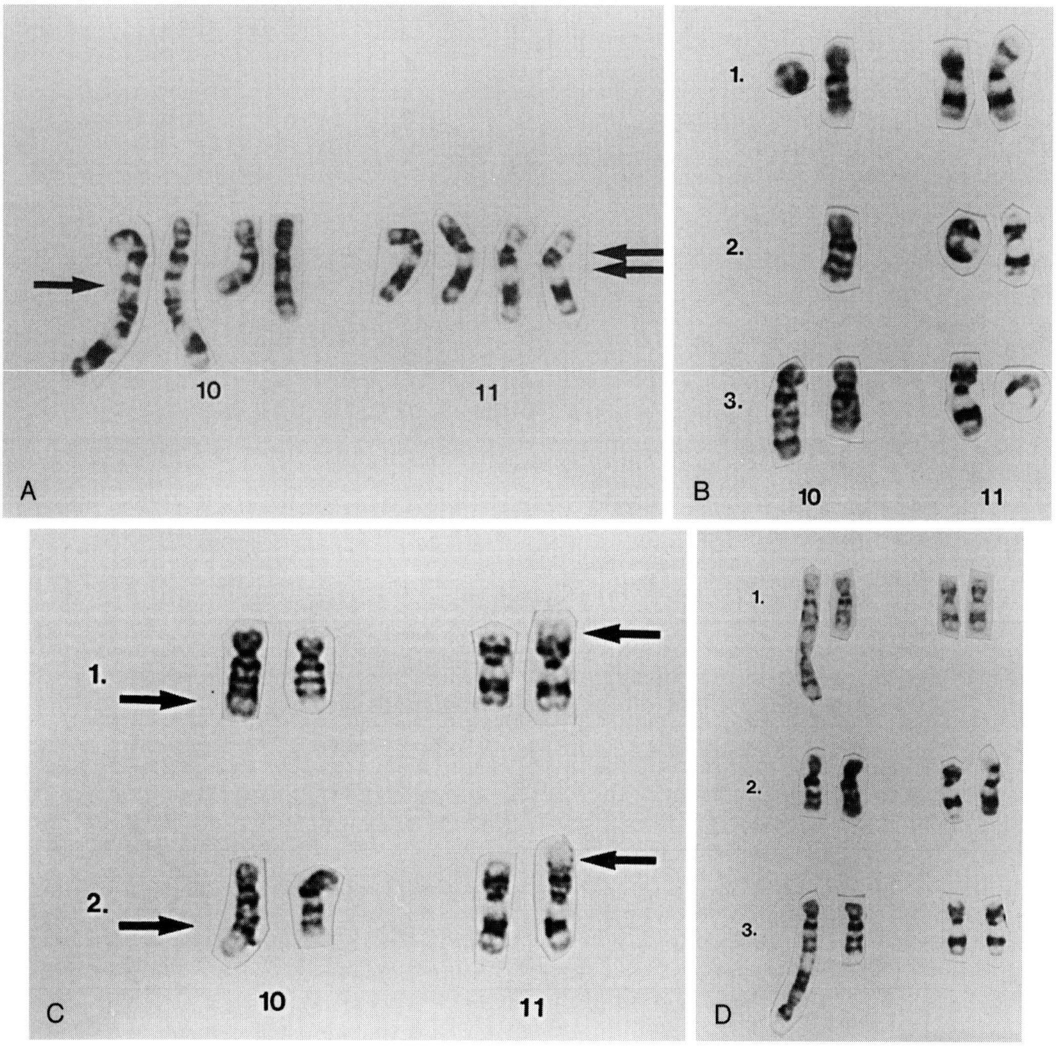

Figure 4–6. Partial karyotypes of different cells from a giant cell tumor of the distal radius of a 34-year-old male. *A*, Tetraploid cell showing the following: t(10;11)(q25;p15)x2,inv(11)(p13q11)x2. *B*, Three different metaphase cells showing the following: (1) r(10)(p15q26); (2) -10,r(11(p15q25); and (3) add(10)(q26), r(11)(p15q13). *C*, Two separate metaphase cells showing the following: add(10)(q26),add(11)(p15). *D*, three different metaphase cells showing the following: (1) tas(8;10)(p23;q26); (2) dic (11;19)(p11;q13); and (3) tas(5;10)(q35;q26). (From Bridge JA, Neff JR, Mouron BJ: Giant cell tumor of bone: Chromosomal analysis of 48 specimens and review of the literature. Cancer Genet Cytogenet 58:2, 1992.)

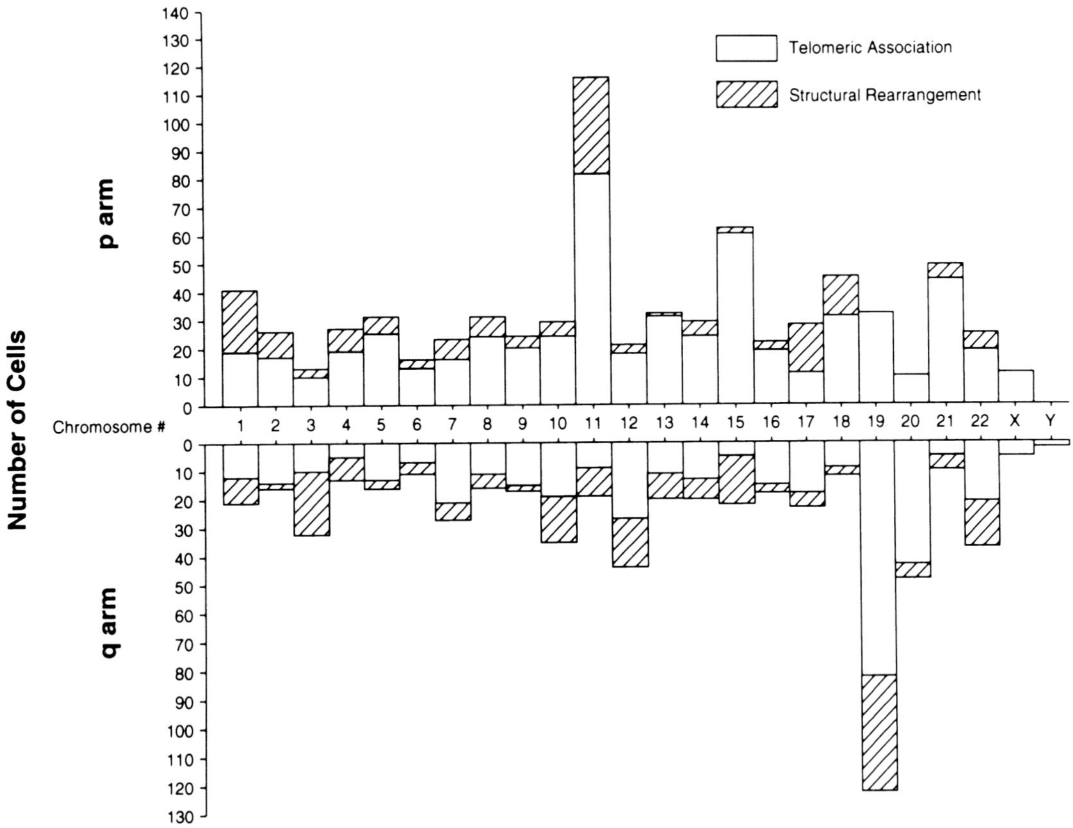

Figure 4–7. Chromosomal short- and long-arm telomeric involvement in giant cell tumor of bone. (From Sandberg AA, Bridge JA: The Cytogenetics of Bone and Soft Tissue Tumors. Austin, RG Landes Co, 1994.)

The biologic behavior of giant cell tumor of bone is unpredictable. Histologic and radiographic grading and staging systems have been developed[39–41] but have proved to be of limited prognostic value (see Chapter 15). Preliminary studies indicate that karyotypic findings may serve as a predictor of clinical behavior. The presence of chromosomal abnormalities appears to be associated with more aggressive behavior. Analysis of 48 specimens of giant cell tumor of bone revealed chromosomal anomalies in all primary lesions in which a recurrence subsequently occurred and in all recurrent lesions.[36] Moreover, the most complex clonal abnormalities were detected in a giant cell tumor of the sacrum that showed malignant transformation.[42] Additional studies must be performed to determine whether chromosomal analysis is a prognostic parameter for giant cell tumor of bone independent of factors such as location and the surgical procedure employed.

Osteosarcoma

Osteosarcoma, the most common primary malignancy of bone, is not a single disease entity (see Chapter 9). Approximately 75% of osteosarcomas arise in the intramedullary cavity and are referred to as *conventional* or *classic* osteosarcoma.[43] Classic osteosarcoma can be further subdivided according to the microscopic appearance of the predominant matrix (osteoblastic, chondroblastic, fibroblastic, telangiectatic, and giant cell rich). Other less common subsets of osteosarcoma include secondary, multifocal, parosteal, and high-grade surface osteosarcoma.

To date, nearly 70 cases of osteosarcoma have been cytogenetically evaluated.[2, 32, 44–49] Most osteosarcomas are characterized by complex karyotypes with multiple numerical and structural abnormalities (Fig. 4–8). Many of the abnormal chromosomes are unidentifiable with standard G-banding (marker chromo-

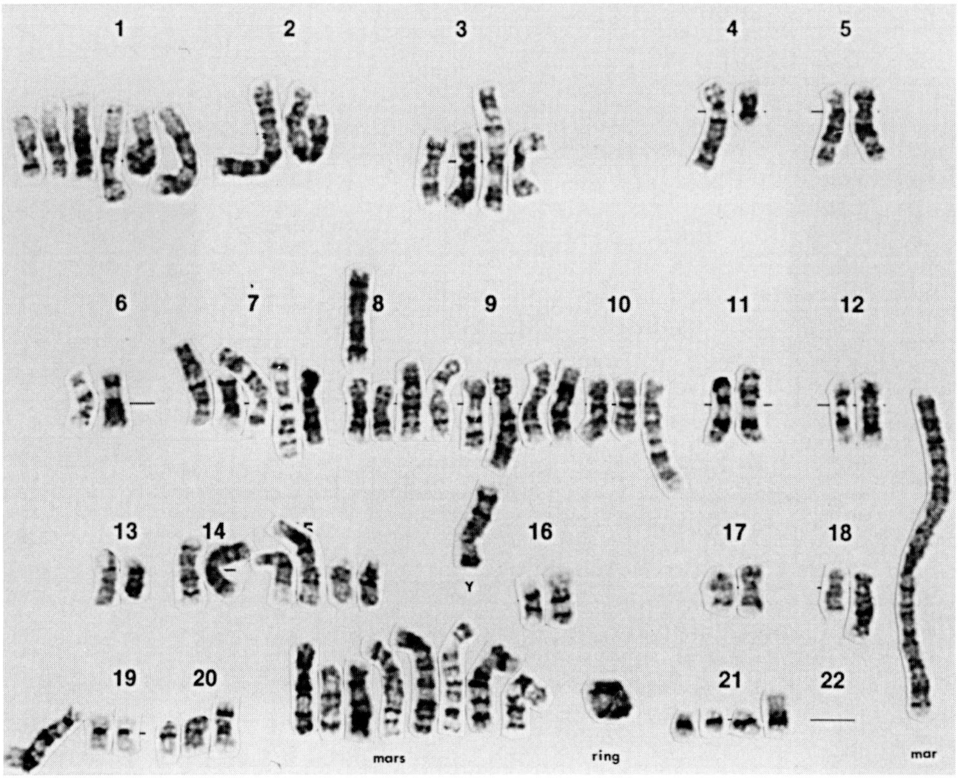

Figure 4–8. Complex karyotype in an osteosarcoma. Multiple numerical aberrations are seen most frequently in this tumor as extra copies of individual chromosomes. The modal number of chromosomes is 71, in contrast to the normal number of 46. Multiple structural abnormalities are also present and include deletions, translocations, unidentifiable chromosomes (so-called marker chromosomes, at the bottom of the karyotype), and a ring chromosome. (From Bridge JA: Cytogenetics and molecular cytogenetic techniques in orthopaedic surgery. Current Concepts Review. J Bone Joint Surg 75A:606, 1993.)

somes) and the modal chromosome number is wide, often in the triploid range. Furthermore, pronounced cell-to-cell variation or heterogeneity is common. All of these factors contribute to the challenge of producing an accurate or complete karyotypic description.

Although a recurrent or tumor-specific chromosomal translocation has not yet emerged for *conventional osteosarcoma,* certain chromosomal regions appear to be repeatedly involved in structural rearrangements (at least six cases each) and include the following: 1q11, 1q21, 3p11, 9p11, 9q34, 12p13, 14p11, 15p11, and 17p12. Additionally, several whole chromosomes or chromosomal regions appear to be lost or deleted nonrandomly. Fletcher et al.[49] described the following nonrandom chromosome losses or deletions in 10 or more high-grade osteosarcomas from a series of 15 patients: 6q21-qter, 9p21-pter, 10, 13, 17p12-pter, and 20. These findings are similar to those published by other investigators. Interestingly, two of the most thoroughly studied chromosomal regions of deletion in osteosarcoma include 13q14 and 17p13, the loci of the tumor suppressor genes RB and TP53, respectively.[50–53]

The development of retinoblastoma is thought to be the result of a loss of function of the RB gene and follows the two-hit kinetic model proposed by Knudson[54] (Fig. 4–9). Several authors have demonstrated that the mutational profiles of the RB gene in osteosarcoma are basically the same as for retinoblastoma, and that mutation of the RB gene plays an essential role in the development of osteosarcoma.[55, 56] These studies apply to sporadic osteosarcomas, as well as to osteosarcomas that have arisen in patients with retinoblastoma.

Deletion or functional inactivation of the p53 gene is a frequent event in sporadic high-grade osteosarcomas. Additionally, p53 germline mutations are seen in a rare familial cancer syndrome in which osteosarcomas are

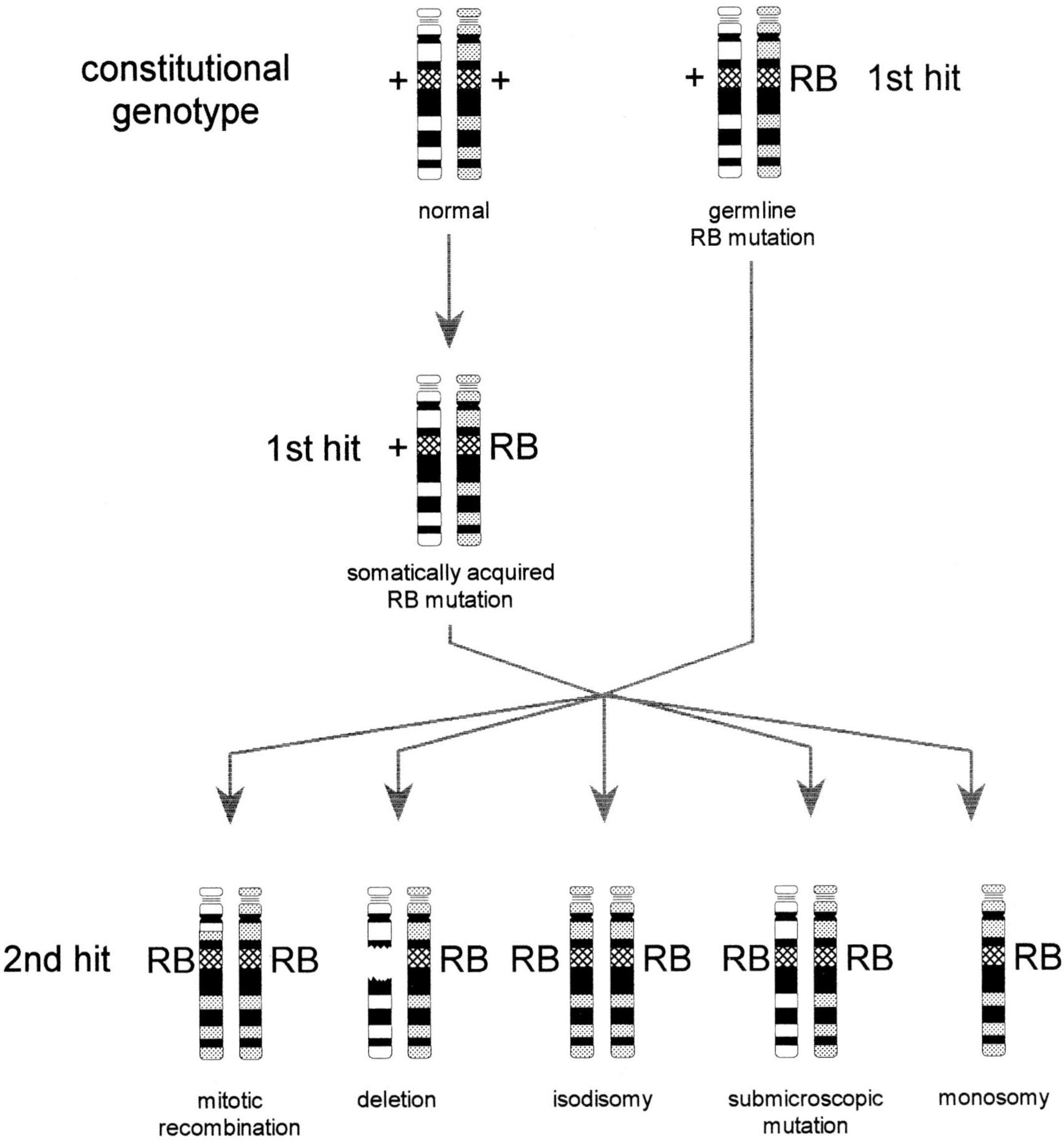

Figure 4–9. Schematic presentation of the two-hit theory proposed by Knudson.[54] In this figure, the gene for retinoblastoma (*RB*) has been used as an example, though a similar mechanism may apply to other tumor types. In the upper left corner are shown two normal homologues of chromosome 13 (as would be expected in a normal individual) and to the right of these, another pair of homologues but with a germline mutation of the *RB* gene at 13q14 (as would be expected in an individual with the inherited form of retinoblastoma: constitutional anomaly). Tumor development (retinoblastoma or osteosarcoma) is not possible until there is loss of both copies of the suppressor gene (+). For individuals with the hereditary form of retinoblastoma, the first mutation is carried in the germline and requires only "one somatic hit" (mutation) for loss of tumor suppression. Normal individuals require "two somatic hits." At the bottom of the figure are examples of the different mechanisms by which loss of tumor suppression may occur.

frequent (Li-Fraumeni syndrome)[57] and also in a subgroup of young patients with osteosarcoma whose family histories are not indicative of the Li-Fraumeni syndrome.[58] Deactivation of the p53 gene has been shown to contribute to genetic instability in several experimental models and may be relevant with respect to the complex cytogenetic heterogeneity observed in osteosarcoma.[49]

Data obtained by molecular cytogenetic techniques has also contributed valuable information regarding the genetic abnormalities in osteosarcoma. Comparative genomic hybridization (CGH) studies have shown amplification of 1q21-23, 3q26, 6p, 8q23-qter, 12q12-13, 17p11-12, and Xq12, and loss of DNA sequences from 2q, 6q, 8p, and 10p as most prominent.[59, 60] Note that losses of 13q or 17p were not recognized as frequent anomalies with this form of analysis. Instead, amplification of 17p11-12, a region not known to harbor any known genes or oncogenes, has been encountered unexpectedly. Forus et al.[59] suggest that loss of heterozygosity at 17p13 and amplification of the 17p11-12 region are independent events in the development of osteosarcoma.

The cytogenetic findings in *parosteal osteosarcoma* differ from other types of osteosarcoma and provide a unique marker for distinguishing this clinicohistopathologic subtype.[61, 62] Parosteal osteosarcoma is characterized cytogenetically by the presence of a supernumerary unidentified ring chromosome, often as the sole karyotypic anomaly (Fig. 4–10). Prognostically, patients with parosteal osteosarcoma fare significantly better than patients with other forms of osteosarcoma. The observation of a ring chromosome in this neoplasm is of interest because other low-grade malignant mesenchymal neoplasms (well-differentiated liposarcoma, dermatofibrosarcoma protuberans, and myxoid malignant fibrous histiocytoma) are also characterized by ring chromosomes.[2] Hence, the observation of a ring chromosome as the sole abnormality in an osteosarcoma may not only be of diagnostic utility but may also serve as an important prognostic indicator of a neoplasm of low-grade malignant potential.

Chondrosarcoma

Chondrosarcoma is second only to osteosarcoma in frequency as a primary malignancy of bone. The histologic diagnosis and classification of chondrosarcoma presents one of the greatest challenges for the surgical pathologist (see Chapter 10). Microscopic features are evaluated subjectively to distinguish between benign and malignant tumors and to grade the latter, with potential sampling problems and site-specific criteria for malignancy.[63–67]

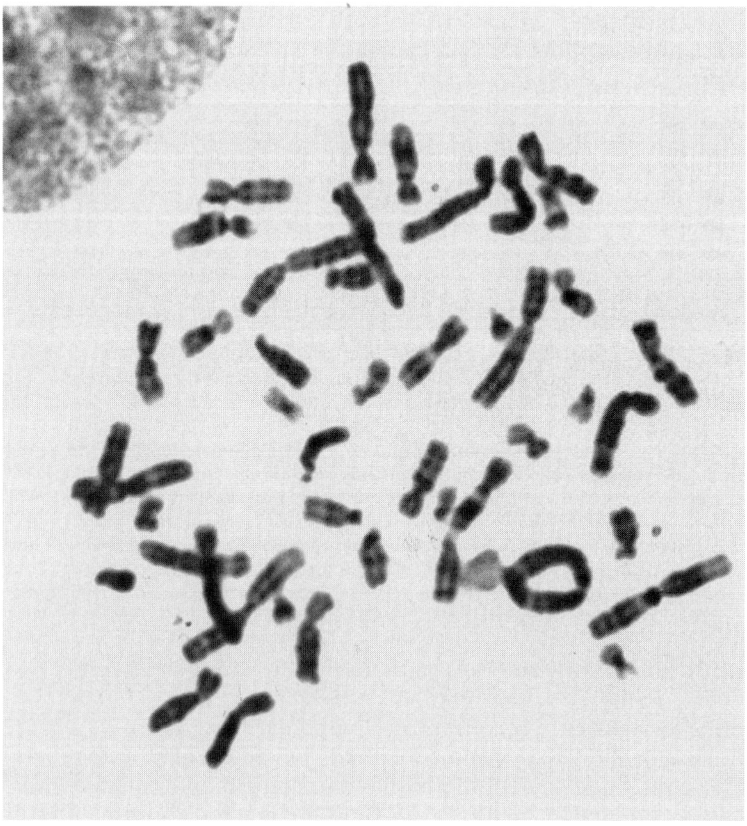

Figure 4–10. Ring chromosome in a parosteal osteosarcoma. The presence of a ring chromosome as the sole anomaly is characteristic of this clinicohistopathologic subtype. (From Orndal C, Mandahl N, Rydholm A, et al: Supernumerary ring chromosomes in five bone and soft tissue tumors of low or borderline malignancy. Cancer Genet Cytogenet 60:170, 1992.)

Cytogenetic studies of chondrosarcoma are relatively few but have shown that certain chromosomal anomalies are recurrent in chondrosarcoma and that these abnormalities can be useful diagnostically and possibly prognostically.[2, 23, 48, 68, 69]

Overall, structural aberrations of chromosomes 1, 12, and 15 and numerical anomalies of chromosomes 5, 7, 8, and 18 appear to be most frequent in classic chondrosarcoma.[68] The anomalies involving chromosome 12 are commonly at the 12q13-15 breakpoint region. This region is also frequently altered cytogenetically in other mesenchymal neoplasms including lipoma, myxoid liposarcoma and clear cell sarcoma. Recently, the genes located on the long arm of chromosome 12 (12q13-15), which are involved in lipoma, myxoid liposarcoma, and clear cell sarcoma, have been defined and include HMGI-C, CHOP, and ATF-1, respectively.[70, 71] Although it has not been determined what gene or genes may be altered at 12q13-15 in cartilaginous lesions, it is of interest that the major component of normal cartilage, type II collagen, has been localized to this same chromosomal region.[72]

Abnormalities that may be useful in distinguishing benign from malignant chondromatous tumors include the observation of primarily structural abnormalities of chromosome 8 in benign tumors and numerical anomalies of chromosome 8 in malignant tumors. Also, abnormalities of chromosomes 1 and 7 have been detected almost exclusively in malignant cartilaginous neoplasms (Fig. 4–11).

Of further diagnostic importance is the observation of a recurrent translocation, t(9;22)(q22-31;q12), in a specific histologic subtype of chondrosarcoma, myxoid chondrosarcoma (Fig. 4–12).[73–76] Myxoid chondrosarcoma may arise as a primary skeletal lesion or as an extraskeletal lesion, often in the deep

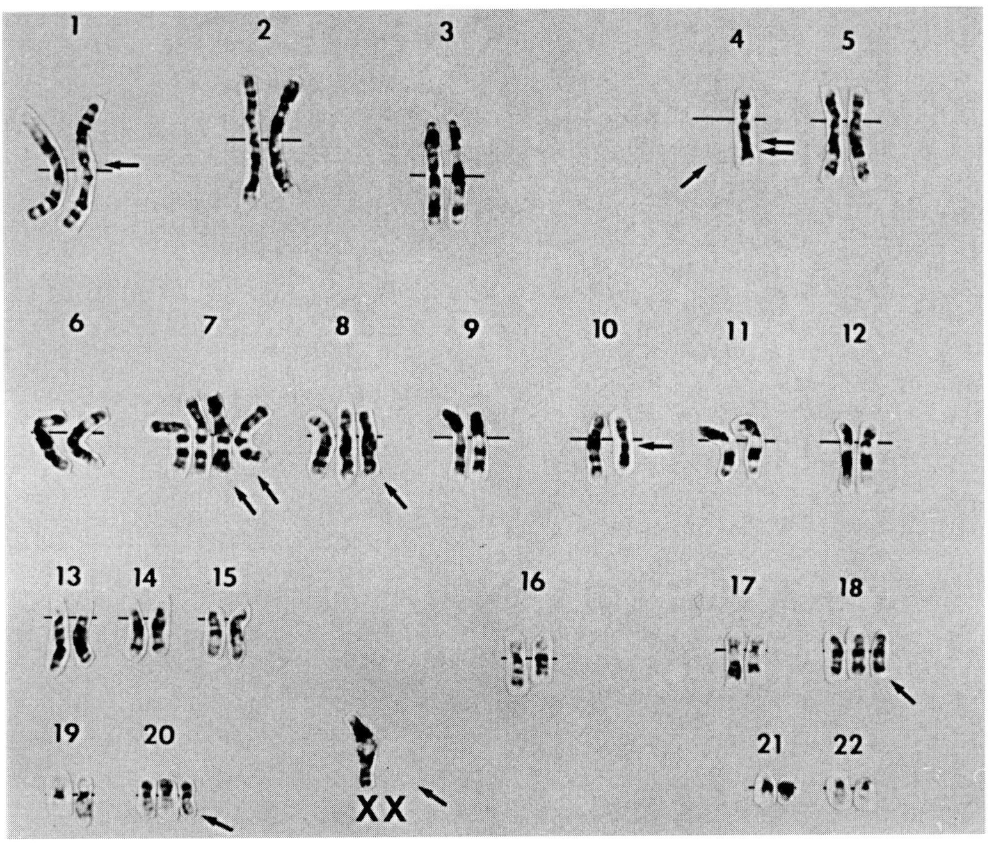

Figure 4–11. Abnormalities of chromosomes 1 and 7 in a Grade III chondrosarcoma. Anomalies involving other chromosomes are also seen in this tumor, characterized by the following abnormal complement: 50,X,-X,i(1)(q10),del(4)-(q27q31),+7,+7,+8,add(10)(q11),+18,+20. The loss of chromosome 4 was a random abnormality detected in this cell only. (From Mandahl N, Heim S, Arheden K, et al: Chromosomal rearrangements in chondromatous tumors. Cancer 65(2):242, 1990. Copyright 1990, American Cancer Society. Reprinted by permission of Wiley-Liss, Inc., a subsidiary of John Wiley & Sons, Inc.)

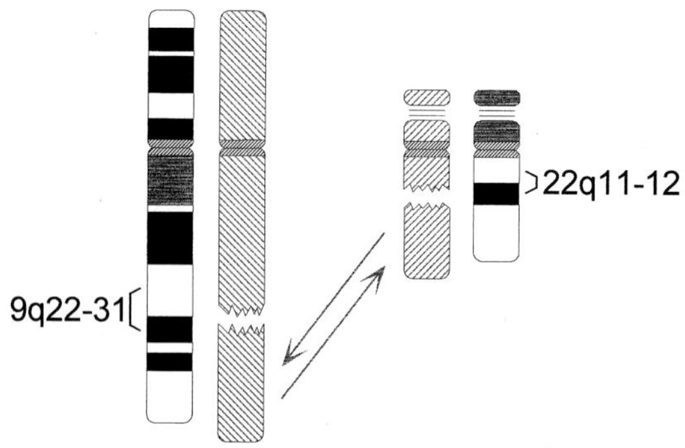

Figure 4–12. Schematic representation of the 9;22 translocation t(9;22)(q22-31;q12) characteristic of myxoid chondrosarcoma.

tissues of the extremities. Fusion of the EWS gene (located on 22q12) to a DNA segment from 9q22-31 has been demonstrated in a skeletal myxoid chondrosarcoma.[77] Involvement of EWS has also been shown to occur in three other types of human sarcoma: Ewing's sarcoma and peripheral PNETs, clear cell sarcoma, and desmoplastic small round cell tumor.[70]

Cytogenetic and molecular cytogenetic evaluation of dedifferentiated chondrosarcoma has provided important histopathogenetic information. Dedifferentiated chondrosarcoma is an aggressive variant that is composed of a low-grade chondrosarcoma with one or more additional malignant mesenchymal elements, such as fibrosarcoma, malignant fibrous histiocytoma, osteosarcoma, and rhabdomyosarcoma. The term *dedifferentiation* implies an ability of the differentiated cell to convert or revert to a primitive, undifferentiated state. The cellular process of dedifferentiation is incompletely understood. A combined approach of interphase cytogenetics and fluorescence immunophenotyping of a dedifferentiated chondrosarcoma with a rhabdomyosarcomatous component revealed that the chondrosarcomatous and rhabdomyosarcomatous elements were derived from the same abnormal clone.[78] These findings support the existence of a common primitive mesenchymal cell progenitor with the ability to differentiate or express features of more than one line of mesenchymal differentiation and indicate that the term "dedifferentiated" may be an inaccurate designation for this neoplasm.

Chordoma

Chordomas represent approximately 1 to 4% of primary malignant bone tumors and occur primarily in the spheno-occipital and sacrococcygeal regions (see Chapter 17).[79] Chondroid chordomas must be distinguished from chondrosarcoma.

To date, fewer than 20 cases of chordoma have been cytogenetically examined,[80–84] however, certain features appear common. Specifically, all but two cases have been hypodiploid or near diploid and all but one have shown an abnormality of chromosome 3. In particular, loss of chromosome 3 is frequent. Both numerical and structural abnormalities of chromosome 21 are also prominent in chordoma. Flow cytometric studies suggest that aneuploidy is more common in chordomas with a malignant spindle cell component than in conventional chordomas.[85] The overall rarity of chordoma and the challenge of successfully culturing the tumor cells may account for the limited number of cytogenetic reports regarding this neoplasm.

Ewing's Sarcoma

Ewing's sarcoma is a malignant neoplasm characterized by uniformly sized, densely packed cells with round nuclei and indistinct cytoplasmic borders (see Chapter 14), which

Table 4–2. Chromosomal Abnormalities in Small Round Cell Tumors

Tumor	Chromosomal Abnormality
Ewing's sarcoma & peripheral PNET	t(11;22)(q24;q12)
Embryonal rhabdomyosarcoma	LOH of 11p*
Alveolar rhabdomyosarcoma	t(2;13)(q37;q14)
Non-Hodgkin's lymphoma	t(14;18)(q32;q21) t(8;14)(q24;q32) +12
Neuroblastoma	del(1)(p31–32) Double minute chromosomes Homogeneously staining regions
Small cell osteosarcoma†	t(11;22)(q24;q12)

PNET, primitive neuroectodermal tumor.

*Loss of heterozygosity for 11p in all informative embryonal rhabdomyosarcomas examined in one study (not reflected cytogenetically) may indicate that this is a primary genetic event in this neoplasm.[86]

†These results are based on a report of only a single case of small cell osteosarcoma.[87]

most commonly arises in bone but can also occur in extraskeletal locations. Ewing's sarcoma belongs to a group of small round cell tumors that also includes PNETs, rhabdomyosarcoma, non-Hodgkin's lymphoma, neuroblastoma, and small cell osteosarcoma. It is often difficult with traditional histologic approaches to classify this group of malignancies because of their similar appearance on light microscopy and their frequent lack of organ specificity. Fortunately, however, separate or distinct chromosomal anomalies have been recognized in most of these tumors (Table 4–2).[86, 87]

Ewing's sarcoma and PNETs differ in their histopathologic criteria (neural differentiation can be demonstrated in PNET) but there is a close histopathogenetic relationship between them as both are characterized cytogenetically by an 11;22 translocation, t(11;22)(q24;q12) (Fig. 4–13),[6] that is present in greater than 90% of lesions evaluated. Some oncologists now use the collective term *Ewing's/PNET* for these neoplasms.[88]

As a consequence of the 11;22 translocation, the 5′ amino terminus of the EWS gene located on chromosome 22 is fused to the 3′ carboxy terminus of the FLI-1 gene on chromosome 11, whereas on chromosome 22, the RNA-binding domain of EWS is replaced by the DNA-binding domain of FLI-1.[89] It is thought that the EWS/FLI-1 fusion contributes to the transformed phenotype of Ewing's sarcoma cells by inducing the deregulated activation of genes, or the unscheduled activation of genes, or both, that are normally responsive to FLI-1 or other members of the ETS family.[3] In addition to the EWS/FLI-1 fusion that occurs with the classic 11;22 translocation, the EWS gene can be fused to ERG, a transcription factor in the same ETS gene family as FLI-1, located on chromosomal breakpoint 21q22.[90] This variant translocation is as follows: t(21;22)(q22;q12).[91] Thus, fusion of EWS to different members of the ETS family may result in the expression of similar disease phenotypes, and oncogenic conversion is achieved by the linking of the two domains with no marked constraint on the connecting peptide (see Chapter 5 for more details).

The 11;22 translocation characteristic of Ewing's sarcoma and peripheral PNETs can be detected by traditional cytogenetic techniques, reverse transcriptase–polymerase chain reaction (RT-PCR) methodologies, and FISH (see Chapter 14, Figures 14–8 and 14–9). FISH can be performed by utilizing cosmids from loci flanking or overlapping the 7-kilobase region called EWSR1 on chromosome 22 and the 40- to 50-kilobase region called EWSR2 on chromosome 11, which allows localization of the two breakpoints of the t(11;22)(q24;q12) within a 10-kilobase resolution.[92] With either the RT-PCR or the FISH approach, cryptic or masked translocations may be seen, thereby increasing the level of sensitivity of detection.

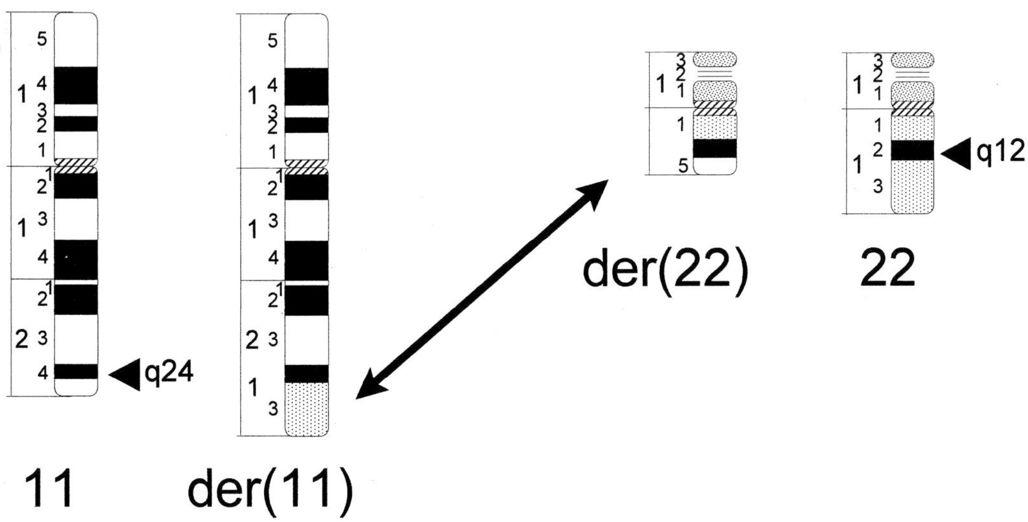

Figure 4–13. The (11;22)(q24;q12) translocation characteristic of Ewing's sarcoma and peripheral primitive neuroectodermal tumor.

REFERENCES

1. Bridge JA: Cytogenetics and molecular cytogenetic techniques in orthopaedic surgery. Current Concepts Review. J Bone Joint Surg 75A:606, 1993.
2. Sandberg AA, Bridge JA: The Cytogenetics of Bone and Soft Tissue Tumors. Austin, RG Landes Co, 1994.
3. Bridge JA: Cytogenetics and experimental models of sarcomas. Curr Opin Oncol 7:333, 1995.
4. Ludecke HJ, Johnson C, Wagner MJ, et al: Molecular definition of the shortest region of deletion overlap in the Langer-Giedion syndrome. Am J Hum Genet 49:1197, 1991.
5. Ahn J, Ludecke HJ, Lindow S, et al: Cloning of the putative tumour suppressor gene for hereditary multiple exostoses (EXT1). Nature Genet 11:137, 1995.
6. Stephenson CF, Bridge JA, Sandberg AA: Cytogenetic and pathologic aspects of Ewing's sarcoma and neuroectodermal tumors. Hum Pathol 23:1270, 1992.
7. Akerman M, Alvegard T, Eliasson J, et al: A case of Ewing's sarcoma diagnosed by fine needle aspiration. Acta Orthop Scand 59:589, 1988.
8. Fletcher JA, Kozakewich HP, Hoffer FA, et al: Diagnostic relevance of clonal cytogenetic aberrations in malignant soft-tissue tumors. N Engl J Med 324:436, 1991.
9. Pandis N, Bardi G, Heim S: Interrelationship between methodological choices and conceptual models in solid tumor cytogenetics. Cancer Genet Cytogenet 76:77, 1994.
10. Orndal C, Rydholm A, Willen H, et al: Cytogenetic intratumor heterogeneity in soft tissue tumors. Cancer Genet Cytogenet 78:127, 1994.
11. Limon J, Dal Cin P, Sandberg AA: Application of long-term collagenase disaggregation for the cytogenetic analysis of human solid tumors. Cancer Genet Cytogenet 23:305, 1986.
12. Mandahl N: Methods in solid tumor cytogenetics. *In* Rooney DE, Czepulkowski BH (eds): Human Cytogenetics: A Practical Approach. Vol 2: Malignancy and Acquired Chromosome Abnormalities. Oxford, IRL Press, 1992, p 155.
13. Sandberg AA, Bridge JA: Techniques in cancer cytogenetics: An overview and update. Cancer Invest 10:163, 1992.
14. ISCN (Mitelman F, ed): An International System for Human Nomenclature. Basel, S. Karger, 1995.
15. Anastasi J: Interphase cytogenetic analysis in the diagnosis and study of neoplastic disorders. Am J Clin Pathol 95:22, 1991.
16. Weber-Matthiesen K, Deerberg J, Muller-Hermelink A, et al: Rationalization of in situ hybridization: Testing up to 16 different probes on a single slide. Cancer Genet Cytogenet 68:91, 1993.
17. Ried T, Baldini A, Rand TC, et al: Simultaneous visualization of seven different DNA probes by in situ hybridization using combinatorial fluorescence and digital imaging microscopy. Proc Natl Acad Sci 89:1388, 1992.
18. Xiao S, Renshaw A, Cibas ES, et al: Novel fluorescence in situ hybridization approaches in solid tumors. Characterization of frozen specimens, touch preparations and cytological preparations. Am J Pathol 147:896, 1995.
19. du Manoir S, Speicher MR, Joos S, et al: Detection of complete and partial chromosome gains and losses by comparative genomic in situ hybridization. Hum Genet 90:590, 1993.
20. Kallioniemi O-P, Kallioniemi A, Piper I, et al: Optimizing comparative genomic hybridization for analysis of DNA sequence copy number changes in solid tumors. Genes Chromosomes Cancer 10:231, 1994.
21. Houldsworth J, Chaganti RSK: Comparative genomic hybridization. An overview. Am J Pathol 145:1253, 1994.
22. Cook A, Raskind W, Blanton SH, et al: Genetic heterogeneity in families with hereditary multiple exostoses. Am J Hum Genet 53:71, 1993.
23. Bridge JA, Bhatia PS, Anderson JR, et al: Biologic and clinical significance of cytogenetic and molecular cytogenetic abnormalities in benign and malignant cartilaginous lesions. Cancer Genet Cytogenet 69:79, 1993.
24. Mertens F, Rydholm A, Kreicbergs A, et al: Loss of chromosome band 8q24 in sporadic osteocartilaginous exostoses. Genes Chromosomes Cancer 9:8, 1994.
25. Hecht JT, Hogue D, Strong LC, et al: Hereditary multiple exostosis and chondrosarcoma: Linkage to chromosome 11 and loss of heterozygosity for EXT-linked markers on chromosomes 11 and 8. Am J Hum Genet 56:1125, 1995.
26. Raskind WH, Conrad EU, Chansky H, et al: Loss of heterozygosity in chondrosarcomas for hereditary multiple exostoses-linked markers on chromosomes 8 and 11. Am J Hum Genet 56:1132, 1995.
27. Springfield DS, Rosenberg AE, Mankin HJ, et al: Relationship between osteofibrous dysplasia and adamantinoma. Clin Orthop 309:234, 1994.
28. Bridge JA, Dembinski A, DeBoer J, et al: Clonal chromosomal abnormalities in osteofibrous dysplasia of the tibia: Implications for histopathogenesis and its relationship with adamantinoma. Cancer 73:1746, 1994.
29. Sozzi G, Miozzo M, DePalma S, et al: Involvement of the region 13q14 in a patient with adamantinoma of the long bones. Hum Genet 85:513, 1990.
30. Mills SE, Fechner RE: The nose, paranasal sinuses and nasopharynx. *In* Sternberg SS (ed): Diagnostic Surgical Pathology. New York, Raven Press, 1994, p 851.
31. Bridge JA, Rosenthal H, Sanger WG, et al: Desmoplastic fibroma arising in fibrous dysplasia. Chromosomal analysis and review of the literature. Clin Orthop 247:272, 1989.
32. Tarkkanen M, Kaipainen A, Karaharju E, et al: Cytogenetic study of 249 consecutive patients examined for a bone tumor. Cancer Genet Cytogenet 68:1, 1993.
33. Dal Cin P, Sciot R, Speleman F, et al: Chromosome aberrations in fibrous dysplasia. Cancer Genet Cytogenet 77:114, 1994.
34. Sawyer JR, Tryka AF, Bell JM, et al: Nonrandom chromosome breakpoints at Xq26 and 2q33 characterize cemento-ossifying fibromas of the orbit. Cancer 76:1853, 1995.
35. Dal Cin P, Sciot R, Fossion E, et al: Chromosome abnormalities in cementifying fibroma. Cancer Genet Cytogenet 71:170, 1993.
36. Bridge JA, Neff JR, Mouron BJ: Giant cell tumor of bone: Chromosomal analysis of 48 specimens and review of the literature. Cancer Genet Cytogenet 58:2, 1992.
37. Schwartz HS, Dahir GA, Butler MG: Telomere reduction in giant cell tumor of bone and with aging. Cancer Genet Cytogenet 71:132, 1993.
38. McComb E, Johansson S, Neff JR, et al: Chromosomal

anomalies exclusive of telomeric associations in giant cell tumor of bone. Cancer Genet Cytogenet 81:1, 1996.
39. Jaffe HL, Lichtenstein L, Portis RB: Giant cell tumor of bone: Its pathologic appearance, grading, supposed variants, and treatment. Arch Pathol 30:993, 1940.
40. Campanacci M, Giunti A, Olmi R: Giant cell tumors of bone: A study of 209 cases with long-term follow-up in 130. Ital J Orthop Traumatol 1:249, 1975.
41. Present D, Bertoni F, Hudson T, et al: The correlation between the radiologic staging studies and histopathologic findings in aggressive stage 3 giant cell tumor of bone. Cancer 57:237, 1986.
42. Bridge JA, Mouron BJ, Neff JR, et al: Significance of chromosomal abnormalities in a malignant giant cell tumor of bone. Cancer Genet Cytogenet 57:87, 1991.
43. Dahlin DC, Coventry MB: Osteogenic sarcoma. A study of 600 cases. J Bone Joint Surg 49A:101, 1967.
44. Mitelman F: Catalog of Chromosome Aberrations in Cancer. 5th ed. New York, Wiley-Liss, 1994.
45. Biegel JA, Womer RB, Emanuel BS: Complex karyotypes in a series of pediatric osteosarcomas. Cancer Genet Cytogenet 38:89, 1989.
46. Mertens F, Mandahl N, Orndal C, et al: Cytogenetic findings in 33 osteosarcomas. Int J Cancer 55:44, 1993.
47. Hoogerwerf WA, Hawkins AL, Perlman EJ, et al: Chromosome analysis of nine osteosarcomas. Genes Chromosomes Cancer 9:88, 1994.
48. Ozisik YY, Meloni AM, Peier AP, et al: Cytogenetic findings in 19 malignant bone tumors. Cancer 74:2268, 1994.
49. Fletcher JA, Gebhart MC, Kozakewich HP: Cytogenetic aberrations in osteosarcomas: Nonrandom deletions, rings and double-minute chromosomes. Cancer Genet Cytogenet 77:81, 1994.
50. Toguchida J, Ishizaki K, Sasaki MS, et al: Chromosomal reorganization for the expression of recessive mutation of retinoblastoma susceptibility gene in the development of osteosarcoma. Cancer Res 48:3939, 1988.
51. Scheffer H, Kruize YCM, Osinga H, et al: Complete association of loss of heterozygosity of chromosomes 13 and 17 in osteosarcoma. Cancer Genet Cytogenet 53:45, 1991.
52. Toguchida H, Yamaguchi T, Ritchie B, et al: Mutation spectrum of the p53 gene in bone and soft tissue sarcomas. Cancer Res 52:6194, 1992.
53. Yamaguchi T, Toguchida J, Yamamuro T, et al: Allelotype analysis in osteosarcomas: Frequent allele loss on 3q, 13q, 17p, and 18q. Cancer Res 52:2419, 1992.
54. Knudson AG: Mutation and cancer: Statistical study of retinoblastoma. Proc Natl Acad Sci 68:820, 1971.
55. Friend SH, Bernards R, Rogelj S, et al: A human DNA segment with properties of the gene that predisposes to retinoblastoma and osteosarcoma. Nature 323:643, 1986.
56. Scholz RB, Kabisch H, Weber B, et al: Studies of the RB1 gene and the p53 gene in human osteosarcomas. Pediat Hematol Oncol 9:125, 1992.
57. Malkin D, Li FP, Strong LC, et al: Germline p53 mutations in a familial syndrome of breast cancer, sarcoma, and other neoplasms. Science 250:1233, 1990.
58. Toguchida J, Yamaguchi T, Dayton SH, et al: Prevalence and spectrum of germline mutations for the p53 gene among patients with sarcoma. N Engl J Med 326:1301, 1992.
59. Forus A, Olde Weghuis D, Smeets D, et al: Comparative genomic hybridization analysis of human sarcomas: II. Identification of novel amplicons at 6p and 17p in osteosarcomas. Genes Chromosomes Cancer 14:15, 1995.
60. Tarkkanen M, Karhu R, Kallioniemi A, et al: Gains and loss of DNA sequences in osteosarcomas by comparative genomic hybridization. Cancer Res 55:1334, 1995.
61. Sinovic JF, Bridge JA, Neff JR: Ring chromosomes in parosteal osteosarcoma. Clinical and diagnostic significance. Cancer Genet Cytogenet 62:50, 1992.
62. Orndal C, Mandahl N, Rydholm A, et al: Supernumerary ring chromosomes in five bone and soft tissue tumors of low or borderline malignancy. Cancer Genet Cytogenet 60:170, 1992.
63. Mirra JM, Gold R, Downs J, et al: A new histologic approach to the differentiation of enchondroma from chondrosarcoma of the bones. A clinicopathologic analysis of 51 cases. Clin Orthop 201:214, 1985.
64. Evans HL, Ayala AG, Romsdahl MM: Prognostic factors in chondrosarcoma of bone. A clinicopathologic analysis with emphasis on histologic grading. Cancer 40:818, 1977.
65. Meachim G: Histological grading of chondrosarcomata. J Bone Joint Surg 61B:393, 1979.
66. Marcove RC, Mik JV, Hutter RVP, et al: Chondrosarcoma of the pelvis and upper end of the femur. An analysis of factors influencing survival time in 113 cases. J Bone Joint Surg 54A:561, 1972.
67. Dahlin DC, Unni KK: Chondrosarcoma. *In* Dahlin DC, Unni KK (eds): Bone Tumors. 4th ed. Springfield, Charles C Thomas, 1986, p 33.
68. Mandahl N, Heim S, Arheden K, et al: Chromosomal rearrangements in chondromatous tumors. Cancer 65:242, 1990.
69. Dijkhuizen T, van den Berg E, Molenaar WM, et al: Cytogenetics as a tool in the histologic subclassification of chondrosarcomas. Cancer Genet Cytogenet 76:100, 1994.
70. Bridge JA: Soft tissue sarcomas. *In* Wolman S, Sell S (eds): Cytogenetic Markers of Human Disease. Clifton, NJ, Humana Press, Inc., 1997, p 425.
71. Ashar HR, Schoenberg Fejzo M, Tkachenko A, et al: Disruption of the architectural factor HMGI-C: DNA-binding AT hook motifs fused in lipomas to distinct transcriptional regulatory domains. Cell 82:57, 1995.
72. Takahashi E, Hori T, O'Connell P, et al: R-banding and non-isotopic in-situ hybridization: Precise localization of the human type II collagen gene (COLqA1). Hum Genet 86:14, 1990.
73. Hinrichs SH, Jaramillo MA, Gumerlock PH, et al: Myxoid chondrosarcoma with a translocation involving chromosomes 9 and 22. Cancer Genet Cytogenet 14:219, 1985.
74. Turc-Carel C, Dal Cin P, Rao U, et al: Recurrent breakpoints at 9q31 and 22q12.2 in extraskeletal myxoid chondrosarcoma. Cancer Genet Cytogenet 30:145, 1986.
75. Orndal C, Carlen B, Akerman M, et al: Chromosomal abnormality t(9;22)(q22;q12) in an extraskeletal myxoid chondrosarcoma characterized by fine needle aspiration cytology, electron microscopy, immunohistochemistry and DNA flow cytometry. Cytopathology 2:261, 1991.
76. Sciot R, Dal Cin P, Fletcher C, et al: t(9;22)(q22-31;q11-12) is a consistent marker of extraskeletal myxoid chondrosarcoma: Evaluation of three cases. Mod Pathol 8:765, 1995.

77. Gill S, McManus AP, Crew AJ, et al: Fusion of the EWS gene to a DNA segment from 9q22-31 in a human myxoid chondrosarcoma. Genes Chromosomes Cancer 12:307, 1995.
78. Bridge JA, DeBoer J, Travis J, et al: Simultaneous interphase cytogenetic analysis and fluorescence immunophenotyping of dedifferentiated chondrosarcoma: Implications for histopathogenesis. Am J Pathol 144:215, 1994.
79. Rich TA, Schiller A, Suit HD, et al: Clinical and pathologic review of 48 cases of chordoma. Cancer 56:182, 1984.
80. Persons DL, Bridge JA, Neff JR: Cytogenetic analysis of two sacral chordomas. Cancer Genet Cytogenet 56:197, 1991.
81. Gibas Z, Miettinen M, Sandberg AA: Chromosomal abnormalities in two chordomas. Cancer Genet Cytogenet 58:169, 1992.
82. DeBoer JM, Neff JR, Bridge JA: Cytogenetics of sacral chordoma. Cancer Genet Cytogenet 64:95, 1992.
83. Mertens F, Kreicbergs A, Rydholm A, et al: Clonal chromosome aberrations in three sacral chordomas. Cancer Genet Cytogenet 73:147, 1994.
84. Bridge JA, Pickering D, Neff JR: Cytogenetic and molecular cytogenetic analysis of sacral chordoma. Cancer Genet Cytogenet 75:23, 1994.
85. Hruban RH, Traganos F, Reuter VE, et al: Chordomas with spindle cell components. A DNA flow cytometric and immunohistochemical study with histogenetic implications. Am J Surg Pathol 137:435, 1990.
86. Whang-Peng J, Knutsen T, Theil K, et al: Cytogenetic studies in subgroups of rhabdomyosarcoma. Genes Chromosomes Cancer 5:299, 1992.
87. Noguera R, Navarro S, Triche T: Translocation (11;22) in small cell osteosarcoma. Cancer Genet Cytogenet 45:121, 1990.
88. Kretschmar CS: Ewing's sarcoma and the "peanut" tumors. N Engl J Med 331:325, 1994.
89. Zucman J, Delattre O, Desmaze C, et al: Cloning and characterization of the Ewing's sarcoma and peripheral neuroepithelioma t(11;22) translocation breakpoints. Genes Chromosomes Cancer 5:271, 1992.
90. Zucman J, Melot T, Desmaze C, et al: Combinatorial generation of variable fusion proteins in the Ewing family of tumors. EMBO J 12:4481, 1993.
91. Sorensen PHB, Lessnick SL, Lopez-Terrada D, et al: A second Ewing's sarcoma translocation, t(21;22), fuses the EWS gene to another ETS-family transcription factor, ERG. Nature Genet 6:146, 1994.
92. Desmaze C, Zucman J, Delattre O, et al: Interphase molecular cytogenetics of Ewing's sarcoma and peripheral neuroepithelioma t(11;22) with flanking and overlapping cosmid probes. Cancer Genet Cytogenet 74:13, 1994.

Chapter

5

MOLECULAR MARKERS IN THE EVALUATION OF BONE NEOPLASMS

R.B. Scholz, H. Christiansen, H. Kabisch, and K. Winkler

Molecular markers indicating mutational events involved in cancerogenesis not only provide valuable information for improving our basic understanding of cancer but are emerging as highly specific diagnostic tools and important prognostic indicators, and will provide key information for designing novel therapeutic modalities. This chapter focuses on the diagnostic and prognostic aspects of genetic markers and comments on some markers that, despite tumor nonspecificity, are highly characteristic and are helpful for clarifying the histogenesis and differential diagnosis of some tumors (Table 5–1).

GENETIC EVENTS IN CANCEROGENESIS

There has been a recent explosion in cancer research accompanying the dramatic advances in cellular and molecular biology. In the past 20 years, many genes that play a key role in the initiation and progression of cancer have been identified, particularly oncogenes, tumor suppressor genes, and, most recently, repair genes.

Oncogenes were first detected as passengers in the genomes of retroviruses.[1] Molecular analysis of these genetic loci revealed that they were not viral genes but cellular genes (proto-oncogenes) processed and taken up into the viral genomes where they confer the host virus with oncogenic potential.[2] Nonphysiologic activation of cellular proto-oncogenes converts them into oncogenes, which are involved in malignant transformation. They may be activated by dominant mutations that stimulate them to produce an oncogenic protein. Such gain of function mutations may result from amplification (*myc, neu, MDM2*, and *SAS*),[3–6] chromosome translocation (*BCR-ABL, FLI-ETS*, Ig-*myc*),[7–9] or from point mutation (*ras, src*), which then destroys the regulation of the proteins (*ras*) and enhances their activity.[1]

In contrast to the oncogenes, the tumor supressor genes (recessive cancer genes) may exert their oncogenic potential by loss of function mutations.[10] A (germline) mutation in one of the alleles results in a predisposition for developing cancer.[10] A mutation in the second, wild-type allele may facilitate or initiate cancer.[11] This combination commonly occurs in one cell or in small numbers of cells, and hence, the inherited predisposition behaves as a dominant trait.

In the third type of genetic defect, the DNA repair system is the target. External factors such as x-rays, ultraviolet (UV) photons and chemicals as well as endogenous factors, cellular processes, and intrinsic properties can produce a spectrum of DNA alterations.[12–14] The errors in the DNA sequence are usually corrected by repair enzymes executing different repair processes, depending on the specific defect: base-excision, nucleotide excision, or

Table 5–1. Synopsis of Chapter

Genetic events in cancerogenesis
Cell cycle as target for cancerogenic events
Genes active in germline cells and embryogenesis as targets for cancerogenesis
Predisposition to cancer
Cancer epidemiology
Histogenesis, differentiation, and prognosis of malignant disease
Detection of unknown mutations
Basic principles of nucleic acid analysis
Detection of large mutations in DNA
Detection of subtle mutations in DNA
Detection of altered RNA expression
Molecular abnormalities in bone tumors
Osteosarcoma
Malignant fibrous histiocytoma of bone
Chondrosarcoma
Ewing's sarcoma and peripheral neuroectodermal tumors
Lymphomas
Nucleic acid analysis
Isolation of nucleic acids
Digestion of DNA with restriction enzymes, Southern hybridization and Northern hybridization
Standard PCR and RT-PCR amplification protocols
Single strand conformational polymorphism analysis
TGGE in p53
Direct sequencing
Fluorescence in situ hybridization
Protein analysis
Immunohistochemistry
Western blotting

recombination repair.[15–18] In general, mutations in the repair system are of the loss-of-function type and may contribute tremendously to a cancer predisposition (e.g., xeroderma pigmentosum, ataxia telangiectasia).[18, 19] A mutation in the repair machinery may lead to an increased number of mutations in oncogenes and tumor suppressor genes, thereby increasing the potential for both categories of oncogenes to initiate and propagate the malignant process.[20] Cancerogenesis is a multistep process that includes several (genetic) events leading to disregulation of a complex cell cycle–regulating system. It seems likely that cancers that develop typically in the fifth or sixth decade of life may require more mutational events than tumors predominantly associated with childhood or adolescence.[21]

Cell Cycle as Target for Cancerogenic Events

To understand the function of cancer-associated genes, the ways in which the cell monitors and regulates its cycle of division need to be understood.[22] In the cell cycle, two major events are easy to observe: the duplication of the cellular genome (the DNA synthesis, or S-phase) and the subsequent separation of the two equal portions destined for each daughter cell (the mitotic, or M-phase). Between these two central phases there are two gap phases, during which the cell generates building blocks for DNA synthesis (G1) and for mitosis (G2).[22]

In many experiments utilizing cell culture, primitive animals such as *Xenopus laevis*,[23] and yeast,[24] as well as germline transfection and knock-out techniques in higher animals,[25] a set of genes and their proteins have been identified that are essential for the decision as to whether cells should rest, divide, or die by apoptosis.

The general concept is that the positive control of the cell cycle is regulated by the proto-oncogenes and the negative control is exerted by the tumor suppressor genes, mainly p53 and *RB*1 (retinoblastoma susceptibility gene) (Fig. 5–1).[22] Additional proteins that are functionally important in the cell cycle are the cyclins. Mammalian cells possess several cyclins, cyclin I and E for the G1 phase, cyclin A for the S-phase, and cyclin B for the G2 and M phases.[22] The cyclins are the target proteins for the cyclin-dependent kinases that positively regulate the cell cycle.

Antagonistic to this positive regulation is the action of the cyclin-dependent kinase inhibitors (mainly p16 and p15 tumor suppressors),[22] which block the progression of the cell cycle. Damage to the genome is normally detected by checkpoint controls leading to an increased level of the p53 gene product.[22] p53 (among other functions) exerts transcription factor activity enhancing the expression of p21 (WAF),[26] which in turn suppresses the activity of cyclin D4. Without this repair mechanism, DNA replication would result in a much higher mutation rate. It seems clear that cells lacking functional p53 protein are more prone to mutations than are cells with normal p53.[27]

Progression in the cell cycle may be stopped in response to external signals or conditions, which are evaluated by specific receptors on the cell surface and transferred via several pathways to the regulators of the cell cycle.[22, 26] Molecules involved in the information cascade may act as oncogenes (*ras, raf, src*) or tumor suppressor genes (*DCC*).[28]

Apoptosis or programmed cell death is a

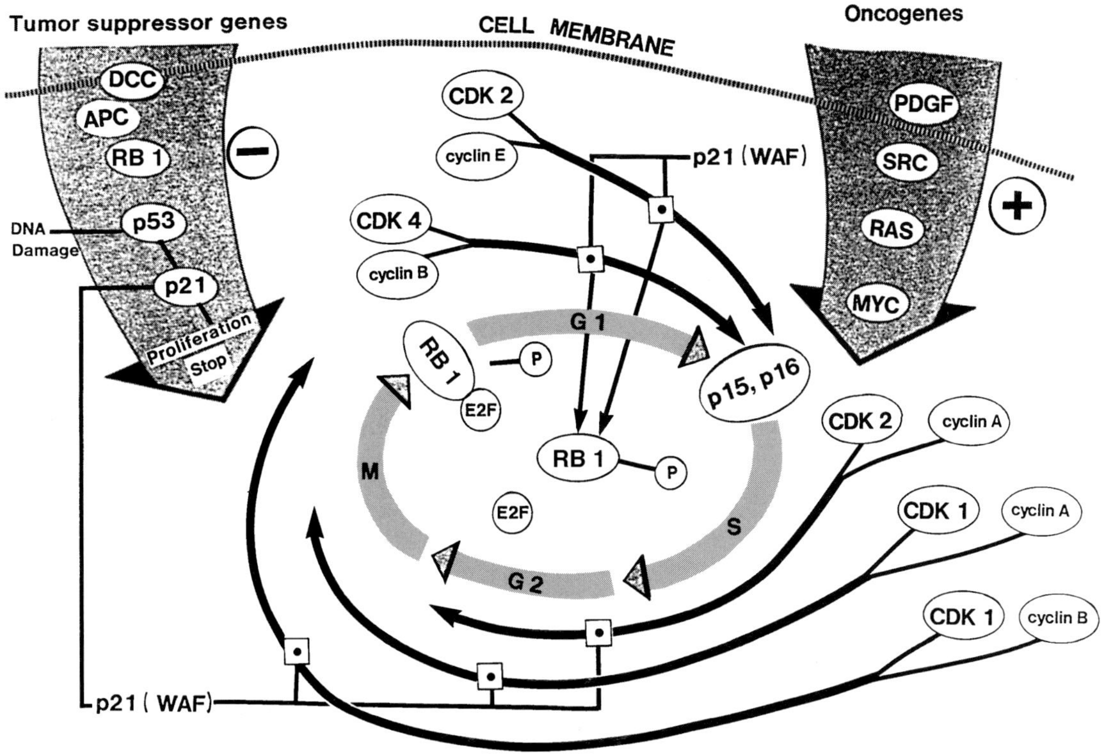

Figure 5–1. Simplified scheme of the cell cycle. + indicates activation of cell proliferation by oncogenes. − indicates suppression of cell proliferation by tumor suppressor genes. APC = adenomatous polyposis gene product; *RB*1 = retinoblastoma susceptibility gene; CDK 1,2,4 = cyclin-dependent kinases; E2F = transcription factor; p15, p16 = closely related cyclin kinase inhibitors; p21 WAF1 = cyclin kinase inhibitor, platelet-derived growth factor.

physiologic process by which the cellular life span is controlled and certain cells are programmed for elimination. The specific morphologic changes that typify apoptosis are cell shrinkage, membrane blebbing, chromatin and cytoplasmic condensation, and, most characteristically, fragmentation of nuclear DNA.[29] Nowadays, it is thought that many cytotoxic drugs exert their activity on the apoptotic machinery of the tumor cell, which may be inhibited by mutations of the p53 protein, the key molecule in positive apoptotic regulation.[27, 29]

Genes Active in Germline Cells and Embryogenesis as Targets of Cancerogenesis

Recent research has brought into focus two oncogene categories that are highly active in germline cells, embryogenesis, and organ development: telomerase and the family of *PAX* (paired *BOX*) and *HOX* (homeo *BOX*) genes.[30–32] It is conceivable that those genes, if expressed nonphysiologically, might destabilize cell cycle regulation and hence contribute to cancerogenesis.[30–34]

Germline cells express telomerase, an enzyme that functions as a reverse transcriptase by virtue of its internal RNA template.[30, 31] The telomerase is critical for replication of chromosomal termini, or telomeres. In the absence of telomerase, the chromosome shortens with each cell division, a mechanism that has been proposed to be the mitotic clock by which cells count their divisions and that contributes to replicative cellular senescence in somatic cells.[30, 31]

It has been postulated that telomerase is inactive in somatic cells but is reactivated in most immortal cells and in cancer.[30, 31] Thus, cancer cells have acquired an activation of a gene whose normal function may be to allow germ cells to avoid the mortality of somatic cells.[30, 31] Recent data suggest that the aberrant expression of telomerase in cancer cells is a rather late event in cancerogenesis and may result from a mutation in sequences (oncogenes or antioncogenes) that normally control its expression.[35]

The proto-oncogenes of the *HOX* and *PAX* family are intimately involved in embryogenic and tissue development.[32–34] They govern complex biologic processes including embryonic segmentation and the development of an eye.[32] Aberrant expression of *HOX* genes has been identified in leukemias and colorectal cancer, whereas *PAX* genes are involved in rhabdomyosarcoma and Wilms' tumor.[32, 36] As early promoters of development, they may influence a wide range of genes directly or indirectly.[33] It is difficult to define their precise position in the oncogenic cascade, or to categorize their function as oncogenic or antioncogenic activity.[32] Truncated sequences of this class of genes are found in a number of fusion genes as *PAX/FHKR*[36] and *PBX/E2A*,[37] and in this context they act as oncogenes.

Predisposition to Cancer

Once a gene that predisposes to cancer has been cloned, it is possible to test for a mutant gene in an individual's (germline) DNA. The first studies were done on the *RB*1 (familial retinoblastoma) and p53 tumor suppressor gene (Li-Fraumeni syndrome).[11] Detailed analysis of three recently isolated tumor suppressor genes—the familiar adenomatous polyposis gene (*APC*) on chromosome 5, the neurofibromatosis-1 gene (*NF*1) on chromosome 17, and the Wilms' tumor gene (*WT*1) on chromosome 11—can often identify individuals at risk for developing the associated tumors in families with an established disease history and allow preventive strategies to be implemented.[38]

Cancer Epidemiology

Viruses

A few viruses have been implicated in childhood and adult cancer.[39] Prenatal or childhood exposure to viruses has especially been associated with cancer later in life. Examples include hepatitis B virus (HBV) and Epstein-Barr (EBV) infections contributing to hepatocellular carcinoma and Burkitt's and Hodgkin's lymphoma in childhood, respectively. Human T-cell leukemia virus I (HTLV I) infection is involved in adult T-cell leukemia (ATL).[39]

Chemical Carcinogens

The analysis of specific mutations in the p53 gene may become a useful tool for carcinogen exposure or defining new cancerogens.[40–42] Lung tumors, for example, harbor unique mutations in codon 157, while codon 249 mutations are common in hepatocellular carcinoma.[43, 44] It is suggested that the codon 157 mutation, a guanidine to thymidine (G-T) transversion, is induced by benzopyrene, an ingredient of cigarette smoke.[45] The codon 249 mutation is also a G-T transversion and seems to be caused by aflatoxin B1, a liver-specific mutagen.[44, 46]

Histogenesis, Differentiation, and Prognosis of Malignant Disease

The detection of a monoclonal rearrangement of immunoreceptor (immunoglobulin and T-cell receptor) genes has proved to be a reliable method for detecting monoclonal cell populations in lymphoid malignancies.[47, 48]

The identification of expression of the myogenic regulatory protein, *MyoD*, is a potential tool in the differential diagnosis of small round cell tumors (see Chapter 14). In this setting, only embryonal and alveolar rhabdomyosarcomas express *MyoD* at the RNA level.[49, 50]

When gene expression is very low, the polymerase chain reaction (PCR) technique permits the detection of even a minimal amount of mRNA. Although *MyoD* is expressed in embryonal and alveolar rhabdomyosarcomas, these tumors can be differentiated further at the molecular genetic level. The embryonal rhabdomyosarcoma harbors a mutation in a putative tumor suppressor gene located on chromosome 11p15, but the alveolar rhabdomyosarcoma is defined by the 2;13 translocation, resulting in fusion gene (*PAX*3/*FHKR*) that can be easily detected by fluorescence in situ hybridization (FISH) or reverse transcriptase–PCR (RT-PCR) (see later discussion).[36]

Ewing's sarcoma and primitive neuroectodermal tumor (PNET) are defined molecularly by the 11;22 (*EWS/FLI*) fusion gene and its variants.[8] The fusion genes in leukemia, such as *BCR-ABL*, not only typify a certain leukemic disease but are of prognostic value, as they may be used to indicate a failure of conventional chemotherapy and the need for bone marrow transplantation.[51, 52]

p53 mutations in breast,[53] lung,[54] and colon carcinomas,[55] as well as in acute and chronic myelocytic leukemias, herald an unfavorable prognosis, but they seem to be a good prognostic sign in some B-cell lymphomas.[56]

Detection of Unknown Mutations

Detection of mutations is a critical step in many studies of cancer genetics. Currently, mutations can be detected by a variety of methods utilizing single or double strand DNA and denaturing or nondenaturing gels, including the PCR technique and sequencing.[57] Mutation detection involves two strategies: scanning mode, in which a stretch of DNA is sequenced for unknown mutations, and a diagnostic mode, in which specific tests are designed to detect known mutations.[58] At present, the detection of mutations is time-consuming and expensive. Much research is devoted to improving this situation,[59] and test systems revealing functional properties of mutations are being introduced into cancer research.[60] This may bring us into the position of being able to describe the complete molecular pattern of the development of neoplasms, including as yet unknown mutations that may be causally related to the malignant phenotype more strongly than those that are already known. Together, these methods may all participate in the implementation of sophisticated gene and gene expression technologies into clinical practice.

BASIC PRINCIPLES OF NUCLEIC ACID ANALYSIS

The identification of gene alterations that are causally involved in carcinogenesis is a stepwise process escalating from simple screening methods to sophisticated, definitive analyses.

Detection of Large Mutations in DNA

Cytogenetic techniques reveal chromosomal alterations affecting more than 1 megabase, including deletions, insertions, translocations, and extra-chromosomal material.[61, 62]

Fluorescent in situ hybridization, using (multiple) fluorescence-labeled DNA probes for hybridization in chromosome spreads, reveals both the copy number of a target gene and the (abnormal) localization within the genome of single cells (see also Chapter 4).[63, 64] Entire genomes,[65] chromosomal regions,[66] and unique sequences,[67, 68] can be specifically visualized in metaphase and in interphase cells by the use of FISH.[69–71] Chromosomal abnormalities, such as deletions,[72] can be visualized, and the chromosomal location of specific genes can be determined. Thus, FISH plays an important role in gene mapping, tumor biology, prenatal diagnosis, and cytogenetics. The analysis of single copy DNA sequences in interphase nuclei by a modified hybridization protocol termed *fluorescent in situ suppression hybridization* (FISSH)[73] has already proved to be of value both for the detection of numerical chromosomal alterations occurring in neoplasia and for the delineation of specific translocations, as t(9;22)(q34;q11) in chronic myeloid leukemia.[74]

Comparative genomic hybridization (CGH) does not need sequence-specific probes and allows rapid screening for deleted or amplified regions within tumor DNA using cohybridization of differently labeled tumor DNA and nontumor reference DNA to normal chromosome spreads.[75]

Southern blot analysis allows the screening of large stretches of genomic DNA for a target gene, even when lacking detailed knowledge of its structure. Restriction enzymes catalyze double-strand cleavage at specific sites of the DNA, resulting in unique sets of fragments that are size-fractionated during agarose gel electrophoresis and transferred as single strands to synthetic membranes. Upon hybridization with a labeled complementary single-stranded DNA or RNA probe, a target gene within the blotted fragments is visualized by fluorescence or radiography. Signal location and intensity reveal (partial) deletions, rearrangements, and increased copy number of genes, and structural alterations of about 500 bp in size can be detected easily (Fig. 5–2*A*).[76, 77]

Loss of heterozygosity (LOH) can be observed if homologous alleles differ in size constitutionally and one allele is lost during tumor formation.[78] Allelic heterozygosity results from physiologic distance variations between restriction enzyme cleavage sites (e.g., due to a variable number of tandem repeats, leading to restriction fragment length polymorphism. LOH is assumed to reflect the loss of one allele of a tumor suppressor gene, and the

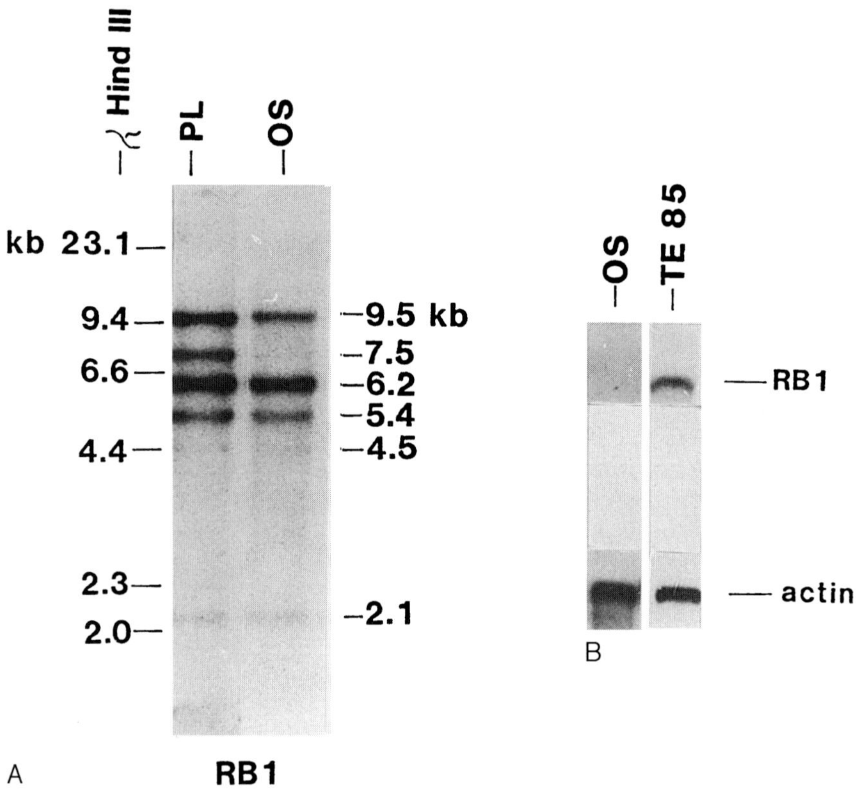

Figure 5–2. DNA and RNA analysis of the retinoblastoma susceptibility gene (*RB*1) in an osteosarcoma. *A*, Southern blot analysis of 10 μg of Hind III digested DNA (hybridized with a ^{32}P-labeled *RB*1 gene-specific probe) shows the normal pattern of the *RB*1 gene in placental DNA (PL) and the complete deletion of the 7.5 kb Hind III fragment in the osteosarcoma. Lambda Hind III DNA serves as size standard. *B*, Nothern blot analysis of 20 μg of total RNA shows no detectable *RB*1 gene transcript in the osteosarcoma compared with the control cell line (TE85). After removal of the *RB*1 gene probe, the filter was rehybridized with an actin-specific gene probe to show comparable loading of intact RNA in both lanes.

remaining one is believed to carry an inactivating (subtle) mutation.[79, 80] Studying LOH can uncover (new) tumor suppressor genes, recessive carriers of predisposing alleles, and the preferential loss of maternal or paternal alleles most probably indicating involvement of genomic imprinting.[80–83]

Detection of Subtle Mutations in DNA

The polymerase chain reaction (PCR) can be applied if the DNA sequences flanking the region of interest on both strands are known so that complementary oligonucleotides can be synthesized. Repeated cycles of heating and cooling denature the double-stranded DNA and allow primer annealing and chain elongation catalyzed by heat-stable DNA polymerases, resulting in an exponentially increasing number of copies.[84] *Multiplex PCR* allows the simultaneous targeting of different regions within the same gene.[85] Through size fractionating of the PCR products, deletions or insertions in the target tumor DNA, as compared to control samples, can be recognized directly.

To detect point mutations, several screening techniques can be applied prior to direct sequencing. *Single-stranded conformational polymorphism* (SSCP) analysis detects 90% of all mutations in fragments up to 200 bp.[86] Single strands have a characteristic three-dimensional conformation, depending on the primary sequence, and sequence alterations lead to a mobility shift during migration within a nondenaturing gel.[87, 88]

Denaturing gradient gel electrophoresis (DGGE) and *temperature gradient gel electrophoresis* (TGGE) examine the migration of double-stranded DNA within an increasing gradient of denaturing agents or temperature.[57, 89–91] Sequence-dependent dissociation of double strands leads to a considerably reduced mobility separating mutant and wild-type homoduplices (Mm, Ww) as well as two heteroduplices (Wm, Mw).[57] The sensitivity of this assay seems to be superior to that of SSCP.[57] New gel matrices have been developed to facilitate heteroduplex analyses (Fig. 5–3A).[92]

Direct sequencing of single-stranded PCR products annealed to a sequencing primer can be performed according to the chain termination reaction.[93] A large number of DNA chains complementary to the PCR template are created either by T7 polymerase (sequenase system) or by Taq polymerase (cycle sequencing). These chains, differing in size from several nucleotides up to full length, are base-specifically (G, A, T, and C respectively) terminated in four separate reactions. After high-resolution polyacrylamide gel electrophoresis, DNA fragments differing in size by only one nucleotide are separated, and the base sequence "ladder" can be read (Fig. 5–3B). Isotopic detection is more time consuming, but automatic fluorescence detection requires more expensive equipment.

Detection of Altered RNA Expression

Northern blot analysis is used to determine the (abnormal) amount and (altered) size of intact mRNA in different tissues and tumors. After denaturing agarose gel electrophoresis and transfer of the RNA to suitable membranes, the target mRNA can be identified by hybridization with a labeled gene-specific probe (see Fig. 5–2B).[77]

In *RT-PCR,* mRNA is enzymatically reverse-transcribed into a complementary DNA, which then serves as template during PCR. Since mRNA corresponds to only the exons of a gene, longer genomic distances can be investigated. Tumor-specific translocations represent an exchange of genetic material between two chromosomes in the early stage of tumorigenesis. The translocations break specific genes in the involved chromosomal regions and fuse them to create novel chimeric genes. These new genes are expressed as chimeric transcripts that encode fusion proteins that combine functional domains usually found in separate proteins. The fusion region of chimeric RNA transcripts from chromosomal translocations (e.g., t(11;22) in Ewing's sarcoma) can be targeted by RT-PCR (see Chapters 4 and 14) using it as a tumor marker and for the detection of minimal residual disease.[8, 48] Increased or decreased gene expression can also be recognized.

MOLECULAR ABNORMALITIES IN BONE TUMORS

Osteosarcoma

Chromosomal Alterations and Loss of Heterozygosity

Aneuploidy and a high fraction of cells in the S-phase are strong indicators of a high-

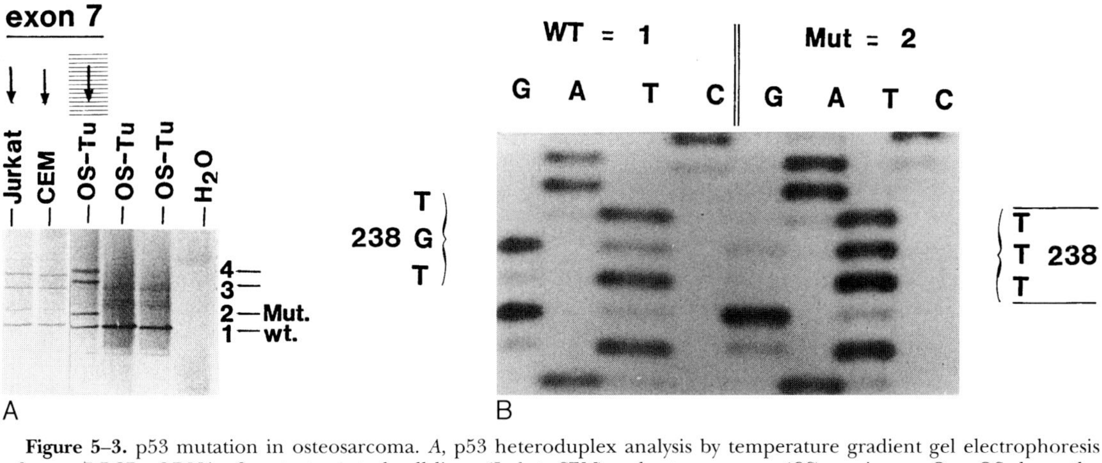

Figure 5–3. p53 mutation in osteosarcoma. *A,* p53 heteroduplex analysis by temperature gradient gel electrophoresis of exon 7 PCR of DNA of mutant control cell lines *(Jurkat, CEM)* and osteosarcoma *(OS)* specimens. One OS shows the formation of heteroduplex bands (3,4) in addition to the wild-type (1) and mutant (2) homodimer band. *B,* Direct sequence analysis after elution and reamplification of the wild-type (*WT,* 1) and mutant (*Mut,* 2) homodimer bands shows a missense mutation at codon 238 of the p53 gene (Cys-Phe).

grade tumor.[94–97] Recurrent abnormalities among complex karyotypic alterations observed in high-grade osteosarcomas are loss of 13q or 17p, suggesting the involvement of the *RB*1 (13q14) and the p53 (17p13) tumor suppressor genes, respectively. No consistent chromosomal translocation has been identified in osteosarcomas so far.[98–100] However, in some small cell osteosarcomas, an 11;22 translocation has been described.[101] In parosteal osteosarcoma, the only consistent karyotypic alteration is the presence of supernumerary ring chromosomes, although one case showed a 5;10 translocation.[98, 99] CGH has shown a high level of amplification at 12q12-13, suggesting the involvement of oncogenes located in this region (e.g., MDM2/SAS) and detected as yet unidentified amplification sites at 17p11-12 and 6p.[102, 103] Allelotype study has revealed LOH at frequencies higher than 60% at chromosome arms 3q, 13q, 17p, and 18q, most probably indicating loss of RB1, p53, and additional tumor suppressor genes.[104] One candidate gene in the region of 18q might be the *DCC* gene (Deleted in Colon Carcinoma),[81, 105] the expression of which is suppressed in the majority of osteosarcomas studied.[106] Interestingly, a tendency is seen toward a primary mutation of the paternally derived *RB*1 allele, followed by loss of the maternally derived allele.[107]

*RB*1 Alterations

The *RB*1 gene was the first tumor suppressor gene associated with osteosarcoma development, since survivors from inherited retinoblastoma have an increased risk for developing osteosarcoma as a second malignancy.[108] The localization of the *RB*1 gene was narrowed to chromosome 13q14, the smallest common region among overlapping deletions in the karyotypes of retinoblastoma patients.[109] Following the development of an *RB*1 cDNA probe,[110] gross gene alterations were demonstrated in about 50% of investigated osteosarcomas (see Fig. 5–2), most frequently partial deletions of DNA (often involving exons 13–17)[111–114] and loss of or aberrant RNA expression.[113, 115, 116] Such alterations occur more frequently in high-grade than in low-grade sarcomas.[113] More subtle *RB*1 mutations were found in 6% of 63 high-grade osteosarcomas, in contrast to a higher frequency in retinoblastomas.[116] The same study showed a correlation with poor prognosis of gross and subtle *RB*1 mutations, and LOH at a polymorphic *RB*1 sequence, respectively.[116] This finding was confirmed by investigating LOH at the *RB*1 gene in biopsy material of 21 osteosarcomas with a defined response to the same preoperative chemotherapy.[117] However, the loss of *RB*1 protein expression (54%) as determined by immunohistochemical analysis (IHC) has not yet been related to a poor prognosis, indicating a more complex influence of the *RB*1 gene on the biology of osteosarcoma, possibly involving *RB*1 gene modulators.[116] The high frequency of *RB*1 gene mutations in osteosarcoma (promoting uncontrolled progression through the cell cycle) may explain why alterations of the p15/p16 tumor suppressor genes, which function in the regulation of *RB*-mediated G1 cell cycle block, are infrequently observed in osteosarcomas, in contrast to other malignancies.[118]

p53 and MDM2 Alterations

Since not all patients who are cured of inherited retinoblastoma develop secondary osteosarcoma, additional factors must be involved.[119] The p53 tumor suppressor gene (17p13) is frequently found to be abnormal (see Fig. 5–3).[115, 120] In about 40% of investigated osteosarcomas, structural p53 alterations occur, half with gross changes and half with subtle mutations.[121–124] The latter were most frequently point mutations within exons 5, 6, 7, and 8 as described in other human malignancies, with a possible predominance of mutations in exons 7 and 8.[45, 125] p53 mutations can increase the normally short half-life of the corresponding protein, allowing its (nuclear) accumulation to be detectable by IHC.[126] Hence, a positive IHC result may indicate p53 protein alteration, although some p53 mutations can lead to lack of p53 protein synthesis, and increased immunohistochemical expression of p53 protein is not always associated with detectable mutations.[127, 128]

Positive p53 IHC staining is reported in 28 to 70% of osteosarcomas.[129, 130] Our own investigations found positive p53 IHC in 9 of 13 osteosarcomas and demonstrated a corresponding gene alteration in six of these positive cases, including one low-grade osteosarcoma with (cytoplasmic) p53 overexpression and amplification of a p53 inhibitor (*MDM2*) (suggesting that the p53 protein in this tumor cannot exert its typical function in the nucleus).[131, 132]

The *MDM2* (Murine Double Minute 2) oncogene was originally isolated from a tumorigenic mouse fibroblast cell line containing double minutes.[132] The human homologue is located at chromosome 12q13-14. A correlation between *MDM2* amplification and marker ring chromosomes has been found in soft tissue sarcomas.[133]

The *MDM2* protein can bind to p53 protein, so that *MDM2* overexpression may inhibit p53 function.[132] Results from several groups show *MDM2* amplification in 5 to 27% of investigated osteosarcomas.[134, 135] In our own study, 3 of 20 osteosarcomas showed *MDM2* amplification, and 8 cases showed gross or subtle mutations of the p53 gene; hence about 50% of osteosarcomas (including two periosteal and one central, low-grade osteosarcoma) showed impaired p53 function according to nucleic acid analysis, and a further 15% of cases according to IHC analysis (Table 5–2).[136] To date, no correlation between p53 mutations and the prognosis of osteosarcoma patients has been shown. One might speculate that p53 dysfunction is obligatory in osteosarcoma development and that a high *MDM2* expression is similar in effect to loss of p53 function, whereas p53 missense mutations could have different functional effects on the biologic behavior of osteosarcoma.[137]

Germline p53 mutations have been detected in 3% of 235 osteosarcoma patients and indicate a generally increased cancer risk that may also be a factor in the development of multifocal osteosarcoma.[138]

Alterations in Other Oncogenes and SV40-Like Sequences

Within the MAR (multiple aberration region) on 12q13-15, additional genes are located that tend to be coamplified in several solid tumors, including some osteosarcomas.[139–143] One of these is the *SAS* gene (Sarcoma Amplified Sequences), which encodes for a transmembrane protein thought to participate in signal transduction and growth control.[6] Amplification of this gene was found in about 10% of investigated osteosarcomas (see Table 5–2). The *CDK4* gene, which is located in this region, encodes for a cyclin-dependent kinase that phosphorylates the *RB* protein (when activated by cyclin D1), resulting in release of the *RB1*-mediated G1 arrest. Hence, its oncogenic activation may contribute to deregulation of the cell cycle control.[144] Overexpression of several genes located in this region may cause synergistic oncogenic effects,[5] and the true target gene of amplification at 12q may still be unidentified.[141] Although mutations of the *ras* oncogenes have not been found in osteosarcoma,[145] increased c-*fos* expression has been shown in the majority of cases[146] and amplification of the c-*myc* gene in some cases of osteosarcoma.[147] One unexplained observation is a highly significant preponderance of s-allele homozygosity of the L-*myc* oncogene in male but not female patients with osteosarcoma and other sarcomas.[148]

The c-*Met* oncogene encodes the receptor for the hepatocyte growth factor (*HGF*), a cytokine that stimulates the invasive growth of cells. The *Met*/*HGF* receptor is overexpressed in 60% of investigated osteosarcoma and may provide osteosarcoma cells with the capacity to invade neighboring tissues.[149]

The c-*erb*B2 (also called *neu* or *HER2*) protooncogene located on chromosome 17q21 encodes for a transmembrane glycoprotein that shows significant structural similarity to epidermal growth factor. Although no gene amplification or any activating mutation has been identified in osteosarcomas so far, increased protein expression in 11 of 26 primary osteosarcomas was correlated with early pulmonary metastasis and poor response to chemother-

Table 5–2. Patterns of Gene Dysfunction in 20 Osteosarcomas

	1	2	3	4	5	6	7	8	9*	10	11	12	13†	14†	15	16	17	18	19	20
RB1	+	+	+	+	+	+	+	+	0	0	0	0	0	0	0	0	0	0	0	0
p53	+	+	+	+	+	+	±	+	+	+	±	±	+	+	0	0	0	0	0	0
MDM2	0	0	0	0	0	0	0	+	+	+	0	0	0	0	0	0	0	0	0	0
SAS	0	0	0	0	0	0	0	0	+	+	0	0	0	0	0	0	0	0	0	0

RB1 +: mutation detected by Southern/Northern blot analysis (SB, NB); p53 +: mutation detected by SB, NB, and TGGE prior to direct sequencing (including *MDM2* amplification); p53 ±: positive IHC result although no confirming genetic alteration has been found; *MDM2* +/*SAS*+: amplification shown by SB; 0: no mutation detected by the methods applied.

*Central low-grade osteosarcoma.

†Periosteal osteosarcoma (all other osteosarcomas are central, high-grade type).

apy. Overexpression of c-*erb*B2 may promote the metastatic potential of osteosarcoma and could be a useful prognostic marker.[150]

Recently, *SV40-like sequences* corresponding to the large T-antigen (Tag) were identified by PCR in about one third of 160 bone tumors, including 126 osteosarcomas, 11 chondrosarcomas, six giant cell tumors, and three Ewing's sarcomas.[151] The Tag sequence contains the domain that can bind and inactivate several cellular tumor suppressors. In particular, the retinoblastoma-binding domain is a highly conserved region of Tag, underlining the key role of *RB*1 gene dysfunction in osteosarcoma development. If the putative causal relationship between viral infection and the development of osteosarcoma could be confirmed, immunization against the viral protein may be of therapeutic benefit.

P-Glycoprotein

Multidrug resistance is mediated by the *MDR*1 gene product, P-glycoprotein, and involves numerous chemically very different agents of plant origin, including doxorubicin, the most effective drug in osteosarcoma therapy.[152, 153] Increased *MDR*1 expression can be induced in osteosarcoma cell lines,[154] and a significantly higher proportion of osteosarcoma metastases are resistant to multiple drugs, as compared with primary tumors.[155] Increased *MDR*1 expression may be associated with chemotherapy resistance and also with tumor aggressiveness (see Chapter 8).[156, 157] Sequence analysis of osteosarcoma DNA suggests a correlation between the type of single base changes in the promoter of the *MDR*1 gene and the in vitro responsiveness to *MDR*-relevant drugs.[158]

Malignant Fibrous Histiocytoma of Bone

Malignant fibrous histiocytoma (MFH) of bone is composed of pleomorphic and fibroblastic components and does not show osteoid formation (see Chapter 12).[159–161] DNA aneuploidy correlates with a high-grade tumor.[96] MFH of bone is much less common than MFH of soft tissues, but the few cytogenetic studies of MFH of bone have shown abnormalities of chromosomes 12, 13, 15, 17, and 19 among other karyotypic changes.[162–164] A giant cell type of MFH of bone showed a chromosomal translocation t(14;22)(q11;p12), as well as breakpoints at 7p22, 8p11, and 19q13, and telomeric associations (*tas*).[165] Interestingly, the same breakpoints on chromosomes 7, 8, and 19 were described in a giant cell tumor of bone with malignant transformation.[166]

Molecular genetic investigations of MFH of bone have not been reported. It may be relevant that a broad spectrum of soft tissue sarcomas (including MFH) shows a high frequency of p53 mutations,[167] *RB*1 gene mutations, and c-*myc* amplification.[113, 114, 168] Also, MFH of soft tissue with a 19p+ marker chromosome have an increased relapse risk, whereas tumors with a ring marker bear a reduced relapse risk.[169] The possible contributions of tumor suppressor genes and cytogenetic abnormalities to the development of MFH of bone need further study.

Increased expression of *HSP*27, a member of the small heat-shock protein family, may correlate with increased cellular resistance to cytotoxic agents, including doxorubicin. In a study of 43 primary MFHs, including three cases of bone origin, there was a significant correlation between *HSP*27 overexpression and decreased overall survival after treatment, independent of tumor size, histologic subtype, and necrosis.[170]

Chondrosarcoma

Chondrosarcoma is a malignant cartilage-forming tumor that does not show osteoid formation (see Chapter 10). The majority are Grade I and II tumors, but dedifferentiation into high-grade tumors has been observed in about 10% of chondrosarcomas.[171, 172] Hyperploidy is related to poor prognosis and may be the best predictor of the clinical course of chondrosarcoma.[173] p53 overexpression and mutations seem to be associated with high-grade tumors.[174, 175] The significance of a worse clinical outcome in four of five chondrosarcomas with increased expression of proliferating cell nuclear antigen (PCNA) and tenascin has to be further elucidated.[176]

Comparison of the karyotypes of benign and malignant tumors suggests that the genes encoding the human cartilage link protein (mapped to chromosome 5), the α_2 chain of collagen type XI (chromosome 6), and type II collagen (chromosome 12) might be of etiologic significance in cartilaginous tumors.[177, 178] Abnormalities of chromosome 7 and most probably also of chromosome 1 are related to high-grade tumors. Furthermore, structural abnormalities of chromosomes 8 and 18 are present only in benign tumors, whereas numerical anomalies of these chromosomes are found exclusively in chondrosarcoma (see Chapter 4).[177]

A deletion of the long arm of chromosome 8 (del8q23-24) contributes to the development of exostoses in hereditary multiple exostoses (EXT) and the Langer-Giedion syndrome.[179, 180] Linkage studies suggested three chromosomal regions for EXT genes: *EXT*1 at 8q24.1,[181] *EXT*2 at the pericentric region of chromosome 11,[182] and *EXT*3 on 19p.[183] There is an increased risk of chondrosarcoma developing in EXT, although most chondrosarcomas occur sporadically, suggesting a possible contribution of tumor suppressor genes to their development.[184–186] Supporting a putative function of *EXT*1 and *EXT*2 as tumor suppressor genes, polymorphic markers linked to both genes often show LOH in sporadic chondrosarcomas, while the 19p markers remain intact in these tumors.[187, 188]

Further cytogenetic abnormalities described repeatedly in chondrosarcoma are losses of chromosomes 6, 10, 11, 13, 18, and 22, gains of chromosomes 7 and 20, and structural alterations at chromosomal bands 5q13, 1q21, 7p11, 12q13, and 20q11.[189, 190] Two cases of grade II chondrosarcoma showed t(6;12) or t(12;19).[191] Aberrations at band 1p36 were seen in three dedifferentiated chondrosarcomas, two of which showed additional identical breaks at 5q11.[189, 192]

Breakpoints on chromosome 22q, cytogenetically indistinguishable from those in Ewing's sarcoma, were observed in several (skeletal and extraskeletal) myxoid chondrosarcomas (t(9;22)(q22-31;q11-12)),[193–195] in one dedifferentiated grade IV chondrosarcoma (t(9;22)(q34;q11-12)),[196] and in two mesenchymal chondrosarcomas (t(11;22)(q24;q12), and add(22)(q13), respectively).[197, 198] The possible importance of the *EWS* gene at 22q12 is underlined by some studies specifically demonstrating a rearranged *EWS* gene.[193, 199]

Ewing's Sarcoma and Primitive Neuroectodermal Tumor

Cytogenetics

An important advance in the investigation of Ewing's sarcoma and PNET has been the identification of consistent chromosomal translocations (see Chapters 4 and 14). The most common translocation in Ewing's sarcoma involves the long arms of chromosome 11 and 22, forming the translocation t(11;22)(q24;q12).[200, 201] An apparently identical translocation has been detected in primitive neuroectodermal and Askin's tumors,[202, 203] and in esthesioneuroblastomas,[204, 205] which may be closely related to Ewing's sarcoma.

In about 90% of Ewing's sarcoma and PNET, t(11;22)(q24;q12) can be observed. The second most common translocation is t(21;22),[206] and other tumors show variant translocations consistently involving chromosome band 22q12.[139, 207–210]

Thus, cytogenetics is an important diagnostic tool in the differential diagnosis of small round cell tumors. The inability to always successfully perform cytogenetic analysis in clinical material can be overcome by the visualization of t(11;22) utilizing in situ hybridization techniques.

In Situ Hybridization

In Ewing's sarcoma and PNET, the translocation t(11;22)(q24;q12) can be detected by means of FISSH on metaphase spreads and interphase nuclei.[63, 71, 211] The high incidence of t(11;22) in Ewing's sarcoma and PNET lines and primary tumors has been confirmed by these investigations, which are a reliable diagnostic tool.

Molecular Genetics

In the t(11;22)(q24;q12), the breakpoint at 22q12 interrupts a novel gene, designated *EWS*, whose function is still unclear.[212, 213] The 11q24 breakpoint lies within the *FLI*-1 gene. This gene is the human counterpart of the murine *fli*-1 gene (Friend Leukemia virus Integration site-1), a member of the *Ets* proto-oncogene family,[214] which includes *ATF*1 (210), and *ERG*,[215, 216] and is characterized by an 85-amino-acid region of similarity, the *Ets* domain, which is essential for sequence-specific binding to DNA and is postulated to regulate the transcription of certain tissue-specific genes.[217] In the translocation t(11;22), a portion of the *FLI*-1 gene (3′-half) coding for a putative sequence-specific DNA binding domain is translocated to chromosome 22, and thereby its expression is placed under the control of regulatory elements in the proximal (5′) portion of the *EWS* gene. A chimeric RNA transcript is produced (*EWS-FLI-*1), encoding a protein consisting of the amino terminal portion of the *EWS* protein and the carboxy terminal portion of the *FLI-*1 protein.[213] This nuclear protein binds DNA with the same sequence specificity as the wild-type parental *FLI-*1 protein. *EWS-FLI-*1 is an efficient sequence-specific transcriptional activator of model promoters containing *FLI-*1 (*Ets*)-binding sites, a property that is strictly dependent on the presence of its *EWS* domain. Comparison of the properties of the N-terminal activation domain of *FLI-*1 with those of the *EWS* domain of the fusion protein indicates that *EWS-FLI-*1 has altered transcriptional activation properties compared with *FLI-*1. Thus, *EWS-FLI-*1 might contribute to the transformed phenotype of tumor cells by inducing the deregulation or unscheduled activation of genes normally responsive to *FLI-*1 or to other close members of the *Ets* family.

The *EWS-FLI-*1 chimeric transcripts can be detected by RT-PCR, which constitutes a powerful diagnostic approach for Ewing's sarcoma and PNET (see Chapter 14). RT-PCR for t(11;22) produces products of different length, which can be explained by a variety of fusion types. Only about half of Ewing's sarcoma and PNET chimeric transcripts result from the junction of exons 1 to 7 of the *EWS* gene to exons 6 to 9 of *FLI-*1.[218] Variant fusion transcripts differ by the presence of additional *EWS* sequences encoded by either exons 8 and 9 or 8, 9, and 10 of *EWS* and always include exons encoding the DNA-binding domain of *FLI-*1 (*Ets*-domain).[212, 213] In about 90% of Ewing's sarcoma and PNET, *EWS-FLI-*1 fusion transcripts resulting from t(11;22) can be detected; most of the remaining cases express a novel protein in which *EWS* sequences are fused to the DNA-binding domain of *ERG,* a close relative of *FLI-*1, resulting from the variant translocation t(21;22).[215]

The c-*myc* oncogene is highly expressed in Ewing's sarcoma and PNET, whereas it is never expressed in neuroblastomas. In contrast, N-*myc* is overexpressed in the majority of neuroblastomas, but is expressed at a low level or not at all in Ewing's sarcoma and PNET.[219] These differences may reflect unique biologic features of the precise cell of origin or the genetic events involved in the development of the respective malignancy. In transient transfection assays, *EWS-FLI-*1 up-regulates the activity of c-*myc* promoter constructs, suggesting that c-*myc* proto-oncogene expression in Ewing's sarcoma and PNET could be controlled by *EWS-FLI-*1.[8]

These results unite cytogenetic and molecular observations in Ewing's sarcoma and PNET: a tumor-specific translocation, a particular pattern of oncogene expression, molecular characterization of the translocation breakpoint on the protein level, and the regulatory influence of this protein on the oncogene expression pattern.

Protein Immunohistochemistry

The diagnosis of Ewing's sarcoma and PNET depends on conventional pathologic examination in conjunction with immunohistology, and will be complemented by karyotype analysis to demonstrate the presence of t(11;22) or variant translocations, and RT-PCR to demonstrate specific transcripts in these tumors and in their metastases (see Chapter 14).

Cell culture studies of Ewing's sarcoma revealed evidence of the neuroectodermal origin of the cells (see Chapter 3). Ganglioside G_{D2}, found to be expressed on neuroblastomas,[220] was also present on the majority of Ewing's sarcoma cell lines.[221] Another neuroectoderm-associated glycolipid was detected in Ewing's sarcoma cells by staining with the *HNK-*1 antibody,[222] and other antigens present on neuroectodermal tumors were detected on Ewing's sarcoma cell lines using antibodies to nerve growth factor receptor,[223, 224] neuron-specific enolase, synaptophysin,[225] and neural cell adhesion molecule.[226]

The *MIC2* antigen (CD99) is a 30 to 32 kD cell-surface glycoprotein encoded by *MIC2,* a gene located in the homologous (pseudoautosomal) portion of chromosomes X and Y.[227] The biologic function and significance of the expression of *MIC2* in Ewing's sarcoma and PNET is unclear. *MIC2* is highly expressed in more than 90% of Ewing's sarcoma and PNET, and IHC studies can detect $p30/32^{MIC2}$ in formalin-fixed, paraffin-embedded tissues, including those that have been decalcified.[228, 229] Other tumors occasionally show *MIC2* immunoreactivity, including rhabdomyosarcoma and lymphoblastic lymphoma. It is therefore essential to use a panel of antibodies in diagnostic work, and/or employ molecular techniques such as RT-PCR to confirm the diagnosis (see also Chapter 14).[230, 231]

Lymphomas

Primary lymphomas are uncommon tumors of bone, and are defined as malignant lymphomas arising within a cavity of a single bone without concurrent regional or visceral involvement within a 6-month period.[232] Primary lymphoma of bone is associated with a better prognosis than that of more disseminated lymphoma or other small round cell malignancies such as Ewing's sarcoma.[232] Therefore, the correct diagnosis has important clinical and therapeutic implications. The group of primary bone lymphomas consists mainly of non-Hodgkin's lymphomas (NHLs),[232] and Hodgkin's lymphomas are very rare.[232, 233]

The NHLs of bone are mostly of centroblastic type, followed by the centroblastic-centrocytic and immunoblastic lymphoma.[232–234] In the last decade, immunohistochemical methods have made a major contribution to the diagnosis and classification of lymphoma[234, 235] and have shown that primary bone lymphomas are negative for T-cell markers but express a variety of B-cell markers, including immunoglobulin heavy and light chains.[236, 237] Therefore, immunophenotyping of lymphoma should cover the B-cell markers, T-cell markers, and markers of the myelomonocytic lineage to exclude acute nonlymphocytic leukemia.

An unique biologic property of the lymphocytes is their ability to rearrange the genes coding for immunoglobulins and the T-cell receptor (TCR) in order to execute their specific function in the immune system.[48, 237] Because these rearrangements are clonal, molecular biologic analysis of the immunoreceptors can be used to confirm the diagnosis of a lymphoma and to track the persistence of malignant clones whose rearrangements were determined at diagnosis.[47] Because the *IgH* gene is rearranged in nearly all B-cell lymphomas, it should be the first target of diagnostic investigations.[236, 237]

In T-cell and B-cell malignancies, similar mechanisms exist that lead to oncogene deregulation.[48, 237] Within the immunoglobulin and TCR loci, the sites of physiologic rearrangement become subject to abnormal breakage, resulting in malignancies. Breaks within switch regions or recombinase sites of the immunoglobulin locus at chromosome 14 have been described for a number of B-cell lymphomas, for endemic and sporadic Burkitt's lymphoma t(8;14) combining part of the *IgH* gene with the c-*myc* oncogene, and for follicular lymphoma (centroblastic-centrocytic) t(14;18).[48, 238] In the latter group of NHL, *BCL2* gene function on 18q21 is disrupted by the t(14q32;18q21) translocation, resulting in the prevention of apoptosis.[237, 238] Other genetic markers in B-cell lymphoma are the *BCL1* on chromosome 11[239] and *BCL6* in the chromosome 3q27 region.[240] In some B-cell malignancies, p53 mutations have been detected.[56] NHL of bone might be diagnosed by conventional histologic and immunologic methods, but the detection of molecular markers seems to be highly useful in understanding its pathogenesis and monitoring the clinical course (see Chapter 14).[47, 48, 237]

SELECTED METHODS IN DETAIL

Nucleic Acid Analysis

Isolation of Nucleic Acids

For analyzing DNA and RNA from small pieces of tumor tissue, we have found it suitable to link a well-proven RNA isolation method with a procedure for DNA isolation.[112, 241] Tissue frozen in liquid nitrogen is pulverized using a micro-dismembrator (Biotech International) followed by gentle homogenization in 4 M guanidinthiocyanate. This lysate is layered on a cushion of 5.7 M CsCl, and the RNA is sedimented by ultracentrifugation and solubilized in diethylpyrocarbonate (DEPC) containing water (to inhibit ribonucleases).[242, 243] The DNA remaining in the cushion is recovered in water followed by extraction (two times) with phenol-chloroform-isoamylethanol (PCI) (25:24:1) and extraction (three times) with chloroform-isoamylethanol. To optimize purification, DNA and RNA are repeatedly precipitated with two volumes of absolute ethanol after the addition of 1/10 of 3 M sodium acetate. Photometric analysis and ethidium bromide staining of size-fractionated aliquots of DNA and RNA during agarose gel electrophoresis serves to determine the quantity and quality of isolated nucleic acids.[244] Rapid isolation kits for the simultaneous preparation of DNA and RNA (and protein) are now available (e.g., Biozym, Gentra Systems, Minneapolis) and should be suitable for bone specimens.

Digestion of DNA with Restriction Enzymes and Southern Hybridization

A reaction mixture of 60 μL (sterile) is set up on ice and contains 5 to 10 μg of genomic DNA; 6 μL of the recommended 10-fold concentrated restriction buffer; usually 5–10 U of the appropriate restriction enzyme/1 μg of DNA; and aqua bidest to 60 μL (1 U is the amount of enzyme needed for complete digestion of 1 μg of lambda DNA under optimal conditions).[245–248] In practice, an excess of enzyme and a prolonged incubation time might be used. For digestion with several enzymes, a single buffer is used (One For All Buffer, Gibco). After overnight incubation at the appropriate temperature (mostly 37°C) a 1/10 aliquot is checked in a mini-gel (2 hours, 50 V) (BioRad MiniSub) to prove complete digestion of DNA.

The digested DNA samples are heat-denaturated (5 minutes, 78°C), immediately chilled on ice to prevent renaturation, mixed with one-sixth volume of a sixfold glycerol-dye loading buffer, and size-fractionated in a 0.8% agarose gel (249) in 1-fold TAE buffer (0.04 M Tris-acetate, 0.001 M EDTA, pH 8.0) containing 0.5 μg/mL ethidium bromide.[249, 250] A size standard is loaded into one outwardly directed slot. After overnight electrophoresis at 20 V in horizontal, standard-sized (20 × 20 cm) electrophoresis systems, the fractionated DNA is visualized by UV light and a photograph of the gel, including a ruler beside the DNA standard, is taken for later size determination of hybridized fragments. Subsequently, the DNA is partially nicked, denaturated, and neutralized by gentle agitation of the gel in the appropriate solution at room temperature (5 minutes in 0.2 N HCl; rinse in water; 45 minutes in 5 M NaCl, 0.5 M NaOH; rinse in water; 2 × 30 minutes in 1 M Tris pH 7.4, 1.5 M NaCl). The capillary transfer of the DNA is performed as described elsewhere,[245] except that Gene Screen Plus Membrane (DuPont) is used. After (overnight) blotting, the membrane is soaked for 45 seconds in 0.4 M NaOH, for 30 seconds in 2-fold concentrated SSC (20-fold concentrated stock solution: 3 M sodium chloride, 0.3 M sodium citrate pH 7.0), 0.2 M Tris, followed by air drying.

Prehybridization of the membrane is performed in a tube by constant rotation (Hybridiser HB-1, Techne) for 4 hours at 65°C in 10 to 20 mL of the hybridization mixture (sterile) containing: 0.5-fold SSPE (20-fold concentrated stock solution: 3 M NaCl, 0.2 M NaH_2PO_4 pH 7.4, 0.02 M Na_2 EDTA), 6% PEG (polyethyleneglycol), 0.5% SDS (sodium dodecylsulphate), and 2.5-fold Denhardt's solution (10-fold concentrated stock solution: 2% bovine serum albumin, 2% polyvinylpyrrolidone, 2% Ficoll 400). To prevent nonspecific hybridization, herring sperm DNA (HS-DNA) is heat-denaturated and immediately cooled on ice to get single strands (ssDNA) and added to a final concentration of 10 μg/mL cocktail. Hybridization is performed overnight at 65°C after the addition of 1 to 2 × 10^6 cpm of the isotopic labeled ssDNA probe. After hybridization, the membranes are washed to remove the nonspecific bound labeled probe: 2 × 5 minutes at room temperature in 2-fold concentrated SSC, 0.1% SDS; 2 × 30 minutes at 65°C (water bath) in 2-fold concentrated SSC, 0.1% SDS; 2 × 30 minutes at 65°C in 1-fold concentrated SSC, 0.1% SDS. If necessary, an additional wash in 0.5-fold concentrated SSC, 0.1% SDS is performed. The stringency of hybridization and washing varies with the gene probe used.

Northern Hybridization

Usually, 20 μg of total cellular RNA or 1 to 3 μg of poly A^+–enriched RNA are size-fractionated during denaturing and 1.2% agarose gel electrophoresis (20 × 20 cm, horizontal) containing 2.2 M formaldehyde, as described elsewhere,[242, 243] and transferred to Gene Screen Plus membrane as described for Southern transfer, except that the gel is placed in the inverted direction for blotting (slots in contact with the filter papers).

Prehybridization is performed at 65°C by constant rotation in 10 to 20 mL hybridization cocktail containing 3-fold concentrated SSC, 10% dextran sulfate, 1% SDS, 10-fold concentrated Denhardt's solution, and 10 μg/mL ssHS-DNA. After 4 hours, 0.5 to 1 × 10^6 cpm/mL of the labeled ssDNA probe is added. After (overnight) hybridization at 65°C, filters are washed, usually in 3-fold concentrated SSC, 2 × 5 minutes at room temperature, 2 × 5 minutes at room temperature in 3-fold concentrated SSC, 1% SDS; 2 × 15 minutes at 65°C in 3-fold concentrated SSC, 1% SDS; 2 × 15 minutes at 65°C in 2-fold concentrated SSC, 1% SDS (if necessary 2 × 15 minutes at 65°C in 1-fold concentrated SSC, 1% SDS).

Because of the toxic vapors, this technique should be performed in a chemical hood. Melt the appropriate amount of agarose in water and cool to 60°C. Mix one part of a 12.3 M formaldehyde stock solution (37%) with 3.5 parts of the cooled agarose and 1.1 parts of 5-fold concentrated formaldehyde gel running buffer to get a final concentration of 2.2 M formaldehyde and 1-fold concentrated running buffer. Cast the gel and allow it to set for at least 30 minutes.

For the preparation of 5-fold concentrated formaldehyde gel running buffer (0.1 M MOPS pH 7.0, 40 mM sodium acetate, 5 mM EDTA pH 8.0), dissolve 20.6 g of MOPS (3-N-morpho-lino-2-propane sulfonic acid) in 800 mL DEPC-treated water and adjust the pH to 7.0 with 2 M NaOH, add 10 mL of DEPC-treated EDTA pH 8.0, and adjust to 1 L with DEPC-treated water. Sterilize by filtration or autoclave and protect it from light. Straw-colored buffer works well; darker buffer does not.

For sample preparation, mix in a sterile tube 4.5 μL of RNA (up to 30 μg) with 2.0 μL of 5-fold concentrated running buffer, 3.5 μL of 12.3 M formaldehyde, and 10 μL of deionized formamide. Incubate the samples at 65°C for 15 minutes and chill them on ice. Add 2 μL of gel loading buffer containing 50% glycerol, 1 mM EDTA pH 8.0, 0.25% bromphenol blue, and 0.25 % xylene cyanol FF. Immediately before loading the samples (including a size standard), prerun the gel for 5 minutes at 5 V/cm. Run the gel in 1-fold concentrated running buffer for about 4 hours until the bromphenol blue dye has migrated approximately 8 cm. After 2 hours, take half of the buffer from each reservoir and return it to the opposite reservoir. Cut the lane containing the RNA standard and stain with ethidium bromide (0.5 μg/mL in 0.1 M ammonium acetate) for 45 minutes and photograph the marker beside a ruler. Rinse the gel with several changes of DEPC-treated water and hydrolyze the RNA for optimal transfer with 0.05 M NaOH for 20 minutes. Rinse it with DEPC-treated water and incubate the gel then in 20-fold concentrated SSC for 45 minutes. After hydrolization, the RNA can be transferred by the identical blotting procedure as for DNA except that the gel is placed in the inverted direction for capillary blotting on the 3MM paper.[242, 243]

Probe Labeling

For probe labeling, 25 ng of the ssDNA template (5 minutes at 100°C, immediately cooled on ice) are labeled with alpha ^{32}dCTP according to the random primed DNA labeling method (e.g., Gibco BRL Life Technologies, Inc.), and unincorporated nucleotides are removed by passing through a Sephadex G 50 spin column.[251]

We used the following gene-specific probes when examining tumors for gross structural alterations, increased gene copy numbers, and altered RNA expression: *RB*1 gene (pRB 3.8 and pRB 0.9),[110] p53 gene (p4.2 R),[252] *MDM*2 gene,[132] *SAS* gene,[140] and an actin control probe.[112]

Analysis of DNA and RNA Filters and Removal of Probes

After exposure to Kodak XAR 5 x-ray films at −80°C with the addition of intensifying screens, the signal intensities can be quantified by densitometric measurement. When the examination with one gene probe is completed, the probe can be removed prior to additional hybridization. Southern filters incubate firstly in 0.4 M NaOH at 42°C for 30 minutes and secondly in 0.1-fold concentrated SSC, 0.1% SDS, 0.2 M Tris HCl pH 7.5; Northern filters rinse several times with a boiling solution of 0.01-fold concentrated SSC, 0.01% SDS.

Standard Polymerase Chain Reaction Amplification Protocol

Typical primers are 18 to 30 nucleotides in length, having about 50% of G+C content, minimal self-complementarity, and low complementarity to each other, particularly at the 3′ end.[253] Complete denaturation of the template DNA is essential for optimal product yield.[254, 255] The annealing temperature (55–80°C) might be empirically optimized starting at 55°C. Stringent annealing temperatures enhance the specificity of the annealing reaction. Usually elongation is carried out at 72°C. The Mg^{2+} concentration is a very crucial point and should be optimized (usually 0.5–10 mM).[253–255] For efficient amplification of difficult templates, it may help to modify the melting behavior of DNA by the addition of dimethylsulfoxide to the PCR reaction, up to a final concentration of 2.5%. Special PCR buffers are now available that should eliminate the need for optimization of individual primer-template systems (e.g., Quiagen PCR buffer systems, Hilden, Germany). A 100 μL standard reaction mixture contains (according to Ampli Taq, Perkin Elmer Cetus) about 500 ng of genomic DNA, 10 μL 10-fold concentrated PCR reaction buffer (500 mM KCl, 100 mM

Tris pH 8.3, 15 mM $MgCl_2$, 0.1% gelatin), 50 pmol primer upstream, 50 pmol primer downstream, and 0.2 mM each dNTP, 2.5 U Taq polymerase enzyme, and aqua bidest to 100 μL. It can be overlaid with 100 μL of light mineral oil to prevent evaporation (not necessary in water-bath thermocycler). After the initial denaturation step for 5 to 10 minutes at 94°C, 25 to 35 cycles are carried out as follows: denaturation at 94°C for 30 to 60 seconds; annealing at 55°C for 30 to 60 seconds; elongation at 72°C for 30 to 60 seconds. A final extension step at 72°C for 5 to 10 minutes is recommended. To reduce the number of pipetting steps, a mixture containing buffer, dNTPs, primers, and Taq polymerase can be used. Avoid carrying over traces of DNA from one reaction tube to another or contaminating stock solutions. Always include DNA-free controls to check for contamination. The efficiency of the reaction can be checked by running 1/10 of the PCR and a suitable DNA size standard on a 2% NuSieve/1% Seakem agarose gel (FMC Corp., Rockland, ME).

Reverse Transcriptase Polymerase Chain Reaction

Total RNA from frozen primary tumors is extracted by first cutting approximately five 5 μm thick sections at −20°C from unfixed frozen tissue. The sections are then placed in precooled autoclaved 1.5 mL microfuge tubes, and RNA is extracted according to standard methods.[256]

Complementary DNA (cDNA) is generated in a 20 μL reaction by first adding 14 μg of total RNA to 50 mM Tris HCl (pH 8.3) containing 75 mM KCl, 3 mM $MgCl_2$, 10 mM dithiothreitol, 1 mM deoxynucleotide triphosphate, and 100 pmol random hexanucleotide primers (Boehringer). This solution is heated to 95°C for 5 minutes and cooled slowly to room temperature. Then 20 U recombinant human placental RNAse inhibitor (Promega) and 100 U Moloney murine leukemia virus (MMLV) reverse transcriptase (Gibco) are added and the solution is incubated at 37°C for 90 minutes. The reverse transcriptase is then inactivated by heating to 95°C for 3 minutes; cDNA is used immediately or stored at −20°C.

Polymerase chain reaction is carried out in a 50 μL reaction containing 1 to 5 μL cDNA template, 200 μM deoxynucleotide triphosphates, 50 pmol of each oligonucleotide primer, and 2.5 U Taq polymerase (Perkin-Elmer Cetus) in a 8 mM Tris HCl buffer (pH 8.3) containing 40 mM KCl, 1.5 mM $MgCl_2$, and 0.0008% gelatin.

Oligonucleotide primers used for RT-PCR t(11;22) are:

(FLI-1) 5′ACT CCC CGT TGG TCC CCT CC 3′
(EWS) 5′TCC TAC AGC CAA GCT CCA AGT C3′

Oligonucleotide primers used for RT-PCR t(21;22) are:

(EWS) 5′TCC TAC AGC CAA GCT CCA AG3′
(ERG) 5′ACT CCC CGT TGG TGC CTT CC3′

Thirty-five cycles of PCR are performed, with each cycle including denaturation at 94°C for 30 seconds, annealing at 65°C for 60 seconds, and extension at 72°C for 120 seconds (Biomed Cycler). PCR is preceded by a 4-minute incubation at 94°C. Amplified products are identified by gel electrophoresis (2% agarose gels) and ethidium-bromide staining.

Single-Strand Conformational Polymorphism Analysis

After 100- to 500-fold dilution of the PCR reaction mixture with loading buffer (90% formamide, 20 mM EDTA, 0.05% xylene cyanol FF, and 0.05% bromphenol blue) and heat denaturation, samples are kept on ice until they are applied to a nondenaturing 6% polyacrylamide gel containing 90 mM Tris-borate, pH 8.3, and 4 mM EDTA. Analysis should be performed in parallel gels with and without 10% glycerol. Electrophoresis is carried out at 30 V for 2 to 10 hours, depending on the size of the PCR product.[257] DNA bands can be visualized at high sensitivity by silver staining of the gel according to the kit instructions (Bio Rad, Munich, Germany); therefore, isotopic labeling can be omitted.[57] For p53 screening, suitable PCR-SSCP primers are described elsewhere.[257]

TGGE for Rapid Screening of the Exons 5, 6, 7, and 8 of the p53 Gene

Sequences not complementary to the template can be added to the 5′ end of the primer and become incorporated into the created double strands by PCR. Hence, restriction sites can be created, or a GC-clamp can be attached, to make sure that the highest melting temperature is located outside the investigated region.[258]

For p53 screening, we set up a 50 μL reaction in a sterile microcentrifuge tube containing 10 mM Tris HCL, pH 8.3; 1.5 mM $MgCl_2$, 50 mM KCl, 200 μM dNTP each, 25 pmol primer upstream and 25 pmol primer downstream, about 500 ng genomic template DNA, 1 U Taq DNA polymerase, and sterile double distillated water.

The following primers were used[57]:

exon 5: forward (GC_{40}) TTCCTCTTCCTACAGTACTC
reverse CTGGGCAACCAGCCCTGTCGT
exon 6: forward (GC_{40}) ACGACAGGGCTGGTTGCCCA
reverse AGTTGCAAACCAGACCTCAG
exon 7: forward (GC_{40}) TCTCCTAGGTTGGCTCTGACTG
reverse GCAAGTGGCTCCTGACCTGG
exon 8: forward CCTATCCTGAGTAGTGGTAATC
reverse (GC_{40}) CCGCTTCTTGTCCTGCTTGCTT
GC_{40}: CGCCCGCCGCGCCCCGCGCCCGGC CCGCCGCCCCCGCCCG.[90]

Polymerase chain reaction is performed under following conditions (usually 35 cycles, with pretreatment at 94°C for 5 minutes as well as post-treatment at 55°C for 60 seconds; 72°C for 7 minutes; and 18°C overnight) in a waterbath thermocycler (Autogene II, Grant):

exon 5: 60°C, 30 seconds; 72°C, 60 seconds; 94,5°C, 30 seconds
exons 6, 8: 55°C, 30 seconds; 72°C, 60 seconds; 94,5°C, 30 seconds
exon 7: 65°C, 30 seconds; 72°C, 60 seconds; 94,5°C, 30 seconds

Samples are purified by extraction with PCI (25:24:1), precipitated with ethanol, and redissolved in 30 μL TGGE running buffer (20 mM MOPS, 1 mM EDTA, pH 8.0) and applied to a 5% polyacrylamide gel (in 4 M urea, 20 mM MOPS, and 1mM EDTA, pH 8.0). Electrophoresis at 250 V is carried out in parallel orientation to the temperature gradient (Quiagen, Hilden, Germany), which is applied after the samples have run into the gel for a distinct run-in time.

The optimal temperature gradient and running conditions for each exon analysis[57] are:

exon 5: run-in time (20°C): 120 minutes, apply temperature gradient: 45°C–75°C, running time: 3 hours
exon 7: run-in time (20°C): 40 minutes, apply temperature gradient: 40°C–75°C, running time: 2h 40 minutes
exon 8: run-in time (20°C): 180 minutes, apply temperature gradient: 40°C–78°C, running time: 3 hours

The DNA bands were visualized by silver staining (Quiagen, Hilden, Germany). Homozygous mutations are indicated by one aberrant band compared with the wild-type control. If mutant and wild-type p53 alleles are present in the tissue sample, four bands are present.[57]

Direct Sequencing

Genomic DNA that shows a mutant pattern during TGGE is sequenced using the exon-specific primers without the GC-clamp. Two primer pairs are created: the forward primer is biotinylated, and to the reverse primer, a M13 sequence is added, and vice versa. After purification of PCR products (Qiaex, Diagen, Hilden) and binding to Dynabeads M-280 (Dynal, Oslo, Norway), strand separation takes place. The biotinylated strand of both reactions is sequenced using Sequenase Version 2.0 (United States Biochemicals) and the M13 universal sequence primer. Hence, the mutation is confirmed on the sense and antisense strand. ^{35}S isotopic labeled products are size-fractionated on a 6% polyacrylamide gel electrophoresis (BRL, Life Technologie SA electrophoresis apparatus). Alternatively, the DNA can be eluted from the homodimer mutant band prior to reamplification and sequencing.

Fluorescent In Situ Suppression Hybridization

DNA probes for in situ hybridization of t(11;22) are cosmid clones 23.2 (D11S374) and 5.8 (D11S372), located centromeric and telomeric to the t(11;22)(q24;q12) breakpoint on chromosome 11q24. Labeled cosmid clones are hybridized to chromosome preparations or nuclei from Ewing's sarcoma and PNET. Detection of labeled DNA is performed with fluorescein-conjugated avidin. Hybridization of repetitive sequences to nontargeted chromosomes is suppressed by a preannealing step with human *ALU* repeat DNA (FISSH). Cohybridization with competitor DNAs has not been performed in the absence of repetitive sequences of the hybridization probe (FISH).

Short-Term Cultures. Fresh tumors are minced into small pieces and incubated for 1 hour at 37°C in 2 mg/mL collagenase type I (Sigma) in phosphate-buffered saline (PBS). The solution is repeatedly vortexed to facilitate the detachment of tumor cells from the stroma. The supernatant is collected and centrifuged at 400 g for 10 minutes. The cell pellet is washed twice in IMDM (Iscove's modified Dulbecco's medium) medium containing 15% fetal calf serum. Cells are seeded in 25 cm^2 flasks previously coated with fibronectin (Collaborative Research), with IMDM supplemented with 15% FCS (Gibco), 1% bovine pituitary extract, and 0.5% mito plus serum extender. Cultures are incubated at 37°C in a humidified atmosphere of 5% CO_2. Cells are harvested by trypsinization within 4 days after the establishment of the culture, washed twice in cold PBS, treated in a hypotonic solution of 0.075 M KCl for 30 minutes, and fixed with three changes of methanol-acetic acid (3:1).

Direct Harvesting for Interphase Nuclei Preparations. Cells obtained from the disaggregation of the biopsy specimen are washed twice in cold PBS, treated in a hypotonic solution of 0.075 M KCl for 30 minutes, and fixed with three changes of methanol-acetic acid (3:1).

Preparation of Metaphase Chromosomes. Metaphase spreads are prepared following standard techniques.

Biotin-Labeling. Twenty-five to 50 ng of DNA are treated for 1 hour at 14°C with a dilution 1:1000 of 1 mg/mL DNAse1. Labeling is performed using a random primer extension reaction.[251] To increase biotin incorporation, dTTP is replaced with bio-11-dUTP, and dCTP is replaced with bio-11-dCTP, each at 20 μm final concentration. The random primer reaction is carried out using a labeling system according to manufacturer's instructions (BRL). After labeling, the cosmid probes are purified from unincorporated nucleotides by passing the reaction mixture through Sephadex G-50 (Pharmacia) in 1 mL spin columns.

Hybridization. Before hybridization, the metaphase chromosomes are treated with RNase (100 μg/mL in 0.3 M NaCl, 30 mM sodium citrate–2-fold concentrated SSC) for 1 hour at 37°C, followed by dehydration in a series of 70%, 85%, and 100% ethanol baths. Proteinase K digestion is then carried out at a concentration of 0.5 μg/mL in 20 mM Tris–2 mM $CaCl_2$ at 37°C for 7 minutes. Slides are fixed in 4% paraformaldehyde in PBS plus 50 mM $MgCl_2$ at room temperature for 10 minutes. To obtain chromosome denaturation, slides are immersed in 70% formamide–2-fold concentrated SSC (pH 7.0) at 75°C for 2 minutes, then dehydrated in an ice-cold 70%, 85%, and 100% ethanol series.

Hybridization is carried out as follows: 25 to 50 ng of biotinylated cosmid DNA is precipitated with 2 μg of human placental DNA, 1 to 2 μg of human *ALU* repeat DNA probe, pBLUR8 and 7 μg of salmon sperm DNA. All competitor DNAs and salmon sperm DNA are ribonuclease-treated, extracted with phenol and chloroform, and sonicated to a final size range of 200 to 400 bp. The biotinylated cosmid probes, coprecipitated with the competitor DNAs, are resuspended in 10 μL of hybridization buffer (50% formamide–2-fold concentrated SSC (pH 7), final concentration, 10% dextran sulfate) and then denaturated at 75°C for 5 minutes. Preannealing of repetitive DNA sequences is carried out for 30 minutes at 42°C before application of the hybridization mixture to the denatured slides.

Hybridization is carried out at 37°C for 16 to 24 hours in a humidified chamber. Posthybridization washes of the slides are carried out as described.[71] The slides are then treated with alternating layers of fluoresceinated avidin and biotinylated goat anti-avidin (Vector), both at 5 μg/mL, until two layers of avidin are applied. The avidin and goat anti-avidin treatments are separated by three washes of 3 minutes each in 4-fold concentrated SSC, 4-fold concentrated SSC–0.1% Triton X, and PN buffer (0.1 M phosphate buffer [pH8]–0.1% Nonidet P-40), respectively. After the final avidin treatment, a fluorescence antifade solution (254) containing 200 μg/L of propidium iodide to stain double-stranded DNA, is applied to the slides under a coverslip.

Microscopy. The slides are evaluated on a Zeiss Axiophot fluorescence microscope. Narrow band pass filters are used to obtain separate images of each fluorochrome (550 nm filter for FITC; 610 nm filter for propidium iodide). The fluorescence signals are quantitated directly. Photographs in epifluorescence mode are taken.

Protein Analysis

Immunohistochemical Staining of Tissue Sections

Sections 5 μm thick are cut from paraffinized tissues, heated at 60°C for 15 minutes, and deparaffinized. For frozen tissues, 4 to 7 μm cryostat sections are cut, dried for 4 to 25 hours at 20°C, fixed in acetone for 30 minutes, and then washed with TBS (0.05 M Tris, 0.1 M NaCl; pH 7.6).

Peroxidase Detection. Tissue sections are rehydrated in PBS solution. Slides are pretreated with 0.05% saponin in distilled water for 30 minutes at room temperature, followed by washes with distilled water and PBS. The tissue is then set in 0.2% Tween20 in PBS for 30 minutes, washed in PBS without Tween20, blocked in 10% normal horse serum with calcium- and magnesium-free PBS (CMF/PBS) for 30 minutes, and then allowed to incubate overnight in a moist chamber with primary antibody (1 μg/mL) in 10% normal horse serum with 0.05% Tween20 at 4°C. Then the tissue sections are washed in PBS with 0.05% Tween20, followed by incubation with biotinylated horse anti-mouse serum (Vector Laboratories, Burlingham, CA) at 1:200 in 10% normal horse serum with 0.05% Tween20 for 30 minutes at room temperature. The endogenous peroxidase is subsequently blocked in 3% H_2O_2 in CMF/PBS, 0.05% Tween20, and 0.1% sodium azide for 30 minutes. The tissues are then washed and stained with use of the Vector Elite avidin-biotin-complex immunoperoxidase kit (Vector Laboratories) for 30 minutes. The final reaction product is revealed by the diaminobenzidine reaction. Finally, the sections are washed, counterstained with hematoxylin blue in PBS, and washed again before being dehydrated through graded alcohols, cleared in xylene, and placed under coverslips. The presence of immunoreactivity for the antigen is indicated by dark brown staining.

APAAP Detection. Tissue sections are incubated with the first antibody (recognizing a specific antigen: e.g. mouse antibody) for 30 minutes at 20°C. After washing with TBS, rabbit anti-mouse IgG is added followed by the APAAP complex (DAKO, Glostrup, Denmark). The APAAP complex is visualized with fast red. Sections are counterstained with Mayer's acid hemalum.

Western Blotting

Polyacrylamide-SDS Gel. Mix 25 mL of deionized 30% acrylamide-bisacrylamide with 15 mL of 4-fold concentrated running gel buffer (1.5 M TrisHCl, 0.4% SDS [pH8.8]) and 100 μL of ammonium persulfate. Bring volume to 60 mL with H_2O. This gives a 12.5% gel; the percentage of acrylamide can be changed, depending on the protein size. Attach clean glass plates to each other, separated by a lightly greased spacer. Add 30 μL TEMED to catalyze polymerization. Pour the 60 mL into the prepared plates and gently layer a few milliliters of 2-fold concentrated stacking gel buffer (0.25 M TrisHCl, 0.2% SDS [pH6.8]) on top to form a flat surface while the acrylamide polymerizes. After 1 hour, pour the upper unpolymerized liquid out. Prepare a top "stacking gel" gel. Mix 1 mL of 30% acrylamide-bisacrylamide (29:1), 4 mL of H_2O, 5 mL 2-fold concentrated stacking gel buffer, 10 μL ammonium persulfate, and 5 μL TEMED. Pour enough of this stacking gel mixture to fill the upper 3 cm of the gel. Insert sample position-forming comb, and allow the stacking gel to polymerize. The addition of the stacking gel sharpens the bands and increases resolution. Attach gel to electrophoresis unit and add approximately 500 mL 1-fold concentrated electrode buffer (30.25 g Tris base [0.25M], 144 g glycine, add H_2O to 850 mL [pH8.3], 100 mL 10% SDS, add 1 L with H_2O) to both top and bottom chambers and check for leaks. Clean sample wells by pipetting electrode buffer in and out of each. Mix 10 μL of sample (1–100 μg protein) with 10 μL of 2-fold concentrated sample buffer (0.125 M TrisHCl, 4% SDS, 10% glycerol, 0.02% bromophenol blue, 4% β-mercaptoethanol). Heat to 95°C for 3 minutes and load samples on gel. Include molecular weight standards in one or two lanes. Run gel until the blue dye front just runs out of the gel. The typical setting is 100 V, for about 4 to 6 hours.

Transfer. The proteins in polyacrylamide gel are transferred electrophoretically to nitrocellulose filter (Electrophoretic Transfer Apparatus, BioRad). First, both the gel and the NC filter are rinsed in transfer buffer (12 g Tris, 57.65 g glycine, 4L H_2O; after Tris and glycine are dissolved, add 1l methanol, pH to 8.3, with HCl). Place NC filter against gel on flat surface. Smooth filter over gel by rolling with a 5 mL glass pipette to remove all air bubbles. Wrap a piece of 3MM filter paper (prewetted with transfer buffer) around the gel and filter to make a sandwich. Keep wet and avoid bubbles. The paper/gel/filter/paper sandwich is placed in the electrophoretic transfer apparatus, with the gel facing the cathode. Place in buffer tank and fill with transfer buffer to cover gel. Connect to power supply and run electrophoretic transfer. After transfer is complete, remove filter and gel from unit and discard gel. Float the filter in amido black until the molecular weight standards become visible; mark standard positions. Wash NC filter briefly in 100 mL H_2O. Incubate filter in blot buffer (5% w/v Carnation nonfat dry milk in PBS) for 1 hour at 37°C. Wash in PBS-Tween buffer (0.05% Tween20 in PBS) for 1 hour at room temperature. Seal filter inside plastic bag (seal as close as possible to filter to keep the inside volume small). Cut corner of bag to use as buffer entry port and close with dialysis clamp.

Antibody Reaction. Mix 100 μL of normal goat serum (NGS) with antibody (dilution will vary) in 10 mL of blot buffer, add to bag with filter and incubate for 2 hours at room temperature with rocking. Wash filter in a shallow dish with four changes of 75 mL of PBS-Tween buffer for a total of 300 mL over 30 minutes. Add biotinylated goat anti-rabbit immunoglobulin G (40 μL in 10 mL blot buffer with 100 μL NGS) (Vector) to bag. Incubate for 1 hour at room temperature with rocking. Wash filter again in a shallow dish with four changes of 7 mL of PBS-Tween buffer for a total of 300 mL over 30 minutes. Add avidin-HRP (40 μL in 10 mL of blot buffer with 100 μL of NGS) (Vector). Incubate for 30 minutes at room temperature with rocking. Wash filter again in a shallow dish with four changes of 75 mL of PBS-Tween buffer for a total of 300 mL over 30 minutes. Make color indicator-substrate (mix 3 mL color indicator stock solution [4-chloro-1-naphtol (3 mg/mL H_2O)] with 9 mL PBS and add 150 μL of 1% hydrogen peroxide). Use immediately. Incubate at room temperature with rocking until purple color develops and background begins to be detectable (1–10 minutes). Transfer filter and wash in another container containing H_2O to halt color development. Air-dry. Store in a plastic bag in the dark.

Acknowledgments

The authors are very grateful to B. Weber, E. Scholten, and S. Torggler for their invaluable help, and to the Elternforderge-meinschaft for the financial support of their work.

REFERENCES

1. Varmus H: An historical overview of oncogenes. *In* Weinberg RA (ed): Oncogenes and the Molecular Origins of Cancer. New York, Cold Spring Harbor, 1989, p 3.
2. Stehlin D, Varmus HE, Biskop JM, et al: DNA related to the transforming genes of avian sarcoma virus is present in normal avian DNA. Nature 260:170, 1976.
3. Schwab M, Alitalo K, Klempnauer K, et al: Amplified DNA with limited homology to myc-cellular oncogene is shared by human neuroblastoma cell lines and a neuroblastoma tumor. Nature 305:245, 1983.
4. Berns EMJC, Klein IGM, Van Putten C, et al: C-myc amplification is a better prognostic factor in primary breast cancer. Cancer Res 52:1107, 1992.
5. Khatib ZA, Matsushime H, Valentine M, et al: Coamplification of the CDK4 gene with MDM2 and GLI in human sarcomas. Cancer Res 53:5535, 1993.
6. Jankowski SA, Mitchell DS, Smith SH, et al: SAS, a gene amplified in human sarcomas encodes a new member of the transmembrane 4 superfamily of proteins. Oncogene 9:1205, 1994.
7. Heisterkamp N, Stephenson IR, Groffen J, et al: Localization of the abl oncogene adjacent to a translocation breakpoint in chronic myelocytic leukemias. Nature 306:239, 1983.
8. Bailly RA, Bosselut R, Zucman J, et al: DNA-binding and transcriptional activation properties of the EWS-FLI-1 fusion protein resulting from the t(11;22) translocation in Ewing sarcoma. Mol Cell Biol 14:3230, 1994.
9. Taub R, Kirsch J, Morton C, et al: Translocation of the myc gene into the immunoglobulin heavy chain locus in human Burkitt's lymphoma and murine plasmacytoma cells. Proc Natl Acad Sci 79:6922, 1982.
10. Weinberg RA: Tumor suppressor genes. Science 254:1138, 1991.
11. Malkin D, Friend SH: The role of tumor suppressor genes in familial cancer. Cancer Biol 3:121, 1992.
12. Ward JF: Biochemistry of DNA lesions. Radiat Res 104:103, 1985.
13. Harris CC: Chemical and physical carcinogenesis: Advances and perspectives for the 1990s. Cancer Res 51(suppl):5023, 1992.
14. Machowich S, de Grujl FR: Skin cancer and UV radiation. Nature 366:23, 1993.
15. Modrich P: Mismatch repair, genetic stability and cancer. Science 266:1959, 1959.
16. Dianov G, Lindahl T: Reconstitution of the base pair excision: Repair pathway. Curr Biol 4:1069, 1994.
17. Pero RW, Johnson DB, Markowitz M, et al: DNA repair synthesis in individuals with and without a family history of cancer. Carcinogenesis 10:6938, 1989.
18. Tanaka K, Miura N, Sotakata I, et al: Analysis of a human excision repair involved in group A xeroderma pigmentosum and containing a zinc finger domain. Nature 348:73, 1990.
19. Kastan MB, Zhon Q, El Diery WS, et al: A mammalian cell cycle checkpoint pathway utilizing p53 and GADD 45 is defective in ataxia telangiectasia. Cell 75:587, 1992.
20. Fishel R, Lesco MK, Rao MRS, et al: The human mutator gene homolog MSH 2 and its association with hereditary non-polyposis colon cancer. Cell 75:1027, 1993.
21. Knudson AG: Pediatric molecular oncology. Cancer 71(suppl):3320, 1993.
22. Toshiyasu H, Koeffler HP: Role of the cyclin-dependent kinase inhibitors in the development of cancer. Blood 86:841, 1995.

23. Paris J, Le Guellec R, Couturier A, et al: Cloning by differential screening of a xenopus cDNA coding for a protein highly homologous to cdc 2 protein. Proc Natl Acad Sci 88:1039, 1991.
24. Suriami V, Nurse P: The cell cycle control gene cdc2+ of fission yeast encodes a protein kinase potentially regulated by phosphorylation. Cell 45:261, 1986.
25. Donehower LA, Haevey M, Slagle BL, et al: Mice deficient for p53 are developmentally normal but susceptible to spontaneous tumors. Nature 356:215, 1992.
26. El-Diery WS, Tokino T, Velculescu VE, et al: WAF 1, a potential mediator of p53 tumor suppression. Cell 75:817, 1993.
27. Lane DP: p53 guardian of the genome. Nature 358:15, 1992.
28. Cho KR, Fearon ER: DCC: A potential link between tumor suppressor genes and altered cell surface interaction in cancer. Opin Gene Dev 5:72, 1995.
29. Fisher DE: Apoptosis in cancer therapy: Crossing the threshold. Cell 78:539, 1994.
30. Kim NW, Piatyszek MA, Prowse KR, et al: Specific association of human telomerase activity with immortal cells and cancer. Science 266:2011, 1994.
31. Holt SE, Skay JW, Wright WE: Defining the telomere: Telomerase hypothesis of aging and cancer. Nature Biotechnol 14:836, 1996.
32. Stuart ET, Yokota Y, Gruss P: PAX and HOX in neoplasia. *In* Hall JC, Dululap JC, (eds): Advances in Genetics. San Diego, Academic Press, 1995, p 255.
33. Blatt C: The betrayal of homeo box genes in normal development: The link to cancer. Cancer Cells 6:186, 1990.
34. Castronovo V, Kusaka M, Chariot A, et al: Homeobox genes: Potential candidates for the transcriptional control of the transformed phenotype and invasive phenotype. Biochem Pharmacol 47:137, 1994.
35. Counter CM, Hirte HW, Bacchetti S, et al: Telomerase activity in human ovarian cancer. Proc Natl Acad Sci 91:2900, 1994.
36. Gallili N, Davis RJ, Fredericks WJ, et al: Fusion of a forkhead domain gene to PAX3 in the solid tumor alveolar rhabdomyosarcoma. Nature Genet 5:230, 1993.
37. Hunger S, Galili N, Carroll AJ, et al: The t(1;19)(q23; p13) results in consistent fusion of E2A and PBX1 coding sequences in lymphoblastic leukemias. Blood 77:786, 1991.
38. Offit K, Brown K: Quantitating familial cancer risk: A resource for clinical oncologists. J Clin Oncol 12:1724, 1994.
39. Howley PM: Viral carcinogenesis. *In* Mendelsohn J, Howley PM, Israel MA, Liotta LA (eds): The Molecular Basis of Cancer. Philadelphia, WB Saunders, 1995, p 38.
40. Chang F, Syrgäenen S, Tervahauta A, et al: Tumourigenesis associated with the p53 tumor suppressor gene. Br J Cancer 68:653, 1993.
41. Vogelstein B, Kinzler KW: Carcinogens have fingerprints. Nature 355:209, 1992.
42. Brash DE, Rudolph JA, Simon JA, et al: A role for sunlight in skin cancer: UV-induced p53 mutations in squamous cell carcinoma. Proc Natl Acad Sci 88:10124, 1991.
43. Miller CW, Simon K, Aslo A, et al: p53 mutations in human lung tumors. Cancer Res 52:1695, 1992.
44. Hsu IC, Metcalf RA, Sun T, et al: Mutational hotspot in the p53 gene in human hepato-cellular carcinoma from southern Africa. Nature 350:427, 1991.
45. Hollstein M, Sidransky I, Vogelstein B, et al: p53 mutations in human cancers. Science 253:49, 1991.
46. Aquilar F, Hussain SP, Cerutti P: Aflatoxin B 1 induces the transversion of G-T in codon 249 of the p53 tumor suppressor gene in human hepatocytes. Proc Natl Acad Sci 90:8586, 1992.
47. Veelken H, Tycho B, Sklar J: Sensitive detection of clonal antigen receptor gene rearrangements for the diagnosis of lymphoid malignancies by a polymerase chain reaction-mediated ribonuclease protection assay. Blood 78:1318, 1991.
48. Gauwerky CE, Croce CM: Molecular genetics and cytogenetics of hematopoietic malignancies. *In* Mendelsohn J, Howley PM, Usrael MA, Liotta LA (eds): The molecular basis of cancer. Philadelphia, WB Saunders, 1995, p 18.
49. Scrable H, Witte J, Shimada H, et al: Molecular differential pathology of rhabdomyosarcoma. Genes Chrom Cancer 1:23, 1989.
50. Dias P, Parham DM, Shapiro DN, et al: Myogenic regulatory protein (Myo D1) expression in childhood solid tumors: Diagnostic utility in rhabdomyosarcoma. Am J Pathol 137:1283, 1990.
51. Thomas ED, Clift RA, Fefer A, et al: Bone marrow transplantation for the treatment of chronic myelogenous leukemia. Ann Intern Med 104:1556, 1986.
52. Forman SJ, O'Donnell MR, Nademance AP, et al: Bone marrow transplantation for patients with Philadelphia chromosome-positive acute lymphoblastic leukemia. Blood 70:587, 1987.
53. Thor AO, Moore DH, Edgerton SM, et al: Accumulation of p53 suppressor protein: Independent marker of prognosis in breast cancer. J Natl Cancer Inst 84:845, 1993.
54. Mitsudomi T, Oyama T, Kusano T, et al: Mutations of the p53 gene as a predictor of poor prognosis in patients with non-small-cell lung cancer. J Natl Cancer Inst 85:2018, 1993.
55. Remvikos Y, Tominaga O, Hammel P, et al: Increased p53 protein content of colorectal cancer correlates with poor survival. Br J Cancer 66:758, 1992.
56. Preudhomme C, Dervit I, Wattel E, et al: Clinical significance of p53 mutations in newly diagnosed Burkitt's lymphoma and acute lymphoblastic leukemia: A report of 48 cases. J Clin Oncol 13:812, 1995.
57. Scholz RB, Milde-Langosch K, Jung R, et al: Rapid screening for Tp53 by temperature gradient gel electrophoresis: A comparison with SSCP analysis. Hum Mol Genet 2:2155, 1993.
58. Grompe M: The rapid detection of unknown mutations in nucleic acids. Nature Genet 5:111, 1993.
59. Forrest S, Cotton R, Landegren U, et al: How to find all those mutations. Nature Genet 10:375, 1995.
60. Ishioka C, Frebourg T, Yan YX: Screening patients for heterozygous p53 mutations using a functional assay in yeast. Nature Genet 5:124, 1993.
61. Jonasson JA: Analysis and interpretation of human chromosome preparations. *In* Rooney DE, Czepulkowski BH (eds): Human Cytogenetics: A Practical Approach. Washington, DC, IRL Press, 1986, p 85.
62. Malcolm S, Cowell KK, Young BD: Specialist techniques in research and diagnostic clinical cytogenetics. *In* Rooney DE, Czepulkowski BH (eds): Human Cytogenetics: A Practical Approach. Washington, DC, IRL Press, 1986, p 197.

63. Taylor C, Patel K, Jones T, et al: Diagnosis of Ewing's sarcoma and peripheral neuroectodermal tumour based on the detection of t(11;22) using fluorescence in situ hybridization. Br J Cancer 67:128, 1993.
64. Pinkel D, Straume T, Gray JW: Cytogenetic analysis using quantitative high-sensitivity fluorescence hybridization. Proc Natl Acad Sci 83:2934, 1986.
65. Joos S, Bergerheim USR, Pan Y, et al: Mapping of chromosomal gains and losses in prostate cancer by comparative genomic hybridisation. Genes Chrom Cancer 14:267, 1995.
66. Cremer T, Lichter P, Borden J, et al: Detection of chromosome aberrations in metaphase and interphase tumor cells by in situ hybridization using chromosome-specific library probes. Hum Genet 80:235, 1988.
67. Bérubé D, Passage E, Mattei MG, et al: Fine mapping of the long arm of human chromosome 11 by in situ hybridization using different translocations, including the t(11;22) of Ewing sarcoma. Cytogenet Cell Genet 54:142, 1990.
68. Cherif D, Julier C, Delattre O, et al: Simultaneous localization of cosmids and chromosome R-banding by fluorescence microscopy: Application to regional mapping of human chromosome 11. Proc Natl Acad Sci 87:6639, 1990.
69. Lichter P, Tang CJC, Call K, et al: High-resolution mapping of human chromosome by in situ hybridization with cosmid clones. Science 247:64, 1990.
70. Trask BJ: Fluorescence in situ hybridization: Application in cytogenetics and gene mapping. Trends Genet 7:149, 1991.
71. Selleri L, Hermanson GG, Eubanks JH, et al: Molecular localization of the (q24;q12) translocation of Ewing's sarcoma by chromosomal in situ suppression hybridization. Proc Natl Acad Sci 88:887, 1991.
72. Christiansen H, Schestag J, Christiansen NM, et al: Clinical impact of chromosome 1 aberrations in neuroblastoma: A metaphase and interphase cytogenetic study. Genes Chrom Cancer 5:141, 1992.
73. Lichter P, Cremer T, Borden J, et al: Delineation of individual human chromosomes in metaphases and interphase cells by in situ suppression hybridization using recombinant DNA libraries. Hum Genet 80:224, 1988.
74. Tkachuk DC, Westbrook CA, Andreeff M, et al: Detection of bcr-abl fusion in chronic myelogenous leukemia by in situ hybridization. Science 250:559, 1990.
75. Kallioniemi A, Kallioniemi O-P, Piper J, et al: Comparative genomic hybridization for molecular cytogenetic analysis of solid tumors. Science 258:818, 1992.
76. Southern EM: Detection of specific sequences among DNA fragments separated by gel electrophoresis. J Mol Biol 98:503, 1975.
77. Darnell J, Lodish H, Baltimore D: Tools of molecular cell biology: Molecular Technology. *In* Darnell J, Lodish H, Baltimore D (eds): Molecular Cell Biology, New York, Scientific American Books, 1986, p 8.
78. Vogelstein B, Fearon ER, Kern SE, et al: Allelotype of colorectal carcinomas. Science 244:207, 1989.
79. Cavanee WK, Dryja TP, Phillips RA, et al: Expression of recessive alleles by chromosomal mechanisms in retinoblastoma. Nature 305:779, 1983.
80. Knudson AG: Mutation and cancer: Statistical study of retinoblastoma. Proc Natl Acad Sci 68:820, 1971.
81. Fearon ER, Cho KR, Nigro JM, et al: Identification of a chromosome 18q gene that is altered in colorectal cancers. Science 247:49, 1990.
82. Wiggs J, Nordenskjld M, Yandell D, et al: Prediction of the risk of hereditary retinoblastoma, using DNA polymorphisms within the retinoblastoma gene. N Engl J Med 318:151, 1988.
83. Feinberg AP: Genomic imprinting and gene activation in cancer. Nature Genet 4:110, 1993.
84. Mullies KB, Falcona FA: Specific synthesis of DNA in vitro via a polymerase catalyzed chain reaction. Meth Enzymol 155:335, 1987.
85. Runnebaum IB, Tong X-W, Moebus V, et al: Multiplex PCR screening detects small p53 deletions and insertions in human ovarian cancer cell lines. Hum Genet 93:629, 1994.
86. Sakar G, Yoon HS, Sommer SS: Screening for mutations by RNA single strand (rSSCP): comparison with DNA-SSCP. Nucl Acids Res 20:871, 1992.
87. Orita M, Iwahana H, Kanazawa H, et al: Detection of polymorphisms of human DNA by gel electrophoresis as single-strand conformation polymorphisms. Proc Natl Acad Sci 86:2766, 1989.
88. Murakami Y, Hayashi K, Hirohashi S, et al: Aberrations of the tumor suppressor p53 and retinoblastoma genes in human hepatocellular carcinomas. Cancer Res 51:5520, 1991.
89. Meyers RM, Fischer SG, Lerman LS, et al: Nearly all single base substitutions in DNA fragments jointed to a GC-clamp can be detected by denaturing gradient gel electrophoresis. Nucl Acids Res 13:3131, 1985.
90. Sheffield VC, Cox DR, Lerman LS, et al: Attachment of a 40 base-pair G+C-rich sequence (GC clamp) to genomic DNA fragments by the polymerase chain reaction results in improved detection of single base changes. Proc Natl Acad Sci 86:232, 1989.
91. Meyer CG, Tannich E, Herders J, et al: Direct sequencing of variable HLA gene segments after in vitro amplification and allele separation by temperature gradient gel electrophoresis. J Immunol Meth 142:251, 1991.
92. Soto D, Sukumar S: Improved detection of mutations in the p53 gene in human tumors as single-stranded conformation polymorphs and double-stranded heteroduplex DNA. PCR Methods Applications 2:96, 1992.
93. Sanger F, Nicklen S, Coulson AR: DNA sequencing with chain-terminating inhibitors. Proc Natl Acad Sci 74:5463, 1977.
94. Hiddemann W, Roessner A, Wörmann B: Tumor heterogeneity in osteosarcomas as identified by flow cytometry. Cancer 59:324, 1987.
95. Bauer HCF, Kreicbergs A, Silfverswärd C: DNA analysis in the differential diagnosis of osteosarcoma. Cancer 61:2532, 1988.
96. Alho A, Skjeldal S, Melvic JE, et al: The clinical importance of DNA synthesis and aneuploidy in bone and soft tissue tumours. Anticancer Res 13:2383, 1993.
97. El-Naggar AK, Hurr K, Tu ZN, et al: DNA and RNA content analysis by flow cytometry in the pathobiologic assessment of bone tumors. Cytometry 19:256, 1995.
98. Mertens F, Mandahl N, Örndal C: Cytogenetic findings in 33 osteosarcomas. Int J Cancer 55:44, 1993.
99. Fletcher JA, Gebhardt MC, Kozakewich HP: Cytogenetic aberrations in osteosarcomas. Cancer Genet Cytogenet 77:81, 1994.
100. Hoogerwerf WA, Hawkins AL, Perlman EJ, et al: Chromosome analysis of nine osteosarcomas. Genes Chrom Cancer 9:88, 1994.

101. Grundmann E, Roessner A, Ueda Y, et al: Current aspects of the pathology of osteosarcoma. Anticancer Res 15:1023, 1995.
102. Tarkannen M, Karhu R, Kallioniemi A, et al: Gains and losses of DNA sequences in osteosarcoma by comparative genomic hybridization. Cancer Res 55:1334, 1995.
103. Forus A, Weghuis DO, Smeets D, et al: Comparative genomic hybridization analysis of human sarcomas: II. Identification of novel amplicons at 6p and 17p in osteosarcomas. Genes Chrom Cancer 14:15, 1995.
104. Yamaguchi T, Toguchida J, Yamamuro T, et al: Allelotypic analysis in osteosarcomas: Frequent allele loss on 3q, 13q, 17p, and 18q. Cancer Res 52:2419, 1992.
105. Rosales C, O'Brien VO, Kornberg L, et al: Signal transduction by cell adhesion receptors. Biochem Biophys Acta 1242:77, 1995.
106. Horstmann MA, Pösl M, Scholz RB, et al: Frequent reduction or loss of the DCC gene expression in human osteosarcoma. Br J Cancer 75:1309, 1997.
107. Toguchida J, Ishizaki K, Sasaki MS, et al: Preferential mutation of the paternally derived RB gene as the initial event in sporadic osteosarcoma. Nature 338:156, 1989.
108. Hansen MF, Koufos A, Gallie BL, et al: Osteosarcoma and retinoblastoma: A shared chromosomal mechanism revealing recessive predisposition. Proc Natl Acad Sci 82:6216, 1985.
109. Sparkes RS, Sparkes MC, Wilson MG, et al: Regional assignment of genes for human esterase D and retinoblastoma to chromosome Band 13q14. Science 208:1042, 1980.
110. Friend SH, Bernards R, Rogeli S, et al: A human DNA segment with properties of the gene that predisposes to retinoblastoma and osteosarcoma. Nature 323:643, 1986.
111. Toguchida J, Ishizaki K, Sasaki MS, et al: Chromosomal reorganization for the expression of recessive mutation of retinoblastoma susceptibility gene in the development of osteosarcoma. Cancer Res 48:3939, 1988.
112. Scholz RB, Kabisch H, Delling G, et al: Homozygous deletion within the retinoblastoma gene in a native osteosarcoma specimen of a patient cured of a retinoblastoma of both eyes. Pediat Hematol Oncol 7:265, 1990.
113. Wunder SJ, Czitrom AA, Kandel R, et al: Analysis of alterations in the retinoblastoma gene in bone and soft-tissue sarcomas. J Natl Cancer Inst 83:194, 1991.
114. Araki N, Uchida A, Kimura T, et al: Involvement of the retinoblastoma gene in primary osteosarcomas and other bone and soft-tissue tumors. Clin Orthop 270:271, 1991.
115. Scholz RB, Kabisch H, Weber B, et al: Studies of the RB1 gene and the p53 gene in human osteosarcomas. Pediat Hematol Oncol 9:125, 1992.
116. Wadayama B, Toguchida J, Shimizu T, et al: Mutation spectrum of the retinoblastoma gene in osteosarcomas. Cancer Res 54:3042, 1994.
117. Feugeas O, Guriec N, Babin-Boilletot A, et al: Loss of heterozygosity of the RB gene is a poor prognostic factor in patients with osteosarcoma. J Clin Oncol 14:467, 1996.
118. Miller CW, Aslo A, Campbell MJ, et al: Alterations of the p15, p16 and p18 genes in osteosarcoma. Cancer Genet Cytogenet 86:136, 1996.
119. Schreck RR: Tumor suppressor gene (Rb and p53) mutations in osteosarcoma. Pediat Hematol Oncol 9:9, 1992.
120. Scheffer H, Kruize YCM, Osinga J, et al: Complete association of loss of heterozygosity of chromosomes 13 and 17 in osteosarcoma. Cancer Genet Cytogenet 53:45, 1991.
121. Miller CW, Aslo A, Tsay C, et al: Frequency and structure of the p53 rearrangements in human osteosarcoma. Cancer Res 50:7950, 1990.
122. Toguchida J, Yamaguchi T, Ritchi B, et al: Mutation spectrum of the p53 gene in bone and soft tissue sarcomas. Cancer Res 52:6194, 1992.
123. Smith-Sorensen B, Gebhardt MC, Kloen P: Screening for Tp53 mutations in osteosarcomas using constant denaturant gel electrophoresis (CDGE). Human Mutation 2:274, 1993.
124. Castresana JS, Rubio M-P, Gomez L, et al: Detection of TP53 gene mutations in human sarcomas. Eur J Cancer 31A:735, 1995.
125. de Fromentel CC, Soussi T: TP53 tumor suppressor gene: A model for investigating human mutagenesis. Genes Chrom Cancer 4:1, 1992.
126. Davidoff AM, Humphrey PA, Iglehart JD, et al: Genetic basis for p53 overexpression in human breast cancer. Proc Natl Acad Sci 88:5006, 1991.
127. Sjögren S, Inganäs M, Norberg T, et al: The p53 gene in breast cancer: Prognostic value of complementary DNA sequencing versus immunohistochemistry. J Natl Cancer Inst 88:173, 1996.
128. Elledge RM: Assessing p53 status in breast cancer prognosis: Where should you put the thermometer if you think your p53 is sick? J Natl Cancer Inst 88:141, 1996.
129. Wadayama B, Toguchida J, Yamaguchi T, et al: p53 expression and its relationship to DNA alterations in bone and soft tissue sarcomas. Br J Cancer 68:1134, 1993.
130. Ueda Y, Dokhorn-Dworniczack B, Blasius S, et al: Immunohistochemical analysis of mutant p53 protein in osteosarcomas and other malignant and benign lesions of bone. J Cancer Res Clin Oncol 3:172, 1993.
131. Scholz RB, Horstmann M, Wittenstein B, et al: p53 mutation and MDM2/SAS-amplification in human osteosarcoma. J Cell Biochem 19A:76, 1995.
132. Oliner JD, Kinzler KW, Meltzer PS, et al: Amplification of a gene encoding a p53-associated protein in human sarcomas. Nature 358:80, 1992.
133. Nilbert M, Rydholm A, Willen H, et al: MDM2 gene amplification correlates with ring chromosomes in soft tissue tumors. Genes Chrom Cancer 9:261, 1994.
134. Ladanyi M, Cha C, Lewis R, et al: MDM2 gene amplification in metastatic osteosarcoma. Cancer Res 53:16, 1993.
135. Nakayama T, Toguchida J, Wadayama B, et al: MDM2 gene amplification in bone and soft tissue tumors: Association with tumor progression in differentiated adipose tissue tumors. Int J Cancer 64:342, 1995.
136. Scholz RB, Horstmann M, Weber B, et al: Mutation pattern of the RB1, p53, MDM2 and SAS genes in osteosarcomas (OS). Med Pediatr Oncol 27:223, 1996.
137. Cho Y, Gorina S, Jeffrey PD, et al: Crystal structure of a p53 tumor suppressor-DNA Complex: Understanding tumorigenic mutations. Science 265:346, 1994.
138. McIntyre JF, Smith-Sorensen B, Friend SH, et al: Germline mutations of the p53 tumor suppressor gene in children with osteosarcoma. J Clin Oncol 12:925, 1995.

139. van de Ven WJM, Schoenmakers EFPM, Wandschura S, et al: Molecular characterization of MAR, a multiple aberration region on human chromosome segment 12q13-15 implicated in various solid tumors. Genes Chrom Cancer 12:296, 1995.
140. Meltzer PS, Jankowski SA, Dal Cin P, et al: Identification and cloning of a novel amplified DNA sequence in human malignant fibrous histiocytoma derived from a region of chromosome 12 frequently rearranged in soft tissue tumors. Cell Growth Different 2:495, 1991.
141. Forus A, Florens VA, Maelandsmo GM, et al: Mapping of amplification unit in the q13-14 region of chromosome 12 in human sarcomas: Some amplica do not include MDM2. Cell Growth Different 4:1065, 1993.
142. Kinzler KW, Bigner SH, Bigner DD, et al: Identification of an amplified, highly expressed gene in a human glioma. Science 235:70, 1987.
143. Roberts MW, Douglass EC, Peiper SC, et al: Amplification of the gli gene in childhood sarcomas. Cancer Res 49:5407, 1989.
144. Maelandsmo GM, Berner J-M, Florenes VA, et al: Homozygous deletion frequency levels of CDK4 and CCND1. Br J Cancer 72:393, 1995.
145. Antillon-Kluesmann F, Garcia-Delgado M, Villa-Elizaga I, et al: Mutational activation of ras genes is absent in pediatric osteosarcoma. Cancer Genet Cytogenet 79:49, 1995.
146. Wu J-X, Carpenter PM, Gresens C, et al: The protooncogene c-fos is over-expressed in the majority of human osteosarcomas. Oncogene 5:989, 1990.
147. Ladanyi M, Park CK, Lewis R, et al: Sporadic amplification of the MYC gene in human osteosarcomas. Diagn Mol Pathol 2:163, 1993.
148. Kato M, Toguchida J, Honda K, et al: Elevated frequency of a specific allele of the L-MYC Gene in male patients with bone and soft-tissue sarcomas. Int J Cancer 45:47, 1990.
149. Ferracini R, Di Renzo MF, Scotlandi K, et al: The Met/HGF receptor is overexpressed in human osteosarcomas and is activated by either a paracrine or an autocrine circuit. Oncogene 10:739, 1995.
150. Onda M, Matsuda S, Higaki S, et al: ErbB-2 expression is correlated with poor prognosis for patients with osteosarcoma. Cancer 77:71, 1996.
151. Carbone M, Rizzo P, Procopio A, et al: SV40-like sequences in human bone tumors. Oncogene 13:527, 1996.
152. Roninson IB, Chin JE, Choi KG, et al: Isolation of human mdr DNA sequences amplified in multidrug-resistant KB carcinoma cells. Proc Natl Acad Sci 83:4538, 1986.
153. Gottesman MM, Pastan I: Biochemistry of multidrug resistance mediated by the multidrug transporter. Ann Rev Biochem 62:385, 1993.
154. Serra M, Scotlandi K, Manara MC, et al: Establishment and characterization of multidrug-resistant human osteosarcoma cell lines. Anticancer Res 13:323, 1993.
155. Serra M, Scotlandi K, Manara MC, et al: Analysis of P-glycoprotein expression in osteosarcoma. Eur J Cancer 68:226, 1995.
156. Baldini N, Scotlandi K, Barbanti-Brodano G, et al: Expression of P-glycoprotein in high-grade osteosarcomas in relation to clinical outcome. N Engl J Med 333:1380, 1995.
157. Pinedo HM, Giaccone G: P-Glycoprotein—A marker of cancer-cell behaviour. N Engl J Med 333:1417, 1995.
158. Stein U, Walther W, Wunderlich V: Point mutations in the mdr1 promoter of human osteosarcomas are associated with In vitro responsiveness to multidrug resistance relevant drugs. Eur J Cancer 30A:1541, 1994.
159. Roessner A, Hobik HP, Grundmann E: Malignant fibrous histiocytoma of bone and osteosarcoma: A comparative light and electron microscopic study. Pathol Res Pract 164:385, 1979.
160. Roessner A, Zwadlo G, Vollmer E, et al: Biological characterization of human bone tumors IX. Occurrence of macrophages. Pathol Res Pract 182:336, 1987.
161. Ballance WA, Mendelsohn G, Carter JA, et al: Osteogenenic sarcoma: Malignant fibrous histiocytoma subtype. Cancer 62:763, 1988.
162. Bridge JA, Sanger WG, Neff JR, et al: Cytogenetic findings in a primary malignant fibrous histiocytoma of bone and the lung metastasis. Pathology 22:16, 1990.
163. Smith S, Fisher C: Chromosome abnormalities in malignant fibrous histocytoma of bone. Pathology 23:275, 1991.
164. Örndahl C, Mandahl N, Carlen B, et al: Near-haploid clones in a malignant fibrous histiocytoma. Cancer Genet Cytogenet 60:147, 1992.
165. Molenaar WM, van den Berg E, Veth RP-H, et al: Tumor progression in a giant cell type malignant fibrous histiocytoma of bone: Clinical, radiologic, histologic, and cytogenetic evidence. Genes Chrom Cancer 10:66, 1994.
166. Bridge JA, Mouron BJ, Neff JR, et al: Significance of chromosomal abnormalities in a malignant giant cell tumor of bone. Cancer Genet Cytogenet 57:87, 1991.
167. Andreassen A, Oyjord T, Hovig E, et al: p53 Abnormalities in different subtypes of human sarcomas. Cancer Res 53:468, 1993.
168. Ozaki T, Ikeda S, Kawai A, et al: Alterations of retinoblastoma susceptibility gene accompanied by c-myc amplifications in human bone and soft tissue tumors. Cell Mol Biol 2:235, 1993.
169. Rydholm A, Mandahl N, Heim S, et al: Malignant fibrous histiocytomas with a 19p+ marker chromosome have increased relapse rate. Genes Chrom Cancer 2:296, 1990.
170. Tetu B, Lacasse B, Bouchard HL, et al: Prognostic influence of HSP -27 expression in malignant fibrous histiocytoma: a clinicopathological study. Cancer Res 52:2325, 1992.
171. Dirix LY, Van Oosterom AT: Chondrosarcoma and other rare bone sarcomas. Curr Sci 3:694, 1991.
172. Evans HL, Ayala AG, Romsdahl MM: Prognostic factors in chondrosarcoma of bone: A clinicopathologic analysis with emphasis on histological grading. Cancer 40:818, 1977.
173. Kreicbergs A, Boquist L, Borssen B, et al: Prognostic factors in chondrosarcoma: A comparative study of cellular DNA content and clinicopathologic features. Cancer 50:577, 1982.
174. Dobashi Y, Sugimura H, Sato A, et al: Possible association of p53 overexpression and mutation with high-grade chondrosarcoma. Diagn Mol Pathol 2:257, 1993.
175. Coughlan B, Feliz A, Ishida T, et al: p53 expression and DNA ploidy of cartilage lesions. Hum Pathol 26:620, 1995.

176. Hasegawa T, Seki K, Yang P, et al: Differentiation and proliferative activity in benign and malignant cartilage tumors of bone. Hum Pathol 26:838, 1995.
177. Bridge JA, Bhatia PS, Anderson JR, et al: Biological and clinical significance of cytogenetic and molecular cytogenetic abnormalities in benign and malignant cartilaginous lesions. Cancer Genet Cytogenet 69:79, 1993.
178. Dijkhuizen T, van den Berg E, Molenaar W, et al: Cytogenetics as a tool in the histologic subclassification of chondrosarcomas. Cancer Genet Cytogenet 76:100, 1994.
179. Fryns JP, Heremanns G, Marien J, et al: Langer-Giedion syndrome and a deletion of the long arm of chromosome 8. Confirmation of the critical segment to 8q23. Hum Genet 64:194, 1983.
180. Langer LO, Krassikoff N, Laxoya R, et al: The tricho-rhino-phalangeal syndrome with exostosis (or Langer-Giedion syndrome): Four additional patients without mental retardation and review of the literature. Am J Med Genet 19:81, 1984.
181. Cook A, Raskind W, Blanton SH, et al: Genetic heterogeneity in families with hereditary multiple exostoses. Am J Hum Genet 53:71, 1993.
182. Wu YQ, Heutink P, deVries BBA, et al: Assignment of a second locus for multiple exostoses to the pericentromeric region of chromosome 11. Hum Mol Genet 3:167, 1994.
183. Le Merrer M, Legeai-Mallet L, Jeannin PM, et al: A gene for hereditary multiple exostoses maps to chromosome 19p. Hum Mol Genet 3:717, 1994.
184. Gitelis S, Bertoni F, Picci P, et al: Chondrosarcoma of bone. J Bone Joint Surg 8:1248, 1981.
185. Gordon SL, Buchanan JR, Ladda RL: Hereditary multiple exostoses: Report of a kindred. J Med Genet 18:428, 1981.
186. Schmale GA, Conrad EU, Raskin WH, et al: The natural history of hereditary multiple exostoses. J Bone Joint Surg 76A:986, 1994.
187. Hecht JT, Hogue D, Strong LC, et al: Hereditary multiple exostoses and chondrosarcoma: Linkage to chromosome 11 and loss of heterozygosity for EXT-linked markers on chromosomes 11 and 8. Am J Hum Genet 56:1125, 1995.
188. Raskind WH, Conrad EU, Chansky H, et al: Loss of heterozygosity in chondrosarcomas for markers linked to hereditary multiple exostoses loci on chromosomes 8 and 11. Am J Hum Genet 56:1132, 1995.
189. Mandahl N, Heim S, Arheden K, et al: Chromosomal rearrangements in chondromatous tumors. Cancer 65:242, 1990.
190. Örndahl C, Mandahl N, Rydholm A, et al: Chromosome aberrations and cytogenetic intratumor heterogeneity in chondrosarcomas. J Cancer Res Clin Oncol 120:51, 1993.
191. Hirabayashi Y, Yoshida MA, Ikeuchi T, et al: Chromosome rearrangements at 12q13 in two cases of chondrosarcomas. Cancer Genet Cytogenet 60:35, 1992.
192. Zalupsky MM, Ensley JF, Ryan J, et al: A common cytogenetic abnormality and DNA content alterations in dedifferentiated chondrosarcoma. Cancer 66:1176, 1990.
193. Gill S, Aidan P, McManus A, et al: Fusion of the EWS gene to a DNA segment from 9q22-31 in a human myxoid chondrosarcoma. Genes Chrom Cancer 12:7, 1995.
194. Hinrichs SH, Jaramillo MA, Gummerlock PH, et al: Myxoid chondrosarcoma with a translocation involving chromosomes 9 and 22. Cancer Genet Cytogenet 14:219, 1985.
195. Turc-Carel C, Dal Cin P, Rao U, et al: Recurrent breakpoints at 9q31 and 22q12.2 in extraskeletal myxoid chondrosarcoma. Cancer Genet Cytogenet 30:145, 1988.
196. Tarkannen M, Wiklund T, Virolainen M, et al: Dedifferentiated chondrosarcoma with t(9;22)(q34;q11-12). Genes Chrom Cancer 9:136, 1994.
197. Sainati L, Scapinello A, Montaldi A, et al: A mesenchymal chondrosarcoma of a child with the reciprocal translocation (11;22) (q24;q12). Cancer Genet Cytogenet 71:144, 1993.
198. Dobin SM, Donner LR, Speights VO: Mesenchymal chondrosarcoma: A cytogenetic, immunohistochemical and ultrastructural study. Cancer Genet Cytogenet 83:56, 1995.
199. Stenman G, Andersson H, Mandahl N, et al: Translocation t(9;22)(q22;q12) is a primary cytogenetic abnormality in extraskeletal myxoid chondrosarcoma. Int J Cancer 62:398, 1995.
200. Aurias A, Rimbaut C, Buffe D, et al: Translocation of chromosome 22 in Ewing's sarcoma. N Engl J Med 309:496, 1983.
201. Turc-Carel C, Philip M, Berger TJ: Chromosomal translocation in Ewing's sarcoma. N Engl J Med 309:497, 1983.
202. Whang-Peng J, Triche TJ, Knutsen T, et al: Chromosome translocation in peripheral neuroepithelioma. N Engl J Med 311:584, 1984.
203. Whang-Peng J, Triche TJ, Knutsen T, et al: Cytogenetic characterization of selected small round cell tumors of childhood. Cancer Genet Cytogenet 21:185, 1986.
204. Whang-Peng J, Freter CE, Knutsen T, et al: Translocation t(11;22) in esthesioneuroblastoma. Cancer Genet Cytogenet 29:155, 1987.
205. Cavazzana AO, Navarro S, Noguera R, et al: Olfactory neuroblastoma is not a neuroblastoma but is related to primitive neuroectodermal tumor (PNET). Prog Clin Biol Res 271:463, 1988.
206. Haas OA, Chott A, Ladenstein R, et al: Poorly differentiated, neuron-specific enolase positive round cell tumor with two translocations t(11;22) and t(21;22). Cancer 60:2219, 1987.
207. Soukup S, Wang-Wuu S, Workman L, et al: Special findings in chromosome analysis of Ewing's sarcoma. Am J Hum Genet 39A:43, 1986.
208. Speleman F, Van Roy N, Wiegant J, et al: Molecular cytogenetic analysis of a complex t(10:22;11) translocation in Ewing's sarcoma. Genes Chrom Cancer 4:188, 1992.
209. Christiansen H, Altmannsberger M, Lampert F, et al: Translocation t(5;22) in an Askin's tumor. Cancer Genet Cytogenet 62:203, 1992.
210. Squire J, Zielenska M, Thorner P, et al: Variant translocations of chromosome in Ewing's sarcoma. Genes Chrom Cancer 8:190, 1993.
211. Giovannini M, Selleri L, Biegel JA, et al: Interphase cytogenetics for the detection of the t(11;22)(q24;q12) in small round cell tumors. J Clin Invest 90:1911, 1992.
212. Zucman J, Delattre O, Desmaze C, et al: Cloning and characterization of the Ewing's sarcoma and peripheral neuroepithelioma t(11;22) translocation breakpoints. Genes Chrom Cancer 5:271, 1992.
213. Delattre O, Zucman J, Plougastel B, et al: Gene fusion with ETS DNA-binding domain caused by chro-

mosome translocation in human tumours. Nature 359:162, 1992.
214. Ben-David Y, Giddens EB, Letwin K, et al: Erythroleukemia induction by Friend murine leukemia virus: insertional activation of a new member of the ets gene family, FLI-1, closely linked to c-ets-1. Genes Dev 5:908, 1991.
215. Zucman J, Delattre O, Desmaze C, et al: EWS and AFT-1 gene fusion induced by t(12;22) translocation in malignant melanoma of soft parts. Nature Genet 4:341, 1993.
216. Sorensen PHB, Lessnick SL, Lopez-Terrada D, et al: A second Ewing's sarcoma translocation, t(21;22) fuses the EWS gene to another ETS-family transcription factor, ERG. Nature Genet 6:146, 1994.
217. Gegonne A, Punyammalee B, Rabault B, et al: Analysis of the DNA binding and transcriptional activation properties of the Ets-1 oncoprotein. New Biol 4:512, 1992.
218. Zucman J, Melot T, Desmaze C, et al: Combinatorial generation of variable fusion proteins in peripheral primitive neuroectodermal tumors. EMBO J 12:4481, 1993.
219. Thiele CJ, McKeon C, Triche TJ, et al: Differential protooncogene expression characterizes histopathologically indistinguishable tumors of the peripheral nervous system. J Clin Invest 80:804, 1987.
220. Schulz G, Cheresh DA, Varki NM, et al: Detection of ganglioside GD2 in tumor tissues and sera of neuroblastoma patients. Cancer Res 44:5914, 1984.
221. Lipinski M, Braham K, Philipp I, et al: Neuroectodermal-associated antigens on Ewing's sarcoma cell lines. Cancer Res 47:183, 1987.
222. McGarry RC, Helfand SL, Quarles RH, et al: Recognition of myelin associated glycoprotein by the monoclonal antibody HNK-1. Nature 306:376, 1987.
223. Herlyn M, Steplewski Z, Herlyn D, et al: Production and characterization of monoclonal antibodies against human malignant melanoma. Cancer Invest 1:215, 1983.
224. Ross AH, Grob P, Bothwell M, et al: Characterization of nerve growth factor receptor in neural crest tumors using monoclonal antibodies. Proc Natl Acad Sci 81:6681, 1984.
225. Cavazzana AO, Ninfe V, Roberts J, et al: Peripheral neuroepithelioma: a light microscopic, immunocytochemical, and ultrastructural study. Mod Pathol 5:71, 1992.
226. Nguyen C, Mattei M, Mattei JF, et al: Localization of the human N-CAM gene to band 11q23 of chromosome 11: The third gene encoding for a cell interaction molecule mapped to the distal portion of the long arm of chromosome 11. J Cell Biol 102:711, 1986.
227. Fellinger EJ, Gain Chesa P, Triche TJ, et al: Immunohistochemical analysis of Ewing's sarcoma cell surface antigen p30/32MIC2. Am J Pathol 139:317, 1991.
228. Fellinger EJ, Garin-Chesa P, Sui SL, et al: Biochemical and genetic characterization of the HBA71 Ewing's sarcoma cell surface antigen. Cancer Res 51:336, 1991.
229. Ambros IM, Ambros PF, Strehl S, et al: MIC2 is a specific marker for Ewing's sarcoma and peripheral primitive neuroectodermal tumors. Cancer 67:1886, 1991.
230. Weidner N, Tjoe J: Immunohistochemical profile of monoclonal antibody O13: Antibody that recognizes glycoprotein p30/32 MIC2 and is useful in diagnosing Ewing's sarcoma and peripheral neuroepithelioma. Am J Surg Pathol 18:486, 1994.
231. Ladanyi M, Lewis R, Garin-Chesa P, et al: EWS rearrangement in Ewing's sarcoma and peripheral neuroectodermal tumor. Molecular detection and correlation with cytogenetic analysis and MIC2 expression. Diagn Mol Pathol 2:141, 1993.
232. Ostrowski M, Kuni K, Banks P, et al: Malignant lymphoma of bone. Cancer 58:2646, 1986.
233. Vasallo I, Roessner A, Vollmer E, et al: Malignant lymphomas with primary bone manifestations. Pathol Res Pract 182:381, 1987.
234. Pettit CK, Zuckerberg LR, Gray MH, et al: Primary lymphoma of bone. Am J Surg Pathol 14:329, 1990.
235. Radaszkiewiecz T, Hansmann ML: Primary high-grade malignant lymphomas of bone. Virch Arch (A) 413:269, 1988.
236. Griesser H: Molekuläre Genetik maligner Non-Hodgkin Lymphome (Molecular genetical analyses of malignant Non-Hodgkin's Lymphomas). Verh Dtsch Ges Path 76:66, 1992.
237. Gaidano G, Dalla-Favera R: Molecular biology of lymphoid neoplasia. *In* Mendelsohn J, Howley PM, Israel MA, Liotta LA, (eds): The Molecular Basis of Cancer. Philadelphia, WB Saunders, 1995, p 251.
238. Korsmeyer SJ: BCL-2 initiates a new category of oncogenes: Regulators of the cell death. Blood 80:879, 1992.
239. Raffeld M, Jaffe ES: BCL-1, t(11;14), and mantle zone lymphomas. Blood 78:493, 1991.
240. Ye BH, Rao PH, Chaganti RSK, et al: Cloning of BCL-6, the locus involved in chromosome translocations affecting band 3q27 in B-cell lymphoma. Cancer Res 53:2732, 1993.
241. Chirgwin JM, Przybyla AE, MacDonald RJ, et al: Isolation of biologically active ribonucleic acid from sources enriched in ribonucleases. Biochem 24:5294, 1979.
242. Harvard Medical School: Preparation and analysis of RNA. *In* Ausubel FM, Brent R, Kingston RE, et al (eds): Short Protocols in Molecular Biology. New York, John Wiley & Sons, 1989, p 139.
243. Sambrook J, Fritsch EF, Maniatis T: Extraction, purification, and analysis of messenger RNA from eukaryotic cells. *In* Ford N, Nolan C, Ferguson M (eds): Molecular Cloning: A Laboratory Manual. 2nd ed. Vol. 2. New York, Cold Spring Harbor Laboratory Press, 1989, p 7.3.
244. Sambrook J, Fritsch EF, Maniatis T: Commonly used techniques in molecular cloning. *In* Ford N, Nolan C, Ferguson M (eds): Molecular Cloning: A Laboratory Manual. 2nd ed. Vol. 2. New York, Cold Spring Harbor Laboratory Press, 1989, p e.5.
245. Sambrook J, Fritsch EF, Maniatis T: Enzymes used in molecular cloning. *In* Ford N, Nolan C, Ferguson M (eds): Molecular Cloning: A Laboratory Manual. 2nd ed. Vol. 2. New York, Cold Spring Harbor Laboratory Press, 1989, p 5.28.
246. Sambrook J, Fritsch EF, Maniatis T: Analysis and cloning of eukaryotic genomic DNA. *In* Ford N, Nolan C, Ferguson M (eds): Molecular Cloning: A Laboratory Manual. 2nd ed. Vol. 2. New York, Cold Spring Harbor Laboratory Press, 1989, p 9.31.
247. Harvard Medical School: Enzymatic manipulation of DNA and RNA. *In* Ausubel FM, Brent R, Kingston RE, et al (eds): Short Protocols in Molecular Biology. New York, John Wiley & Sons, 1989, p 87.

248. Perbal B: Useful enzymes for molecular cloning. *In* Perbal B (ed): A Practical Guide to Molecular Cloning. New York, John Wiley & Sons, 1984, p 13.
249. Sambrook J, Fritsch EF, Maniatis T: Gel electrophoresis of DNA. *In* Ford N, Nolan C, Ferguson M (eds): Molecular Cloning: A Laboratory Manual. 2nd ed. Vol. 2. New York, Cold Spring Harbor Laboratory Press, 1989, p 6.3.
250. Perbal B: Separation of DNA fragments by electrophoresis. *In* Perbal B (ed): A Practical Guide to Molecular Cloning. New York, John Wiley & Sons, 1984, p 196.
251. Feinberg AP, Vogelstein B: A technique for radiolabeling DNA restriction endonuclease fragments to high specific activity. Anal Biochem 132:6, 1983.
252. Harlow ED, Williamson NM, Ralston R, et al: Molecular cloning and in vitro expression of a cDNA clone for human cellular tumor antigen p53. Mol Cell Biol 1601:1610, 1985.
253. Innis MA, Gelfand DH: Optimization of PCRs. *In* Inis MA, Gelfand DH, Sninsky JJ, White TJ (eds): PCR Protocols: A Guide to Methods and Applications. San Diego, Academic Press, 1990, p 3.
254. Saiko RK: Amplification of genomic DNA. *In* Inis MA, Gelfand DH, Sninsky JJ, White TJ (eds): PCR Protocols: A Guide to Methods and Applications. San Diego, Academic Press, 1990, p 13.
255. Taylor GR: Polymerase chain reaction: Basic principles and automation. *In* McPherson MJ, Quirke P, Taylor GR (eds): PCR: A Practical Approach. New York, Oxford University Press, 1991, p 1.
256. Chomczynski P, Sacchi N: Single-step method of RNA isolation by acid guanidinium thiocyanate-phenol-chloroform extraction. Anal Biochem 162:156, 1987.
257. Murakami Y, Hayashi K, Sekiya T: Detection of aberrations of the p53 alleles and the gene transcript in human tumor cell lines by single-strand conformation polymorphism analysis. Cancer Res 51:3356, 1991.
258. Sheffield VC, Cox DR, Myers RM: Identifying DNA polymorphisms by denaturing gradient gel electrophoresis. *In* Inis MA, Gelfand DH, Sninsky JJ, White TJ (eds): PCR Protocols: A Guide to Methods and Applications. San Diego, Academic Press, 1990, p 206.

Chapter

6

IMAGING STUDIES IN BONE NEOPLASIA

DAVID A. RITCHIE and A. MARK DAVIES

In recent years, the management of bone tumors has improved dramatically. Substantial progress in treatment, including chemotherapy and limb-salvage surgery, has been matched by important advances in imaging. The introduction of computed tomography (CT) and, more recently, magnetic resonance imaging (MRI) has had a major impact in tumor imaging, particularly for tumor staging and follow-up. The optimal outcome requires specialized physicians with a particular interest in orthopedic oncology, and a close liaison between radiologist, pathologist, and surgeon is extremely important. When analyzing the imaging studies, the clinical data including history, examination, and laboratory investigations should be available. Most patients with bone tumors will present to a district hospital where they will have plain radiographs and often some form of cross-sectional imaging. For primary malignant bone tumors especially, further management including biopsy is best performed at the hospital where definitive treatment will be undertaken.

This chapter is an overview of the role of imaging in tumor management. There are brief descriptions of the technical aspects of the different imaging modalities, but emphasis is placed on the appropriate use of various imaging techniques in the detection, diagnosis, further management, staging, and follow-up of patients with bone tumors.

DETECTION OF BONE TUMORS

Although the majority of bone tumors can be detected by plain radiography, some occult lesions may be detected only by bone scintigraphy or MRI.

Plain Radiographs

Plain radiographic films are inexpensive, reproducible, easily obtainable, and universally available and should be the first imaging technique for a suspected bone tumor. Occasionally, bone tumor pain may be referred and, therefore, when the plain films are normal, bone scintigraphy may be more helpful. In the child, a pathologic process of the hip with pain referred to the knee is a classic example.

Radiographic technique is critical; if the film is overexposed or underexposed, or if the coning or positioning is suboptimal, then a lesion may easily be overlooked. The plain film detection of bone tumors depends to a degree on the size and location of the lesion. Large lesions arising in cancellous bone may be radiographically invisible, whereas very small tumors in the dense cortical bone may be easily detected. Similarly, once a lesion in the cancellous bone extends to the cortex, the resultant endosteal scalloping or infiltration is then often recognized. On the other hand, it should also be noted that some aggressive tumors (e.g., Ewing's sarcoma) may cause a permeative pattern of bone destruction that may be difficult to visualize on the plain radiograph (Fig. 6–1). In such cases, however, there is often evidence of a periosteal reaction or an associated soft tissue mass.

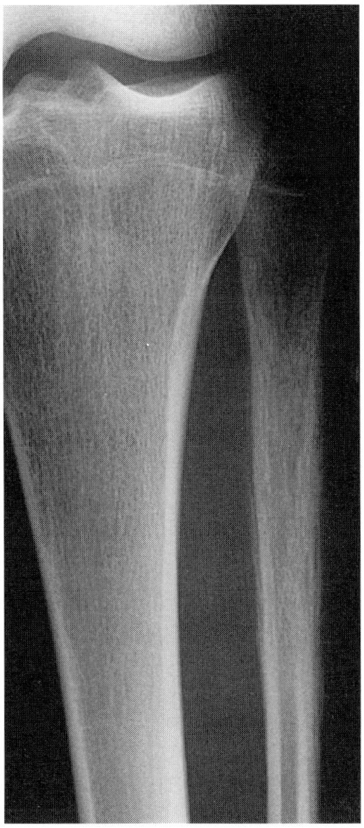

Figure 6–1. Ewing's sarcoma. Anteroposterior radiograph of the lower leg showing a permeative pattern of bone destruction in the proximal fibula.

Bone Scintigraphy

Bone scintigraphy is a valuable investigation in the assessment of suspected bone tumors and is usually performed with the intravenous injection of one of the technetium-labeled phosphate analogues, commonly ^{99m}Tc methylene diphosphonate (Tc-MDP). In addition to the standard 3-hour static images, dynamic images can be acquired, and the addition of single-photon emission computed tomography (SPECT) has increased sensitivity, particularly when imaging complex bony structures. The intensity of skeletal uptake reflects the rate of osteoblastic activity and in a normal scan should be uniform and symmetrical. Abnormalities are manifest as areas of either increased or, less commonly, reduced uptake. In clinical practice, the bone scan is a highly sensitive but relatively nonspecific technique.

Although scintigraphy is of limited value in the assessment of benign bone tumors, it plays a significant role in the detection of suspected and occult osteoid osteomas, especially in the axial skeleton and for the less common intramedullary and subperiosteal types. In such lesions the scan may reveal the "double density sign" in which the central nidus shows greater uptake than the inflammatory response from the surrounding bone (Fig. 6–2). Although this sign is present in less than 50% of cases, it is highly suggestive of an osteoid osteoma and differentiates the lesion from chronic infection. In malignant bone tumors, the main role for scintigraphy is in the detection of suspected metastatic disease and is discussed in the section on staging. Some malignant bone tumors (e.g., Ewing's sarcoma) may be radiographically occult and only detected by scintigraphy. It is important to stress that bone scintigraphy is indicated in a patient with unexplained bone pain and normal radiographs.

Magnetic Resonance Imaging

Although its main role is in staging, MRI may also contribute to the detection and diagnosis of tumors. The physics of MRI are complex, but it is worthwhile discussing some basic technical aspects that are important for optimal imaging. The signal obtained is dependent on certain physical properties of protons in a magnetic field. When a body is placed inside a strong magnetic field, some protons will align with the field. When a radiofrequency pulse is passed across the field, some of the protons will temporarily move away from the main field direction, generating a signal in a nearby detector. The signal itself is complex, containing information that is dependent not only on the density of protons within the tissue itself but also on the relaxation times specific for the tissues observed. Furthermore, the image intensity is also dependent on the pulse sequences selected by the operator. MRI of musculoskeletal tumors requires spin-echo and short tau inversion recovery (STIR) sequences. By altering the parameters of these pulse sequences, the sequences can be described as T1-weighted spin-echo (T1WSE), T2-weighted spin-echo (T2WSE), or proton density–weighted, each reflecting different properties of the tissue.

Most MRI protocols would include T1WSE, T2WSE, and STIR sequences in at least two orthogonal planes. The T1WSE and T2WSE images are complementary in defining the relationship between tumor and surrounding structures. The T1WSE sequence distinguishes

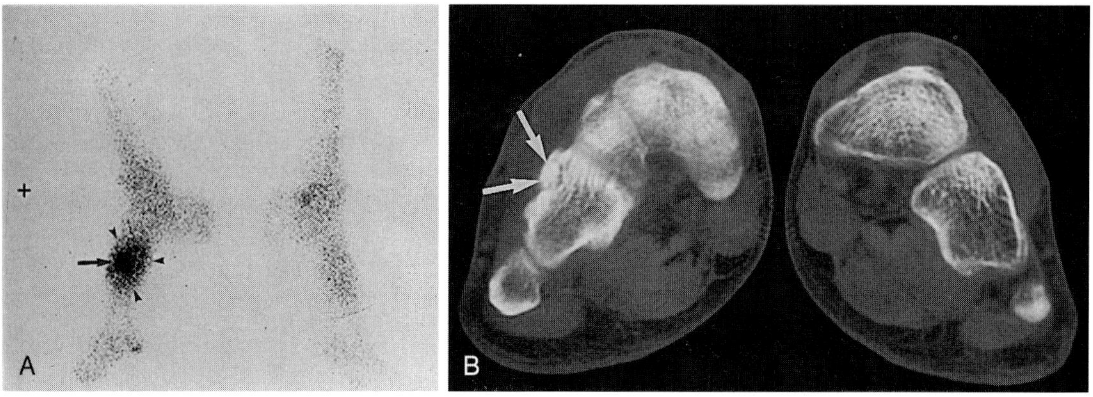

Figure 6–2. Osteoid osteoma. A 35-year-old woman presented with a 12-month history of right foot pain that was worse at night. Radiographs were normal. *A*, Bone scintigraphy shows a "double density" pattern of increased uptake in the right midfoot with the central component (*arrow*) showing greater uptake than the surrounding inflammatory response (*arrowheads*). *B*, Coronal CT scan shows a 6-mm mineralized density on the surface of the superolateral aspect of the right cuboid (*arrows*) in keeping with the ossified nidus of a subperiosteal osteoid osteoma.

tumor from bone marrow and fatty tissue, and the T2WSE sequence allows the tumor to be differentiated from muscle. Because fat and tumor may have similar signal intensity on T2WSE sequences, fat suppression is useful to facilitate tumor recognition. This can be achieved by using the STIR sequence or by applying fat-selective presaturation with the spin-echo sequence. Additional contrast medium–enhanced sequences may be performed by using the paramagnetic contrast medium gadopentetate dimeglumine (Gd-DTPA) and magnetic resonance angiography. The latter relies on the physical properties of flowing blood within the magnetic field and does not require a contrast medium.

Careful patient positioning is important in reducing motion artifacts, and appropriate coil selection is essential for optimal lesion coverage and maximizing spatial resolution. Spatial resolution and area coverage are inversely proportional so that surface coils, commonly used in the extremities, give better spatial resolution but smaller area coverage. Body coils, on the other hand, give greater area coverage but lower spatial resolution. Although an aggressive lesion in an extremity may be well covered by an extremity surface coil, a sequence using the longer body coil will still be required to exclude a skip lesion in another part of the bone (Fig. 6–3).

MRI is the most sensitive imaging technique for the detection of marrow disorders, greater even than bone scintigraphy.[1, 2] For this reason MRI will, on occasion, define radiographically occult lesions. This is due to several factors, including the increased spatial and contrast resolution and the multiplanar facility of MRI. However, bone scintigraphy is more appropriate as a screening test for evaluating the whole skeleton. Although extremely sensitive in detecting abnormalities, the MRI appearances of the majority of bone tumors are not specific and can be found in other processes, including infection, infarction, and trauma.[3] It is also worth noting the detection rate of tumors with different MRI sequences. In the spine, on standard spin-echo sequences, metastases are shown better on T1-weighted rather than T2-weighted sequences, because the signal from tumor on T2 weighting is often isointense with that of fatty marrow. Where appearances are inconclusive, the STIR or contrast-enhanced, fat-suppressed T1WSE sequences are more sensitive for tumor detection (Fig. 6–4).[4] Although protocols vary for different clinical problems, in our institutions, when vertebral malignancy is suggested, then a sagittal STIR sequence is routine.

DIAGNOSIS OF BONE NEOPLASIA

Of all the imaging techniques, the plain radiograph remains the most reliable predictor of the histologic nature of a tumor or tumor-like lesion of bone.[5] Careful analysis of the site, location within the bone, and the morphologic features of the lesion is essential but must be undertaken with a knowledge of the age and clinical presentation of the lesion, of the various diseases that may mimic bone neoplasia, and of the need, in some circumstances, to undertake other investigations to reach a diagnosis.

Age, Multiplicity, Tumor Location

The age of the patient is an important consideration in establishing the diagnosis of a bone tumor and is discussed in more detail in Chapter 1. The peak age incidence and common age range of most tumors are often confined to either two or sometimes three decades, although osteosarcoma has two peaks, one in adolescence and one in late adult life, the latter in association with underlying Paget's disease. In the differential diagnosis of a grossly expansile bone lesion at the end of a long bone, an aneurysmal bone cyst would be more likely than a giant cell tumor in an adolescent, whereas a giant cell tumor is more likely in a patient aged 30–50 years. Other lesions appear to arise in different locations depending on age. Simple bone cysts in the immature skeleton are most often found in the proximal humerus or femur, whereas after maturity they appear in other locations (e.g., calcaneus and pelvis). In general, benign tumors are more common than malignant tumors in childhood and young adults, whereas in older adults the reverse is true.

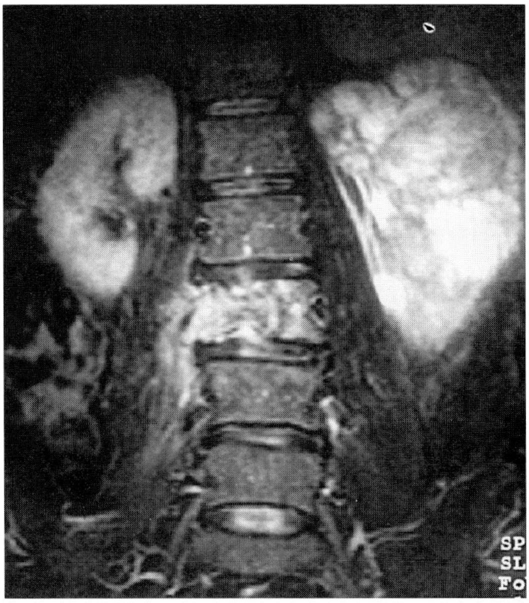

Figure 6–4. Metastasis from adenocarcinoma. Coronal STIR MR image of a metastasis in the third lumbar vertebra from a primary adenocarcinoma that is replacing the left kidney.

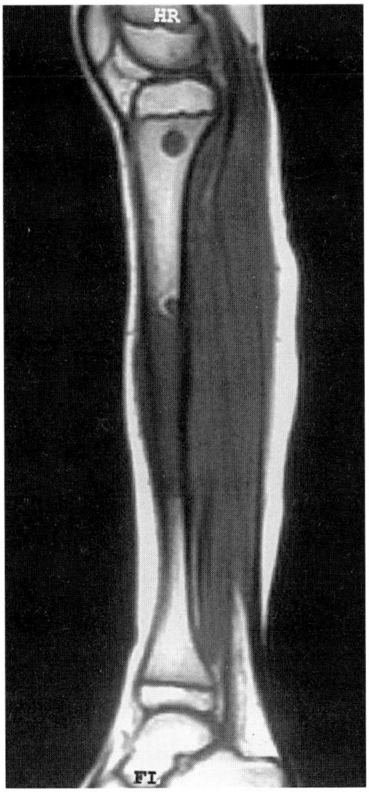

Figure 6–3. Osteosarcoma. Sagittal T1-weighted MR image of a mid-diaphyseal tumor of the tibia with a histologically proven skip metastasis in the proximal metaphysis.

Although age is important, the incidence of tumors in different age groups should also be considered. Metastases are by far the most common malignant tumors in patients older than 40 years of age. Therefore, an aggressive tumor appearing in late adulthood, even if solitary and with bizarre features, is more likely to be due to a metastasis rather than primary bone tumor. Of the bony malignancies encountered in childhood, metastatic neuroblastoma and leukemia should be considered in the first decade of life and osteosarcoma and Ewing's sarcoma in the second decade.

Multiple bone lesions are found in both benign and malignant conditions. In an older adult, the presence of multiple lesions usually indicates metastatic disease, multiple myeloma, or lymphoma. In childhood, multiple lesions are more likely to be benign, and the differential diagnosis includes polyostotic fibrous dysplasia, histiocytosis, multiple enchondromatosis (Ollier's disease), and multiple exostoses (diaphyseal aclasis) (Fig. 6–5).

A knowledge of the locations within the skeleton at which particular neoplasms typically occur helps to narrow the differential diagnosis. Some tumors including metastases, myeloma, lymphoma, and Ewing's sarcoma predominate in areas of hematopoietic marrow, whereas others almost always arise at a specific location (e.g., adamantinoma in the mid tibia and chordoma in the clivus or sacrum) (Fig. 6–6).

Pattern Recognition and Analysis of Bone and Bone Tumor–like Lesions

When assessing neoplasms and tumor-like lesions of bone, it is helpful to differentiate between pattern recognition and pattern analysis. Pattern recognition refers to the "Aunt Minnie" approach in which the radiologic diagnosis is based on the memory of a similar previous case. Reliance on familiarity with the overall appearance of the tumor ignores the fact that many different tumors show similar features and that tumors of the same histologic type may appear dissimilar. This approach is therefore discouraged. Particular problems with this approach occur when a tumor exhibits atypical features or arises at an unusual site. The prudent radiologist will only venture a radiologic diagnosis after a systematic analysis of both the clinical and radiologic findings.

Much of the precise analysis of the morphology of bone and joint tumors in the literature can be attributed to the work of Lodwick, who applied the principles to the computer-assisted analysis of plain radiographs.[6–8] Evaluation of the morphologic features usually provides an accurate assessment of the tumor growth rate and allows differentiation of slow growing from more aggressive lesions. Prediction of histologic diagnosis is less accurate. Analysis of tumor and tumor-like lesions of bone requires the assessment of the location of a lesion within a bone, as well as its morphologic features.

Location of a Lesion in a Single Bone

The location of a tumor refers to its position within the bone and can be described in both

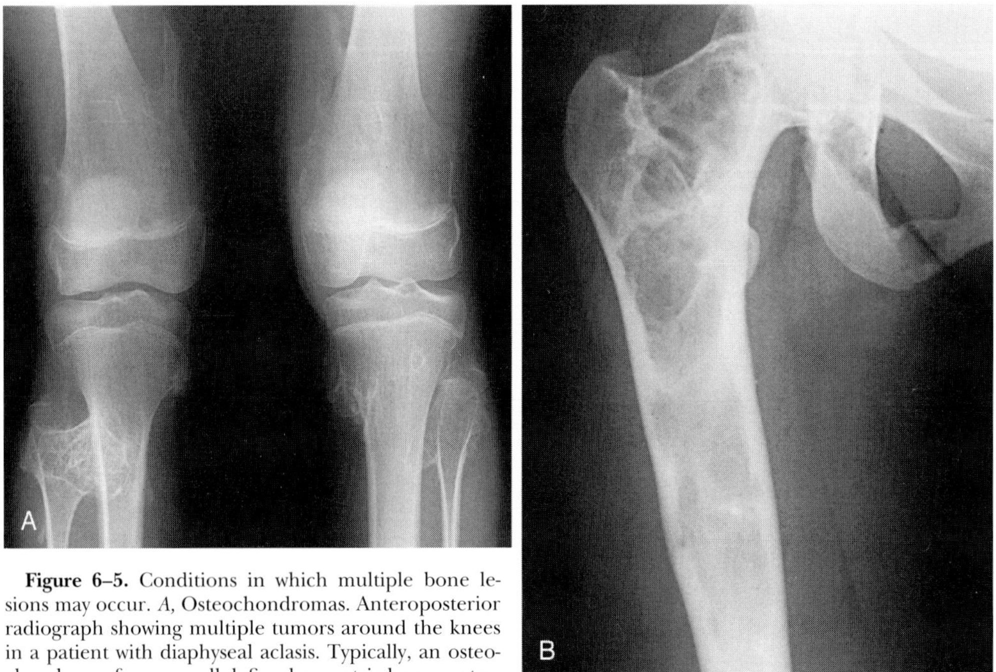

Figure 6–5. Conditions in which multiple bone lesions may occur. *A*, Osteochondromas. Anteroposterior radiograph showing multiple tumors around the knees in a patient with diaphyseal aclasis. Typically, an osteochondroma forms a well-defined eccentric bony protrusion continuous with the cortical and trabecular components of the parent bone. Sessile lesions have a wide base, whereas pedunculated lesions have a narrow base and long stalk. *B*, The upper femoral metaphysis is expanded by a lytic lesion with well-defined edges accompanied by endosteal erosion and a "ground glass" appearance to the lesional tissue. Diagnosis: fibrous dysplasia.

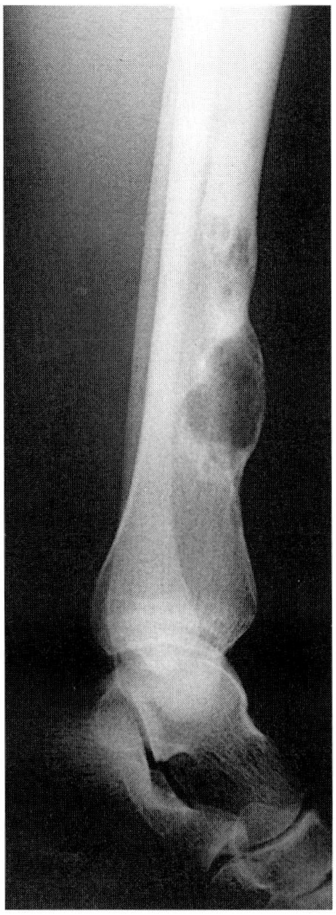

Figure 6–6. Adamantinoma. Lateral radiograph of lower tibia showing an eccentric (mainly cortically based) lytic lesion with reactive sclerosis. This location is classic for this type of tumor.

the transverse and longitudinal planes. In the transverse plane, it is important to establish whether the epicenter of the lesion is central, eccentric, cortical, or juxtacortical (Fig. 6–7*A* through *D*) or is within the soft tissues. Although this classification works in most cases, there are several situations in which lesions may be difficult to categorize: those in which components may arise from various locations (see Fig. 6–6), where the morphology may change (e.g., myositis ossificans; see later), or exophytic type lesions (see Fig. 6–5*A*).

In the longitudinal plane, lesions in the immature skeleton are described by their position relative to the epiphysis, physis (growth plate), metaphysis, and diaphysis, whereas in the mature skeleton lesions are described with reference to the articular end and the shaft of the bone. In the growing skeleton the metaphysis is an area of primary growth with a rich vascular supply; and most primary neoplasms, both benign and malignant, develop at this site. An epiphyseal lesion is very suggestive of either chondroblastoma (Fig. 6–8) or infection, although cases of epiphyseal osteoid osteoma and eosinophilic granuloma have been recorded. In adults, the differential diagnosis for subarticular lesions would include metastasis, ganglion cyst, giant cell tumor, and clear cell chondrosarcoma. If there is transarticular spread, usually across joints of limited mobility, then this is suggestive of a malignant lesion, although benign lesions crossing limited movement joints have been recorded.[9] The diaphysis is often the site of origin of the malignant round cell tumors, including Ewing's sarcoma. Benign lesions at this site would include fibrous dysplasia, nonossifying fibromas, and simple and aneurysmal bone cysts.

Morphology

Patterns of Bone Destruction

The nature of bone destruction caused by a tumor is a measure of its growth rate. Lodwick recognized three patterns of bone destruction: geographic, moth-eaten, and permeative.[6] Determination of the pattern type requires analysis of the margin between the tumor and host bone. Geographic bone destruction refers to well-defined lysis with a narrow zone of transition, with or without a sclerotic rim (see Fig. 6–7*A*). This pattern denotes a slow-growing, indolent lesion that typically is benign. The thicker the sclerotic margin, the greater the likelihood of the tumor being benign. A moth-eaten pattern with a wider zone of transition indicates a moderately aggressive lesion of intermediate growth rate (Fig. 6–9), whereas a permeative pattern with a wide zone of transition, such that the tumor margins are difficult to identify, indicates a locally aggressive lesion with a rapid rate of growth (see Fig. 6–1). Within the spectrum of bone tumors, malignant lesions tend to have an aggressive (moth-eaten or permeative) pattern and benign lesions an indolent (geographic) pattern. Clearly, there can be some overlap of destructive patterns between benign and malignant lesions, and some tumors may show more than one pattern due to variable growth rate. An important differential diagnosis from malignancy of a permeative lesion is osteomyelitis, which, in the acute stages, can behave aggressively.

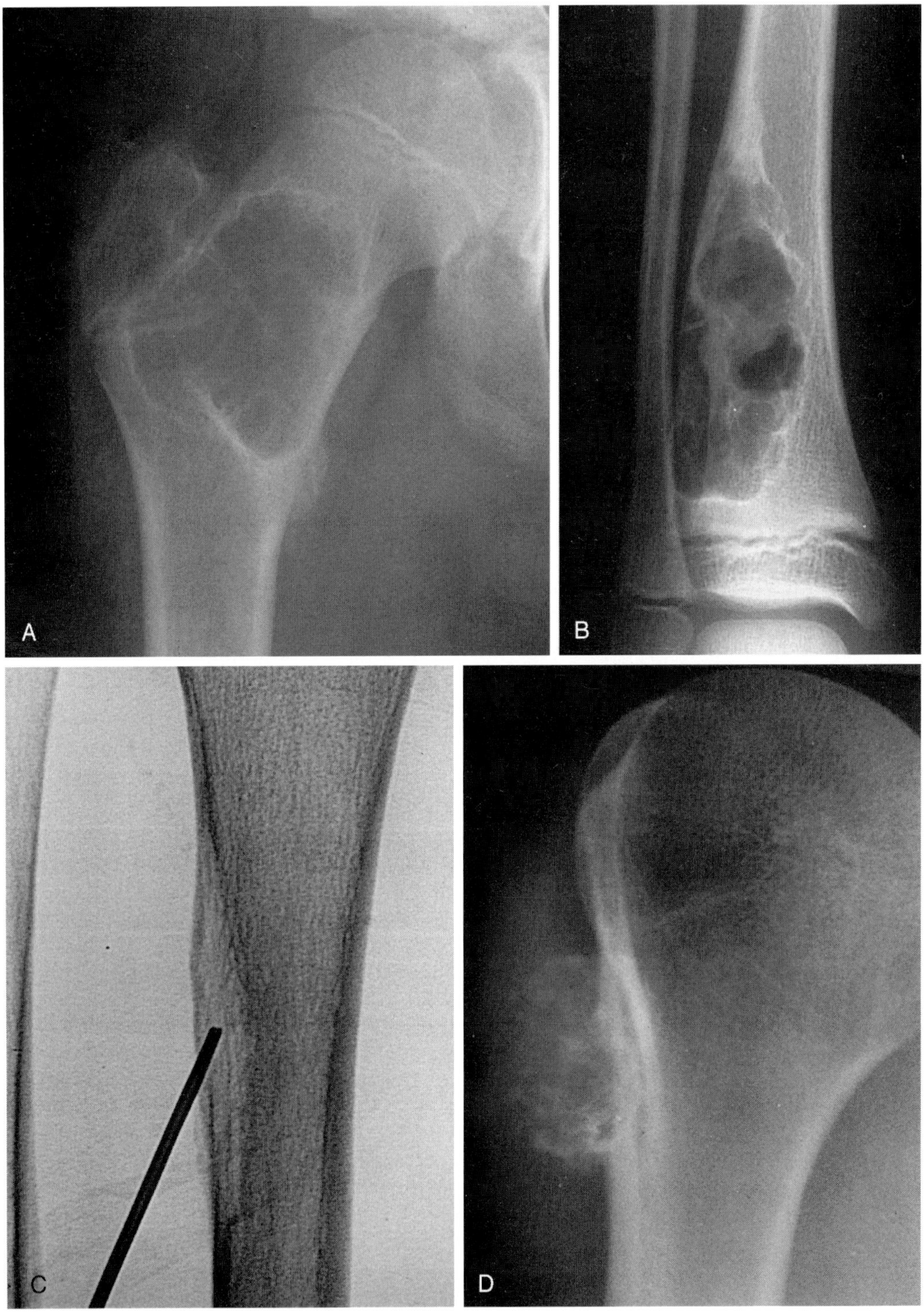

Figure 6–7. Locations of neoplasms within bone. *A,* Well-defined, slightly expansile, centrally located, lytic lesion in the right femoral neck with sclerotic margins typical of geographic bone destruction. Diagnosis: simple bone cyst. *B,* Eccentric expansile lesion of the distal tibia with well-defined rim bordered by a fine sclerotic rim. Diagnosis: nonossifying fibroma. *C,* A 65-year-old woman who had a mastectomy 20 years previously presented with a painful right lower leg. Plain radiography of the right upper tibia revealed an ill-defined, elongated, 5-cm intracortical lesion shown to be solitary on bone scintigraphy. Under fluoroscopic guidance, this lesion was sampled using a disposable Jamshidi needle, and histology revealed metastatic breast carcinoma. *D,* A 30-year-old woman presented with a painful lump in her right upper arm. The radiograph reveals a well-mineralized 2-cm juxtacortical lesion with mild saucerization of the cortical surface. These appearances are typical of a periosteal chondroma.

Tumor Matrix

Although the varied tissue components of bone tumors may reveal remarkably different histologic appearances, the majority will exhibit a radiodensity approximating that of water and are indistinguishable from one another on plain radiography. Only if the radiodensity is significantly different from water will any differentiation of the components be possible. Fat appears radiolucent to water, but appreciation of this feature only applies to imaging of the soft tissues. The matrix of fibrous dysplasia can appear of fractionally greater radiodensity than water to give the classic ground-glass appearance (see Fig. 6–5*B*). Mineralization in the form of calcification or ossification is the most easily identified radiographic evidence of the histologic nature of the tumor matrix. Many tumors will produce relatively nondescript reactive, reparative, or dystrophic mineralization, but it is the bone- and cartilage-forming tumors that exhibit typical mineralization patterns.

Organized bone is characteristic of the benign bone-forming lesions such as ossifying fibroma, osteoma, and osteoblastoma. Malignant osteoid, typified by fluffy, ill-defined, amorphous, and cloud-like densities, indicates an aggressive bone lesion such as osteosarcoma (Fig. 6–10*A*). Mineralized cartilage is variously described as having flocculent, stippled, annular, comma-shaped, or popcorn calcification. Identification of mineralized cartilage suggests the histologic nature of the tissue but does not distinguish between a benign and a malignant tumor (Fig. 6–10*B*). CT is a radiographic technique and, therefore, demonstrates matrix mineralization. In complex bony areas, such as the spine and pelvis, CT will reveal mineralization that is not easily appreciated on the conventional radiograph. Bony trabeculae may be modified or displaced as a result of the neoplasm. Giant cell tumors and aneurysmal bone cysts tend to have delicate trabeculae, whereas chondromyxoid fibroma and desmoplastic fibroma show coarser thicker trabeculae.

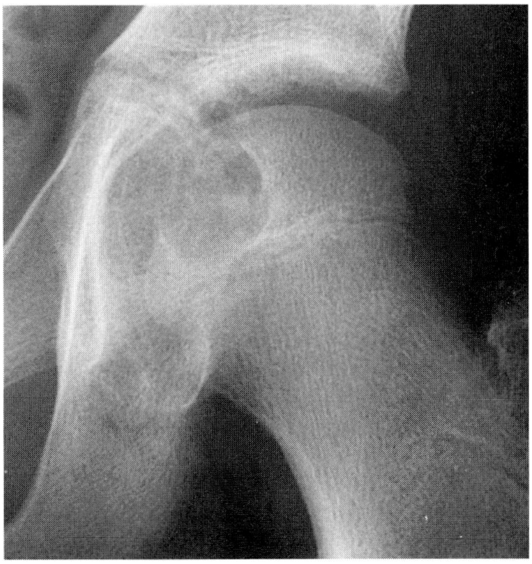

Figure 6–8. Chondroblastoma. Well-defined lytic lesion with a thin sclerotic margin in the femoral capital epiphysis.

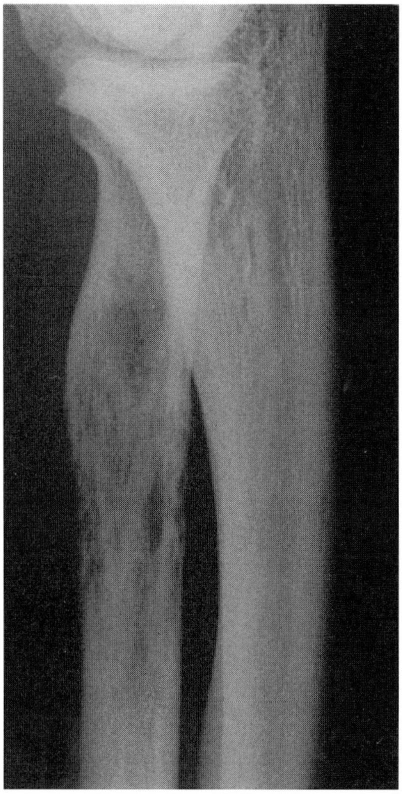

Figure 6–9. Metastatic malignant fibrous histiocytoma. Lateral radiograph of proximal right radius showing a moth-eaten pattern of bone destruction. Note the ill-defined margins and medullary and cortical destruction.

Host Bone Response and Periosteal Reaction

The host response to a tumor can be assessed to a certain extent by its effect on the bony cortex. The cortex may be an effective barrier to further lateral growth of some tumors, whereas in others the neoplasm may

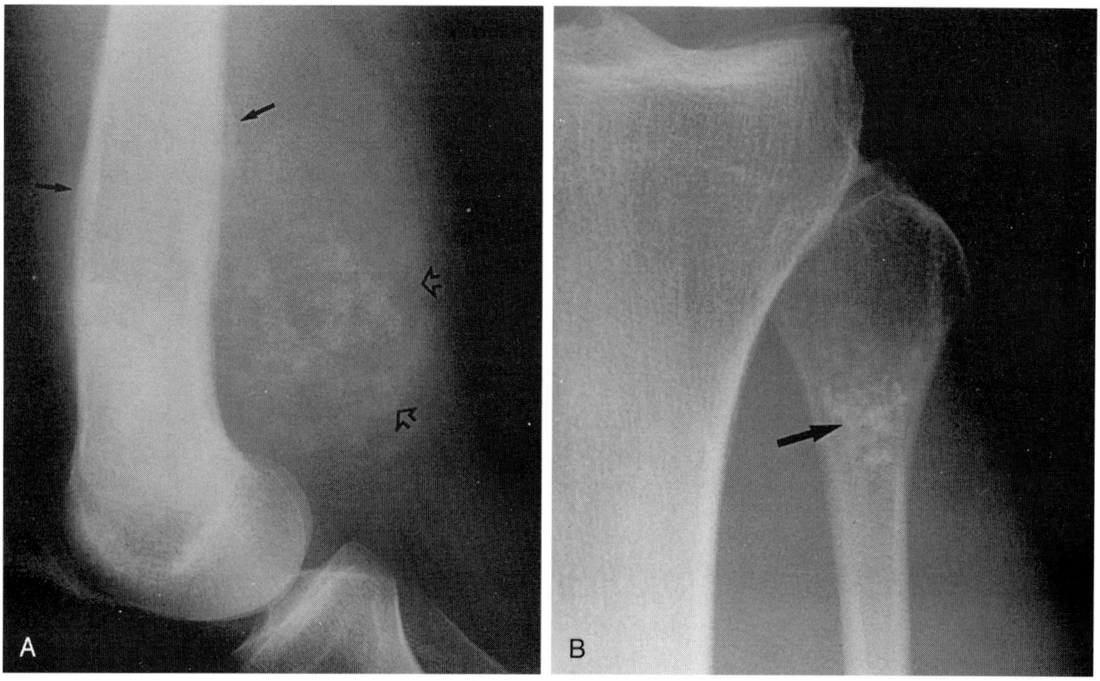

Figure 6–10. Patterns of matrix mineralization. *A*, Fluffy, cloud-like densities (*open black arrows*) within a large mass arising from the posterior aspect of the distal femur typical of an aggressive osteoblastic lesion of the distal femur. Diagnosis: osteosarcoma. Note also the periosteal reaction around the distal femur (*black arrows*). *B*, Small 2-cm lytic lesion in the neck and head of the left fibula. The lesion contains punctate mineralization (*black arrow*) but no malignant features, characteristic of an enchondroma.

penetrate the cortex partially or completely. Involvement of the cortex by a slow-growing intramedullary lesion tends to cause endosteal erosion or scalloping and may be associated with a smooth periosteal reaction. The periosteum itself is not radiopaque but if stimulated will produce reactive bone. If the lesion continues to grow, the process of endosteal resorption and periosteal reaction will be repeated, resulting in an expansile lesion. Therefore, the resultant thickness of the cortical bone depends on the amount of endosteal erosion and periosteal reaction.

The various patterns of periosteal response adjacent to lesions have been classified by Ragsdale.[10] Benign tumors tend to have smooth, solid, uninterrupted periosteal reactions, whereas more aggressive lesions have more ill-defined, irregular, interrupted, and complex reactions. The apparent "cortical shell" of expansile lesions actually represents a thin periosteal reaction that may have a lobulated or ridged appearance. At the junction between an expanded "cortical shell" and normal bone there is often solid periosteal bone, termed *buttressing* (Fig. 6–11*A*), which is often observed in aneurysmal bone cysts. At the periphery of a tumor, where it has extended through the cortex and into the parosseous soft tissues, a triangular elevation of the periosteum may be identified, known as *Codman's triangle* (Fig. 6–11*B*). This is commonly found with primary bone sarcomas such as osteosarcoma, although other patterns such as the "sunburst" or "hair-on-end" patterns are also found. It should be appreciated that the majority of periosteal reactions identified on radiographs will be of traumatic or inflammatory origin and not due to tumor.

Soft Tissue Involvement

Involvement of the soft tissues by a primary bone tumor is usually an ominous sign because it implies cortical breaching and an aggressive or malignant lesion. Soft tissue involvement due to an infective or inflammatory lesion results in the fat planes being obliterated rather than displaced (as occurs with a tumor); however, this is not a reliable sign. In some tumors, such as Ewing's sarcoma, the soft tissue mass may be very large, mimicking a primary soft

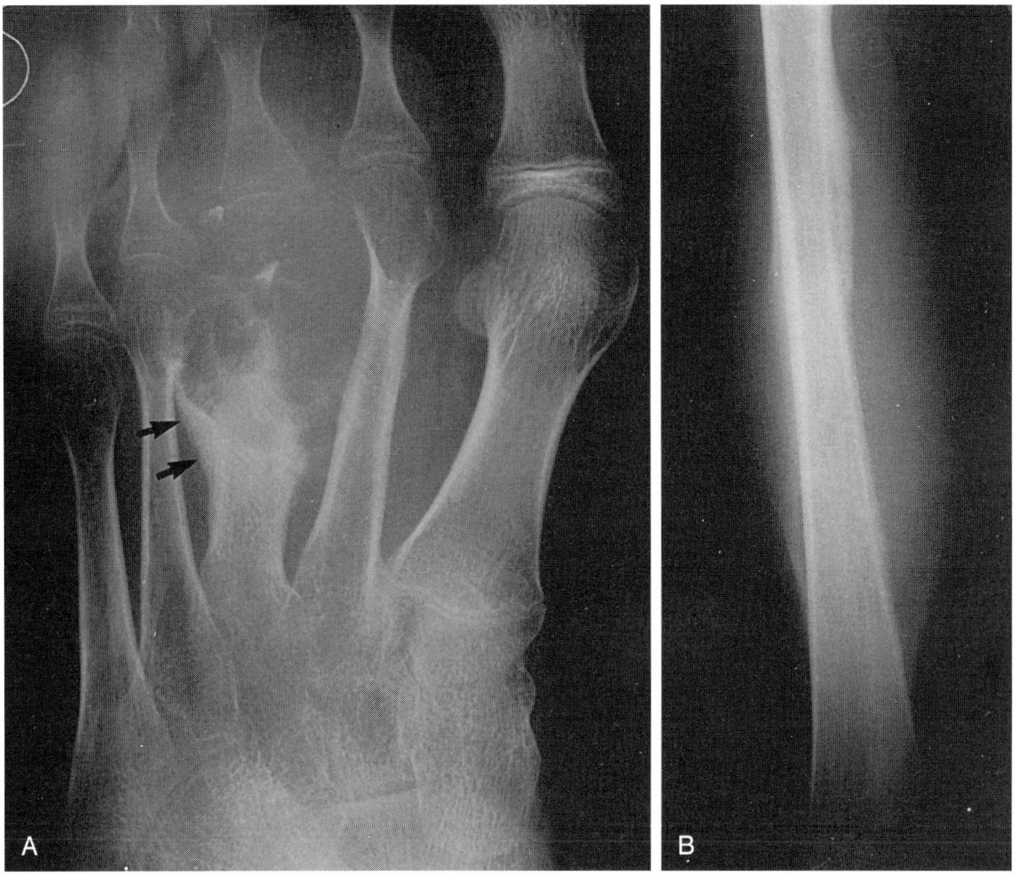

Figure 6–11. Periosteal reactions to bone neoplasms. *A,* Grossly expansile aneurysmal bone cyst of the distal third metatarsal bone. Note the well-formed periosteal bone formation or "buttressing" at the junction of normal cortex and expanded cortical shell (*arrows*). *B,* Extensive Ewing's sarcoma of the right femoral diaphysis showing Codman's triangles due to subperiosteal new bone formation.

tissue lesion. However, primary soft tissue lesions tend to erode rather than infiltrate bone, although there are several exceptions, including synovial sarcoma and fibromatosis.

Benign Versus Malignant Determination

Although it is sometimes difficult to distinguish benign from malignant bone lesions on the basis of radiography alone, certain characteristic features favor one group more than the other. In suggesting a differential diagnosis, the radiologist must weigh the various features that characterize the radiographic image. Benign tumors typically present as well-defined sclerotic borders, a geographic type of bone destruction, an uninterrupted solid periosteal reaction, and no soft tissue mass. Malignant lesions, on the other hand, tend to demonstrate a moth-eaten or permeative pattern of destruction, poorly defined borders with a wide zone of transition, an interrupted periosteal reaction of the sunburst or onion-skin type, and a soft tissue mass. However, most bone metastases do not provoke a periosteal reaction and some malignant tumors, usually of low grade, may have a benign-like appearance (e.g., clear cell chondrosarcoma). Conversely, there are benign lesions that may have aggressive features, including osteoblastoma, desmoplastic fibroma, aneurysmal bone cyst, osteomyelitis, and eosinophilic granuloma. Several benign lesions have the potential for malignant transformation (Table 6–1).

Bone Tumor Mimics

There are numerous non-neoplastic lesions that can have similar appearances to bone tu-

Table 6–1. Benign Bone Lesions That May Be Complicated by the Development of Malignancy

Benign Bone Lesion	Malignancy
Enchondroma/Ollier's disease	Central chondrosarcoma
Osteochondroma/diaphyseal aclasis	Peripheral chondrosarcoma
Fibrous dysplasia	Malignant fibrous histiocytoma, osteosarcoma
Bone infarct	Malignant fibrous histiocytoma
Paget's disease	Osteosarcoma, chondrosarcoma, malignant fibrous histiocytoma
Osteomyelitis	Squamous cell sarcoma, fibrosarcoma

mors. What constitutes a tumor mimic depends on the experience of the radiologist. The majority can be categorized as post-traumatic, inflammatory, or metabolic in origin.

Stress Fractures

Stress fractures can be divided into two types: (1) fatigue fractures that occur when repetitive stresses are applied to normal bone (often affecting adolescents) and (2) insufficiency fractures that occur when normal or physiologic stresses are placed on weakened bone (often affecting the elderly). Fatigue fractures present as bone pain, and the radiograph often shows a periosteal reaction along the shaft of a long bone (e.g., tibia). These findings by themselves are nonspecific and also raise the possibility of a sarcoma (e.g., Ewing's sarcoma[11]) or infection. However, a history of previous trauma, the location in a typical site, the uninterrupted nature of the periosteal reaction, and the absence of a soft tissue mass and associated bone destruction should suggest a fatigue fracture. Often bone scintigraphy, and sometimes CT, are performed for confirmation. Of the insufficiency fractures around the pelvis, parasymphyseal fractures typically show delayed healing with areas of lysis and callus formation simulating malignancy.[12] Such injuries may occur in isolation but are more commonly associated with occult sacral fractures. They can be confirmed on bone scintigraphy by the classic pattern of isotope uptake in the sacrum, termed the *Honda sign* (Fig. 6–12).[13] If there is still doubt, then a CT scan will be diagnostic.

Healing apophyseal avulsion injuries in the adolescent, often due to repetitive stress, can be confused with an osteosarcoma. In the early stages of avulsion injury, amorphous bone forms between the parent bone and avulsed fragment. This should not pose a problem at the lower pole of the patella (Sinding-Larsen disease) or the tibial tuberosity (Osgood-Schlatter disease), where the appearances are classic but could be confusing in the pelvis, particularly at the ischial tuberosity (hamstring insertion) if the sites of the pelvic apophyses are not known. The avulsive cortical irregularity, otherwise known as the periosteal desmoid, arising in the posteromedial metaphysis of the distal femur at the insertion of the adductor magnus muscle, is another lesion occasionally confused with an osteosarcoma. However, this lesion is now well recognized and should no longer be mistaken for an osteosarcoma (see Chapter 11).[14, 15]

Bone Infarcts

Bone infarcts, in their healing phase, present with calcifications in the marrow cavity that are often surrounded by a well-defined, hyalinized fibrotic or sclerotic border. The main differential diagnosis for this lesion is an enchondroma, and at times these infarcts can be difficult to differentiate. The lack of sclerotic rim, endosteal scalloping, and an associated lucency surrounding the calcifications (which may have typical chondroid punctate or ring-like appearances) would be far more suggestive of an enchondroma. It is possible, however, to get an expansile lytic lesion containing calcifications with endosteal scalloping in an encysted bone infarct that can resemble an enchondroma, an intraosseous lipoma, or even a chondrosarcoma.

Enostosis (Bone Island)

An enostosis represents a hamartomatous proliferation of bone and is a common incidental finding in the spine and pelvis. Radiologically, it is a small (< 2 cm), round, sclerotic intramedullary lesion, the margins of which blend in with the surrounding trabeculae. Although considered a stable lesion, it

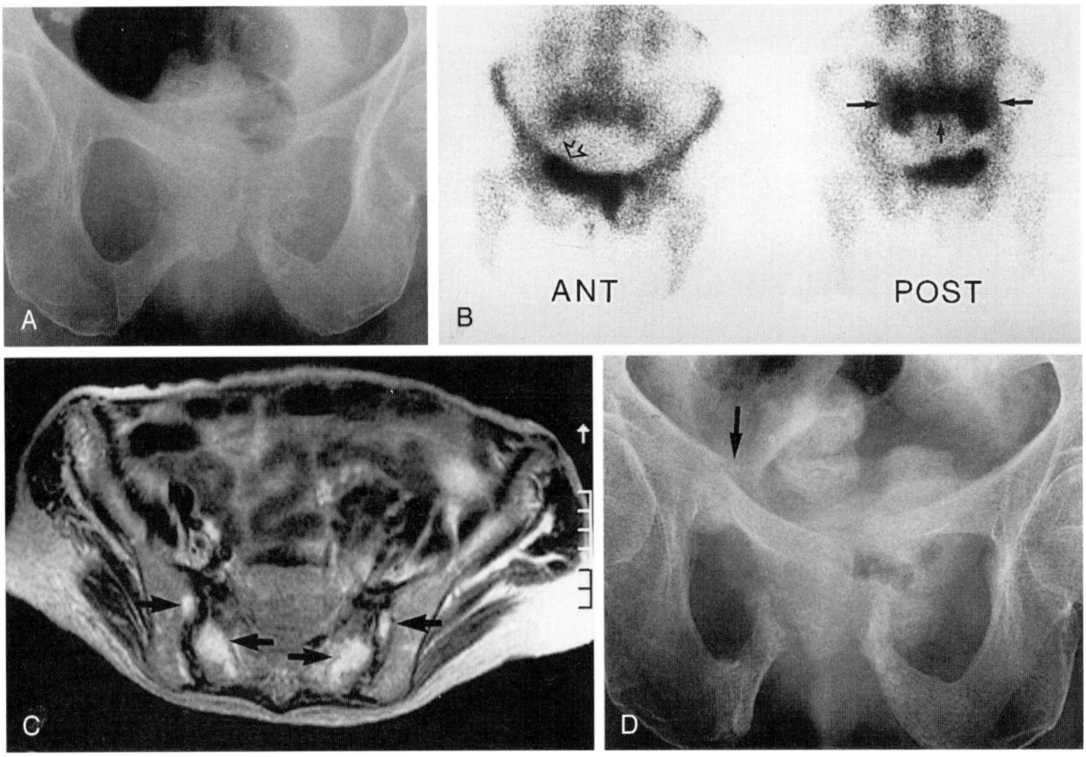

Figure 6–12. Insufficiency fractures in an elderly woman with pelvic pain for several weeks. *A,* Plain radiography shows an apparent pathologic fracture of the left pubic bone with some aggressive features and ill-defined mineralization that can simulate underlying malignancy. There is also a more recent fracture of the right inferior pubic ramus. *B,* Bone scintigraphy reveals areas of increased tracer uptake not only in the pubic bones but also in the sacral ala bilaterally with an H-shaped pattern (*arrows*)—the "Honda" sign. This indicates a horizontal sacral fracture joining two vertically oriented lateral sacral fractures. The scintigram also shows a further developing insufficiency fracture of the right superior pubic ramus (*open arrow*). *C,* The pattern of fractures is confirmed on the axial T2-weighted MR image. *D,* A plain radiograph taken several weeks later shows further development of the developing insufficiency fracture of the right superior pubic ramus (*arrow*) initially detected by the scintigram *(B)*.

may increase or decrease in size or disappear completely.[16] The differential diagnosis includes a dense osteoid osteoma or a sclerotic metastasis, but enostoses are usually painless and show little or no uptake on bone scintigraphy. Furthermore, in osteopoikilosis (multiple epiphyseal enostoses) the lesions tend to be of similar size with a centrifugal distribution, a pattern unlike that of metastases.

Myositis Ossificans

This relatively common condition usually occurs after trauma and is due to the heterotopic formation of non-neoplastic bone and cartilage in soft tissue (see Chapter 11). As the lesion evolves and matures histologically, there are corresponding changes in the radiographic features. Initially, a painful nonspecific soft tissue mass is present, but by 3 to 4 weeks flocculated densities appear within the lesion. At this stage, the lesion can be confused with an osteosarcoma, typically parosteal, both radiologically and histologically. However, the lesion demonstrates a centrifugal pattern of maturation with the periphery demarcated by initial immature bone about a cellular center. Ultrasonography is useful in demonstrating this zonal phenomenon before the typical peripheral ossification is detected radiographically at 6 to 8 weeks (Fig. 6–13).[17] By 5 to 6 months, the lesion becomes more organized, reducing in size as it reaches full maturity. Correlation of clinical information and radiologic findings is important to avoid potentially confusing biopsy results. Furthermore, surgical resection before maturation results in a high rate of recurrence and should also be avoided.

Infection

Osteomyelitis is an important consideration in the differential diagnosis of bone tumors,

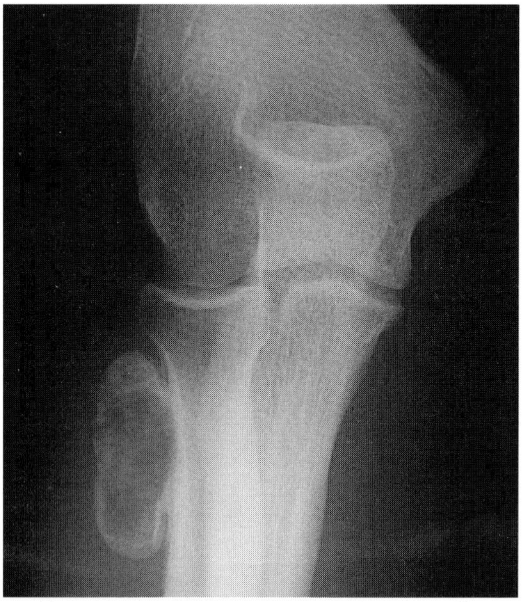

Figure 6–13. Periostitis ossificans. Well-defined ossified lesion contiguous with proximal radius typical of periostitis ossificans. This condition differs from myositis ossificans only in site.

and in its acute form in the younger patient it may mimic Ewing's sarcoma. In both, patients commonly present with pain and swelling in an extremity; radiographically, the conditions may be identical. Although an elevated erythrocyte sedimentation rate, fever, and leukocytosis might seem highly suggestive of infection, such findings may also be found in patients with Ewing's sarcoma, especially in the 10 to 30% of patients who have metastases at presentation.[18] However, acute osteomyelitis tends to have a shorter history (weeks rather than months), and the associated soft tissue swelling noted on the radiographs tends to obliterate rather than displace the fascial planes.

Subacute osteomyelitis (Brodie's abscess) is a more indolent process that can mimic benign neoplasms. Patients present with localized pain and tenderness but without any constitutional upset. The lesion is typically geographic with a well-defined sclerotic rim often in the metaphyseal region (Fig. 6–14). The differential diagnosis includes eosinophilic granuloma and other benign metaphyseal lesions. When present, irregular serpentine channels should suggest the correct diagnosis of infection. Occasionally, a bone abscess can be cortically based and can resemble an osteoid osteoma. Bone abscess can be difficult to diagnose and may require bone scintigraphy, including white blood cell–labeled studies.

Subchondral Cysts

The differential diagnosis of subarticular cystic lesions would include intraosseous ganglion, degenerative cyst, pigmented villonodular synovitis, and bone abscess and is discussed in more detail in Chapter 18.

Brown Tumors of Hyperparathyroidism

Brown tumors are localized accumulations of osteoclasts and fibrous tissue that can produce expansile lytic lesions often within long bones in patients with hyperparathyroidism (see Chapter 13). The name derives from its macroscopic appearance and is due to the breakdown of blood to the brown pigment hemosiderin. The lesions are more commonly found in primary rather than secondary hyperparathyroidism and may be difficult to differentiate from other expansile lesions of bone (e.g., giant cell tumor). If suspected, then the blood biochemistry and the other radiographic manifestations of hyperparathyroidism including osteoporosis, chondrocalcinosis, and subperiosteal bone resorption should give the diagnosis. It should also be noted that after resection of the parathyroid adenoma, "healed" brown tumors may give the appearances of osteoblastic metastases.

Other Imaging Techniques in Determining Diagnosis

Plain film assessment of some tumors may be difficult owing to the nature of the lesion (e.g., permeative bone destruction) or anatomic site (e.g., sacrum). In such cases, cross-sectional imaging helps to further characterize the lesion. Matrix mineralization in cartilage tumors is more easily detected by CT than plain radiography, especially in anatomically complex areas such as the pelvis where the lesion may be obscured. CT also allows differentiation of cystic, solid, and fatty lesions (Fig. 6–15) and may help in the diagnosis of intraosseous lipomas[19] and simple bone cysts, although the latter usually have characteristic plain film appearances. Fluid–fluid levels are often detected in aneurysmal bone cysts (Fig. 6–16), and the superior cortical detail of CT

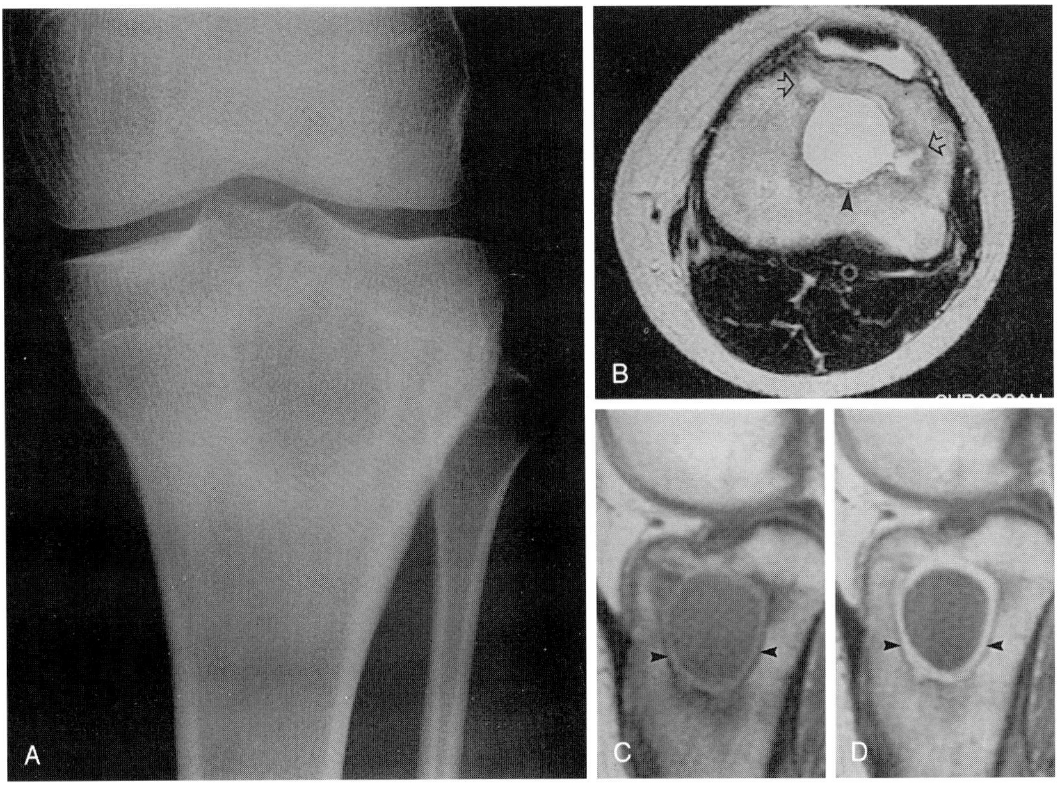

Figure 6–14. Subacute osteomyelitis. A 28-year-old woman presented with a 12-month history of nonmechanical pain in her left knee. *A,* Plain radiographs show an ill-defined 3-cm lytic lesion in the upper end of the tibia with some reactive sclerosis in the surrounding bone. *B,* On MRI the axial T2-weighted image shows the central portion is hyperintense and the peripheral rim slightly less hyperintense (*arrowheads*). Focal lateral and medial extensions are also noted (*open arrows*). *C* and *D,* The sagittal T1-weighted images before *(C)* and after *(D)* intravenous injection of gadolinium show no enhancement from the central fluid component but peripheral enhancement from the rim. These features are compatible with Brodie's abscess (subacute osteomyelitis). After aspiration, *Staphylococcus aureus* was cultured.

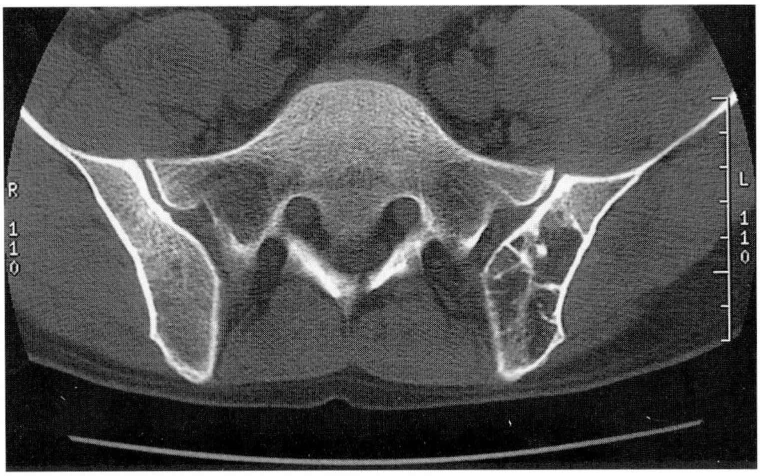

Figure 6–15. Intraosseous lipoma. A 33-year-old man presented with an incidental lesion in the left iliac bone. CT shows the lesion is slightly expansile and is mainly composed of low-density fat with some central ossification.

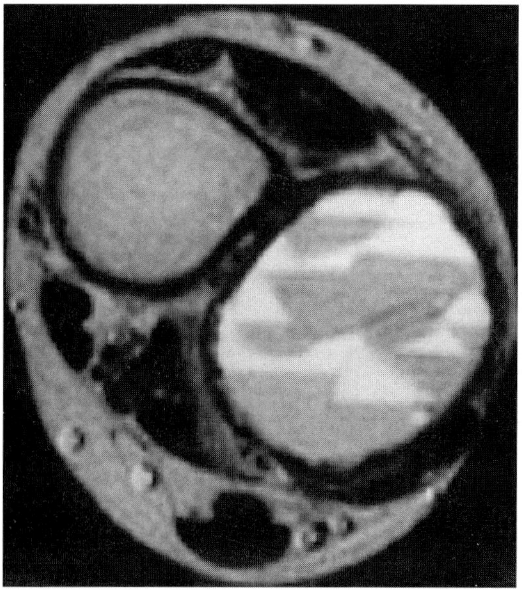

Figure 6–16. Aneurysmal bone cyst. Axial T2-weighted MR image showing multiple fluid–fluid levels in a grossly expansile lesion arising from the distal fibular metaphysis.

over MRI makes it more accurate in the diagnosis of occult osteoid osteomas (see Fig. 6–2).

In the majority of cases, tissue characterization of bone tumors based on signal intensities by MRI has not been successful. Most tumors are of low signal intensity (similar to muscle) on T1 weighting and high signal intensity on T2 weighting. However, the signal intensity and homogeneity vary with the type of tumor matrix (chondroid, osteoid, fibrous) as well as the presence of hemorrhage and necrosis. In general, benign lesions tend to be intracompartmental, well defined, and homogeneous, whereas malignant lesions are often poorly defined, inhomogeneous, and extracompartmental. However, there is a large overlap in the appearances of some benign and malignant tumors. Furthermore, because the same type of tumor may have variable appearances, tumor differentiation is not usually possible on MRI appearances alone. For example, aneurysmal bone cysts may have variable signal intensity because of the presence of both solid components and blood-filled cavernous spaces, which might in some cases be regarded as suggestive of a more aggressive lesion. Although the presence of fluid–fluid levels should suggest an aneurysmal bone cyst, they are not specific and can occasionally be found in giant cell tumors, chondroblastomas, and telangiectatic osteosarcomas.[20]

FURTHER MANAGEMENT AND STAGING OF BONE NEOPLASMS

Further management depends on a careful analysis of the radiographic features in conjunction with patient age and clinical presentation. In most cases, it is possible to characterize the aggressiveness of the tumor from the plain radiograph and thus offer an appropriate radiologic differential diagnosis. Many benign tumors such as fibrous cortical defects, nonossifying fibroma, periosteal desmoid, hemangioma, and fibrous dysplasia are often discovered incidentally and can be regarded as "leave me alone" lesions that do not require further imaging, biopsy, or follow up. Some lesions such as a simple bone cyst in an upper humerus might be followed by periodic radiographic examination, whereas a large expansile simple bone cyst in a femur would probably require treatment (see Fig. 6–7*A*).

When radiographs suggest a malignant or indeterminate lesion, further imaging is required before a biopsy is performed. This should include chest radiography and bone scintigraphy. If scintigraphy reveals multiple lesions, and there is no known primary site or evidence of extraskeletal tumor, then a biopsy of one of the involved bones is required for histologic diagnosis. In middle-aged and older adults, if scintigraphy is negative, then a radiographic skeletal survey and plasma electrophoresis should be performed to exclude myeloma. If the lesion is solitary, local staging will be required to assess tumor extent and thus guide further management. If amputation is the only curative surgical option, then only the proximal extent of the lesion is important.

Imaging Techniques for the Staging of Neoplasms

The objective of surgical staging is to define the tumor in terms of histologic grade and anatomic extent. Staging is performed according to the system of the Musculoskeletal Tumour Society[21] (discussed in more detail in Chapter 1). Stage 1 lesions are classified as low-grade lesions, whereas stage 2 lesions are high grade. The stages are subdivided according to whether the lesion is intracompartmental (A) or extracompartmental (B). Patients with metastases at presentation are classified as stage 3, irrespective of histologic grade.

Magnetic Resonance Imaging

For local staging, MRI is undoubtedly superior to CT for the definition of medullary and extracortical spread and of the relationship of the tumor to critical neurovascular structures. This makes MRI the cross-sectional imaging method of choice for staging lesions with extracompartmental spread. Further advantages of MRI include a direct multiplanar facility, a wide field of view, superb contrast and improving spatial resolution, and the avoidance of bony streak artifacts and ionizing radiation. It is not good policy or cost effective to perform both CT and MRI on patients with bone tumors. The choice of technique depends on the probable nature and likely management of the lesion. If the lesion is likely to be aggressive, then MRI will be required for local staging. More indolent, intraosseous lesions can be staged by either technique, although the superior ability of CT in detecting matrix mineralization and a cortical shell may be advantageous in some cases.

In routine spin-echo imaging, the T1-weighted sequences are better for demonstrating the extent of marrow involvement, and T2-weighted sequences are better for evaluating cortical and juxtacortical soft tissue involvement (Fig. 6–17). Benign and aggressive periosteal reactions can be demonstrated on MRI, although they are best assessed by plain radiography or CT. Fat-suppressed, Gd-DTPA–enhanced T1-weighted images may make a tumor more conspicuous, may distinguish between tumor and edema, and may demonstrate viable tumor (Fig. 6–18). Because the location of viable tumor is important when considering the optimal site for biopsy, the routine use of gadolinium in staging the primary tumor would seem indicated. The use of

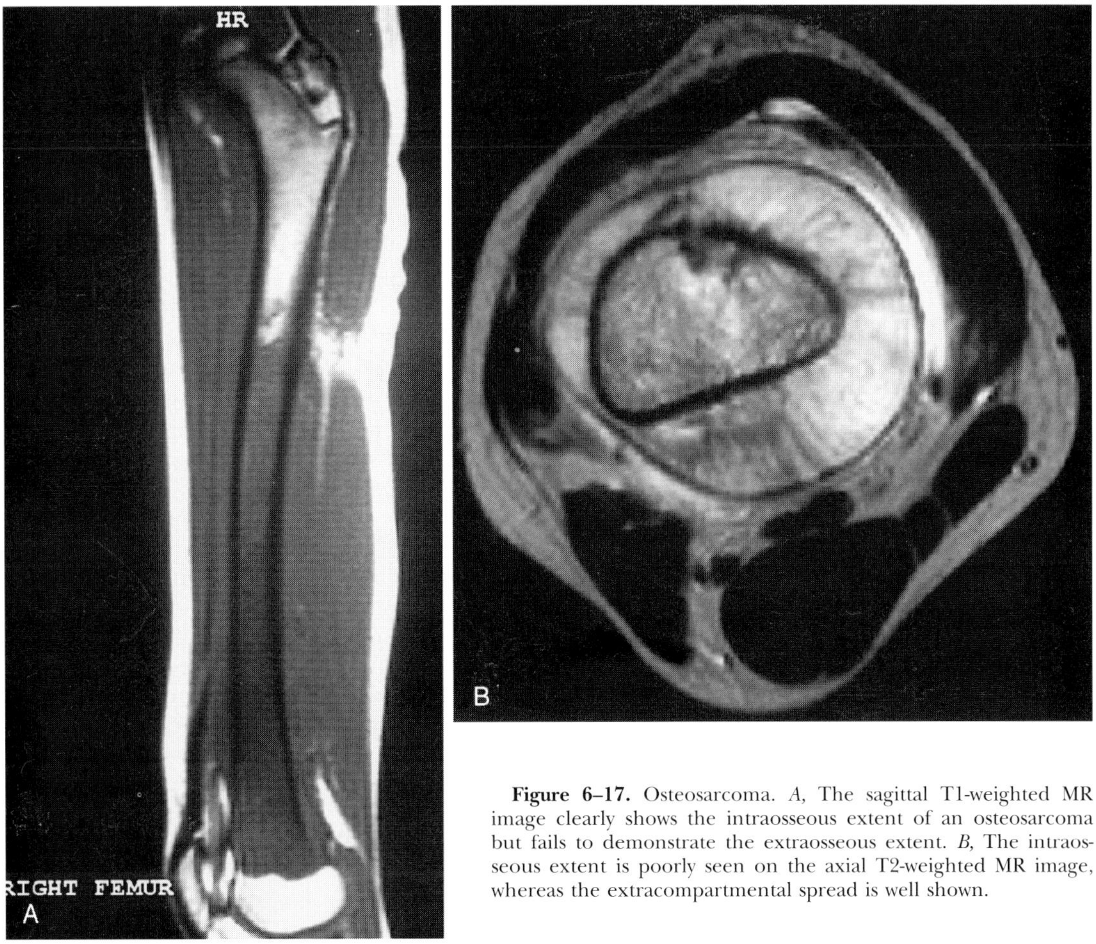

Figure 6–17. Osteosarcoma. *A,* The sagittal T1-weighted MR image clearly shows the intraosseous extent of an osteosarcoma but fails to demonstrate the extraosseous extent. *B,* The intraosseous extent is poorly seen on the axial T2-weighted MR image, whereas the extracompartmental spread is well shown.

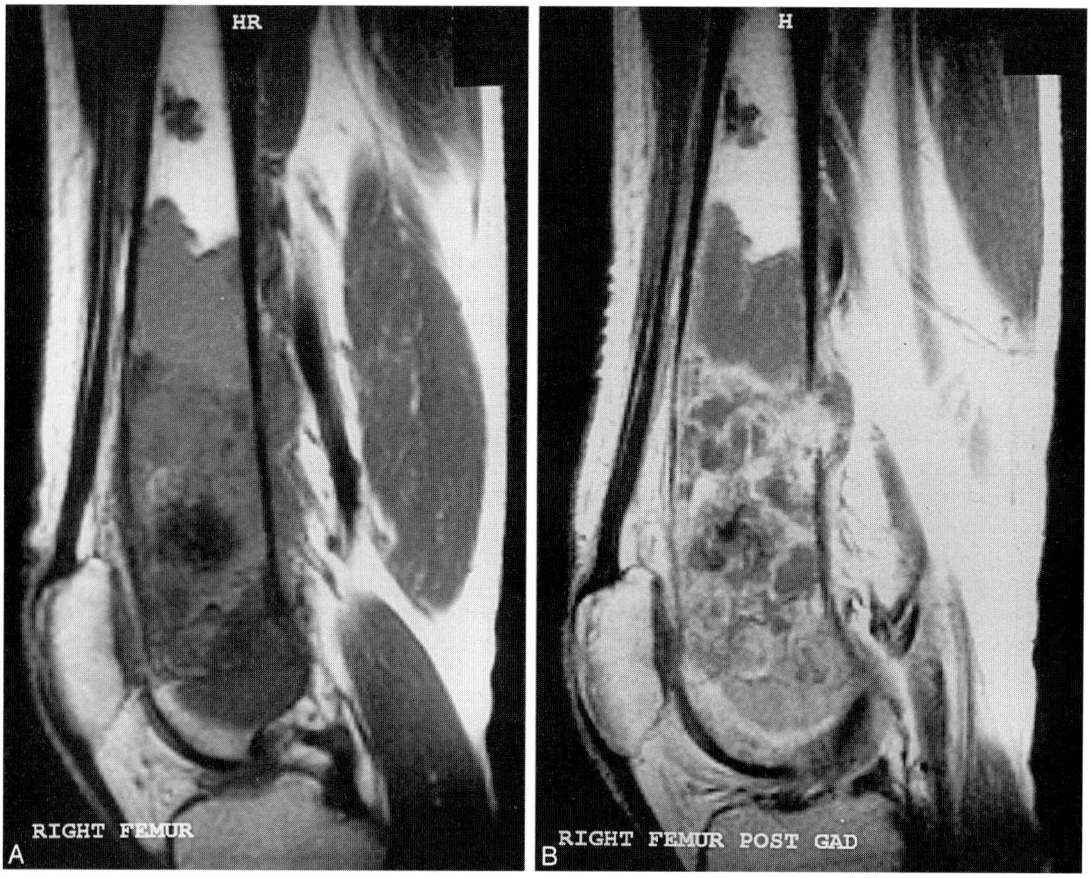

Figure 6–18. Gadolinium enhancement of osteosarcoma. Sagittal T1-weighted MR images before *(A)* and after *(B)* gadolinium enhancement of a distal femoral osteosarcoma. The enhancing areas are viable tumor, whereas the areas that fail to enhance are necrotic. A small skip metastasis is present in the proximal bone.

dynamic Gd-DTPA studies in trying to differentiate between benign and malignant lesions is more controversial and is probably not justified routinely.[22, 23]

Angiography

Although angiography was used in the past to outline the extraosseous extent of bone tumors, it is now rarely used as a diagnostic or staging tool. A prospective study[24] has confirmed the superiority of conventional MRI to CT and angiography in visualizing the relationship between tumor and large vessels (Fig. 6–19). Sufficient progress has now been made with MR angiography in demonstrating tumor neovascularity that it will probably replace conventional arteriography for preoperative planning.[25, 26] Conventional or intra-arterial digital subtraction arteriography remains useful before embolization and intra-arterial chemotherapy.[27]

Computed Tomography

Computed tomography is the best technique at present for detecting early pulmonary metastases and should be performed routinely in the initial staging of bone sarcomas.

Bone Scintigraphy

Isotope scintigraphy is of little value in the primary lesion but is essential for the detection of bony metastases. Of the primary malignant tumors of bone in childhood, scintigraphy of osteosarcoma and Ewing's tumors at presentation reveals bony metastases in approximately 3% and 12%, respectively.[18]

BIOPSY OF BONE NEOPLASMS

Although some surgeons would contend that open biopsy has a higher success rate

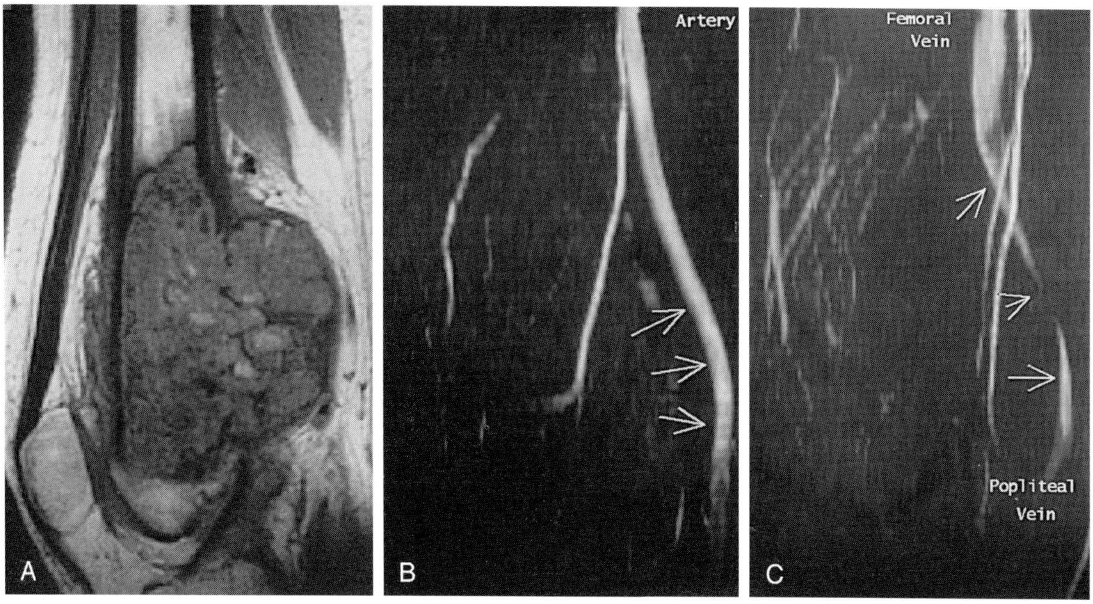

Figure 6–19. Vascular relationships of osteosarcoma. *A,* Sagittal T1-weighted MR image showing an extensive osteosarcoma of the distal femoral metadiaphysis. The tumor extends into the soft tissues posteriorly and into the knee joint inferiorly along the cruciate ligaments. *B* and *C,* The MR angiograms show posterior displacement of the popliteal vessels.

(and is therefore preferable) than percutaneous needle biopsy, this has to be balanced against other factors. Mankin et al., in a study of 597 biopsies of which 512 were open and 85 percutaneous, found diagnostic error in 24% of open biopsies and 40% of needle biopsies.[28] However, the poor results in the percutaneous group were mainly due to fine-needle aspiration biopsy—a technique that is known to be inaccurate in the diagnosis of some primary musculoskeletal tumors (see Chapter 7 for a more detailed discussion of the advantages and limitations of fine-needle aspiration cytology). Furthermore, the complication rate for the open biopsy group was significantly higher than that for the percutaneous biopsy group. Alterations in treatment plan and altered outcome for the open biopsy group occurred in 20% and 11% of the patients, respectively, whereas for the percutaneous group the corresponding figures were 8% and 2%. In a study of 55 open biopsies, Waldron et al.[29] obtained a diagnostic accuracy of 92% but also described complications, including infection, hematoma, inappropriate biopsy excision site, problems with the drain exit site, and tumor seeding.

Percutaneous biopsy is now accepted by many authorities as the biopsy technique of choice. With imaging guidance and local anesthetic, the technique is relatively straightforward, quick, safe, and repeatable and has a low risk of tumor seeding. It is also possible to extract material from tumor at different depths and to reach sites that are otherwise only accessible by major surgery. Percutaneous biopsy has an accuracy rate of over 90% in tumors with uniform cytologic pattern, including metastases, myeloma, lymphoma, Ewing's sarcoma, and solitary plasmacytoma. It is less accurate in bone tumors with a complex pathologic architecture and cell pleomorphism, such as giant cell tumor, aneurysmal bone cysts, osteoblastoma, and most bone sarcomas. However, in most series, positive results are obtained in over 75% of cases,[30] and in some centers the accuracy rates rise to 97% or over.[31] The overall complication rate for needle biopsy is very low (0.6%), and complications tend to be minor.

Discussion between the radiologist and orthopedic surgeon is important in choosing the biopsy site. A biopsy should be taken from the most aggressive and viable part of the lesion as determined by imaging. In aggressive lesions, this part is usually peripherally located because the center is often necrotic. The biopsy should be made within a single compartment through an approach that avoids neurovascular structures and that can be resected at the definitive surgical procedure. There are several imaging modalities that can assist biopsy, including fluoroscopy, CT, and ultrasonography. Fluoroscopy has been the traditional method and has several advantages, including permanent control of the biopsy needle position and availability. A fluoroscopic unit with a C-arm is especially valuable because it allows visualization of the needle in multiple planes without moving the patient. CT allows intermittent but precise control of needle position and is especially useful when lesions are not clearly seen on fluoroscopy or when lesions are close to vital anatomic structures. CT is particularly useful in the percutaneous treatment of osteoid osteomas.[32] Both CT and ultrasonography can assist in obtaining biopsy samples of the soft tissue components of malignant bone tumors.

Although the soft tissue component of a bone tumor can be sampled with a Trucut needle (Travenol Labs, Deerfield, IL), a trephine cutting needle is required for most bone tumors. The choice of biopsy needle depends on personal preference and on the type of bone for biopsy. Some needles, including the Ackerman and Craig needles, include an external cannula that is advanced to the bone and a separate, serrated, trephine bone-cutting needle introduced through the external cannula for sampling. The Jamshidi needle (Fig. 6–20) is different in that its external cannula, which is advanced to the bone with an internal obturator, is also used to remove the bone specimen due to its cutting edge. One of the major difficulties in the past has been trying to sample through thick cortical bone. However, there are now new biopsy needles, including strengthened and serrated biopsy tips, mechanical rotating devices,[33] and a metallic hammer to ensure an adequate specimen is obtained.

Careful handling and processing of the biopsy specimen is important in ensuring a diagnostic study. In all suspected bone tumors, a sample of tissue or aspirated fluid should be sent for culture and sensitivity study and the remainder of the specimen (including any aspirated blood) should be sent for pathologic analysis. Many clinicians perform a combined cytologic study, making a simple imprint either from the fresh biopsy core[34] or from the paraffin-embedded material.[30] Although cytology can be useful in differentiating Ewing's sarcoma from osteomyelitis and eosinophilic granuloma, in many cases cytology is not sufficient for diagnosis.

Where possible, biopsy should not be performed until the imaging staging studies have been completed because the trauma of the biopsy may exaggerate the true extent of the tumor.

ASSESSMENT OF THE EFFECTS OF TREATMENT

Once the diagnosis of a bone tumor has been confirmed by histologic examination, together with the radiologic correlation, the definitive management can be instituted. For benign tumors, this may involve curettage, with or without the use of bone grafting. The optimum treatment for a malignant bone tumor, where practical, is limb salvage surgery. Before surgery, however, the majority of patients un-

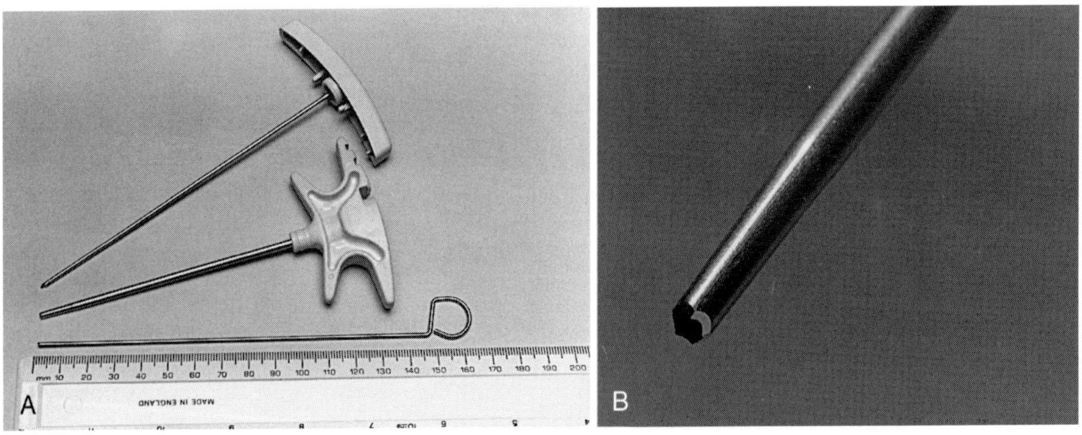

Figure 6–20. Example of biopsy needle. *A*, Disposable Jamshidi-type needle—Biomid (Gallini SRL, Modena, Italy). *B*, Magnified view of the serrated cutting edge and a narrowed tapered end, which avoids crushed specimens.

dergo an intensive regimen of adjuvant chemotherapy, the exception being patients with a chondrosarcoma that is not sensitive to chemotherapy. Radiation therapy is largely reserved for palliative purposes and for tumors in surgically inaccessible areas.

After a course of approximately 10 weeks of chemotherapy, the patients are restaged with a repeat CT scan of the chest and an MRI of the primary tumor. The purpose of restaging is to assess the response of the primary tumor to the chemotherapy and to ensure that the intended surgery remains appropriate. Various imaging parameters show moderate correlation with the percentage necrosis on histology, which in turn correlates well with disease-free survival (see Chapter 8). These parameters include the degree of mineralization in osteosarcoma, changes in size of the extraosseous component, particularly in Ewing's sarcoma, and alterations in the rate of tumor enhancement with Gd-DTPA using a dynamic MRI technique.[35]

Curative limb-salvage surgery is usually possible in approximately 80% of cases with a primary bone sarcoma. The surgery employs either an endoprosthetic replacement or an allograft, depending on the preference and expertise of the treatment center. In those patients in whom limb-salvage surgery is not possible, the options include palliative surgery or amputation. After surgery, the role of imaging focuses on the identification of the development of metastatic disease, local tumor recurrence, and complications of the treatment itself.

The vast majority of bone sarcomas will metastasize to the lungs. Routine follow-up chest radiographs are performed every 3 months for 2 years and every 6 months thereafter. If the chest radiograph suggests the presence of pulmonary metastases, a CT scan of the chest is required. This will accurately document the full extent and distribution of the metastasis, which is necessary if excision through a thoracotomy is being considered.

The introduction of chemotherapy for the treatment of osteosarcoma has altered the pathogenesis of the disease such that a minority of patients will develop bone metastases in the absence of visible pulmonary metastases. In this situation, bone scintigraphy is required to assess the extent of skeletal involvement.

Local recurrence is a problem that has arisen since the introduction of limb-salvage surgery. The risks are greatly increased the more marginal the surgical resection. Recurrence is usually first observed by the patients themselves as pain or swelling. If the tumor mineralizes, this may be detected as calcification or ossification on a radiograph (Fig. 6–21) or as increased activity on bone scintigraphy. The most accurate method for detecting local recurrence is cross-sectional imaging. If the recurrence is greater than 15 mL in volume, both CT and MRI are of comparable accuracy.[36] For smaller tumors, MRI is the technique of choice. Although there will be some image artifact from the metallic endoprosthesis, sufficient detail is usually achieved to detect recurrences as small as 1 to 2 cm in diameter (Fig. 6–22). Enhancement with Gd-DTPA is useful in distinguishing between postoperative fluid collections and recurrent tumor.

The treatment of patients with a primary bone sarcoma is necessarily protracted, and it is not unusual for complications to arise. These include infections associated with the immunosuppressive and toxic effects of chemotherapy, mechanical loosening of endo-

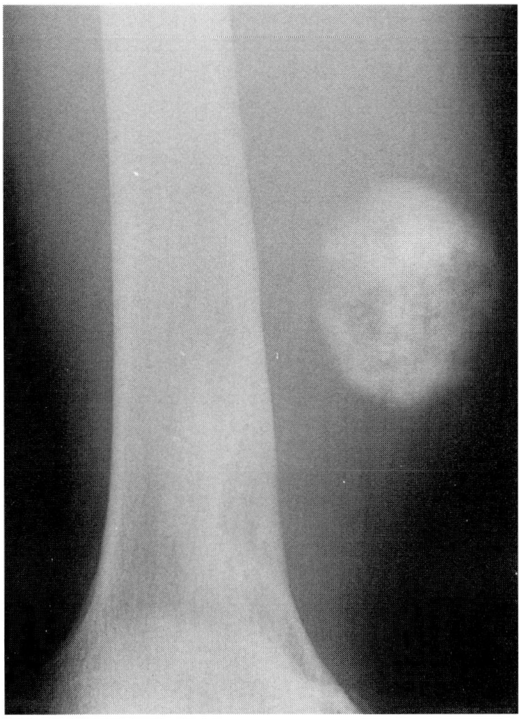

Figure 6–21. Recurrent parosteal osteosarcoma. Mineralized tumor recurrence within the soft tissues of the medial thigh. Appearance is in keeping with recurrence of a previously excised parosteal osteosarcoma. Note the previous excision site in the medial femoral metaphysis.

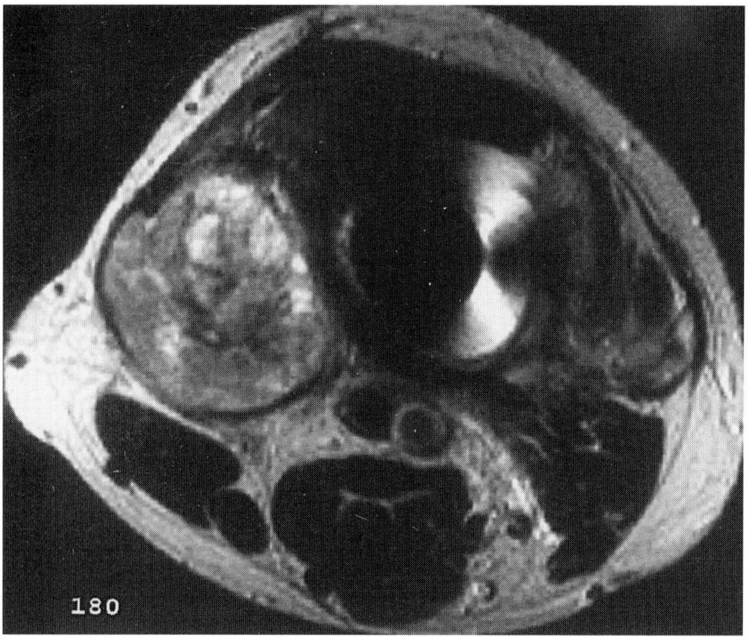

Figure 6–22. Recurrent osteosarcoma and metallic artifact. Axial T2-weighted MR image of the distal thigh showing a 5-cm recurrence of osteosarcoma in the vastus medialis muscle. There is a central signal void with surrounding high signal artifact from the titanium distal femoral endoprosthesis.

prostheses, and the specter of a radiation-induced sarcoma where radiation therapy has been used. Clearly, imaging has a role to play in the detection, diagnosis, and management of any of these complications.

REFERENCES

1. Frank JA, Ling A, Patronas NJ, et al: Detection of malignant bone tumours: MR imaging vs scintigraphy. AJR Am J Roentgenol 155:1043, 1990.
2. Algra PR, Bloem JL, Tissing H, et al: Detection of vertebral metastases: Comparison between MR imaging and bone scintigraphy. Radiographics 11:219, 1991.
3. Erdham WA, Tamburro F, Jayson HT, et al: Osteomyelitis: Characteristics and pitfalls with MR imaging. Radiology 180:533, 1991.
4. Mirowitz SA, Apicella P, Reinus WR, et al: MR imaging of bone marrow lesions: Relative conspicuousness on T1-weighted, fat suppressed T2-weighted and STIR images. AJR Am J Roentgenol 162:215, 1994.
5. Sundarum M, McLeod RA: MR imaging of tumour and tumour-like lesions of bone and soft tissue. AJR Am J Roentgenol 155:817, 1990.
6. Lodwick GS: The bones and joints. *In* Hodes PJ (ed): Atlas of Tumour Radiology. Chicago, Year Book Medical Publishers, 1971.
7. Lodwick GS, Wilson AJ, Farrell C, et al: Determining growth rates of focal lesions of bone from radiographs. Radiology 134:577, 1980.
8. Lodwick GS, Wilson AJ, Farrell C, et al: Estimating rate of growth in bone lesions: Observer performance and error. Radiology 134:585, 1980.
9. Abdelwahab IF, Miller TT, Hermann G, et al: Transarticular invasion of joints by tumours: Hypothesis. Skeletal Radiol 20:279, 1991.
10. Ragsdale BD, Madewell JE, Sweet DE: Radiologic and pathologic analysis of solitary bone lesions: II. Periosteal reactions. Radiol Clin North Am 19:749, 1981.
11. Davies AM, Evans NS, Grimer RJ: Fatigue fractures of the proximal tibia simulating malignancy. Br J Radiol 61:903, 1988.
12. Davies AM, Evans NS, Struthers GR, et al: Parasymphyseal and associated insufficiency fractures of the pelvis and sacrum. Br J Radiol 61:103, 1988.
13. De Smet AA, Neff JR: Pubic and sacral insufficiency fractures. AJR Am J Roentgenol 145:601, 1985.
14. Bufkin AC: The avulsive cortical irregularity. AJR Am J Roentgenol 112:487, 1971.
15. Resnick D, Greenway G: Distal femoral cortical defects, irregularities and excavations: A critical review of the literature with the addition of histologic and palaeolithic data. Radiology 143:345, 1982.
16. Onitsuka H: Roentgenologic aspects of bone islands. Radiology 123:607, 1977.
17. Thomas EA, Cassar-Pullicino VN, McCall IW: The role of ultrasound in the early diagnosis and management of heterotopic bone formation. Clin Radiol 43:190, 1991.
18. Horowitz ME, Tsokos MG, Delaney TF: Ewing's sarcoma. Cancer 42:300, 1992.
19. Williams CE, Close PJ, Meaney J, et al: Intraosseous lipomas. Clin Radiol 47:348, 1993.
20. Burr BA, Resnick D, Syklawer R, et al: Fluid-fluid levels in a unicameral bone cyst: CT and MR findings. J Comput Ass Tomogr 17:134, 1993.
21. Enneking WF: Staging of musculoskeletal neoplasms. Skeletal Radiol 13:183, 1985.
22. Erlemann R, Reiser MF, Peters PE, et al: Musculoskeletal neoplasms: Static and dynamic Gd-DTPA-enhanced MR imaging. Radiology 171:767, 1989.
23. Geirnaerdt MJ, Bloem JL, Eulderink F, et al: Cartilaginous tumours: Correlation of gadolinium-enhanced

MR imaging and histopathologic findings. Radiology 186:813, 1993.
24. Bloem JL, Taminian AH, Eulderink F, et al: Radiologic staging of primary bone sarcoma: MR imaging, scintigraphy, angiography and CT correlated with pathologic examination. Radiology 169:805, 1988.
25. Lang P, Grampp S, Vahlensieck M, et al: Primary bone tumours: Value of MR angiography for preoperative planning and monitoring response to chemotherapy. AJR Am J Roentgenol 165:135, 1995.
26. Swan JS, Grist TM, Sproat IA, et al: Musculoskeletal neoplasms: Preoperative planning with MR angiography. Radiology 194:519, 1995.
27. Bilbao JI, Martin Algarra S, Martinez de Negri J, et al: Osteosarcoma: Correlation between radiological and histological changes after intra-arterial chemotherapy. Eur J Radiol 11:98, 1990.
28. Mankin HJ, Mankin CJ, Simon MA: The hazards of biopsy, revisited. J Bone Joint Surg Am 78:656, 1996.
29. Waldron B, Moran RM, Hurson BJ: Biopsy problems in patients with musculoskeletal tumours. Ir J Med Sci 159:246, 1990.
30. Schajowicz F: Current trends in the diagnosis and treatment of malignant tumours. Clin Orthop 180:22, 1983.
31. Stoker DJ, Cobb JP, Pringle JS: Needle biopsy of musculoskeletal lesions: A review of 208 procedures. J Bone Joint Surg 158B:641, 1991.
32. Mazoyer JF, Kohler R, Bossaro D: Osteoid osteoma: CT-guided percutaneous treatment. Radiology 181: 269, 1991.
33. Ahlstrom KH, Astrom KGO: CT-guided bone biopsy performed by means of a coaxial biopsy system with an eccentric drill. Radiology 188:549, 1993.
34. Stoker DJ, Kissin CK: Percutaneous vertebral biopsy: A review of 135 cases. Clin Radiol 36:569, 1985.
35. Van der Woude HJ, Bloem JL, Verstraete KL, et al: Osteosarcoma and Ewing's sarcoma after neoadjuvant chemotherapy: Value of dynamic MRI in detecting viable tumor before surgery. AJR Am J Roentgenol 165:593, 1995.
36. Reuther G, Mutschler W: Detection of local recurrent disease in musculoskeletal tumours: MRI versus CT. Skeletal Radiol 19:85, 1990.

Chapter

7

FINE NEEDLE ASPIRATION OF BONE AND JOINT NEOPLASMS

LESTER J. LAYFIELD and LESLIE G. DODD

Newly discovered lesions of bone require investigation to determine their clinical significance. Although radiographic study often provides a limited differential diagnosis, the majority of lesions suspicious for a neoplasm will require biopsy before appropriate clinical management can proceed. Selection of the appropriate biopsy technique and operative approach are vital to the success of subsequent therapy.[1-3] There are clear indications for, and advantages associated with, needle, trocar, and open biopsy techniques[2] as well as for fine needle aspiration biopsy. The biopsy technique and site must be selected to ensure adequate sampling to optimize the chances for accurate pathologic diagnosis. Incision sites must be selected to optimize the outcome of subsequent definitive procedures.[1] Specifically, tumor bed contamination must be avoided and biopsy defects must not compromise the load-bearing properties of the bone if limb-salvage surgery is being considered.

ADVANTAGES, LIMITATIONS AND ACCURACY OF FINE NEEDLE ASPIRATION CYTOLOGY

Fine needle aspiration cytology (FNA) offers an attractive alternative to traditional open or cutting needle biopsy. Advantages of FNA include its speed of diagnosis, minimal patient discomfort and morbidity, little or no disruption of tumor bed, no recovery time required, lessened risk of wound infection, and little or no effect on the functional integrity of the bone. Acceptance of FNA has been limited by concerns over diagnostic accuracy and the inherit physical limitations of the technique itself. Because FNA uses a small-caliber needle, many predominantly sclerotic or osteoblastic lesions cannot be effectively entered and generally yield little or no material at the time of aspiration. Cystic lesions, when aspirated, may yield large amounts of blood or fluid but few diagnostic cellular elements. An important limitation of FNA is its inability to accurately subclassify certain types of lesions. For example, many high-grade sarcomas cannot be classified further than "high-grade spindle cell sarcoma."

The majority of bone tumors are metastatic deposits, with a 25:1 ratio between metastases and primary bone neoplasms.[4] Over 80% of metastatic deposits arise from primary tumors within the breast, prostate, lung, kidney, or thyroid. Metastases may be osteolytic or osteoblastic, and, although the radiographic appearance of the lesion usually suggests the diagnosis, a significant number of metastases undergo tissue sampling. FNA represents a rapid and highly accurate technique for such sampling, and most series of bone lesions investigated by aspiration cytology contain a high percentage of metastatic neoplasms.[5-18] Accuracy rates for the diagnosis of metastatic disease have varied from 78[5] to 95%.[9] This compares favorably with diagnostic accuracy rates obtained with core needle biopsy.[19] Because of the high degree of accuracy and the relatively low complication rate associated with the aspiration technique, FNA has become the preferred biopsy method for presumed metastatic lesions involving bone.

Fine needle aspiration cytology as a diagnostic technique for the work-up of a primary bone neoplasm is more controversial and less widely used. Accuracy rates for FNA have varied widely within the literature. In experienced hands, FNA has a diagnostic accuracy of between 62%[20] and 90%.[5] This is similar to the diagnostic accuracy rates of 73 to 96% reported for core needle biopsy.[19, 20] Careful comparison of published accuracy rates for open, core needle, and aspiration biopsy supports the value of FNA for the diagnosis of many bone neoplasms. Mankin et al.[3] studied the accuracy and incidence of complications associated with open or core biopsy in a series of 222 bone lesions. Eighteen per cent of biopsies were associated with a major error in diagnosis, and the optimal treatment plan had to be altered in a similar percentage of cases because of problems related to the biopsy. In 4.5% of cases, an unnecessary amputation had to be performed because of complications resulting from the biopsy. These complication rates are higher than those associated with FNA. Layfield et al.[20] reported a 10% rate of error in diagnosis and a 7% rate of negative impact on therapy due to diagnostic errors associated with FNA.

DIAGNOSTIC APPROACH AND CYTOLOGIC CRITERIA FOR THE DIAGNOSIS OF PRIMARY OSSEOUS NEOPLASMS

The rate of success for the FNA diagnosis of bone lesions can be optimized by careful study of prebiopsy radiographs and selection of cases in which FNA is most likely to succeed. Certain lesions are poor candidates for cytologic diagnosis. A prerequisite for successful aspiration is the ability for a thin needle to enter the diagnostic area of the lesion. Bone tumors with intact surrounding cortices or sclerotic rims are generally not suitable for FNA diagnosis. Similarly, densely sclerotic, calcified, or ossified lesions such as osteoblastoma and osteoid osteoma make poor candidates for needle aspiration cytology. Markedly cystic lesions (aneurysmal bone cyst, telangiectatic osteosarcoma, and unicameral bone cyst) may yield only blood or clear fluid with little or no lesional tissue, making cytologic diagnosis impossible. The cytologic separation of aneurysmal bone cyst from telangiectatic osteosarcoma may be particularly treacherous because of the low cellularity of the aspirated material. A final category of lesions in which FNA is not likely to yield satisfactory results is that of cartilaginous neoplasms. The architectural clues that are extremely important in the separation of low-grade chondrosarcomas from enchondromas are lacking in aspirated material, so that it is frequently impossible to cytologically separate enchondromas from Grade I and some Grade II chondrosarcomas. Many Grade II and all Grade III chondrosarcomas can be recognized as malignant by FNA. Needle aspiration cytology can establish the presence of a cartilage forming neoplasm and hence may be of diagnostic value despite these limitations.

Once these limitations of the FNA technique are appreciated, and an appropriate selection of cases for aspiration is made, aspiration cytology can achieve a high degree of diagnostic accuracy in a shorter time than is required for more conventional methods of diagnosis, thus ultimately improving the management of patients with primary neoplasms of the bone.

Nowhere else in aspiration cytology is clinical-radiographic-cytologic correlation more important than in the diagnosis of bone tumors. Bone lesions frequently have characteristic sites of origin and ages in which they occur. Because the matrix of bone is calcified, radiographs are particularly helpful in defining the gross anatomy of these lesions, the pattern of growth, and interaction with surrounding host bone. This allows the formulation of a reasonably narrow radiographic differential diagnosis. Correlation of clinical and radiographic data is imperative for the accurate cytologic diagnosis of bone tumors.

The diagnosis of primary bone neoplasms by FNA can be facilitated by a systematic approach to their study. The majority of bone lesions can be categorized into one of eight smear patterns: osteoid-containing lesions, myxoid-chondroid–containing lesions, giant cell–rich lesions, small cell lesions, inflammatory cell–containing lesions, spindle cell–predominant lesions, epithelioid lesions, and cystic- or blood-rich lesions. Recognition of each category can be achieved at low to medium magnification, and subsequent study of cytologic detail, immunocytochemical, and clinical-radiographic findings usually allows further classification into specific entities.

OSTEOID-CONTAINING LESIONS

Aspiration of bone tumors characterized by osteoid production will usually yield fragments of a hard, waxy-appearing substance that stains pink-orange with hematoxylin and eosin (H&E) and mauve or magenta with a Romanovsky stain (e.g., Diff-Quik) (Fig. 7–1*A*). This material represents osteoid and, while usually scant in amount, is very useful in defining the nature of the tumor. Fragments of osteoid are often surrounded by cells, but it is rare to see cells trapped within the matrix substance itself. At times, it may be extremely difficult to distinguish osteoid from chondroid or heavy collagen. Characteristically, chondroid has a more mucoid or myxoid appearance and frequently contains cells embedded within its substance (Fig. 7–1*B*). Osteoid is generally present in smaller amounts than chondroid and has a more well-defined aggregated appearance. Lesions characterized by osteoid that is demonstrable in cytologic smears include fracture callus, myositis ossificans, osteoid osteoma, osteoblastoma, and osteosarcoma.

Fracture Callus

Fracture callus rarely undergoes needle aspiration and subsequently there are few reports of its appearance.[21] Cytologic smears contain a small number of oval to spindle-shaped osteoblasts with reactive features (Fig. 7–2). The nuclei are slightly to moderately enlarged and lie eccentrically within an abundant pale cytoplasm. Perinuclear pale zones may be present. The background is frequently bloody. Occasional short, spindle-shaped cells with wispy cytoplasm are a feature of these smears, and

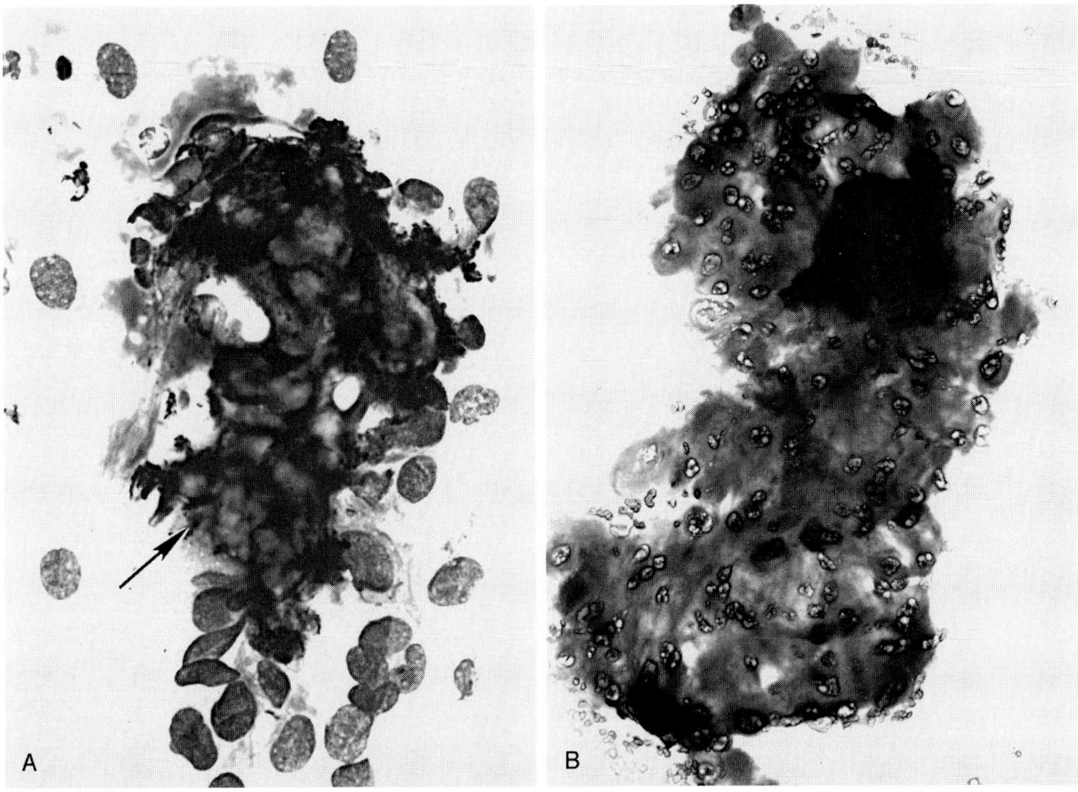

Figure 7–1. Cytologic features of osteoid and chondroid. *A*, Osteoblasts surrounding a fragment of osteoid *(arrow)* in a smear obtained from an intramedullary osteosarcoma (MGG). *B*, Fragment of chondroid with lacunae and small chondrocytes embedded in the matrix (MGG).

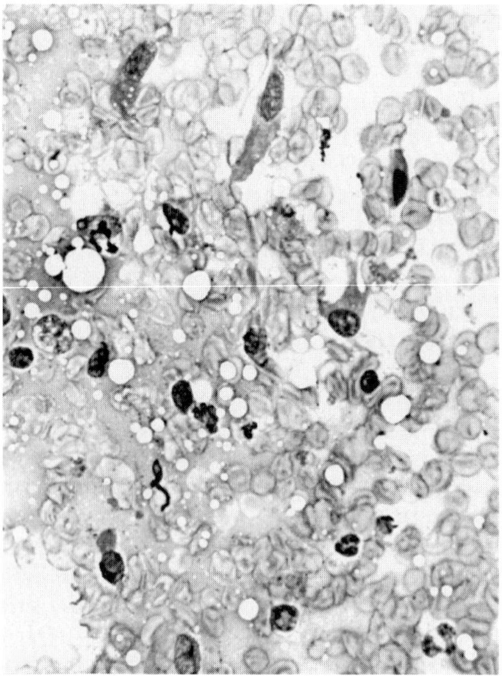

Figure 7–2. Aspirate from an early fracture callus showing reactive spindle cells in a bloody background (MGG).

probably represent endothelial cells. Very rare fragments of osteoid may be seen, and reactive osteoblasts occasionally lie along one surface of these fragments. While reactive atypia may be prominent, true anaplasia and non-mirror–image mitotic figures are not seen in aspirates of fracture callus. Correlation with radiographs is necessary for accurate diagnosis.

Myositis Ossificans

While not strictly a neoplasm of bone, this soft tissue lesion has many features in common with fracture callus and osteosarcoma. Myositis ossificans usually presents as a rapidly enlarging mass within a muscle, often near a bone (see Chapter 11). While radiographic and clinical features are usually characteristic, these lesions frequently undergo biopsy or aspiration for diagnosis. Smears of myositis ossificans vary in appearance with the age of the lesion. In the early stages, the FNA smears show a proliferation of immature stellate and spindle-shaped cells lying in a proteinaceous or myxoid background. The cytoplasm frequently has a vacuolated appearance (Fig. 7–3). As the lesion matures, increasing amounts of osteoid are formed, which finally calcify and develop into well-formed bone of the peripheral shell. Aspirates obtained during the midphase of development of myositis ossificans display a significant number of recognizable osteoblasts having a polygonal shape with eccentric nuclei and a pale blue–staining cytoplasm with Diff-Quik. Mitotic figures are generally easily found but are always of typical form. Besides oval osteoblasts, cells may have an oblong, racquet-shaped, or triangular appearance. Although there is generally only mild variation in size, binucleate cells may be seen. As with osteoblasts of fracture callus, the osteoblasts in myositis ossificans often contain a prominent cytoplasmic hof, which is best seen with Giemsa-based stains. Occasionally, fragments of degenerating muscle or fibrous tissue are seen within the smears. The presence or absence of osteoid within smears of myositis ossificans has been a point of debate. Most authorities believe that little osteoid matrix is found in smears obtained from myositis ossificans.[22–24]

Distinction of myositis ossificans from fracture callus may be difficult, if not impossible, although the absence of stainable osteoid in myositis ossificans may be a point of distinction between myositis ossificans and fracture

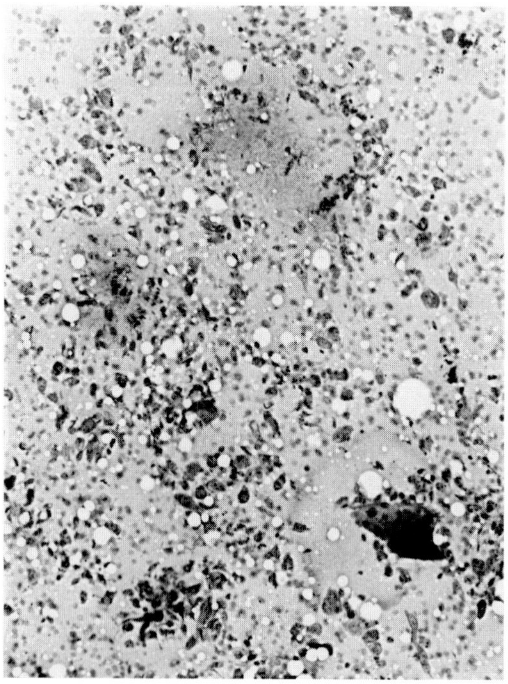

Figure 7–3. Smear obtained from myositis ossificans. Cells appear stellate or spindled and have vacuolated cytoplasm (MGG).

callus. The distinction of myositis ossificans from osteosarcoma is generally achieved by recognition of the reactive rather than anaplastic nature of the atypia in myositis ossificans. High grade intramedullary osteosarcomas almost invariably have greater degrees of nuclear atypia, more osteoid and higher cellularity than is seen in myositis ossificans. In addition, they have a destructive x-ray pattern with origination of the lesion in the medulla of bone. Myositis ossificans, on the other hand, is a soft tissue lesion with reactive, more minor degrees of atypia. Cytologic separation of myositis ossificans from parosteal osteosarcoma may not be possible because both are relatively low-grade lesions. Radiographic findings should be helpful in distinguishing those two lesions. Periosteal osteosarcoma is generally a chondroblastic lesion with smears containing considerable amounts of chondroid, which is not seen in myositis ossificans.

Osteoid Osteoma and Osteoblastoma

Osteoid osteoma and osteoblastoma have many histologic and cytologic features in common (see Chapter 9), and some authors believe it may be impossible to distinguish these two lesions except on the basis of size and radiographic appearance.[25, 26] Sanerkin and Jeffree[27] have described and illustrated the cytologic appearances of osteoid osteoma and osteoblastoma.

The clinical and radiologic features of osteoid osteoma are distinctive. Because of the intense border of sclerosis around the central nidus, aspiration of osteoid osteomas may be very difficult and lesional tissue is infrequently sampled. Smears, when obtainable, contain an almost pure population of osteoblasts with a small number of fibroblasts, endothelial cells, and osteoclast-type giant cells. The osteoblasts have a bland cytologic appearance with moderately abundant pale cytoplasm and eccentric round nuclei. A paranuclear hof is characteristic of these cells. Mitoses are not seen. Occasional binucleate osteoblasts can be found. Small amounts of heavy, waxy-appearing osteoid are present and may be surrounded by osteoblasts. The background may be clean or bloody.

The cytologic appearance of osteoblastoma is quite similar to that of osteoid osteoma. Osteoblastomas can vary in cellularity, and cellular forms are reported. Although the basic cell type is identical to that of osteoid osteoma and has the characteristic osteoblastic morphology, the cells may vary more in nuclear size. Mitotic figures are seen in smears obtained from osteoblastomas. True benign osteoblastomas, however, lack significant nuclear atypia, and the mitotic figures are always typical in form.

Separation of osteoid osteoma and osteoblastoma from osteosarcoma on purely cytologic grounds may be difficult, and clinical-radiographic-cytologic correlation is mandatory. Analysis of radiographs generally distinguishes these lesions. Cytologic features of aid in this differential diagnosis include the greater cellularity of osteosarcoma. Occasional osteoblastomas will be cellular, but in these cases, nuclear atypia is significantly less than that seen in the vast majority of osteogenic sarcomas. Osteogenic sarcomas also display greater degrees of mitotic activity, including atypical mitotic figures. When doubt exists in the cytologic diagnosis, open biopsy is required.

Osteosarcoma

Osteosarcoma is a malignant tumor of bone that forms osteoid. Several clinicopathologic forms occur, including high-grade intramedullary (conventional type), parosteal, periosteal, low-grade intramedullary, and telangiectatic osteosarcomas (see Chapter 9). The high-grade intramedullary type is the most common, and may have a range of microscopic appearances, with sclerosing, chondroblastic, fibroblastic, malignant fibrous histiocytoma-like, and small cell patterns being the most frequently recognized. Cytologic correlates exist for each pattern.

Conventional Osteosarcoma

Smears may vary widely in cellularity, but most reported cases have moderate to high cellularity.[28–30] In our experience, many aspirates are characterized by low cellularity, with individual cells and clusters of cells being dispersed in a bloody background. White et al.[29] described a wide morphologic spectrum for aspirates of osteosarcoma, and divided aspirates into five cytologic patterns: pleomorphic, epithelioid, chondroblastic, small cell, and mixed.

The pleomorphic type is by far the most common (58% of cases). In this form, varying proportions of anaplastic spindle-shaped, round, polygonal, and multinucleated pleomorphic giant cells are present in the smears, lying singly or in small clusters. The anaplastic spindle cells dominate but are not distinctive and resemble those found in malignant fibrous histiocytoma and high-grade fibrosarcomas. The atypical polygonal and round cells are less frequent, but are more characteristic, and recapitulate osteoblasts. These cells have one or, less commonly, two large round or irregular nuclei, with large, prominent nucleoli, lying eccentrically within the cell. A perinuclear hof may be present, and most cells have moderate amounts of well-circumscribed cytoplasm, which may contain clear vacuoles or small pink granules (Diff-Quik). The multinucleated cells have between 2 and 10 large, bizarre nuclei surrounded by dense cytoplasm. When the spindle, oval, and round cells form clusters, they often aggregate around fragments of pink (Diff-Quik or H&E) stromal material (Fig. 7–4). When this material has a dense appearance, it is identifiable as osteoid, but when a fibrillary appearance is present, it is impossible to separate osteoid from collagen. The osteoid matrix is poorly seen on Papanicolaou (Pap)–stained material.[28] Mitotic figures, including atypical forms, are plentiful in the smears.[31] A variable number of bland-appearing, osteoclast-like giant cells are dispersed throughout the background (Fig. 7–5*A*), and many smears show extensive necrosis.[31]

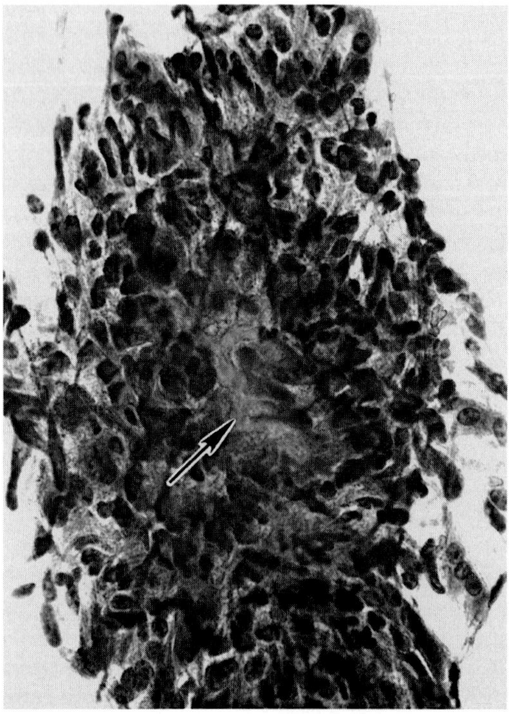

Figure 7–4. A small fragment of osteoid *(arrow)* is visible in the center of this aggregate of malignant cells from an aspirate of osteosarcoma (MGG).

The epithelioid pattern is dominated by the round or polygonal cell type. These cells closely resemble reactive osteoblasts but are larger and have greater degrees of nuclear atypia. The nuclei lie eccentrically and are associated with an abundant dense cytoplasm. A perinuclear hof is often present. Intracytoplasmic red-purple granules are often present and may correspond to primary matrix granules forming immature osteoid.[30] As with the pleomorphic type, osteoid might be present and is often surrounded by the neoplastic osteoblasts.[31]

Some osteosarcomas have prominent areas of chondroid differentiation. Aspirates from these neoplasms will contain large amounts of a gelatinous myxoid-chondroid matrix,[29] which stains blue to magenta with Diff-Quik. This material has a slimy texture and in air-dried preparations can have a feathery appearance with clear vacuoles (Fig. 7–5*B*). When large sheets of chondroid are present, occasional cells will lie within halos of lacunae. The neoplastic cells are round to oval in most cases, but spindle-shaped cells may be found. Separation of these "chondroid" areas from chondrosarcoma is not usually possible cytologically, but occasionally other aspirates demonstrate the characteristic features of osteosarcoma (osteoid).

Small cell osteosarcomas are rare lesions that may present in the differential diagnosis of Ewing's sarcoma (see Chapter 14). The individual neoplastic cells are three to four times the size of a mature lymphocyte, with oval or spindle nuclei, scanty cytoplasm, and fragments of osteoid matrix.[29]

Mixed-pattern aspirates of osteosarcoma contain two or more of the patterns just described, with the epithelioid and pleomorphic appearances being the most frequent. Others have classified osteosarcomas into five types determined by the presence or absence of osteoid, giant cells, and myxoid background substance.[31]

Parosteal Osteosarcomas

Parosteal osteosarcomas are histologically and cytologically low-grade neoplasms that

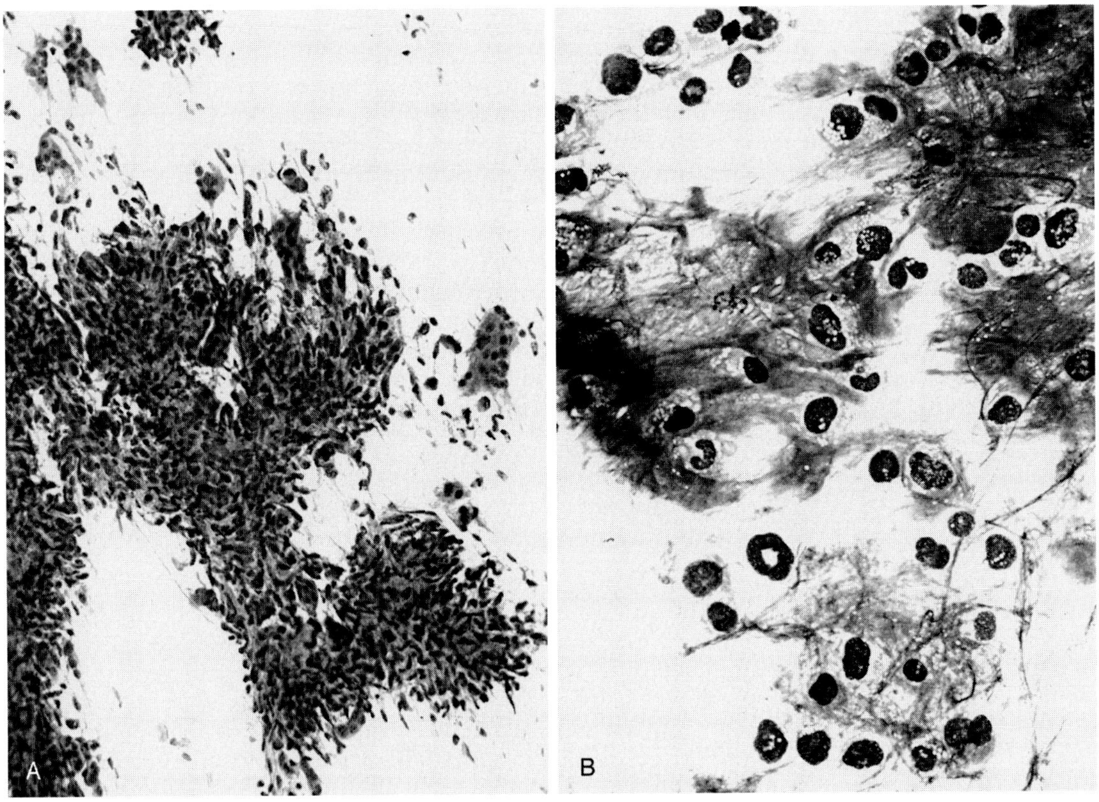

Figure 7–5. Osteosarcoma. *A*, Aspirate from an osteosarcoma containing numerous osteoclast-like giant cells (MGG). *B*, Smear from a chondroblastic osteosarcoma. The matrix has a myxoid and feathery appearance, which is characteristic of chondroid (MGG). Chondroblastic osteosarcomas and chondrosarcomas may be indistinguishable on smears if osteoid is not sampled.

contain well-formed trabeculae of bone lying in a relatively hypocellular fibroblastic stroma (see Chapter 11). Minimal cytologic atypia is present, making diagnosis difficult. Because of the densely sclerotic nature of these neoplasms, they are difficult to smear and the smears may be of very low cellularity.[27]

Experience with the cytologic appearance of these neoplasms is limited. The case described by Walaas and Kindblom[28] is similar to one we have reviewed. The smears are of moderate or low cellularity. The cells lie singly and in clusters. The individual cells are spindle-shaped, mildly polymorphous, and angulated. Scattered fragments of osteoid and chondroid are present, as are occasional osteoclast-like giant cells. Mitotic figures are not found. The low degree of nuclear atypia makes diagnosis of parosteal osteosarcomas very difficult, and great reliance must be placed on the radiographic and clinical findings in order to diagnose these lesions. Purely cytologic separation of parosteal osteosarcoma from fracture callus is often impossible.

Periosteal Osteosarcoma

Periosteal osteosarcomas have abundant chondroid matrix, with bone or osteoid spicules within the chondroid component (see Chapter 11). The cells show mild nuclear atypia, and mitotic activity is low. Cytologic smears of periosteal osteosarcomas show a mixed chondroblastic and osteoblastic appearance. Small clusters of atypical spindle-shaped or oval cells are found. There usually is a prominent cartilaginous matrix component as well as some osteoid.

Telangiectatic Osteosarcoma

Telangiectatic osteosarcoma is an uncommon variant of osteosarcoma (see Chapter 9), that is composed, histologically, of anaplastic cells and slivers of osteoid surrounding an extensive network of anatomizing dilated vascular channels.[27, 32] Anaplastic giant cells and abnormal mitotic figures are usually prominent.[27] Occasionally, telangiectatic osteosarcomas contain only a few anaplastic cells, and separation of these neoplasms from aneurysmal bone cysts is very difficult.[32]

Aspiration smears are dominated by blood, in which are scattered atypical polygonal or spindle-shaped cells along with benign-appearing osteoclast-like giant cells.[27] Telangiectatic osteosarcomas characterized by large numbers of anaplastic stromal cells are usually easily recognized as malignant and clinical-radiologic-cytologic correlation will establish the correct diagnosis. When anaplastic cells are absent, separation from aneurysmal bone cyst is impossible by cytologic examination.

Problems in the Diagnosis of Osteoid-Producing Neoplasms

In general, adequately sampled high-grade osteosarcomas are easily recognized as malignant on cytologic examination. They appear as high-grade anaplastic malignancies with a high mitotic rate.[28] The diagnostic problem lies in the separation of osteosarcoma from other high-grade malignancies involving bone.[29] Clinical and radiographic findings usually suffice for establishing this specific diagnosis. When such correlation is not definitive, documentation of osteoid is necessary to establish a diagnosis of osteosarcoma. Some authors believe it is impossible to conclusively establish the presence of osteoid by FNA, and have been unable to separate osteoid from dense collagen.[29] Other investigators, including ourselves, believe that osteoid can be recognized in aspirated material.[27, 28, 31] In air-dried smears, it has a thick, heavy, amorphous appearance and is often surrounded by neoplastic cells (see Figs. 7–1 and 7–4). It lacks the myxoid or mucoid appearance of cartilage and does not surround cells forming lacunae as seen with cartilage. Walaas and Kindblom[28] used an embedding technique along with ultrastructural analysis to document osteoid in several cases. The smears from these examples contained a pinkish-red coarsely fibrillar matrix (May-Grünwald-Giemsa [MGG]) lying between tumor cells or freely in the background. Unfortunately, osteoid is not found in all smears obtained from osteosarcomas, and, in these cases, separation from malignant fibrous histiocytoma is not possible on cytologic grounds.

Osteoid is often absent from smears obtained from chondroblastic osteosarcomas, and these neoplasms are difficult to separate from high-grade chondrosarcomas (see Fig. 7–5*B*). Cell block preparations can be helpful in the identification of osteoid formation by the malignant cells.[33] Clinical features, including age and radiographic appearance may separate chondroblastic osteosarcoma from chondrosarcoma.

Small cell osteosarcoma must be distinguished from lymphoma and Ewing's sarcoma (see Chapter 14). Small cell osteosarcomas will contain rare fragments of osteoid, and immunocytochemical and periodic acid–Schiff staining and ultrastructural analysis are helpful in the diagnosis. The tissue fragments in small cell osteosarcomas are usually larger and more cohesive than those obtained from Ewing's sarcomas or lymphomas. The cells of small cell osteosarcoma are more irregular or spindle-shaped than the uniformly round cells of Ewing's sarcoma and lymphoma.

Conventional osteosarcomas are generally easily separable from osteoblastomas by the greater nuclear anaplasia and mitotic activity seen in the former. Well-differentiated osteosarcomas may be difficult or impossible to cytologically separate from osteoblastomas, particularly aggressive osteoblastomas or osteoblastomas with degenerative atypia.[29] Finally, the cytologic findings in well-differentiated intramedullary osteosarcoma have not been described, but one would expect that these would be difficult to distinguish cytologically from osteoblastomas and fracture callus.

Osteosarcomas must be separated from metastatic carcinomas. This is usually straightforward, but occasional sarcomatoid carcinomas arising in the kidney, breast, stomach, or pancreas may give rise to significant problems in diagnosis. Immunocytochemistry using antibodies directed against cytokeratins and other epithelial-related antigens can be of great help in solving these diagnostic problems.

The major limitations of FNA for the diagnosis of osteosarcoma are its limited ability to obtain adequate samples in densely osteoblastic tumors and its arguable accuracy in the identification of osteoid.[28, 29] Electron microscopic examination of cell block preparations may be useful in reducing the impact of this latter limitation.[28]

CARTILAGINOUS NEOPLASMS

Cartilaginous neoplasms demonstrate considerable cytologic and histologic overlap between lesions with markedly different clinical behaviors (see Chapters 10 and 11). Enchondromas, low-grade chondrosarcomas, and cases of synovial chondromatosis can have similar if not identical cytologic appearances but follow significantly different clinical courses. Smear cellularity often corresponds to clinical aggressiveness, but the correlation is imperfect and some neoplasms yielding low cellularity aspirates follow an aggressive course. In no other area of needle aspiration diagnosis is the correlation of clinical and radiographic findings with the cytologic picture more important.

Cytologic study may be useful in the management of cartilaginous lesions, even when definitive separation of benign and low-grade malignant neoplasms cannot be achieved. In some cases, the identification of a neoplasm as cartilaginous is sufficient pathologic information, when combined with radiographic and clinical findings, to allow institution of appropriate therapy.

The identification of a myxoid-chondroid matrix surrounding and entrapping round to ovoid cells should give rise to the differential diagnosis of synovial chondromatosis, enchondroma, periosteal chondroma, osteochondroma, chondrosarcoma, and chordoma. Myxoid-chondroid matrix is best identified in air-dried material (Diff-Quik stain), where it stains a pale blue to deep magenta in color and has a slimy to somewhat fibrillar appearance (Fig. 7–6). This material stains green with the Pap technique and pale blue to pink with H&E. Cytologic detail is often obscured in Diff-Quik–stained smears and is best seen in alcohol-fixed, Pap-stained material.[34]

Synovial Chondromatosis

Primary synovial chondromatosis is an uncommon lesion (see Chapter 18), the cytologic features of which have been rarely reported. Saint-Martin et al.[35] describe a single case in which the smears contained large cohesive clusters of "cartilaginous" material. There is a scanty myxoid background in which are scattered occasional mesenchymal cells and rare round chondrocytes. Nuclear atypia is not identified and the cartilage appears mature. These features contrast with the myxoid background and greater cellularity and atypia of chondrosarcomas and many chondromas.

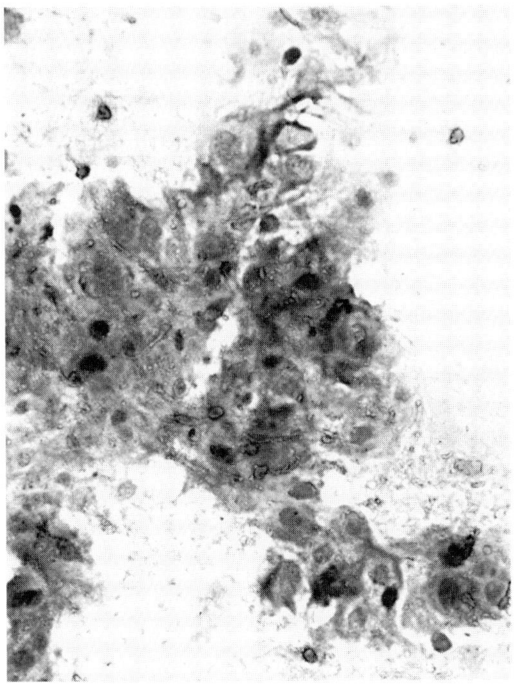

Figure 7–6. Appearance of myxoid-chondroid matrix in air-dried aspirates (MGG). Matrix edges are characteristically feathery or fibrillary.

Enchondroma and Periosteal Chondroma

The histologic and cytologic appearance of these neoplasms can vary considerably. The degree of cellularity, nuclear atypia, and pattern of interaction between the host bone and the neoplasm are important features used to distinguish histologically between chondromas and chondrosarcomas.[36] Cytologic diagnosis is hampered by the inability to evaluate architectural features in aspirated specimens, so clinical and radiographic correlation is important.

Walaas et al.[37] and Sanerkin and Jeffree[38] have described the needle aspiration cytologic features of chondromas. Smears obtained from chondromas contain fragments of cartilage with small cells lying within lacunae. While fragments of thick hyaline cartilage often dominate the smears, some aspirates contain significant quantities of myxoid material in the background. The individual chondrocytes are small, with bland, dark, round condensed nuclei and modest amounts of cytoplasm that often contain glycogen. The glycogen appears as multiple clear vacuoles in Diff-Quik–stained smears. Binucleated cells and mitotic figures are not seen in most cases.

Actively growing chondromas show relatively high cellularity and mild degrees of nuclear atypia requiring radiographic study for their separation from chondrosarcoma. In some cases, such separation is impossible by cytologic study.

Osteochondroma

Smears obtained from the cartilaginous cap of osteochondroma resemble those obtained from enchondromas. Large fragments of hyaline cartilage with bland chondrocytes are characteristic. Cellularity and nuclear atypia are low. Material obtained from osteochondromas with sarcomatous transformation will resemble aspirate smears from chondrosarcomas. Chondrosarcoma should be strongly considered when the cartilage cap of an osteochondroma is greater than 2 cm in thickness.[39]

Chondroblastoma

Reports documenting the FNA cytologic appearance of these predominately epiphyseal neoplasms have described smears with widely varying cellularity.[40–44] The majority of aspirates have been cellular,[29, 43] containing mononuclear round chondroblasts, multinucleated osteoclast-like giant cells, and variable amounts of chondroid matrix.[42] The amount of chondroid matrix within the area sampled will, to a large extent, determine the cellularity of the smears. The chondroblasts are diagnostic of this lesion. These cells are of moderate size, with round to oval nuclei containing longitudinal grooves (Fig. 7–7*A*). The cytoplasm is dense and well-defined, and present in moderate amounts. The nucleus may lie centrally or be polarized to one side. The nuclear chromatin is fine and even, nucleoli are small or absent, and nuclear pseudoinclusions are occasionally seen.[40] Occasional binucleated chondroblasts are seen. Many chondroblasts lay singly, while others form small clusters. Mitotic figures are present in the majority of cases.[42]

Multinucleated osteoclast-like giant cells are intimately admixed with the chondroblasts in all cases and may be prominent.[44] These osteoclasts contain between 10 and 40 bland oval nuclei, with a fine uniform chromatin associated with small but distinct nucleoli. Their cytoplasm is dense and usually well-defined.

Variable amounts of chondroid matrix are present in the smears. In most cases, it is very scant or absent but, in occasional cases, it is a prominent component, and may calcify.

The differential diagnosis includes giant cell tumor, chondromyxoid fibroma and giant cell–rich osteogenic sarcoma. Clinical and radiographic features are helpful in the separation of these neoplasms (see Chapter 15). Giant cell tumors of bone usually occur in a slightly older age group and the stromal cells are more spindle-shaped or elongated than the round mononuclear chondroblasts. The giant cells of giant cell tumors frequently have greater numbers of nuclei than those seen in chondroblastoma. Separation of chondroblastoma from giant cell–rich osteosarcoma depends on radiographic features and the recognition of significant nuclear atypia in osteosarcoma, which is not a feature of chondroblastoma.

Chondromyxoid Fibroma

Aspiration of these neoplasms yields a small amount of gelatinous material, which, when smeared, has a moderately to highly cellular appearance.[45] In the reported cases, there is a mixture of chondroid cells, giant cells, stellate cells, and spindle cells lying in a myxoid-chondroid background.[45, 46] The chondroid cells are usually single and entrapped within the chondroid matrix (Fig. 7–7*B*). These cells are generally mononuclear, but occasional multinucleated or binucleated forms are found. The nuclei may show considerable nuclear pleomorphism and often show degenerative changes with dark condensed chromatin, but mitotic figures are not present.[27]

A second population of cells has a stellate appearance with multiple cytoplasmic extensions and enlarged, often smudged nuclei. Mitotic figures are not seen in these cells. A population of bland fibroblast-like spindle cells is also present in most smears, as are occasional multinucleated osteoclast-like giant cells irregularly scattered in a chondromyxoid background.

Diagnosis requires separation of chondromyxoid fibroma from chondrosarcoma.[46] Both have a chondroid-myxoid background and may contain cells showing nuclear pleomorphism. The nuclei of chondromyxoid fibromas are smudgy and condensed, while those of chondrosarcomas are usually sharp with an irregular chromatin. Mitotic figures are not

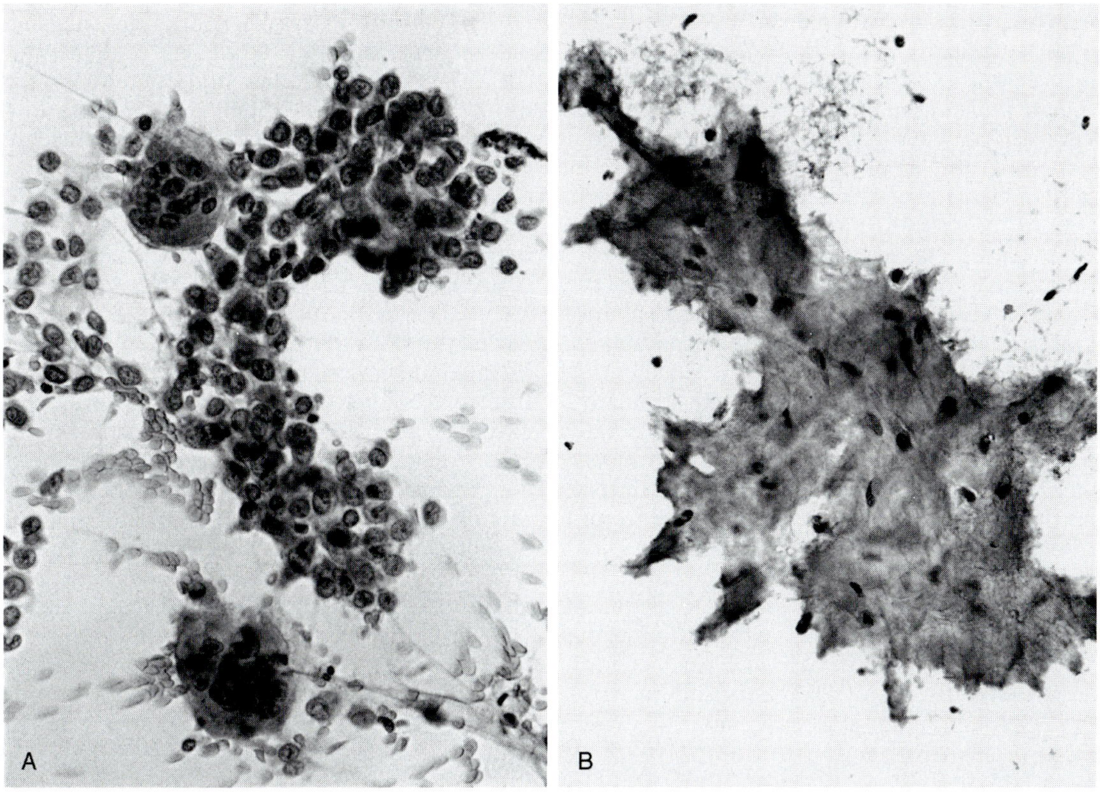

Figure 7–7. Benign chondroid lesions. *A*, Aspirate of chondroblastoma composed of numerous grooved chondroblasts and multinucleated giant cells (Pap). Chondroid matrix is inconspicuous in this example. *B*, Fragment of chondroid matrix from aspirate of chondromyxoid fibroma (CMF). Unlike most chondrosarcomas, chondrocytes of CMF are small, single, and embedded in matrix (Pap).

seen in chondromyxoid fibromas but may be found in Grade II or III chondrosarcomas. Clinical and radiographic features are also helpful in distinguishing these two neoplasms.

Chondrosarcoma

The diagnosis of chondrosarcoma and its separation from other chondroid-producing neoplasms is one of the most difficult areas in aspiration cytology. Clinical-radiologic-cytologic correlation is critical in the diagnosis of these neoplasms (see Chapter 10). Conventional chondrosarcomas are divided into three grades based on cellularity and nuclear atypia. Grading of chondrosarcomas by cytologic evaluation can be difficult, but increasing grade is associated with higher cellularity, larger numbers of binucleated and multinucleated chondrocytes, mitotic activity, increasing nuclear atypia, and a reduction in the amount of dense hyaline cartilage containing distinct lacunar spaces. In addition, several subtypes have been described, including mesenchymal, dedifferentiated, and clear cell chondrosarcomas. Conventional chondrosarcomas are the most frequent, and their cytologic appearance has been described in several reports.[27, 34, 47–49]

The cytologic recognition of a chondrosarcoma depends on finding round to oval vacuolated cells (chondrocytes) associated with fragments of dense hyaline cartilage or myxoid-chondroid stroma. At times, the chondrocytes will have the appearance of "ring cells" owing to the lacunar space surrounding them. Small calcified tissue fragments can be found in all cases.

Fine needle aspirates obtained from Grade I chondrosarcomas yield smears closely resembling those obtained from chondromas, but which tend to be more cellular and contain more binucleate cells. Fragments of chondroid matrix are scattered throughout the smears and on H&E staining have a glassy pink appearance, with individual chondrocytes seen in lacunar spaces of the matrix. The cellularity of these fragments is usually modest, but at times highly cellular areas are detected. Most lacunar spaces contain cells with single nuclei, but occasional binucleate cells are observed. Individual, and small clusters of, chondrocytes are seen lying free in the smears. Some smears demonstrate a pale blue (Diff-Quik) myxoid background. The individual chondrocytes are oval or polygonal with distinct cell borders.[48] The cytoplasm is present in moderate to abundant amounts and has a foamy appearance with many small vacuoles.[49] The nuclei are usually small with a bland, finely granular chromatin pattern. Many cells have only small or absent nucleoli. Mitotic figures are not present. These features are not significantly different than the cytologic features of immature or cellular chondromas, and clinical and radiographic features have to be used to resolve the differential diagnosis.[48]

Grade II chondrosarcomas yield smears with higher cellularity, more atypical nuclei, and larger amounts of myxoid-chondroid matrix than Grade I neoplasms. Fragments of well-circumscribed, well-formed hyaline cartilage are present, but the degree of cellularity in the fragments is higher, and the nuclei are more closely crowded than in Grade I chondrosarcoma, with binucleate and trinucleate cells in the lacunar spaces. Loose, watery myxoid-chondroid matrix is distributed through the background of the smears and surrounds neoplastic chondrocytes and the fragments of heavier hyaline cartilage. The individual cells are oval or polygonal with moderate to abundant cytoplasm (Fig. 7–8*A*), and lie singly or in small clusters (Fig. 7–8*B*). The cytoplasm is finely vacuolated, but at times large vacuoles may displace the nucleus to one side of the cell.[49] Most cells are mononuclear, but binucleate and multinuclear cells are occasionally identified. The nuclei have evenly distributed chromatin of variable coarseness. Occasionally, the chromatin displays prominent margination. Many nuclei have distinct nucleoli. Mitotic figures are not seen.

The finding of oval or polygonal neoplastic cells with vacuolated cytoplasm, an amorphous myxoid-chondroid background matrix, and oc-

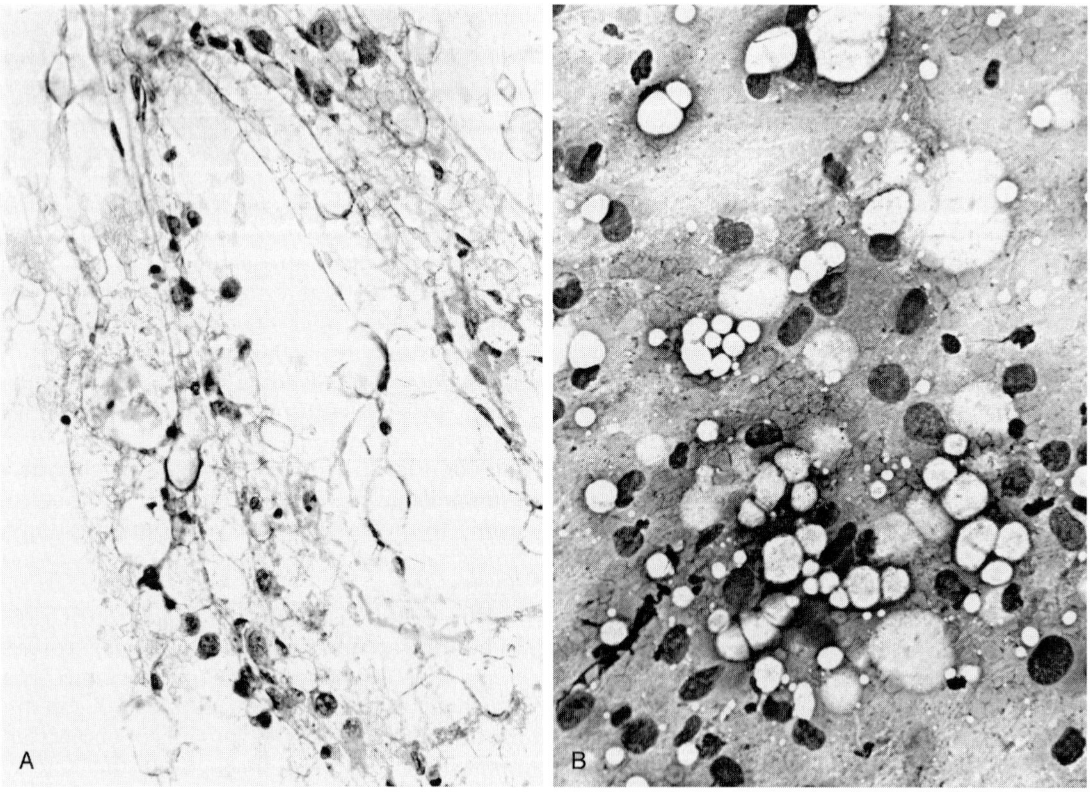

Figure 7–8. Chondrosarcoma, Grade II. *A*, Aspirate showing atypical chondrocytes associated with vacuolated chondroid matrix (Pap). *B*, Air-dried smear showing vacuolated cytoplasm of chondrocytes and watery myxoid matrix in the background (MGG).

casional fragments of hyaline cartilage establishes the diagnosis of a chondroid neoplasm. The cellularity and nuclear atypia confirm the diagnosis of chondrosarcoma.

Grade III chondrosarcomas are characterized by greater cellularity and nuclear atypia, and mitotic figures can be identified.[37] The nuclei are enlarged and hyperchromatic with an uncondensed chromatin. Nucleoli are often prominent when the smears are stained with the H&E or Pap methods. Fragments of hyaline cartilage are rare or not seen, and the majority of the matrix is myxoid-chondroid, which can obscure the nuclear detail of the malignant cells. As with lower grade lesions, multinucleated osteoclast-like giant cells can be found. Necrotic debris is often present in Grade III chondrosarcomas.

Dedifferentiated Chondrosarcoma

Smears are moderately to abundantly cellular with many pleomorphic spindle-shaped cells with elongated cytoplasmic extensions.[50] Nuclei are enlarged, irregular, and hyperchromatic, and irregular nucleoli are prominent. Multinucleated polygonal cells and spindle-shaped cells are seen. In the reported examples of this neoplasm, myxoid or granular matrix is not seen.[50] Separation of dedifferentiated chondrosarcoma from malignant fibrous histiocytoma or fibrosarcoma does not appear possible by purely cytologic study unless the areas of lower grade chondrosarcoma are sampled.[50]

Mesenchymal Chondrosarcoma

Aspirates obtained from mesenchymal chondrosarcomas are grossly gelatinous and often bloody.[51] The smears are cellular and frequently contain necrotic debris associated with neutrophils. The individual neoplastic cells are either small, primitive-appearing round cells or larger, round or oval cells resembling chondrocytes (Fig. 7–9). Both cell types are enmeshed in a myxoid matrix, which stains red-purple in air-dried material and blue in alcohol-fixed smears.

The small cells lie singly or in loose aggregates that are globular in shape.[51] The small cell component has moderate amounts of granular cytoplasm with distinct cellular margins but at times presents as "naked" nuclei. When the cells are intact, the nuclei are centrally located, generally round to oval, and sometimes clefted. The nuclear membranes

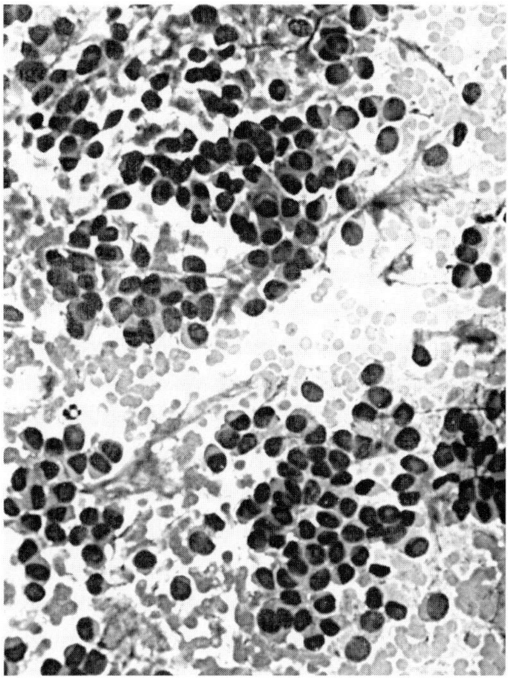

Figure 7–9. Aspirate from mesenchymal chondrosarcoma showing numerous small round cells in aggregates and singly. Chondroid matrix appears as wisps of material between cells in this air-dried preparation (MGG).

are thick and the chromatin is coarsely granular. Chromocenters are seen with Pap staining but nucleoli are small and eosinophilic.

The larger cells are more frequently embedded in the myxoid-chondroid matrix. These cells have more abundant cytoplasm, which is vacuolated.[51] The nuclei are usually eccentrically located with a coarse chromatin, large nucleoli, and irregular nuclear membrane. Binucleated and multinucleated cells are common. Both cell populations are highly mitotically active.

Clear Cell Chondrosarcoma

Clear cell chondrosarcomas yield smears containing small round cells with clusters of large epithelial-like cells. The background contains myxoid matrix and occasional fragments of dense cartilage. The large neoplastic cells have abundant pale blue (Diff-Quik) cytoplasm, which has a vacuolated or foamy appearance. The nuclei of these cells are enlarged hyperchromatic and contain prominent nucleoli.

Chondroblastic Osteosarcomas

Some osteosarcomas will be dominated by the production of neoplastic cartilage and only show rare foci of direct production of neoplastic osteoid. Because FNA sampling is limited, these neoplasms may be inseparable cytologically from chondrosarcomas unless osteoid is present (see Fig. 7–5*B*). Cell block preparations may be helpful in this distinction.[33] Clinical and radiographic features are critical to the accurate identification of chondroblastic osteosarcomas.

Chordoma

The cytologic findings in chordoma have been well described and are considered in detail in the section on the cytologic diagnosis of epithelioid neoplasms.[52–61] On low-power examination of smears, large fragments of a myxoid-chondroid or mucoid material frequently associated with, or engulfing, clusters of polygonal cells are seen.[52, 54, 58, 59] The cells may be large and vacuolated, smaller with granular cytoplasm, or spindle-shaped. The vacuolated, physaliphorous cells, together with the myxoid stroma, help to separate chordomas from chondrosarcomas and chondromas.

SMALL CELL LESIONS

Ewing's Sarcoma

Smear preparations obtained from Ewing's sarcomas are highly cellular with both large, three-dimensional tissue fragments and many noncohesive individual cells (Fig. 7–10*A*).[62–64] Although they appear monomorphous on low-power examination, high-power examination discloses two cell types; a population of small, dark cells with little cytoplasm surrounding nuclei-containing condensed chromatin, and a second population of cells with slightly larger, less dark nuclei and more abundant cytoplasm that contains distinct clear vacuoles that correspond to glycogen on electron microscopic examination.[62] The nuclei of both cell types appear round and only occasionally possess faint nucleoli.[62] Rarely, pseudorosettes

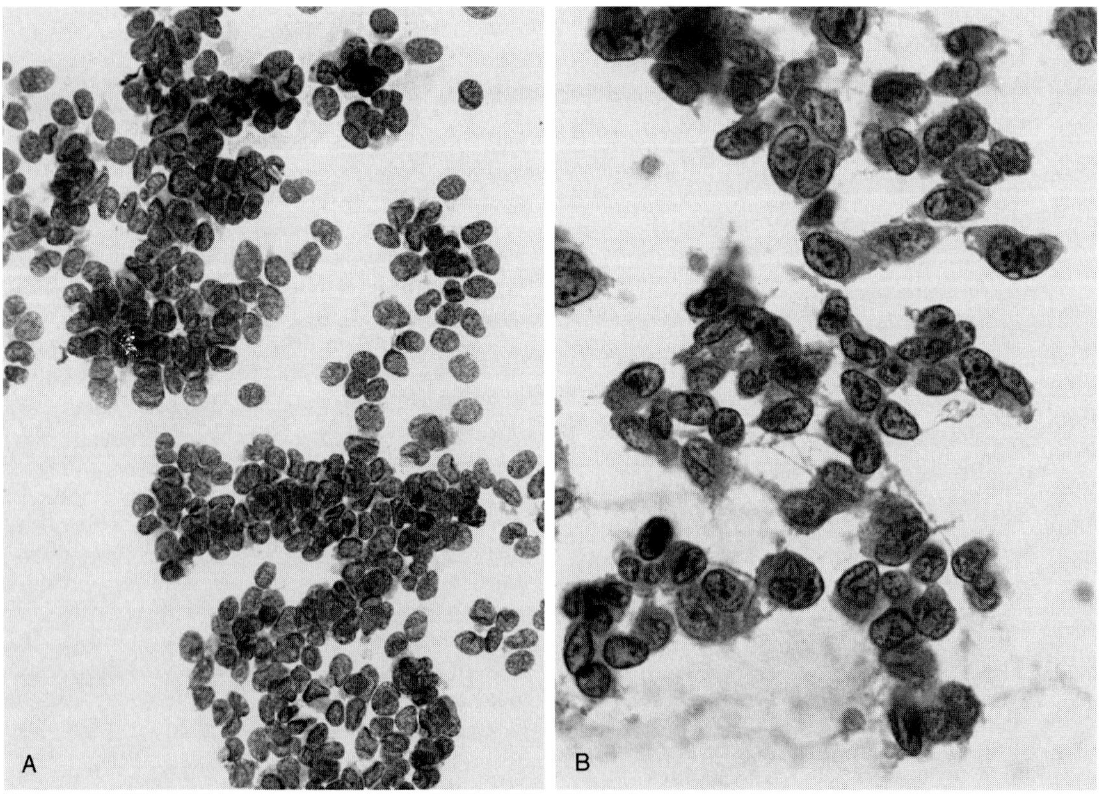

Figure 7–10. Ewing's sarcoma. *A*, Air-dried preparation of an aspirate reveals scanty cytoplasm associated with these small round cells (MGG). A vague, rosetting pattern is present. *B*, Nuclear detail in a large cell variant of Ewing's sarcoma. Nuclear outlines are distinct, and one or more chromocenters are present (H&E).

have been identified in smears obtained from cases of Ewing's sarcoma.[62, 63] Necrotic debris is often present. The demonstration of glycogen by histochemical techniques is unreliable, with many cases disclosing little stainable glycogen despite numerous cytoplasmic vacuoles.

A large cell variant of Ewing's sarcoma has been described cytologically.[64] Smears made from aspirates of these neoplasms are highly cellular. The individual cells have nuclei of round or oval shape two to three times the size of an erythrocyte. The nuclear membranes are prominent and surrounded by a coarse chromatin (Fig. 7–10*B*). Nucleoli are commonly present, often with two per nucleus. The cytoplasm is more abundant than in conventional Ewing's sarcoma, and periodic acid–Schiff (PAS)–positive granules are present in a high percentage of cells.

The characteristic t(11;22) of Ewing's sarcoma can be demonstrated in needle-aspiration material.[65]

Non-Hodgkin's Lymphoma

There are few reports describing the cytologic appearance of primary lymphoma of bone.[66–68] Most primary lymphomas of bone are of large cell type,[69] and the precise cytologic appearance depends on the type of lymphoma. Smears containing a large number of noncohesive, monomorphous round cells lying in a background with numerous lymphoglandular bodies should suggest the diagnosis of lymphoma. Immunohistochemical staining or flow cytometric analysis may then be used to establish the monoclonality of the proliferation and the diagnosis of lymphoma.[70] Some lymphomas yield very scanty material on aspiration, making diagnosis difficult.[68]

Smears of a lymphoblastic lymphoma[67] are characterized by numerous medium-sized to large, round, noncohesive cells lying in a background containing many small cytoplasmic fragments (lymphoglandular bodies). The nuclei are round with a finely stippled chromatin. A small percentage of nuclei are irregular in shape or contain nuclear grooves that are best seen in Pap-stained material.[67] The cytoplasm is restricted to a thin rim around the nucleus and may occasionally contain vacuoles.

The cytologic findings in a primary large cell lymphoma of bone have been described.[66] At low power, the cell population appeared monomorphic, but high-power examination disclosed variation in cell size and shape. Some artifactual cell clumping with nuclear pseudomolding was present. The individual cells are two to three times the size of a small mature lymphocyte. The nuclei are round with a regular contour and a coarsely granular chromatin with areas of chromatin clearing. Rare cleaved cells with prominent nucleoli are observed. The amount of cytoplasm varies from abundant to a scanty rim of cytoplasm around the nucleus.

Plasma Cell Myeloma

The cytologic appearance of material obtained from examples of plasma cell myeloma has varied considerably. The smears are almost always cellular with large numbers of noncohesive oval, round, or polygonal cells (Fig. 7–11).[71–73] Because the degree of differentiation can vary considerably, the cytologic appearance of the individual cells ranges from that of mature plasma cells to cells showing marked nuclear anaplasia resembling high-grade lymphoma or poorly differentiated adenocarcinoma.

Examples of well-differentiated plasma cell

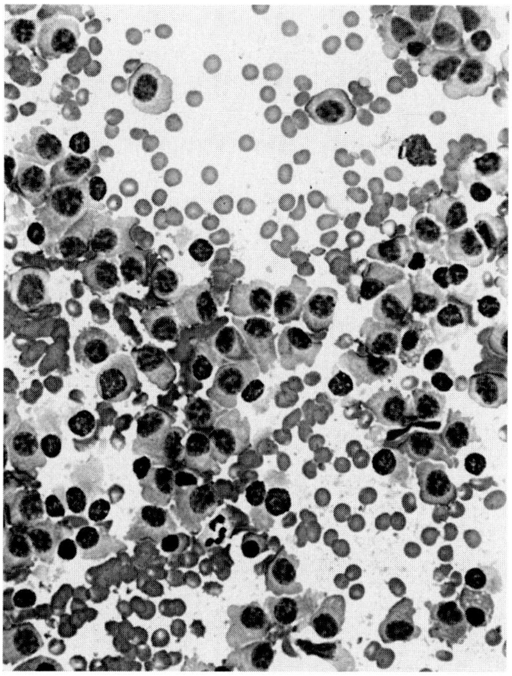

Figure 7–11. Aspirate from plasma cell myeloma showing uniform population of relatively mature plasma cells (MGG).

myeloma contain cells resembling mature plasma cells. These cells have slightly eccentric round nuclei with a coarsely clumped nuclear chromatin in a cartwheel-like distribution. The cells have moderately abundant deep blue (Diff-Quik) or red-purple (H&E) cytoplasm. A paranuclear hof is present in most cells.

More poorly differentiated examples have cells with prominent nucleoli, a finely stippled chromatin, and less distinct paranuclear hofs. These cells may look like poorly differentiated carcinoma but fail to demonstrate the cell-cell cohesion characteristic of most carcinomas. Other poorly differentiated plasma cell myelomas show marked pleomorphism with hyperchromatic nuclei, including bizarre giant multinucleated cells. These cases must be distinguished from large cell pleomorphic lymphomas. The pyroninophilia of the cytoplasm is helpful in this distinction.

Small Cell Osteosarcoma

Small cell osteosarcomas are rare neoplasms and the cytologic appearance of these malignancies has been rarely reported. White et al.[29] described the cytologic findings from two cases and Kumar et al.[31] reported a third. In the reported cases, the smears are cellular, with occasional cohesive cellular fragments that tend to be larger than those seen in Ewing's sarcomas. The majority of the neoplastic cells are noncohesive and dispersed throughout the smear. The individual cells are three to four times the size of a mature lymphocyte.[29] Cytoplasm is scanty and forms a rim around the nucleus, which shows finely dispersed chromatin. The neoplastic cells of small cell osteosarcoma are larger and more irregular and have more oval or spindle-shaped nuclei than those of Ewing's sarcoma. Rarely, fragments of osteoid may be seen in the smears of small cell osteosarcoma.

Cytogenetic studies demonstrating the complex abnormal karyotype of osteosarcoma may be helpful in distinguishing it from Ewing's sarcoma (see Chapters 4 and 14).[65]

FIBROUS AND FIBROBLASTIC LESIONS

Fibrous Dysplasia

Smears obtained from cases of fibrous dysplasia are usually of low or moderate cellularity. The individual cells are bland spindle cells, often with faint wispy cytoplasm (Fig. 7–12). Frequently, the nuclei are stripped of cytoplasm. The nuclei are plump and bacillary-shaped, with an even, fine chromatin pattern. Mitotic activity is not seen. In the examples we have seen, osteoid is not present in the smears.

Non-Ossifying Fibroma

Smears from these lesions are of low to moderate cellularity and contain a mixture of oval or spindle-shaped cells, with wispy cytoplasm and bland nuclei with a fine chromatin pattern, along with larger round or polygonal monocyte-like cells. Osteoclast-like giant cells are usually present, as are foamy (lipid laden) histiocytes. The relative proportions of these cell types varies considerably in the smears. At times, the histiocytic component will dominate, but usually the short or fusiform cell population is predominate. Mitotic figures are usually absent.

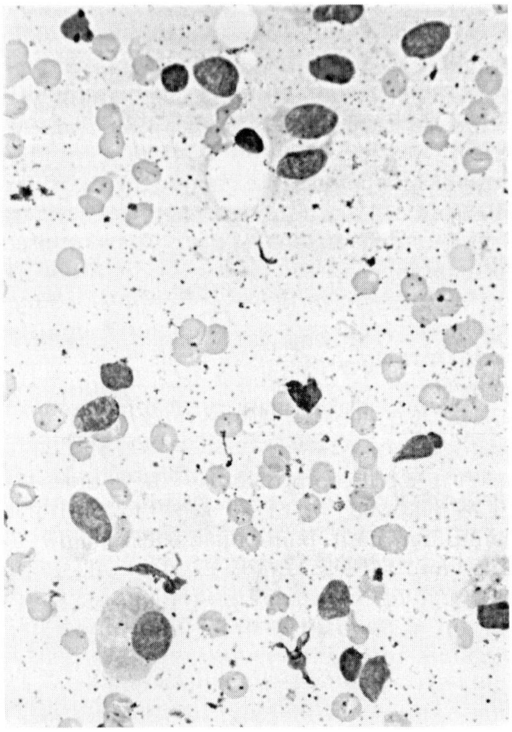

Figure 7–12. Aspirate from a case of fibrous dysplasia showing occasional bland spindle cells and osteoblasts (MGG).

Fibroblastic Osteosarcoma

These neoplasms yield smears with large anaplastic spindle cells, occasional pleomorphic osteoblastic cells, and rare fragments of pink or magenta osteoid. They are further discussed in the section on osteosarcoma.

Fibrosarcoma

Smears of these malignancies are usually of low or moderate cellularity. The major cell type is an atypical spindle cell with bipolar cytoplasmic extensions surrounding an enlarged irregular and hyperchromatic nucleus. Mitotic figures are usually present. Not infrequently, the trauma of aspiration will cause these cells to "round up" and produce a polygonal cell appearance. Despite this artifact, some true spindle cells will remain, allowing the diagnosis to be made. Separation from fibroblastic osteosarcoma may be impossible, although the absence of osteoid cytologically and the absence of matrix product on radiographs support the diagnosis of fibrosarcoma. Low-grade fibrosarcomas do not show cellular pleomorphism and may not be separable from fibromatoses on cytologic examination, although nuclear size is greater in the fibrosarcomas.[74]

Malignant Fibrous Histiocytoma

Aspirates obtained from malignant fibrous histiocytomas are usually cellular with a background of blood, necrotic, or myxoid material.[75–79] The majority of cells are spindle-shaped or polygonal, and are very atypical with significant nuclear pleomorphism, and anaplastic multinuclear giant cells are frequent (for further discussion see the section on giant cell–containing lesions).

Adamantinoma

Only a few reports describe the cytologic findings in adamantinoma.[80–83] Smears are moderately cellular and contain loosely cohesive sheets and bundles of medium-sized spindle cells, in additional to a population of polygonal, epithelial-like cells. The cytologic appearances are discussed in more detail in the section on epithelioid neoplasms.

GIANT CELL–CONTAINING LESIONS OF BONE

Lesions of bone that contain benign, osteoclast-like giant cells or multinucleate, malignant cells are reasonably common. Benign, osteoclast-like giant cells can occur nonspecifically in a variety of neoplasms with widely divergent biologic behaviors, including giant cell tumor, chondroblastoma, chondromyxoid fibroma, osteosarcoma, and aneurysmal bone cyst. The giant cells in malignant fibrous histiocytoma are usually anaplastic and of diagnostic aid. In the presence of osteoclast-like giant cells, differential diagnosis is achieved by analysis of the mononuclear component rather than the giant cell population (see Chapter 15). Nevertheless, the presence of giant cells serves as an important marker for this category of lesions.

Giant Cell Tumor of Bone

Aspirates from giant cell tumors of bone produce smears of moderate to high cellularity with a checkerboard-like appearance due to the presence of a mixture of oval or spindle-shaped mononuclear cells and large multinucleated osteoclast-like giant cells.[84–87] The mononuclear cells form tight clusters, often centered around small vessels. A small number of the mononuclear cells will lie individually. These cells have round, oval, or slightly elongated nuclei that are moderately hyperchromatic with a fine chromatin pattern. The nuclear membrane is well defined and surrounds a single nucleolus. The associated cytoplasm is scanty to moderate in amount and has a syncytial character when the cells form clusters.[84] Occasionally, the cytoplasm will have a vacuolated appearance. Mitotic figures are rarely seen in the mononuclear cell population.[84]

The osteoclast-like giant cells can lie singly but more frequently are adherent to or part of the large cell clusters.[84, 87] The multinucleated giant cells are round or polygonal with more than 20 nuclei per cell (Fig. 7–13*A*). The nuclei are oval and contain one or more nucleoli.

The mononuclear component is diagnostically distinctive. The mononuclear cells of giant cell tumor are oval to elongated (Fig. 7–13*B*), unlike the round chondroblasts of chondroblastoma, and lack the nuclear anaplasia seen in the stromal cells of osteosarcoma. The stromal and giant cells seen in

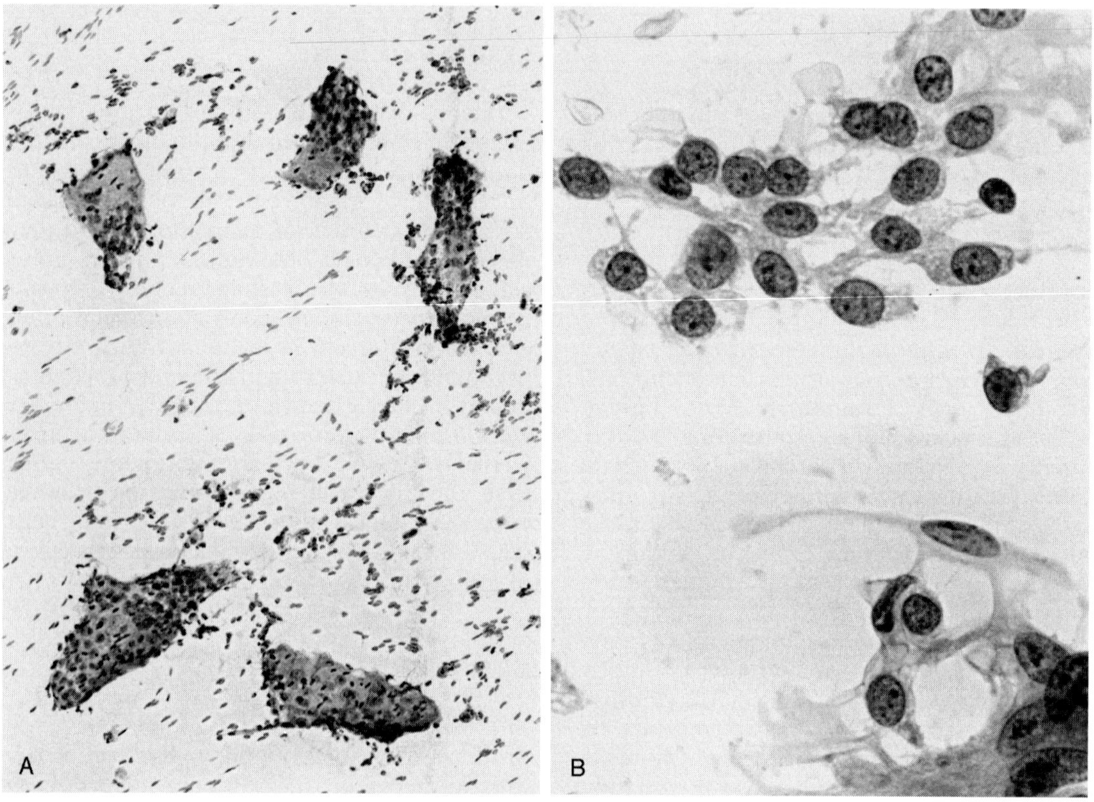

Figure 7–13. Giant cell tumor of bone. *A*, Aspirate showing the characteristic multinucleated cells, which have a syncytial appearance, polygonal shape, and usually numerous (>40) nuclei (Pap). The mononuclear cells are oval or spindle-shaped. *B*, Aspirate demonstrating the spindle-shaped mononuclear cells characteristic of giant cell tumor of bone (MGG).

some aspirates from aneurysmal bone cysts appear identical to those of giant cell tumor. Radiographic features and the large amount of blood present in aneurysmal bone cysts help to distinguish the two lesions.

Occasional giant cell tumors of bone will follow an aggressive coarse. Cytologic smears obtained from the intraosseous component of these neoplasms will appear identical to the classic form described earlier, but aspirates from the soft tissue extension are characterized by freely dispersed mononuclear cells that have some mitotic figures but display little or no nuclear atypia.[87] Multinucleate giant cells are seen in lesser numbers than in the classic intraosseous giant cell tumor.

Chondroblastoma

Many chondroblastomas contain a prominent number of multinucleated osteoclast-like giant cells (see Chapter 15). Separation from giant cell tumor is achieved by recognizing the round nuclear morphology of the chondroblasts, which differs from the spindle-cell morphology of the mononuclear cells in giant cell tumor (see Fig. 7–7*A*), and the presence of thick fragments of chondroid. Chondroblastoma is further discussed and illustrated in the section on chondroid lesions.

Aneurysmal Bone Cyst

Aneurysmal bone cysts are histologically characterized by a spongelike meshwork of open blood-filled spaces lined by septa composed of slivers of osteoid, osteoblasts, fibroblasts, histiocytes, and osteoclast-like giant cells (see Chapter 16). Aspiration yields predominately peripheral blood with few, if any, stromal cells in the smears. Occasionally, smears will contain fragments of the septal walls, containing the cell populations described earlier. The cytologic pattern is nonspecific, and the findings are at best consistent with the diagnosis of aneurysmal bone cyst. Similar findings can be seen in inadequate FNA samplings from a wide variety of bone lesions,[88] including telangiectatic osteosarcomas, which represent an important diagnostic pitfall. Adequate diagnostic aspirates from these osteosarcomas will contain anaplastic cells.

Hyperparathyroidism

We have seen cytologic material from a single case representing a "brown tumor" of hyperparathyroidism. The cytologic material appeared identical to that of giant cell tumor bone. The smears had a bloody background in which are dispersed clusters of short spindle-shaped and ovoid cells. Admixed with these mononuclear cells are prominent multinucleated giant cells imparting a checkerboard-like pattern to the clusters. The stromal cells and giant cells also occur singly in the background. The component cells display nuclear enlargement and nucleoli, but nuclear anaplasia is not seen. Correlation with radiographic and biochemical findings is necessary to establish the diagnosis.

Chondromyxoid Fibroma

Aspirates from these neoplasms can contain prominent osteoclast-like giant cells. The presence of fragments of myxoid-chondroid stroma together with the radiographic findings should suggest the diagnosis of this neoplasm. Chondromyxoid fibroma is discussed in more detail in the section on chondroid-containing lesions (see Fig. 7–7*B*).

Giant Cell–Rich Osteosarcomas

The majority of osteosarcomas have a small component of benign, osteoclast-like giant cells, but smears from occasional osteosarcomas contain very large numbers of these cells.[89] These osteoclasts usually contain fewer than 20 nuclei that are round or, more commonly, ovoid, with a vesicular chromatin pattern and small but distinct nucleoli. Admixed with these cells are atypical osteoblastic and fibroblastic cells with enlarged atypical nuclei and fragments of osteoid. Except for the large number of osteoclast-like giant cells, smears from these sarcomas appear identical to smears obtained from conventional osteosarcomas.

Malignant Fibrous Histiocytoma

There are several reports of the cytologic appearance of soft tissue malignant fibrous histiocytomas,[75–79] but few reports of the cytologic features of malignant fibrous histiocytoma primary in bone.[90] The cytologic findings in primary malignant fibrous histiocytoma of bone appear identical to those of its soft tissue counterpart. The smears are cellular, with many singly dispersed, plump, spindle-shaped or polygonal cells (Fig. 7–14*A*), including irregular bizarre forms.[90] The nuclei are greatly enlarged. Some cells have abundant foamy cytoplasm. A number of multinucleated neoplastic giant cells with large irregular hyperchromatic and markedly atypical nuclei are scattered throughout the smear (Fig. 7–14*B*). Mitotic figures, including atypical forms, are found within the mononuclear cell component.

Pigmented Villonodular Synovitis (Giant Cell Tumor of Tendon Sheath)

Pigmented villonodular synovitis is a relatively common neoplasm (see Chapter 18), but few reports of its cytologic appearance exist.[91, 92] In our experience and in the reported cases, the smears have been cellular, containing predominantly isolated round or oval cells with abundant pale cytoplasm (Fig. 7–15). Cell borders are distinct, and the nuclei are bland with a regular nuclear membrane surrounding a finely granular and evenly distributed chromatin. Nucleoli, when present, are small and indistinct. The cytoplasm is frequently foamy and vacuolated, and coarse granular deposits of hemosiderin-like pigment are seen in some of the oval cells. Multinucleated osteoclast-like giant cells are common and contain from 3 to 50 bland oval nuclei. A second population of bland, small, spindle-shaped mononuclear cells has small oval regular nuclei with an evenly distributed chromatin, pale cytoplasm, and long bipolar wispy cytoplasmic processes. Nuclear atypia is not seen in any of the cells. A few lymphocytes are seen in the background.

LESIONS DOMINATED BY INFLAMMATORY CELLS

Osteomyelitis

The cytologic appearance of smears obtained from cases of osteomyelitis depends on

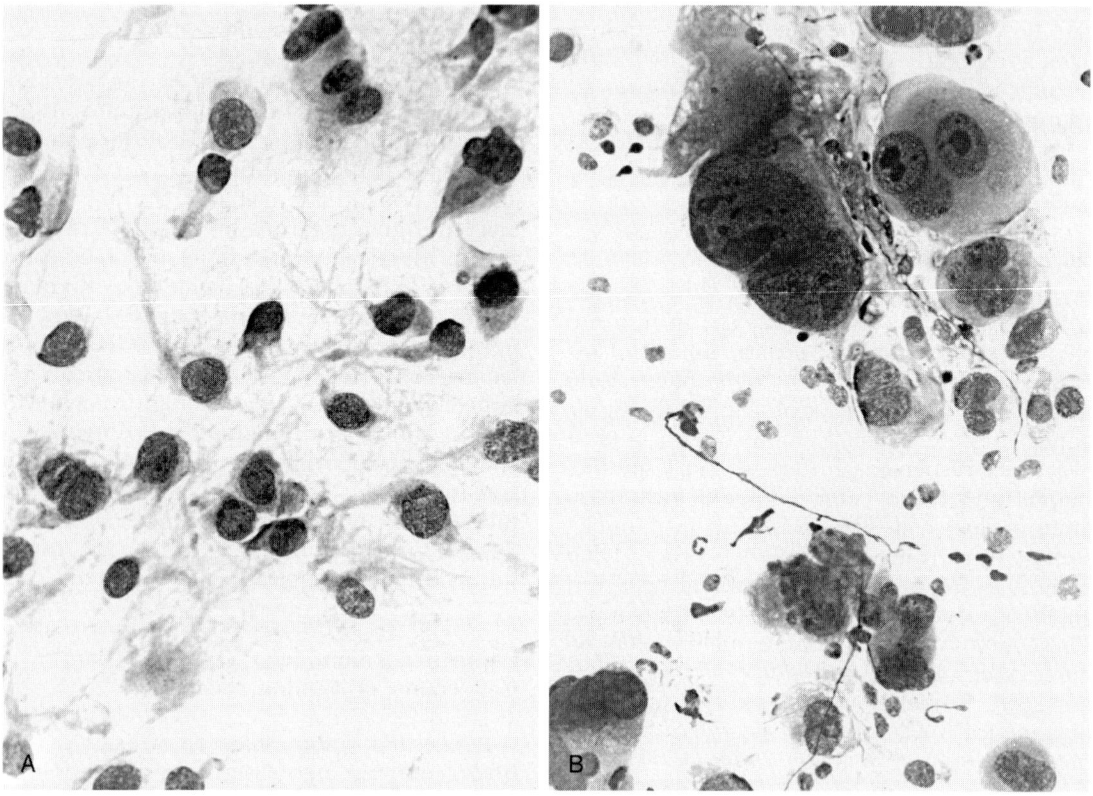

Figure 7–14. Malignant fibrous histiocytoma. *A*, Spindle cells demonstrating significant nuclear atypia (MGG). *B*, Multinucleated anaplastic giant cells (MGG).

the inciting organism and the stage of the disease. Aspirates obtained from acute osteomyelitis yield smears dominated by neutrophils, and culture of the aspirated material often establishes the causative organism.[93] In subacute cases, a prominent number of lymphocytes and histiocytes will be seen in addition to the polymorphonuclear leukocytes. Gram stain of the aspirated material may reveal bacteria.

Smears from cases of chronic osteomyelitis are often of low or moderate cellularity and contain a mixture of lymphocytes, plasma cells, and histiocytes. The findings are rather nonspecific in most cases, but occasionally special stains will reveal bacteria. In some cases, plasma cells will dominate the smears to the point of suggesting multiple myeloma.

Silverman et al.[94] reported the cytologic findings in a case of tuberculous disease of the spine (Pott's disease). The smears contain large numbers of small confluent and cohesive tissue fragments representing granulomas. The fragments are composed of spindle-shaped cells with long wavy nuclei (epithelioid cells). The cytoplasm of these cells is frequently pale and granular, with a syncytial arrangement of the cells. Multinucleated benign giant cells are present in small numbers. Necrotic granular material is scattered in the background. A large number of polymorphonuclear leukocytes is present in the smears. Organisms are not identified by special stains.

Other investigators have reported the FNA cytologic findings in bone infection by cryptococcus[95] and actinomycosis.[96] Frable[96] has emphasized the importance of obtaining cultures of aspirated material in suspected cases of osteomyelitis.

Langerhans' Cell Histiocytosis (Eosinophilic Granuloma)

Smears obtained from cases of eosinophilic granuloma are usually cellular and contain many noncohesive large oval or polygonal cells with a lesser number of eosinophils.[97, 98] The histiocytic component (Langerhans' cells) has abundant cytoplasm in most cases, but it may

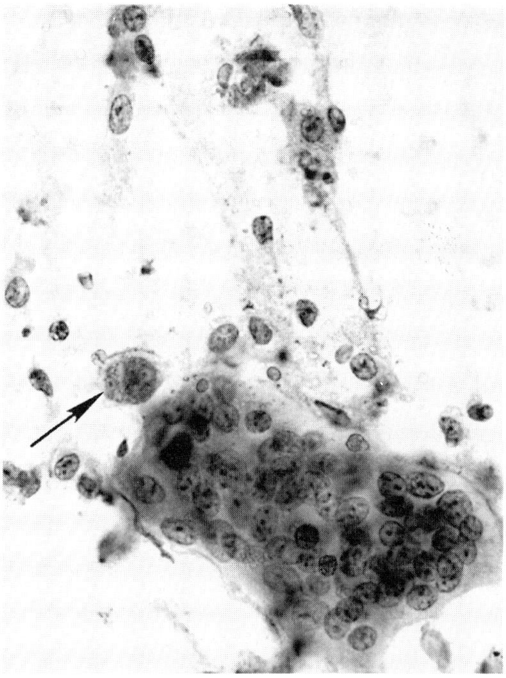

Figure 7–15. Aspirate of pigmented villonodular synovitis showing biphasic population of cells (MGG). Coarse granular pigment is present in the cytoplasm of some of the large cells *(arrow)*.

be scant in amount or entirely stripped away. The oval or reniform nuclei are best seen when stained by H&E or the Pap technique. Many of the nuclei show prominent lobulation or grooving (Fig. 7–16). The chromatin is finely granular and the nucleoli are inconspicuous. Air-dried, Diff-Quik–stained material highlights the eosinophils, but the histiocytes are less well seen. The Langerhans' cells in air-dried smears have a plasmacytoid appearance, and nuclear grooves cannot be seen.

The majority of Langerhans' cells are mononuclear, but occasional binucleated and multinucleated cells will be seen. Slight nuclear pleomorphism is usually present, as are occasional mitotic figures. The background contains small numbers of neutrophils, osteoclast-like giant cells, and foamy histiocytes. The Langerhans' cells will stain positively in cell block preparations with antibodies directed against S-100 protein, and Birbeck granules can be demonstrated on ultramicroscopy (see Chapter 14).[99]

Pigmented Villonodular Synovitis

Smears obtained from pigmented villonodular synovitis contain large numbers of foamy or hemosiderin-like pigment-laden histiocytes along with a prominent number of multinucleated giant cells. These neoplasms are further discussed in the section describing giant cell–containing lesions.

CYSTIC OR BLOOD-RICH LESIONS OF BONE

Predominately cystic lesions, or those composed primarily of blood-filled spaces, are difficult or impossible to diagnose by fine-needle aspiration cytology and make poor candidates for investigation by FNA. When radiographs suggest one of these lesions, open biopsy is preferred to FNA for diagnosis. Despite these limitations, some morphologic data exist for the cytologic appearance of these lesions.

Simple (Unicameral) Bone Cyst

Aspiration of simple bone cysts yields clear yellow or white fluid that is nearly acellular on microscopic examination. Grossly, the fluid is viscous but thinner than that obtained from

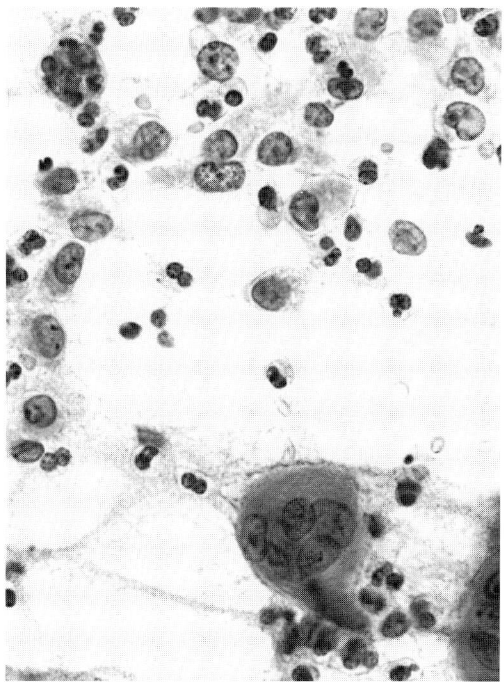

Figure 7–16. Cytologic features of eosinophilic granuloma include multinucleated giant cells, histiocytes with a distinctive nuclear groove, and numerous eosinophils (MGG).

most ganglion cysts. Microscopic examination reveals a dirty granular or mucoid background in which are scattered rare histiocytes. Recognizable lining cells are almost never seen.

Ganglion Cyst (Intraosseous and Articular)

Soft tissue ganglion cysts are common, but their intraosseous counterparts are rare. The two are histologically and cytologically identical. Aspirates obtain a few drops of very thick, viscous, clear gray-white material. Microscopic examination discloses rare scattered histiocytes with a foamy or vacuolated cytoplasm and round or reniform nuclei. The background will have a pale blue granular or myxoid appearance (Diff-Quik) and may contain rare lymphocytes in addition to the histiocytes.

Hemangioma

Like their soft tissue counterpart, intraosseous hemangiomas yield predominately blood on aspiration. Rarely, small three-dimensional clusters of oval endothelial cells and short spindle cells are seen in the extensively bloody background.[100, 101] Little or no nuclei atypia is seen.

Aneurysmal Bone Cyst

Aspiration of these lesions yields predominately blood. Rare multinucleated osteoclast-like giant cells may be seen along with rare polygonal or round cells representing osteoblasts or primitive stromal cells and histiocytes. No significant nuclear atypia is present. Aneurysmal bone cysts may be engrafted on other lesions including chondroblastoma and giant cell tumor, and the cytology from these complex lesions will reflect the primary lesion. The appearance of aneurysmal bone cyst is also discussed in the section on giant cell–containing lesions.

Telangiectatic Osteosarcoma

Fine-needle aspirates of telangiectatic osteosarcomas are very bloody and may contain little diagnostic material, making their cytologic separation from aneurysmal bone cyst and hemangioma very difficult, if not impossible. Diagnostic material, if present, contains large atypical osteoblasts and spindle-shaped cells, along with rare fragments of osteoid. The cytologic appearance is similar to that of conventional osteosarcoma material markedly diluted by blood. Bloody smears must be carefully searched for such atypical cells when there is radiographic evidence for telangiectatic osteosarcoma or aneurysmal bone cyst. Telangiectatic osteosarcoma is further discussed in the section on osteoid-containing lesions.

Angiosarcoma

Angiosarcomas of bone are rare neoplasms and we are aware of only a single case report of the cytologic features,[102] although the appearance is similar to cases from the soft tissues.[103] The smear background is very hemorrhagic, with single cells and small clusters of atypical cells scattered throughout the smear (Fig. 7–17). Cellularity aside from red cells is low. The single cells are large and polygonal or spindle-shaped. The spindle-shaped cells have abundant cytoplasm with elongated cytoplasmic processes. The large central nuclei are

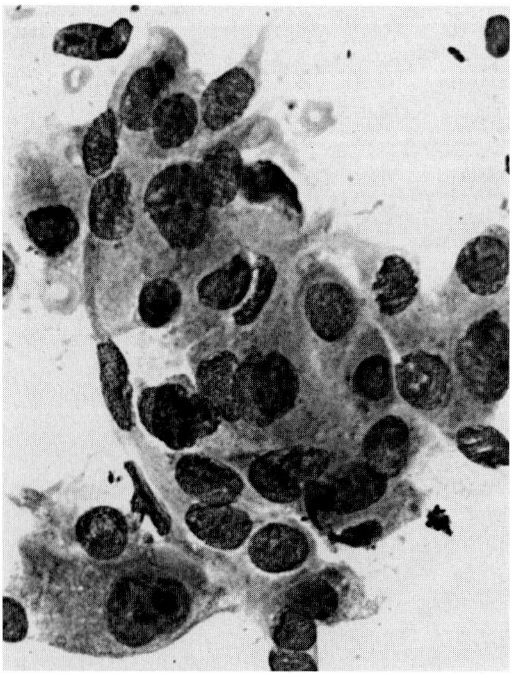

Figure 7–17. Aspirate from an angiosarcoma demonstrating anaplastic, plump endothelial cells in a bloody background (MGG).

hyperchromatic with an irregular nuclear membrane and coarse chromatin clumping. Nuclear atypia is usually marked. The cell clusters are three-dimensional and composed of tightly packed polygonal cells often lining a slitlike structure.[102] The nuclei of these cells have a coarse chromatin pattern with irregular chromocenters but not true nucleoli. Some cells have cytoplasmic tails.

EPITHELIOID LESIONS OF BONE

The majority of lesions containing cells with an epithelioid appearance represent metastatic deposits of carcinoma, but some primary lesions may have cells and cell clusters with an epithelioid appearance.

Adamantinoma

Adamantinomas are rare lesions occurring almost exclusively within the tibia (see Chapter 17), for which there are only a few reports of the cytologic findings.[80–83] Aspirates from these neoplasms are moderately cellular and contain many loosely cohesive sheets and bundles of medium-sized spindle cells that may take on the appearance of anastomosing cords with apparent nuclear palisading (Fig. 7–18).[80]

Three cell types have been described: (1) polygonal cells with large round nuclei showing chromatin clearing and one or more nuclei and a well-defined abundant vacuolated or finely granular cytoplasm; (2) small cells with poorly defined cytoplasm and round nuclei with dark condensed chromatin; and (3) fusiform cells with poorly defined cytoplasm.[81, 83] The background has a granular or fibrillar appearance.[83] The first two cell types appear epithelial and, when present in cell block preparations, can stain with antibodies directed against cytokeratin. These epithelial cells often lie in cords with peripheral palisading and are crucial for the diagnosis of adamantinoma (see Fig. 7–18). The individual spindle-shaped cells have oval to bacillary-shaped nuclei surrounded by ill-defined cytoplasm. The chromatin pattern within the nuclei is fine and evenly distributed. Micronucleoli, nuclear folds, and cytoplasmic nuclear pseudoinclusions are all identified in some populations of spindle-shaped cells. A small number of osteoblasts and osteoclast-like giant cells are scattered throughout the smears.

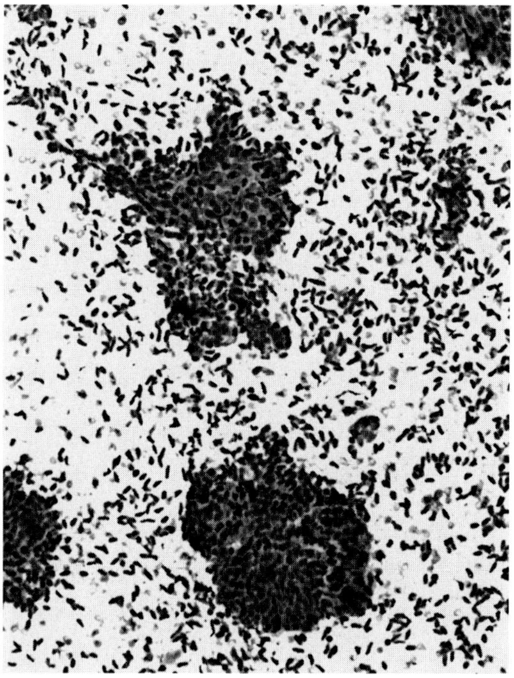

Figure 7–18. Smears from adamantinoma showing aggregates of cells with peripheral palisading as well as a loose, dispersed spindle cell component (MGG).

Chordoma

The cytologic findings in chordoma have been well described.[52–62] Low-power examination of smears reveals large fragments of a myxoid-chondroid or mucoid material frequently associated with, or engulfing, clusters of polygonal cells.[52, 54, 58, 59] Single cells are also dispersed throughout the background. The matrix material stains red-purple with Diff-Quik or MGG,[54] light red with H&E,[58] and eosinophilic with the Pap method.[55] The overall cellularity has been described as moderate in most reports.[52, 59] Cell clusters are numerous,[54] with most being of an irregular shape, although occasionally, papillary-like cell clusters have been observed.[52]

Three types of cells are described in chordomas. The most frequent is a relatively large, round or oval cell that contains prominent cytoplasmic vacuoles or has granular cytoplasm (Fig. 7–19).[52] Some of these cells display a single large vacuole displacing the nuclei to one side and resembling ‘‘signet ring’’ cells.[54] Unlike true signet ring cells, these cells possess a band of cytoplasm between the nucleus and the cell border opposite the vacuole.[54] Other large cells contain multiple large vacuoles

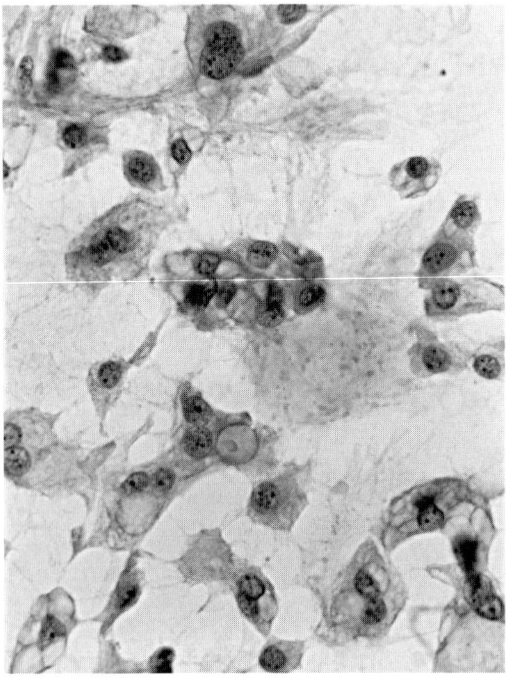

Figure 7–19. Aspirate from chordoma showing numerous signet ring–type cells as well as smaller, nonvacuolated cells with abundant bubbly cytoplasm (MGG).

yielding a spider-web appearance, many of which have a triangular shape with the base along the cytoplasmic membrane and the apex touching the nucleus.[53] The nuclei of these cells are round or oval and at times display intranuclear vacuoles or cleaves.[52] Nucleoli are variably present.[52, 53] Generally, the nuclei are bland with smooth, thin, and regular nuclear membranes,[53, 54] but considerable nuclear pleomorphism can occur.[60] Occasional mitotic figures are present in the majority of reported cases.[52–59]

The second population of cells is smaller and lacks vacuoles. Usually these cells form a minor population, but at times are the only cells present.[61] These cells are monotonous, bland, and relatively equal in size.[61] Although moderate anisonucleosis is present, mitotic figures are absent in this population. These cells have been found to have a granular cytoplasm present in scanty to moderate amounts. The nuclei are round or oval and have small or indistinct nucleoli.

Spindle cells are a small minority of cells in most specimens. Their nuclei are usually bland with pointed ends. Cytoplasm is granular and lacks vacuoles. Occasional bizarre multinucleated giant cells are seen, as are rare osteoclast-like giant cells. Occasional chordomas demonstrate marked nuclear atypia,[60] suggesting the diagnosis of malignant fibrous histiocytoma or high-grade liposarcoma. Careful attention to the presence of more classic physaliferous cells and the abundant myxoid-mucoid stroma should result in the correct diagnosis.

Separation of chordoma from adenocarcinoma may at times be extremely difficult due to the "signet ring" appearance of some cells and the papillary shape to some tissue fragments found in many examples of chordoma. In general, chordomas show the following features that are not seen in adenocarcinomas[54]: the "signet ring" cells in chordomas have a rim or band of cytoplasm extending beyond the nucleus on the side opposite the vacuole; chordomas contain numerous cytoplasmic bubbles, giving a spider-web appearance to many of the large cells; and most cells of chordomas have smooth nuclear contours. The papillary structures in chordomas do not have the sharp borders that characterize true papillae of adenocarcinoma.

Metastatic Carcinoma

The majority of bone neoplasms are metastatic rather than primary lesions of bone.[5–19] Carcinomas account for the greater proportion of metastases and the most common primary tumors (e.g., breast, prostate, lung) constitute the most commonly encountered bone metastases. In the clinical setting of a well-documented, advanced-stage, primary carcinoma, recovery of malignant cells in an aspirate should pose no diagnostic dilemma. In instances of an unknown primary tumor or history of multiple primary tumors, the aspiration cytologist may be pressured to suggest an origin for the lesion based on cytomorphologic characteristics. With the exception of renal, prostatic, and thyroid carcinomas, an unequivocal statement of the origin for a metastatic lesion cannot be made on the cytologic appearance alone.

Renal cell carcinoma is characterized by clusters of cells with clear or granular cytoplasm on FNA (Fig. 7–20). Well-differentiated renal cell carcinomas may closely resemble normal histiocytes or macrophages and may be difficult to separate from them. The presence of a central nucleolus confirms that the cell in question represents metastatic carcinoma. Prostate carcinoma commonly metasta-

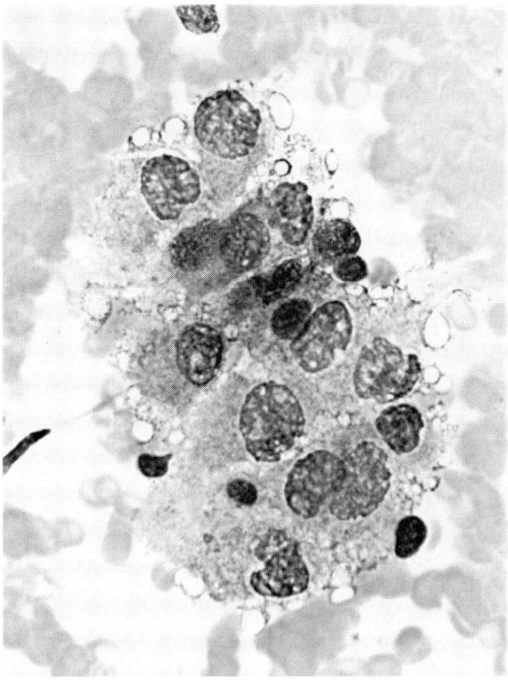

Figure 7–20. Aspirate of metastatic renal cell carcinoma showing characteristic foamy cytoplasm (MGG).

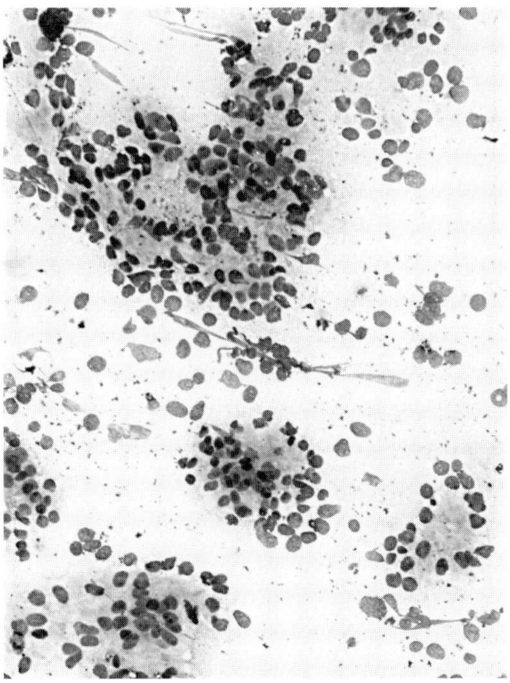

Figure 7–21. Aspirate from a metastatic prostatic carcinoma showing a population of poorly preserved cells. Many retain an acinar pattern, which recapitulates the histology of the primary tumor (MGG).

sizes to bone and can form densely sclerotic or blastic lesions. Aspirates from metastatic prostate carcinoma are characterized by a relatively monomorphous, poorly differentiated cell type with ill-defined cytoplasm that often retains the glandular pattern of the original carcinoma (Fig. 7–21). Metastatic thyroid carcinomas, particularly of the follicular variant, can form acini in metastatic lesions. Like prostate cancers, the origin of thyroid carcinoma can be documented with specific immunohistochemical markers, making this lesion one of the few that can be definitively identified in metastatic form.

A more detailed description of the cytologic appearances of the common carcinomas is available in other texts.[104–107]

REFERENCES

1. Simon MA: Biopsy of musculoskeletal tumors. J Bone Joint Surg 64A:1253, 1982.
2. Enneking WF: Editorial: The issue of the biopsy. J Bone Joint Surg 64A:1119, 1982.
3. Mankin HJ, Lange TA, Spanier SS: The hazards of biopsy in patients with malignant primary bone and soft tissue tumors. J Bone Joint Surg 64A:1121, 1982.
4. Mirra JM: Bone Tumors: Clinical, Radiologic and Pathologic Correlations. Philadelphia, Lea & Febiger, 1989, p 1498.
5. Akerman M, Berg NO, Persson BM: Fine needle aspiration biopsy in the evaluation of tumor-like lesions of bone. Acta Orthop Scand 47:129, 1976.
6. deSantos LA, Lukeman JM, Wallace S, et al: Percutaneous needle biopsy of bone in the cancer patient. AJR Am J Roentgenol 130:641, 1978.
7. El-Khoury GY, Terepka RH, Mickelson MR, et al: Fine-needle aspiration biopsy of bone. J Bone Joint Surg 65A:522, 1983.
8. Legge D, Ennis JT, Dempsey J: Percutaneous needle biopsy in the management of solitary lesions of bone. Clin Radiol 29:497, 1978.
9. Murphy WA, Destouet JM, Gilula LA: Percutaneous skeletal biopsy 1981: A procedure for radiologist—Results, review and recommendations. Radiology 139:545, 1981.
10. Ottolenghi CE, Schajowicz F, De Schant FA: Aspiration biopsy of the cervical spine: Technique and results in thirty-four cases. J Bone Joint Surg 46A:715, 1964.
11. Rabinov K, Goldman H, Rosbash H, et al: The role of aspiration biopsy of focal lesions in lung and bone by simple needle and fluoroscopy. AJR Am J Roentgenol 101:932, 1967.
12. Robertson RC, Ball RP: Destructive spine lesions: Diagnosis by needle biopsy. J Bone Joint Surg 17:749, 1935.
13. Mazet R Jr, Cozen L: The diagnostic value of vertebral body needle biopsy. Ann Surg 135:245, 1952.
14. Frankel CJ: Aspiration biopsy of the spine. J Bone Joint Surg 36:69, 1954.
15. Lalli AF: Roentgen-guided aspiration biopsies of skeletal lesions. J Can Assoc Radiol 21:71, 1970.

16. Pepe RG, Lalli AF: Percutaneous aspiration bone biopsy by fluoroscopic guidance. Cleve Clin Q 43:77, 1976.
17. Thommesen P, Frederiksen P: Fine needle aspiration biopsy of bone lesions: Clinical value. Acta Orthop Scand 47:137, 1976.
18. Adler O, Rosenberger A: Fine needle aspiration biopsy of osteolytic metastatic lesions. Am J Roentgenol 133:15, 1979.
19. Stoker DJ, Cobb JP, Pringle JAS: Needle biopsy of musculoskeletal lesions: A review of 208 procedures. J Bone Joint Surg 73B:498, 1991.
20. Layfield LJ, Armstrong K, Zaleski S, et al: Diagnostic accuracy and clinical utility of fine needle aspiration cytology in the diagnosis of clinically primary bone lesions. Diagn Cytopathol 9:168, 1993.
21. Sanerkin NG, Jeffree GM: Cytology of Bone Tumors: A Color Atlas with Text. Philadelphia, JB Lippincott, 1980, p 19.
22. Popok SM, Naib ZM: Fine-needle aspiration cytology of myositis ossificans. Diagn Cytopathol 1:236, 1985.
23. Rööser B, Herrlin K, Rydholm A, et al: Pseudomalignant myositis ossificans: Clinical, radiologic, and cytologic diagnosis in 5 cases. Acta Orthop Scand 60:457, 1989.
24. Layfield LJ, Glasgow BJ, Anders KH, et al: Fine-needle aspiration cytology of primary bone lesions. Acta Cytol 31:177, 1987.
25. Byers PD: Solitary benign osteoblastic lesions of bone: Osteoid osteoma and benign osteoblastoma. Cancer 22:43, 1968.
26. Schajowicz F, Lemos C: Osteoid osteoma and osteoblastoma. Closely related entities of osteoblastic derivation. Acta Orthop Scand 41:272, 1970.
27. Sanerkin NG, Jeffree GM: Cytology of Bone Tumours: A Color Atlas with Text. Philadelphia, JB Lippincott, 1980, p 26.
28. Walaas L, Kindblom L-G: Light and electron microscopic examination of fine-needle aspirates in the preoperative diagnosis of osteogenic tumors: A study of 21 osteosarcomas and two osteoblastomas. Diagn Cytopathol 6:27, 1990.
29. White VA, Fanning CV, Ayala AG, et al: Osteosarcoma and the role of fine-needle aspiration: A study of 51 cases. Cancer 62:1238, 1988.
30. Xiaojing P, Xiangcheng Y: Cytodiagnosis of bone tumors by fine needle aspiration. Acta Cytol 29:570, 1985.
31. Kumar RV, Rao CR, Hazarika D, et al: Aspiration biopsy cytology of primary bone lesions. Acta Cytol 37:83, 1993.
32. Mirra JM: Bone Tumors. Clinical, Radiologic, and Pathologic Correlations. Philadelphia, Lea & Febiger, 1989, p 316.
33. Ellison DA, Silverman JF, Strausbach PS, et al: Fine-needle aspiration of chondroblastic osteosarcoma of the skull: Report of a case in an 11 year old girl. Diagn Cytopathol 14:51, 1996.
34. Stanfield BL, Powers CN, Desch CE, et al: Fine-needle aspiration cytology of an unusual primary lung tumor, chondrosarcoma: Case report. Diagn Cytopathol 7:423, 1991.
35. Saint-Martin M, Castelli MJ, Gattuso P: Fine-needle aspiration biopsy of synovial chondromatosis of the temporomandibular joint. Diagn Cytopathol 11:93, 1994.
36. Ganjei P, Evans DA, Moezzi M: Differential diagnosis of chondroid lesions of bone by fine needle aspiration cytology. Acta Cytol 33:717, 1989.
37. Walaas L, Kindlblom L-G, Gunterberg B, et al: Light and electron microscopic examination of fine-needle aspirates in the preoperative diagnosis of cartilaginous tumors. Diagn Cytopathol 6:396, 1990.
38. Sanerkin NG, Jeffree GM: Cytology of Bone Tumours: A Color Atlas with Text. Philadelphia, JB Lippincott, 1980, p 53.
39. Mirra JM: Bone Tumors: Clinical, Radiologic, and Pathologic Correlations. Philadelphia, Lea & Febiger, 1989, p 1661.
40. Ascoli V, Facciolo F, Muda AO, et al: Chondroblastoma of the rib presenting as an intrathoracic mass: Report of a case with fine needle aspiration biopsy immunocytochemistry and electron microscopy. Acta Cytol 36:423, 1992.
41. Fanning CV, Sneige N, Carrasco CH, et al: Chondroblastoma: Fine needle aspiration cytology. Acta Cytol 31:658, 1987.
42. Fanning CV, Seige NS, Carrasco CH, et al: Fine needle aspiration cytology of chondroblastoma of bone. Cancer 65:1847, 1990.
43. Pohar-Marinsek Z, Us-Krasovec M, Lamovec J: Chondroblastoma in fine needle aspirates. Acta Cytol 36:367, 1992.
44. Kilpatrick SE, Pike EJ, Geisinger KR, et al: Chondroblastoma of bone: Use of fine-needle aspiration biopsy and potential diagnostic pitfalls. Diagn Cytopathol 16:65, 1997.
45. Gupta S, Dev G, Marya S: Chondromyxoid fibroma: A fine-needle aspiration diagnosis. Diagn Cytopathol 9:63, 1993.
46. Layfield LJ, Ferreiro JA: Fine-needle aspiration cytology of chondromyxoid fibroma: A case report. Diagn Cytopathol 4:148, 1988.
47. Drut R, Pollono D: Chondrosarcoma of bone as second tumor after diffuse anaplastic Wilms' tumor: Diagnosis by fine-needle aspiration cytology. Diagn Cytopathol 9:205, 1993.
48. Abdul-Karim FW, Wasman JK, Pitlik D: Needle aspiration cytology of chondrosarcoma. Acta Cytol 37:655, 1993.
49. Olszewski W, Woyke S, Musiatowicz B: Fine needle aspiration biopsy cytology of chondrosarcoma. Acta Cytol 27:345, 1983.
50. Dee S, Meneses M, Ostrowski ML, et al: Pleomorphic ("dedifferentiated") chondrosarcoma: Report of a case initially examined by fine needle aspiration biopsy. Acta Cytol 35:467, 1991.
51. Doria MI Jr, Wang HH, Chinoy MJ: Retroperitoneal mesenchymal chondrosarcoma: Report of a case diagnosed by fine needle aspiration cytology. Acta Cytol 34:529, 1990.
52. Apaja-Sarkkinen M, Väänänen K, Curran S, et al: Carcinomatous features of cervical chordoma in a fine needle aspirate. Acta Cytol 31:769, 1987.
53. Carvalho G, Coelho LHMR: Chordoma of rhinopharynx: Report of a case. Acta Cytol 18:425, 1974.
54. Clark SA, Bloch T, Edwards MK, et al: Diagnosis of cervical chordoma by fine needle aspiration biopsy. Acta Cytol 31:765, 1987.
55. Finely JL, Silverman JF, Dabbs DJ, et al: Chordoma: Diagnosis by fine needle aspiration biopsy with histologic, immunocytochemical and ultrastructural confirmation. Diagn Cytopathol 2:330, 1986.
56. Lefer LG, Rosier RP: The cytology of chordoma. Acta Cytol 22:51, 1978.
57. Nijhawan VS, Rajwanshi A, Das A, et al: Fine needle aspiration cytology of sacrococcygeal chordoma. Diagn Cytopathol 5:404, 1989.

58. Perasole A, Infantolino D, Spigariol F: Aspiration cytology and immunocytochemistry of sacral chordoma with liver metastases: A case report. Diagn Cytopathol 7:277, 1991.
59. Plaza JA, Ballestin C, Pérez-Barrios A, et al: Cytologic, cytochemical, immunocytochemical and ultrastructural diagnosis of a sacrococcygeal chordoma in a fine needle aspiration biopsy specimen. Acta Cytol 33:89, 1989.
60. Rone R, Ramzy I, Duncan D: Anaplastic sacrococcygeal chordoma. Fine needle aspiration cytologic findings and embryologic considerations. Acta Cytol 30:183, 1986.
61. Thompson SK, Callery RT: Cytologic diagnosis of a chordoma without physaliferous cells. Diagn Cytopathol 4:144, 1988.
62. Akhtar M, Ali MA, Sabbah R: Aspiration cytology of Ewing's sarcoma: Light and electron microscopic correlations. Cancer 56:2051, 1985.
63. Kontozoglou T, Krakauer K, Qizilbash AH: Ewing's sarcoma: Cytologic features in fine needle aspirates in two cases. Acta Cytol 30:513, 1986.
64. Dahl I, Akerman M, Angervall L: Ewing's sarcoma of bone: A correlative cytological and histological study of 14 cases. Acta Pathol Microbiol Immunol Scand (A) 94:363, 1986.
65. Akerman M, Dreinhöfer K, Rydholm A, et al: Cytogenetic studies on fine-needle aspiration samples from osteosarcoma and Ewing's sarcoma. Diagn Cytopathol 15:17, 1996.
66. Ascoli V, Facciolo F, Nardi F: Cytodiagnosis of a primary non-Hodgkin's lymphoma of bone. Diagn Cytopathol 11:168, 1994.
67. Niemann TH, Thomas PA: Primary lymphoma of bone: Diagnosis by fine needle aspiration biopsy in a pediatric patient. Diagn Cytopathol 12:165, 1995.
68. Htwe WM, Lucas DR, Bedrossian CWM, et al: Fine-needle aspirate of primary lymphoma of bone. Diagn Cytopathol 15:421, 1996.
69. Pettit CK, Zukerberg LR, Gray MH, et al: Primary lymphoma of bone: A B-cell with a high frequency of multilobulated cells. Am J Surg Pathol 14:329, 1990.
70. Levitt S, Cheng L, Dupuis MH, et al: Fine needle aspiration diagnosis of malignant lymphoma with confirmation by immunoperoxidase staining. Acta Cytol 29:895, 1985.
71. Das DK, Gupta SK, Sehgal S: Extramedullary plasma cell tumors: Diagnosis by fine needle aspiration cytology. Diagn Cytopathol 2:248, 1986.
72. Hajdu SI, Melamed MR: The diagnostic value of aspiration smears. Am J Clin Pathol 59:530, 1973.
73. Orell SR, Sterett GF, Walters MNI, et al: Manual and Atlas of Fine Needle Aspiration Cytology. Edinburgh, Churchill Livingstone, 1992, p 324.
74. Sanerkin NG, Jeffree GM: Cytology of Bone Tumours: A Color Atlas with Text. Philadelphia, JB Lippincott, 1980, p 75.
75. Nguyen GK, Jeannot A: Cytopathologic aspects of pulmonary metastasis of malignant fibrous histiocytoma, myxoid variant: Fine needle aspiration biopsy of a case. Acta Cytol 26:349, 1982.
76. Walaas L, Angervall L, Hagmar B, et al: A correlative cytologic and histologic study of malignant fibrous histiocytoma: An analysis of 40 cases examined by fine needle aspiration cytology. Diagn Cytopathol 2:46, 1986.
77. Hong IS: Cytologic findings in a case of malignant fibrous histiocytoma. Acta Cytol 22:519, 1978.
78. Lindholm K, Nordgren H, Akerman M: Electron microscopy of fine needle aspiration biopsy from malignant fibrous histiocytoma: Report of a case. Acta Cytol 23:399, 1979.
79. Kim K, Goldblatt PJ: Malignant fibrous histiocytoma: Cytologic, light microscopic and ultrastructural studies. Acta Cytol 26:507, 1982.
80. Laucirica R, Mody D, MacLeay L, et al: Adamantinoma: A case report with aspiration cytology and differential diagnostic and immunohistochemical considerations. Acta Cytol 36:951, 1992.
81. Tabei SZ, Abdollahi B, Nili F: Diagnosis of metastatic adamantinoma of the tibia by pulmonary brushing cytology. Acta Cytol 32:579, 1988.
82. Hales MS, Ferrell LD: Fine-needle aspiration biopsy of tibial adamantinoma: A case report. Diagn Cytopathol 4:67, 1988.
83. Galera-Davidson H, Fernandez-Rodriquez A, Torres-Olivera FJ, et al: Cytologic diagnosis of a case of recurrent adamantinoma. Acta Cytol 33:635, 1989.
84. Vetrani A, Fulciniti F, Boschi R, et al: Fine needle aspiration biopsy diagnosis of giant-cell tumor of bone: An experience with nine cases. Acta Cytol 34:863, 1990.
85. Szyfelbein WM, Schiller AL: Cytologic diagnosis of giant cell tumor of bone metastatic to lung: A case report. Acta Cytol 23:460, 1979.
86. Sneige N, Ayala AG: Fine needle aspiration cytology of giant-cell tumor of bone. Acta Cytol 28:649, 1984.
87. Rios-Martin JJ, Otal-Salaverri C, González-Cámpora R, et al: Fine needle aspiration diagnosis of aggressive giant cell tumor of bone: A case report. Acta Cytol 39:550, 1995.
88. Sanerkin NG, Jeffree GM: Cytology of Bone Tumours: A Color Atlas with Text. Philadelphia, JB Lippincott, 1980, p 146.
89. Mirra JM: Bone Tumors: Clinical, Radiologic and Pathologic Correlations. Philadelphia, Lea & Febiger, 1989, p 326.
90. Kannan V, von Ruden D: Malignant fibrous histiocytoma of bone: Initial diagnosis by aspiration biopsy cytology. Diagn Cytopathol 4:262, 1988.
91. Dawiskiba S, Eriksson L, Elner A, et al: Diffuse pigmented villonodular synovitis of the temporomandibular joint diagnosed by fine needle aspiration cytology. Diagn Cytopathol 5:301, 1989.
92. Wakely PE, Frable WJ: Fine-needle aspiration biopsy cytology of giant cell tumor of tendon sheath. Am J Clin Pathol 102:87, 1994.
93. Sanerkin NG, Jeffree GM: Cytology of Bone Tumours: A Color Atlas with Text. Philadelphia, JB Lippincott, 1980, p 144.
94. Silverman JF, Larkin EW, Carney M, et al: Fine needle aspiration cytology of tuberculosis of the lumbar vertebrae (Pott's disease). Acta Cytol 30:538, 1986.
95. Ganjei P, Evans DA, Fischer ML: Diagnosis of cryptococcal osteomyelitis by fine needle aspiration cytology: A case report. Acta Cytol 26:224, 1982.
96. Frable WJ: Thin needle aspiration biopsy. *In* Bennington JL (ed): Major Problems in Pathology. Vol. 14. Philadelphia, WB Saunders, 1983, p 289.
97. Elsheikh T, Silverman JF, Wakely PE, et al: Fine needle aspiration cytology of Langerhans' cell histiocytosis (eosinophilic granuloma) of bone in children. Diagn Cytopathol 7:261, 1991.
98. Thommesen P, Bartholdy N, Anderson MJF: Histiocytosis X: IX. Fine needle aspiration biopsy for differentiation between histiocytosis X and spondylitis. Acta Radiol Oncol 22:349, 1983.

99. Layfield LJ, Bhuta S: Fine-needle aspiration cytology of histiocytosis X: A case report. Diagn Cytopathol 4:140, 1988.
100. Kaw YT, Esparza AR: Cytologic diagnosis of a cavernous hemangioma of the liver with fine-needle biopsy. Diagn Cytopathol 7:628, 1991.
101. Willems JS: Aspiration biopsy cytology of soft tissue tumors. *In* Linsk JA, Franzen S (eds): Clinical Aspiration Cytology. Philadelphia, JB Lippincott, 1983, p 334.
102. Khiyami A, Green LK, Gyorkey F, et al: Primary angiosarcoma of the cuboidal bone: A case report. Diagn Cytopathol 7:520, 1991.
103. Cohen MB, Layfield LJ: Fine needle aspiration biopsy of soft tissue tumors. *In* Schmidt W, Miller T, Katz R, et al (eds): Cytopathology Annual. Chicago, ASCP Press, 1994, p 115.
104. Frable WJ: Thin-needle aspiration biopsy. *In* Bennington JL (ed): Major Problems in Pathology. Vol 14. Philadelphia, WB Saunders, 1983, p 20.
105. Koss LG, Woyke S, Olszewski W: Aspiration Biopsy Cytologic Interpretation and Histologic Bases. 1st ed. New York, Igaku-Shoin, 1984, p 53.
106. Linsk JA, Franzen S: Clinical Aspiration Cytology. 1st ed. Philadelphia, JB Lippincott, 1983, p 61.
107. Orrel SR, Sterrett GF, Walters MNI, et al: Manual and Atlas of Fine Needle Aspiration Cytology. 2nd ed. Edinburgh, Churchill Livingstone, 1992, p 96.

Chapter

8

ASSESSMENT OF THE EFFECTS OF TREATMENT ON BONE NEOPLASMS

PIERO PICCI and NICOLA BALDINI

The development and implementation of primary (neoadjuvant) chemotherapy has dramatically changed treatment options and led to longer survival and better quality of life for patients with osteosarcoma and Ewing's sarcoma. Before the introduction of primary chemotherapy, more than 80% of patients with osteosarcoma were treated by amputation of a limb immediately after diagnosis, and then received a standard chemotherapeutic regimen.[1–4]

In osteosarcoma, the extent of necrosis after primary chemotherapy was soon discovered to be correlated to prognosis. These data were used to plan postoperative treatment, by either intensifying or modifying chemotherapy in patients with poor response. Major institutions in which these more advanced protocols are applied are now showing an improvement in disease-free survival from 50 to 70%,[5–8] together with a dramatic reduction in amputations, from 80% to less than 20%.[9–12]

A correlation between chemotherapy-induced necrosis and prognosis has also been demonstrated for Ewing's sarcoma,[13–15] and the evaluation of the effects of primary chemotherapy has become one of the major steps in the treatment strategy for bone tumors.

OSTEOSARCOMA

Evaluation of Chemotherapy-Induced Necrosis

Histology

Evaluation of chemotherapy-induced necrosis requires an accurate histologic examination of the entire specimen. An entire tumor section along its major axis plus another section along the transversal axis are prepared. These sections are then photographed and successively divided into several numbered blocks for staining.[16] A tumor map may thus be reconstructed, the percentage of necrosis calculated, and areas where viable tumor is most likely to persist ("sanctuary" areas) described. Another method is to stain macrosections of the tumor without dividing it into blocks, but with this method, the evaluation of the cytologic details may often be difficult.

The extent of chemotherapy-induced necrosis is generally expressed as a percentage of viable tumor compared with the entire tumoral mass. This evaluation is possible because osteosarcoma generally produces an abundant intercellular osteoid matrix that persists after complete cellular necrosis, thus retaining the pretreatment volume of the tumor.

Several classifications, involving from three to six different grades, have been suggested to quantify necrosis.[7, 8, 16, 17] An exact standardization of grading is unrealistic and probably not necessary. It is, in fact, impossible to count each viable cell, calculating the precise percentage as compared with the necrotic ones. Only an estimate is possible, and the major criterion is the experience of the pathologist who, on the basis of multiple observations, can assess the efficacy of treatment without quantifying the number of viable and nonviable cells. A nonresponse (necrosis below 50% or 60%), an intermediate (necrosis up to

90%), or a good response (necrosis greater than 90%), is generally stated.

By consulting the reconstructed maps, it is possible to evaluate the preferential sites of persistent viable tumor after preoperative chemotherapy. These "sanctuary" areas are consistently found in the invaded soft tissues, the cortex and the subcortex, zones in contact with cartilage (both epiphyseal and articular), invaded ligaments and other articular structures, and areas surrounding necrotic-hemorrhagic lacunae. In contrast, necrosis appears to be more concentrated in the central medullary areas.[16]

One of the major explanations for the presence of "sanctuary" areas is vascularization. Areas adjacent to cartilage, cortex, and ligaments are poorly vascularized and, although tumor in the soft tissues is nourished by a network of new vessels, this may be insufficient to permit an adequate drug concentration. Moreover, necrotic-hemorrhagic lacunae within the tumor may impede permeation of drugs. When planning definitive surgery with adequate and safe margins, the surgeon must keep in mind the existence of these areas, which very often are at the periphery of the tumor.

Radiology

The radiographic evidence of a good tumor response is most often observed as a rim of reactive bone (see later discussion). The diminished neovascularity observed on post-chemotherapy angiograms, when compared to the pre-chemotherapy ones, is another indication of a good tumor response. The techniques under investigation that give useful information regarding the extent of necrosis include pre-chemotherapy and post-chemotherapy gallium and quantitative bone scintigraphy,[18, 19] magnetic resonance angiography,[20] and dynamic magnetic resonance imaging.[21, 22] This last technique seems to offer the best results; however, the interpretation of changes seen on pre-chemotherapy and post-chemotherapy magnetic resonance is not completely reliable.

Correlation with Prognosis

The importance of chemotherapy-induced necrosis lies in its correlation with prognosis. From the start, it was evident that the greater the effect of the drugs on the tumor, the longer the disease-free survival. Based on these observations, in most cases postoperative chemotherapy is planned according to the grade of necrosis; that is, the grade of necrosis is used as an "in vivo" chemosensitivity test. Postoperative chemotherapy may either be changed or increased in patients without a satisfactory grade of necrosis, or may be reduced in patients with a good response to aggressive preoperative chemotherapy.

With the adoption of more aggressive and effective protocols for neoadjuvant chemotherapy, the achievement of total (100%) necrosis may become of prognostic significance.

Evaluation of the Effects on Local Aggressiveness

For many decades, amputation was the most frequent surgical treatment for osteosarcoma. Only after the adoption of primary chemotherapy did the percentages of amputations decrease below 20% in major centers, while maintaining a low local recurrence rate.[23–28] It is therefore evident that preoperative chemotherapy plays an important role in controlling the local aggressiveness of this disease and, consequently, in reducing the risk of local recurrence.[29] The change in surgical strategy from amputation to local resection means that the distance between the tumor and surgical margin is less. This is why the pathologist must study the specimen not only to assess necrosis, but also to evaluate tumor aggressiveness and the real surgical margins achieved.

Histology and Radiology

The radiographic appearance that is equivalent to extensive tumor necrosis is most often observed as a rim of histopathologically proven reactive bone (Figs. 8–1 and 8–2). This correlates well with the softening of the surrounding soft tissues observed clinically. The techniques used to investigate the effects of chemotherapy are described earlier, and a reliable radiographic method of evaluating tumor necrosis would be of great assistance in indicating the minimal surgical margins required for appropriate local control.

A close collaboration between the pathologist and the surgeon is essential to obtain useful information on the adequacy of local excision. During surgery, the surgeon should mark with methylene blue those areas on the surgical specimen where the margins are uncertain.

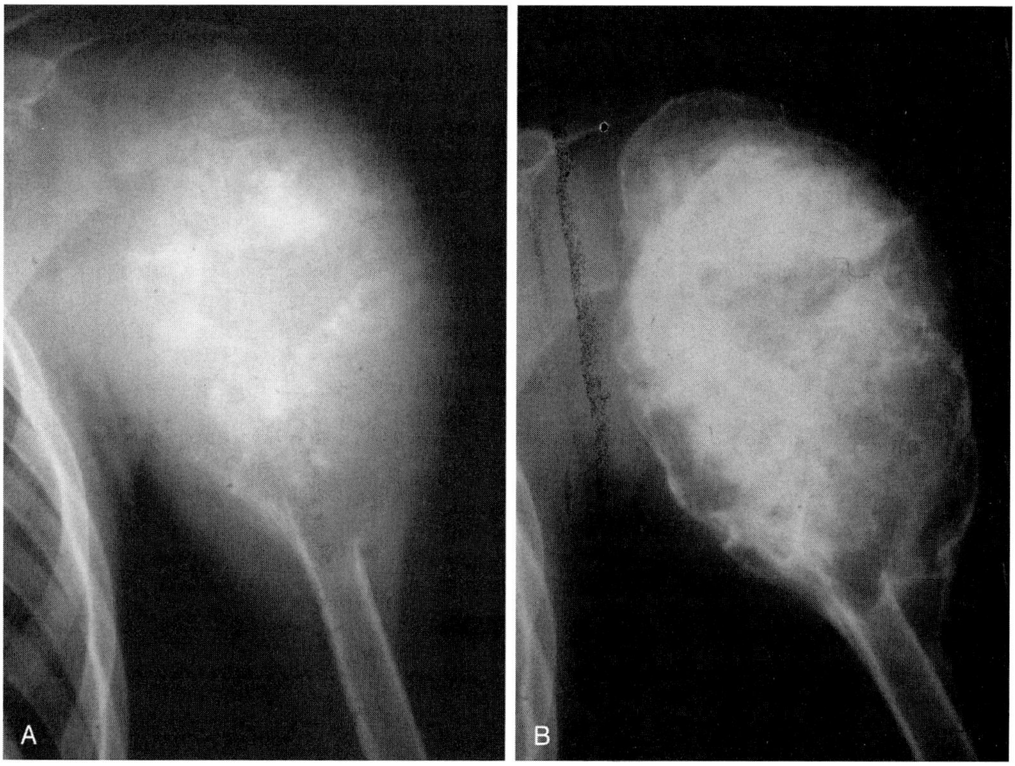

Figure 8–1. Radiographs of a conventional osteosarcoma of the left proximal humerus. *A*, Before chemotherapy there is a large, aggressive osteoblastic lesion in the metaphysis and diaphysis of the humerus, with epiphyseal extension superiorly. Codman's angles are present inferiorly and there is extensive soft tissue infiltration. *B*, After chemotherapy, there is an increase in mineralization in the medullary cavity and at the periphery of the sarcoma, in keeping with a favorable response.

Intramedullary canal curettages from the shaft of the retained stump have to be submitted for microscopic evaluation. In the pathology laboratory, the surgical specimen is inspected, and all margins previously marked by the surgeon plus any additional areas thought to be in question are marked with India ink and evaluated microscopically. Samples from the medullary canal are also evaluated.

Following the guidelines of the Musculo-Skeletal Tumor Society,[30] the overall surgical margin is defined as the single least adequate margin microscopically identified on the entire surgical specimen. Margins may be described as intralesional, marginal, wide, radical, or contaminated (Table 8–1).

In untreated osteosarcoma, as well as in patients without a chemotherapeutic response, a poorly formed, loosely arranged pseudocapsule is generally observed. This pseudocapsule is formed in part by compressed normal structures and in part by reactive tissues (i.e., periosteal reaction, reactive fibrous proliferation with few inflammatory cells, and small immature vessels). It is frequently penetrated by finger-like projections of tumor tissue (Fig. 8–3*A*) (see also color Figure 8–3), and satellite tumor nodules may develop in fat and muscle well beyond the pseudoencapsulation.

In contrast, the pathologic findings in patients with a chemotherapy response are quite striking. The pseudocapsule becomes an almost true capsule made of mature collagen bundles or mature bone. The tumor is delimited by highly collagenized fibrous tissue that is variable in width but continuous around the neoplasm (Fig. 8–3*B*). This presumably is related to an arrest in tumor growth, which gives the host sufficient time to respond by developing a well-differentiated fibrous or bony capsule, or both. The apparent histopathologic maturation of the capsule associated with a good tumor response may be seen clinically as decreased local swelling and edema. In some cases, probably associated with the periosteum, mature bone trabeculae may

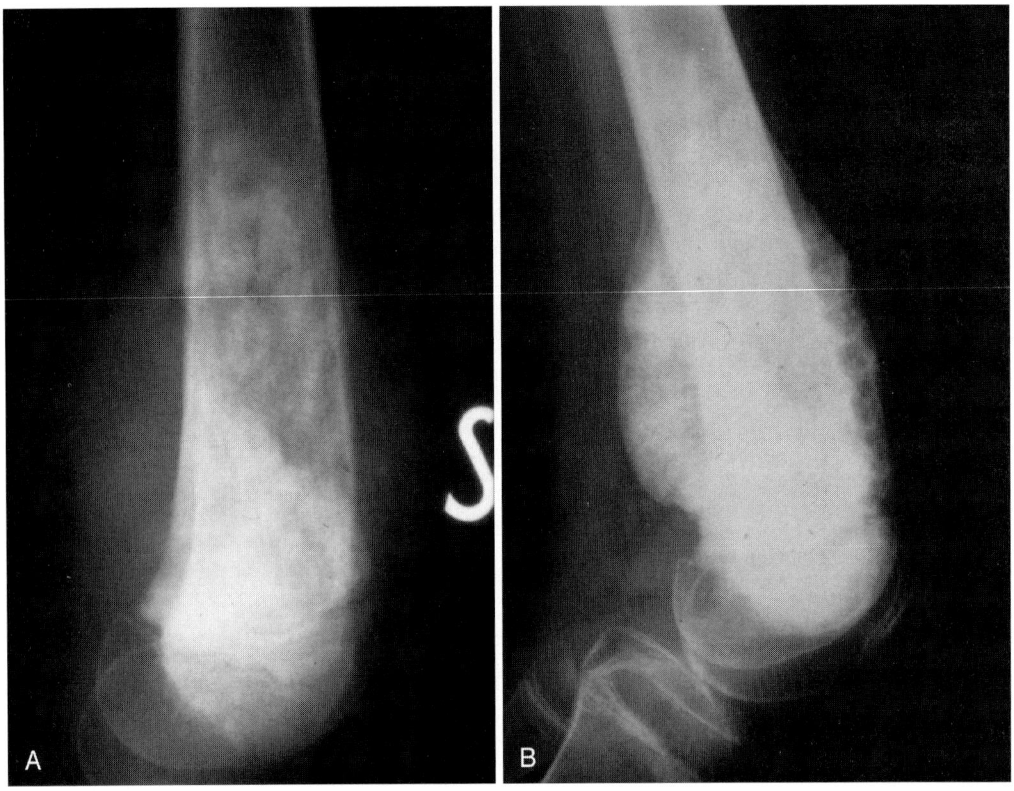

Figure 8–2. Radiographs of a conventional osteosarcoma of the distal femur. *A*, Before chemotherapy there is an aggressive osteoblastic lesion in the metaphysis that extends into the diaphysis and epiphysis. Codman's angles are present, and there is soft tissue infiltration. *B*, After chemotherapy, there is a marked increase in medullary and peripheral mineralization, suggesting a favorable response.

form in combination with the fibrous capsule. Cartilaginous tumor lobules of osteosarcoma may also ossify peripherally (Fig. 8–3*C*). The vascularity present in the poorly formed pseudocapsule is no longer observed, and inflammatory cells are also uncommon after a good response. The strands of tumor penetrating the compressed reactive tissues and pseudocapsule are destroyed, and the surrounding mature collagenized tissue now appears to encapsulate the underlying necrotic tumor tissue. When satellite nodules are observed in specimens having a good response, they too are encapsulated (Fig. 8–3*D*).

Surgical margins as defined by the Musculo-Skeletal Tumor Society remain applicable also after preoperative chemotherapy.[30] The terms intralesional, marginal, wide, and radical correlate appropriately to the quality of the tissues dividing the surgical dissection planes and the tumor. Preoperative chemotherapy does not change the anatomic description of the margins, but it may change the quality and therefore their adequacy. It is our opinion that the histopathologic quality of surgical margins is more important than the quantitative description of the thickness of the tissues surrounding the tumor specimen.

EWING'S SARCOMA

Evaluation of Chemotherapy-Induced Necrosis

As for osteosarcoma, the last decade has seen important advances in the treatment of Ewing's sarcoma. However, as survival has improved, so late complications from local radiation treatment (secondary tumors and local recurrences) have become more common.[2, 7–9] In the attempt to avoid some of these complications, surgery, when feasible, has been combined with neoadjuvant chemotherapy.[31–34]

The increased use of surgical resection in the primary treatment of Ewing's sarcoma has permitted the histopathologic analysis of tumor response to preoperative chemotherapy.

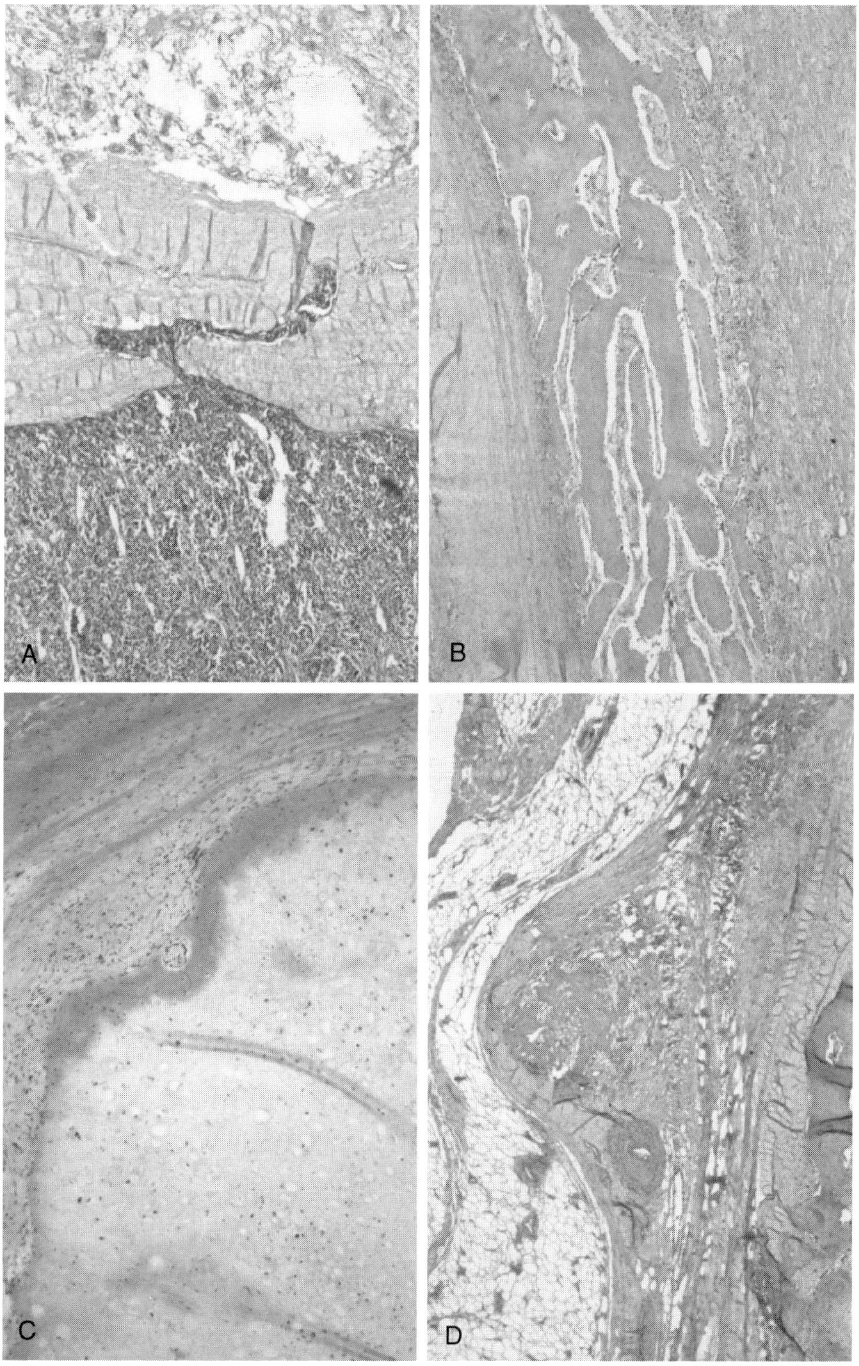

Figure 8–3. Osteosarcoma before *(A)* and after *(B,C,D)* chemotherapy. *A*, In untreated tumors, the reactive pseudocapsule is often penetrated by finger-like projections. *B*, When the tumoral cells are destroyed by chemotherapy *(right)*, the pseudocapsule matures and becomes a true capsule. Mature bone trabeculations, probably associated with the periosteum, may be seen. *C*, Cartilaginous tumor lobules ossify peripherally. *D*, Satellite nodules, when present, appear to be encapsulated. (See also color figure.)

Table 8–1. Terminology Used to Describe Surgical Margins of Excision

Description	Interpretation
Intralesional	The surgical plane of dissection passes through tumor tissue.
Marginal	The surgical plane of dissection passes through the reactive tissue zone, i.e., pseudocapsule, without microscopic evidence of tumor.
Wide	The surgical plane of dissection passes outside the reactive zone and through normal tissue.
Radical	The surgical margins are all wide and include the entire anatomic compartments involved by the tumor.
Contaminated	A margin obtained by the surgical re-excision of the wound previously found to be microscopically intralesional in the same operative procedure.

The histopathologic grading system for necrosis commonly utilized for patients with osteosarcoma cannot be applied appropriately to patients with Ewing's sarcoma. As previously described, osteosarcomas produce a collagenous, osseous, and cartilaginous framework that remains intact and maintains the tumor volume despite the complete necrosis of tumor cells after chemotherapy. Therefore, an estimate of the percentage of tumor necrosis compared with the pre-chemotherapy mass is possible. However, Ewing's sarcoma cells do not produce a framework in response to chemotherapy, but tend to disappear completely, so that a dramatic decrease in tumor volume is observed (Fig. 8–4).[35] Due to this important reduction in tumor volume, estimations of necrosis cannot be based on viable cells per unit area of residual "tumor." We therefore suggest a different histopathologic approach in which the absolute quantity of viable tumor cells after preoperative chemotherapy is calculated independently from any tumor mass variation.[13]

The specimen is prepared as for osteosarcomas, and then graded from I to III for tumor necrosis:

Grade I defines the chemotherapy response when a surgical specimen contains at least one residual macroscopic nodule of viable tumor. Macroscopic nodules are defined as individual nodules larger than one 10× magnification field, or scattered microscopic nodules that individually are smaller than one 10× field, but collectively exceed one 10× field.

Grade II defines the chemotherapy response when only isolated microscopic nodules of viable tumor cells are identified. These individually are less than the size of one 10× magnification field, and the sum of the areas of these nodules does not exceed one 10× field (Fig. 8–5).

For *Grade III,* no viable nodules of tumor cells are identified within the specimen. A specimen with scattered, individual tumor cells that are not distinguishable from nontumorous cells could be included within this group as long as no clusters of tumor cells are present.

Correlation with Prognosis

By grading necrosis in this way, a strict correlation with prognosis was found in 108 cases.[14] Disease-free survival was 94% in patients with total necrosis (Grade III), in comparison to 69% in those with persistence of microscopic

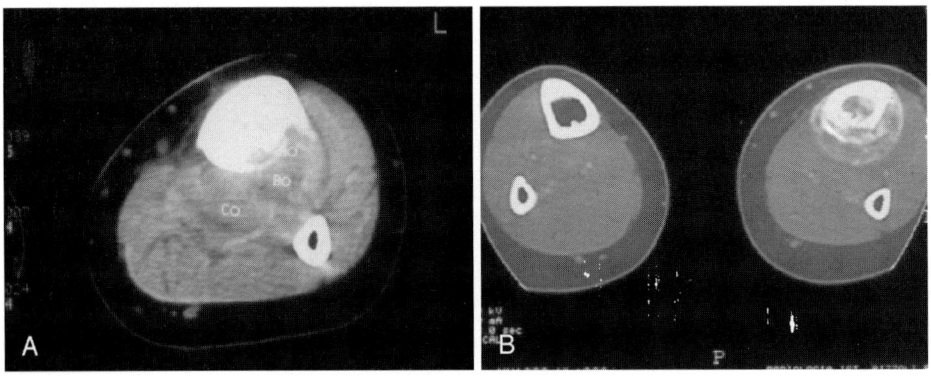

Figure 8–4. Computed tomography scans of Ewing's sarcoma of the tibial shaft. *A,* Before chemotherapy there is a large soft tissue mass within the calf muscles. *B,* After chemotherapy, the tumor volume is greatly reduced and there is peripheral mineralization.

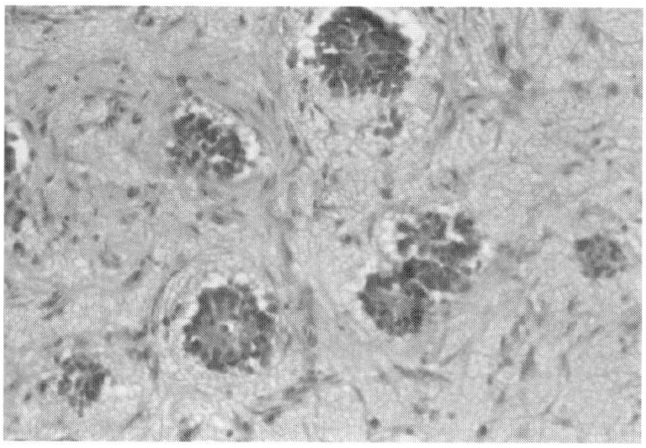

Figure 8–5. Scattered, isolated microscopic nodules of viable cells after preoperative chemotherapy in Ewing's sarcoma.

foci (Grade II) and 41% for those patients with persistence of macroscopic foci (Grade I). Patients with Ewing's sarcoma of the extremities who are given primary chemotherapy and surgery (without preoperative radiation) can have their postoperative chemotherapy regimens designed in accordance with the grading data.

The histopathologic analysis of these 108 cases revealed the existence of "sanctuary" areas for Ewing's sarcoma. Fifty-four per cent of patients had residual nodules of viable tumor in the subperiosteal space, whereas 70% of patients had residual tumor in the soft tissues and 65% in areas of hemorrhage. The intramedullary canal had evidence of residual tumor in 46% of patients.

These data reinforce the message that to obtain local control, wide surgical margins are necessary both in the soft tissues and in bone, especially in patients with Grade I tumor necrosis. Adjunctive postoperative radiation therapy should be considered in these patients, even when apparently wide surgical margins are obtained.

EXPRESSION OF THE MULTIDRUG RESISTANCE GENE, *MDR*1

The heterogeneous response of bone sarcomas to chemotherapy may be partially attributed to inherent drug resistance of the tumor. At the cellular level, the lack of responsiveness to cytotoxic drugs may be caused by a variety of mechanisms. The best known, termed *multidrug resistance,* is characterized in vitro by cross-resistance to a wide spectrum of structurally and functionally unrelated lipophilic anticancer agents following exposure to one of them.[36] The *MDR*1 gene product, P-glycoprotein, is an ATP-dependent plasma membrane protein involved in the active efflux of cytotoxic molecules out of the cell, and plays a central role in multidrug resistance.[37] Increased amounts of P-glycoprotein may confer multidrug resistance on cells by preventing the intracellular accumulation of a variety of cytotoxic drugs,[38] including doxorubicin, the most effective agent for the treatment of sarcomas.[39]

An altered expression of the *MDR*1 gene has been reported to play an important role in a number of human tumors.[40, 41] Several authors have included sporadic observations of cases of osteosarcoma and Ewing's sarcoma in their studies,[42–45] but only recently have a few papers specifically addressed the issue of the clinical significance of multidrug resistance in primary malignant bone tumors[46–52] (see Chapter 5).

Osteosarcoma

In a series of bone and soft tissue sarcomas, Stein and colleagues,[48] at the Free University of Berlin, included 11 cases of osteosarcoma, the majority of which (91%) showed *MDR*1 overexpression. In a consecutive series of 15 cases of osteosarcoma, Wunder and colleagues,[46] at the Mount Sinai Hospital of Toronto, observed *MDR*1 overexpression in nine patients (60%) and found a trend toward a worse outcome in cases exhibiting high levels of *MDR*1 expression. At the Hospital for Sick Children of Toronto, Chan and colleagues[49] collected samples from 62 patients with osteosarcoma, reporting an incidence of P-glycoprotein overexpression at diagnosis in 44% of cases. In 47 cases, the histologic response to chemotherapy was significantly lower for the group of patients with P-glycoprotein overexpression than for the P-glycoprotein–negative group. Moreover, the disease-free and the overall survival were both associated with the P-glycoprotein status, with only 2 of the 35 patients in the group negative for P-glycoprotein having relapsed, compared with 25 of the 27 patients in the P-glycoprotein–positive group.

We have analyzed P-glycoprotein expression in two different series of patients with osteosarcoma observed at the Istituti Ortopedici Rizzoli. In both investigations, multidrug-resistant cell variants derived from human osteosarcoma cell lines[53] were used as controls for low levels of multidrug resistance. A retrospective study of 92 patients with high-grade osteosarcoma of the extremities, who had undergone the same therapeutic program of surgery and chemotherapy, examined P-glycoprotein expression in the biopsy specimens obtained before chemotherapy and preserved in paraffin-embedded tissue blocks.[52] P-glycoprotein immunoreactivity was found in 28 tumors (30%), whereas the remaining 64 tumors were P-glycoprotein–negative (Fig. 8–6) (see also color figure). In this series, no relationship was found between the presence of P-glycoprotein expression and the extent of tumor necrosis after preoperative chemotherapy. However, increased levels of P-glycoprotein in the biopsy specimen were significantly associated with a decreased probability of event-free and overall survival at a 5-year minimum follow-up. In a multivariate analysis, P-glycoprotein status and the extent of tumor necrosis after preoperative chemotherapy were independent predictors of clinical outcome. In particular, patients with increased levels of P-glycoprotein in tumor cells at the time of diagnosis had a more than threefold increased risk of adverse events compared with patients with P-glycoprotein–negative tumors. In this series, the patients had been treated both with multidrug resistance related (doxorubicin, etoposide) and unrelated (methotrexate, cisplatin, ifosfamide) drugs, so that the absence of a relationship between the level of P-glycoprotein and the extent of tumor necrosis might reflect the killing of a majority of tumor cells by drugs that act independently of P-glycoprotein.

In a prospective investigation of 105 cases of osteosarcoma, these observations were substantially confirmed. P-glycoprotein overexpression was present in 23% of primary osteosarcomas. In 38 patients treated with surgery and chemotherapy and followed for at least 2 years, overexpression of the P-glycoprotein was associated with a higher relapse rate and a worse outcome. Interestingly, the incidence of P-glycoprotein overexpression among metastatic lesions occurring before chemotherapy was similar to that observed in primary, untreated

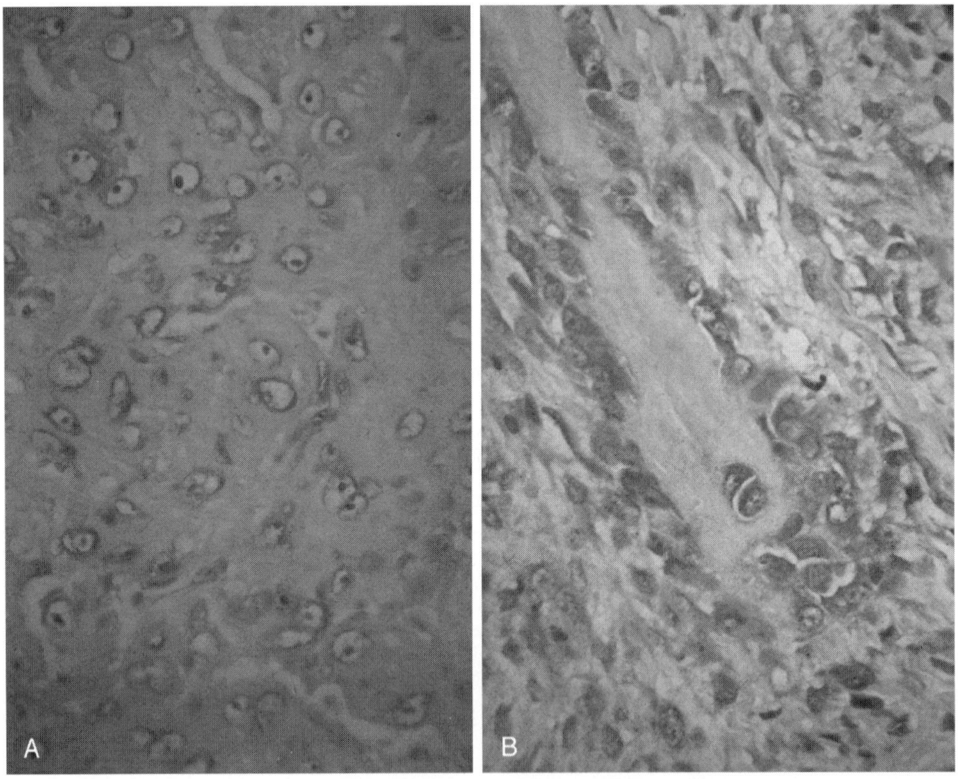

Figure 8–6. Different patterns of P-glycoprotein immunoreactivity in human osteosarcoma. *A*, In this osteosarcoma, the malignant cells do not show detectable labeling for the P-glycoprotein. *B*, In a different osteosarcoma, there is strong cytoplasmic labeling in most malignant cells for P-glycoprotein. (Avidin-biotin-peroxidase immunostaining using JSB-1 monoclonal antibody at 1:20 dilution.) (See also color figure.)

lesions (20%), whereas metastases occurring after chemotherapy were associated with a significantly higher incidence of P-glycoprotein overexpression (57%). These data suggest that multidrug resistance may be an inherent feature of osteosarcoma and that the presence of multidrug resistant clones may be enhanced during the course of the disease, possibly under the pressure of anti-cancer agents. This effect was actually observed in the few cases in which both primary and metachronous secondary lesions were available for analysis. However, it cannot be excluded that in osteosarcoma, as in other tumors, the observed overexpression of P-glycoprotein may also be associated with a progression of malignancy.[54]

Ewing's Sarcoma

Evidence for a role for P-glycoprotein in Ewing's sarcoma is much less than for osteosarcoma, with only two published reports to date. At the University of Münster, Roessner and colleagues[47] found P-glycoprotein overexpression in 57% of cases of Ewing's sarcoma analyzed either before or after chemotherapy. In patients with a poor response to chemotherapy, 77% were positive for P-glycoprotein, whereas only 25% of patients with a good histologic response were P-glycoprotein–positive. Death occurred in 33% of P-glycoprotein-negative cases, and in 58% of P-glycoprotein-positive cases. These data suggest that the immunodetection of P-glycoprotein in Ewing's sarcoma is associated with a poor histologic response to chemotherapy and a worse clinical outcome. More recently, Hijazi and colleagues,[50] from the National Cancer Institute in Bethesda, analyzed the expression of P-glycoprotein in 35 cases of Ewing's sarcoma and peripheral primitive neuroectodermal tumors. P-glycoprotein expression was found to be inherently expressed in about one-half of the cases, with no difference in the prevalence of expression between Ewing's sarcoma and peripheral primitive neuroectodermal tumors. Interestingly, among those cases that were initially negative for P-glycoprotein, one-half showed immunoreactivity for P-glycoprotein in recurrent tumors. In this small series, however, no difference was found in the relapse-free survival rate based on the expression of P-glycoprotein at diagnosis.

Assessment in Practice

Despite the fact that chemotherapy for osteosarcoma and Ewings's sarcoma is partly based on agents that are not involved in the multidrug-resistant phenotype, these observations are highly suggestive of a key role for the biochemical resistance mechanisms in determining the clinical outcome of these malignancies. Multidrug resistance may be an inherent feature of both osteosarcoma and Ewing's sarcoma, and this should be taken into account when scheduling highly toxic, potentially lethal chemotherapeutic programs that, based on this evidence, are unlikely to be successful. The analysis of *MDR*1 expression should be carried out in all tumor samples at the time of biopsy both in osteosarcoma and in Ewing's sarcoma. This can be easily accomplished at a low cost by immunohistochemistry on paraffin-embedded material in any pathology laboratory. To enhance the reproducibility of the data obtained by different laboratories that use different techniques, standard materials and methods have been outlined.[55] In particular, for immunohistochemistry, both the intensity of labeling and the percentage of P-glycoprotein–positive cells should be assessed. The intensity of labeling is reported as negative, low (+), intermediate (++), high (+++), or ultrahigh (++++). The use of adequate controls for the quality of the specimen (for example, by using anti-vimentin antibodies), for the specificity of the immunostaining (for example, by using renal tissue, which shows a strong positivity for the P-glycoprotein in the proximal tubules and negative immunostaining in the glomeruli), and for the sensitivity of the immunoreaction (for example, by using multidrug-resistant cell lines with defined levels of resistance) may help to increase the reliability of the assay. The use of more than one monoclonal antibody directed against different epitopes of the P-glycoprotein is advisable.[56] The adoption of different approaches, for example by combining immunohistochemistry with reverse transcriptase polymerase chain reaction (RT-PCR) or in situ hybridization for the detection of *MDR*1 mRNA may be of additional help,[57] although, at the present time, these tools are not available for a routine diagnostic use in most laboratories.

It is evident that additional prospective, well-controlled, and preferably multimethodology studies of *MDR*1 expression are needed[58] for the evaluation of the role of multidrug resistance in bone sarcomas to confirm the observed association of multidrug resistance with response to treatment and outcome, to understand the relationship of the multidrug-resistant phenotype with the metastatic behavior, to analyze the possible relevance of alternative mechanisms of multidrug resistance that are not mediated by the P-glycoprotein,[59] and to investigate therapeutic strategies to stably reverse the multidrug-resistant phenotype, not only in vitro, but also in clinical settings.[60, 61]

REFERENCES

1. Rosen G, Suwansirikul S, Kuon C, et al: High-dose methotrexate with citrovorum factor rescue and Adriamycin in childhood osteogenic sarcoma. Cancer 33:1151, 1974.
2. Sutow WW, Gehan EA, Vietti TJ, et al: Multidrug chemotherapy in primary treatment of osteosarcoma. J Bone Joint Surg 58A:629, 1976.
3. Jaffe N, Frei E, III, Watts H, et al: High-dose methotrexate in osteogenic sarcoma: A 5 year experience. Cancer Treat Rep 62:259, 1978.
4. Campanacci M, Bacci G, Bertoni F, et al: The treatment of osteosarcoma of the extremities: Twenty year experience at the Istituto Ortopedico Rizzoli. Cancer 48:1569, 1981.
5. Rosen G, Marcove RC, Caparros B, et al: Primary osteogenic sarcoma: The rationale for preoperative chemotherapy and delayed surgery. Cancer 43:2163, 1979.
6. Rosen G, Caparros B, Huvos AG, et al: Preoperative chemotherapy for osteogenic sarcoma: Selection of postoperative adjuvant chemotherapy based on the response of the primary tumor to preoperative chemotherapy. Cancer 49:1221, 1982.
7. Jaffe N, Knapp J, Chuang VP, et al: Osteosarcoma: Intraarterial treatment of the primary tumor with cis-diamine-dichloroplatinum II. Angiographic, pathologic, and pharmacologic studies. Cancer 51:402, 1983.
8. Winkler K, Beron G, Delling G, et al: Neoadjuvant chemotherapy of osteosarcoma: Results of a randomized cooperative trial (COOS 82) with salvage chemotherapy based on histologic tumor response. J Clin Oncol 6:329, 1988.
9. Rosen G: Preoperative (neoadjuvant) chemotherapy for osteogenic sarcoma: A ten year experience. Orthopedics 8:658, 1985.
10. Benjamin RS, Chawla SP, Carrasco C, et al: Arterial infusion in the treatment of osteosarcoma. *In* Ryan J, Baker L (eds): Recent Concepts in Sarcoma Treatment. Boston, Kluwer Academy Publishers, 1988, p 269.
11. Bacci G, Picci P, Ruggieri P, et al: Primary chemotherapy and delayed surgery (neoadjuvant chemotherapy) for osteosarcoma of the extremities. The Rizzoli's experience in 127 patients treated preoperatively with methotrexate i.v. (high vs moderate dose) and cisplatinum i.a. Cancer 65:2539, 1990.
12. Bacci G, Picci P, Ferrari S, et al: Primary chemotherapy and delayed surgery for non-metastatic osteosarcoma of the extremities. Results in 164 patients preoperatively treated with high dose of methotrexate (iv) followed by cisplatinum (ia) and Adriamycin (iv). Cancer 72:3227, 1993.
13. Picci P, Rougraff BT, Bacci G, et al: Prognostic significance of histopathologic response to chemotherapy in nonmetastatic Ewing's sarcoma of the extremities. J Clin Oncol 11:1763, 1993.
14. Picci P, Bacci G, Ferrari S, et al: Chemotherapy-induced necrosis and prognosis in Ewing's sarcoma. A study on 108 cases (abstract). Proc Am Soc Clin Oncol 14:437, 1995.
15. Meyers PA, Wunder J, Healey J, et al: Ewing's sarcoma/primitive neuroectodermal tumor of bone: Histological response to pre-operative chemotherapy predicts event-free survival (abstract). Proc Am Soc Clin Oncol 14:441, 1995.
16. Picci P, Bacci G, Campanacci M, et al: Histologic evaluation of necrosis in osteosarcoma induced by chemotherapy. Regional mapping of viable and nonviable tumor. Cancer 56:1515, 1985.
17. Huvos AG, Rosen G, Marcove RC: Primary osteosarcoma: Pathologic aspects in 20 patients after treatment with chemotherapy, en bloc resection and prosthetic replacement. Arch Pathol Lab Med 101:14, 1977.
18. Chuang VP, Benjamin RS, Jaffe N, et al: Radiographic and angiographic changes in osteosarcoma after intraarterial chemotherapy. AJR Am J Roentgenol 139: 1065, 1982.
19. Yeh SDJ, Rosen G, Caparros B, et al: Semiquantitative gallium scintigraphy in patients with osteogenic sarcoma. Clin Nucl Med 9:175, 1984.
20. Lang P, Grampp S, Vahlensieck M, et al: Primary bone tumors: Value of MR angiography for preoperative planning and monitoring response to chemotherapy. AJR Am J Roentgenol 165:135, 1995.
21. Holscher HC, Bloem JL, van der Woude HJ, et al: Can MRI predict the histopathological response in patients with osteosarcoma after the first cycle of chemotherapy? Clin Radiol 50:384, 1995.
22. van der Woude HJ, Bloem JL, Verstraete KL, et al: Osteosarcoma and Ewing's sarcoma after neoadjuvant chemotherapy: Value of dynamic MR imaging in detecting viable tumor before surgery. AJR Am J Roentgenol 165:593, 1995.
23. Jaffe N, Smith D, Jaffe MR, et al: Intraarterial cisplatinum in the management of IIB osteosarcoma in the pediatric and in the adolescent age group. Clin Orthop 270:15, 1991.
24. Glasser DB, Lane JM: Stage IIB osteosarcoma. Clin Orthop 270:29, 1991.
25. Marsden FW, Stephens FO, McCarthy SW, et al: IIB osteosarcoma: Current management, local control, and survival statistics: The Australian experience. Clin Orthop 270:113, 1991.
26. Eckardt JJ, Eilber FR, Rosen G, et al: Endoprosthetic replacement for stage IIB osteosarcoma. Clin Orthop 270:202, 1991.
27. Petrilli AS, Gentil FC, Epelman S, et al: Increased survival, limb preservation, and prognostic factors for osteosarcoma. Cancer 68:733, 1991.
28. Rougraff BT, Simon MA, Kneisl JS, et al: A long-term oncologic, functional, and quality of life study of limb salvage versus amputation for osteosarcoma of the distal femur. J Bone Joint Surg 76A:649, 1994.
29. Picci P, Sangiorgi L, Rougraff BT, et al: Relationship of chemotherapy-induced necrosis and surgical mar-

gins to local recurrence in osteosarcoma. J Clin Oncol 12:2699, 1994.
30. Enneking WF, Spanier SS, Goodman MA: Current concepts review: The surgical staging of musculoskeletal sarcoma. J Bone Joint Surg 62A:1027, 1980.
31. Bacci G, Toni A, Avella M, et al: Long-term results in 144 localized Ewing's sarcoma patients treated with combined therapy. Cancer 63:1477, 1989.
32. Wilkens R, Pritchard DJ, Burgert E, et al: Ewing's sarcoma of bone: Experience with 140 patients. Cancer 58:2551, 1986.
33. Neff JR: Nonmetastatic Ewing's sarcoma of bone: The role of surgical therapy. Clin Orthop 204:111, 1986.
34. Sauer R, Jurgens H, Burgers J, et al: Prognostic factors in the treatment of Ewing's sarcoma. Radiother Oncol 10:101, 1987.
35. Jaffe N: Chemotherapy for malignant bone tumors. Orthop Clin North Am 20:487, 1989.
36. Ling V, Thompson LH: Reduced permeability in CHO cells as a mechanism of resistance to colchicine. J Cell Physiol 83:103, 1974.
37. Endicott JA, Ling V: The biochemistry of P-glycoprotein-mediated multidrug-resistance. Ann Rev Biochem 58:137, 1989.
38. Gottesman MM, Pastan I: Biochemistry of multidrug resistance mediated by the multidrug transporter. Ann Rev Biochem 62:385, 1993.
39. Blaney SM, Smith MA, Grem JL: Doxorubicin: role in the treatment of osteosarcoma. *In* Humphrey GB, Koops HS, Molenaar WS, Postma A (eds): Osteosarcoma in Adolescence and Young Adults: New Developments and Controversies. Boston, Kluwer Academic, 1993, p 55.
40. Goldstein LJ, Galski H, Fojo A, et al: Expression of a multidrug resistance gene in human cancers. J Natl Cancer Inst 81:116, 1989.
41. Cordon-Cardo C, O'Brien JP, Boccia J, et al: Expression of the multidrug resistance gene product (P-glycoprotein) in human normal and tumor tissues. J Histochem Cytochem 38:1277, 1990.
42. Fojo AT, Ueda K, Slamon DJ, et al: Expression of a multidrug-resistance gene in human tumors and tissues. Proc Natl Acad Sci USA 84:265, 1987.
43. Gerlach JH, Bell DR, Karakousis C: P-glycoprotein in human sarcomas: Evidence for multidrug resistance. J Clin Oncol 5:1452, 1987.
44. Noonan KE, Beck C, Holzmayer TÅ, et al: Quantitative analysis of MDR1 (multidrug resistance) gene expression in human tumors by polymerase chain reaction. Proc Natl Acad Sci U S A 87:7160, 1990.
45. Vergier B, Cany L, Bonnet F, et al: Expression of MDR1/P-glycoprotein in human sarcomas. Br J Cancer 68:1221, 1993.
46. Wunder JS, Bell RS, Wold L, et al: Expression of the multidrug resistance gene in osteosarcoma: A pilot study. J Orthop Res 11:396, 1993.
47. Roessner A, Ueda Y, Bockhorn-Dworniczak B, et al: Prognostic implication of immunodetection of P glycoprotein in Ewing's sarcoma. J Cancer Res Clin Oncol 119:185, 1993.
48. Stein U, Wunderlich V, Haensch W, et al: Expression of the mdr1 gene in bone and soft tissue sarcomas of adult patients. Eur J Cancer 29A:1979, 1993.
49. Chan HSL, Thorner PS, Haddad G, et al: Multidrug resistance in sarcomas of children. *In* Novak JF, McMaster JM (eds): Frontiers in Osteosarcoma Research. Seattle, Hogrefe & Huber, 1993, p 51.
50. Hijazi YM, Axiotis CA, Navarro S, et al: Immunohistochemical detection of P-glycoprotein in Ewing's sarcoma and peripheral primitive neuroectodermal tumors before and after chemotherapy. Am J Clin Pathol 102:61, 1994.
51. Serra M, Scotlandi K, Manara MC, et al: Analysis of P-glycoprotein expression in osteosarcoma. Eur J Cancer 12:1998, 1995.
52. Baldini N, Scotlandi K, Barbanti-Brodano G, et al: Expression of p-glycoprotein in high-grade osteosarcomas in relation to clinical outcome. N Engl J Med 333:1380, 1995.
53. Serra M, Scotlandi K, Manara MC, et al: Establishment and characterisation of multidrug-resistant human osteosarcoma cell lines. Anticancer Res 13:323, 1993.
54. Pinedo HM, Giaccone G: P-glycoprotein: A marker of cancer-cell behavior. N Engl J Med 333:1417, 1995.
55. Beck WT, Grogan TM, Willman CL, et al: Methods to detect P-glycoprotein-associated multidrug resistance in patients' tumors: Consensus recommendations. Cancer Res 56:3010, 1996.
56. Grogan T, Dalton W, Rybski J, et al: Optimisation of immunocytochemical P-glycoprotein assessment in multidrug-resistant plasma cell myeloma using three antibodies. Lab Invest 63:815, 1990.
57. Kandel RA, Campbell S, Noble Topham S, et al: Correlation of P-glycoprotein detection by immunohistochemistry with mdr-1 mRNA levels in osteosarcomas. Pilot study. Diagn Mol Pathol 4:59, 1995.
58. Triche TJ: Multiple-drug resistance in Ewing's sarcoma and peripheral primitive neuroectodermal tumors. Am J Clin Pathol 102:1, 1994.
59. Cole SPC, Bhardwaj G, Gerlach JH, et al: Identification of a novel ATP-binding cassette transporter gene overexpressed in a multidrug resistant human lung cancer cell line. Science 258:1650, 1992.
60. Sikic BI: Modulation of multidrug resistance: At the threshold. J Clin Oncol 11:1629, 1993.
61. Baldini N, Scotlandi K, Serra M, et al: Nuclear immunolocalisation of P-glycoprotein in multidrug-resistant cell lines showing similar mechanisms of doxorubicin distribution. Eur J Cell Biol 68:226, 1995.

Chapter

9

BONE-FORMING NEOPLASMS ARISING WITHIN BONE

JEAN A.S. PRINGLE

Bone-forming tumors account for approximately 20% of all primary bone neoplasms, and the vast majority arise in a central, intramedullary location (Table 9–1). Surface bone-forming tumors are very rare. Osteosarcoma is approximately four times as common as benign bone-forming tumors and, within the benign group, osteoid osteoma is four times more common than osteoblastoma.

BENIGN BONE-FORMING TUMORS

Osteoma of Long Bones

Osteoma of the long bones is typically situated on the bone surface and is discussed in Chapter 11.

Osteoid Osteoma

Clinical and Radiologic Features

This unusual tumor is small and, by definition, should not exceed 1 cm or 1.5 cm in diameter.[1] Osteoid osteomas affect mainly children, adolescents, and young adults and occur more commonly in males. The symptoms are disproportionately severe for the small tumor size; night pain relieved by nonsteroidal anti-inflammatory drugs is typical of osteoid osteoma. The femur and tibia are the most common sites, and the majority of lesions arise within cortical bone, associated with an extensive zone of reaction that may render the central tumor nidus difficult to identify. There is some confusion in terminology, as some authors refer to the *nidus* as the whole lesion, whereas others use *nidus* to describe only the small area of central mineralization seen in many osteoid osteomas. A few osteoid osteomas arise in cancellous bone where they are associated with less intense reactive bone formation. Osteoid osteomas may occur close to the articular surface of a joint and induce a severe inflammatory synovitis that may obscure the presence of the tumor. A proportion of juxta-articular osteoid osteomas extrude into the joint space.

The main clinical and radiologic differential diagnosis is a localized form of osteomyelitis, Brodie's abscess. Occasionally the pattern of reactive bone may raise the possibility of Ewing's sarcoma. On plain radiographs, it may be difficult to identify the small lucent lesion, but there is intense uptake on technetium 99m scans. Precise localization is best achieved by fine/close-cut computer tomography (CT) scanning of the affected area.

Pathologic Features

It is accepted practice to perform excision biopsy in a suspected osteoid osteoma, and the pathologist often receives a large amount of the surrounding reactive bone. It may be difficult to identify the lesion within large areas of granite-hard, reactive bone, and many levels through multiple blocks may be required. It is

Table 9–1. Bone-Forming Neoplasms Arising Within the Medullary Cavity of Bone

Benign	Osteoid osteoma Osteoblastoma Ossifying cementicular fibroma
Intermediate	Aggressive osteoblastoma
Low-Grade Malignancy	Osteoblastoma-like osteosarcoma Central osteosarcoma
High-Grade Malignancy	Central osteosarcoma

helpful to perform a fine detail radiograph using a Faxitron before decalcification in order to locate the osteoid osteoma by the delicate trabecular pattern in the lesional tissue (Fig. 9–1*A*). When the osteoid osteoma is identified on macroscopic examination of the tissue fragments, it appears like a small red cherry because of its relative vascularity.

The histologic features of osteoid osteoma are fairly uniform, with some variation in the degree of mineralization. The lesion, if removed intact, is often round in cross section and, although well defined, the peripheral trabeculae merge imperceptibly into the surrounding reactive bone (Fig. 9–1*B*). The lesion consists of delicate, sometimes irregular, purple spiculated bone and osteoid with intervening vascular areas containing osteoblasts, osteoclasts, and spindle cells. A proportion of the trabeculae may contain prominent cement lines (Fig. 9–1*C* and *D*). Sometimes sheets of osteoid are present. The degree of inflammatory infiltrate in the reactive zone of an osteoid osteoma may be so great that the pathologist may be convinced that the differential diagnosis of osteomyelitis is the correct diagnosis. In some cases, the distinction from osteoblastoma is difficult and depends on knowledge of the size of the tumor.

Treatment and Prognosis

The current trend in surgery for osteoid osteoma is to minimize the amount of bone sacrificed; this is a logical approach as the reactive bone gradually resolves once the osteoid osteoma is removed. Some believe that the tumor is self-limiting and will eventually "burn out" if treated conservatively with nonsteroidal anti-inflammatory drugs. More often an attempt is made to mark the tumor under CT control to enable the surgeon to identify it at operation and distinguish it from the reactive bone. Another method is the intra-operative use of the Coulston probe, which identifies the area of maximum uptake of a radioactive isotope that is associated with the osteoid osteoma. These methods preserve bone and reduce morbidity. An even more conservative method is the drilling-out of the lesion under x-ray control. Sometimes the specimen is so affected by artefact due to the drilling that histologic confirmation of the diagnosis is impossible.[2]

In some cases the pathologist fails to find an osteoid osteoma in the bone removed. It is helpful in this instance to check with the surgeon if the patient's pain has been relieved postoperatively. This is a reliable guide to removal of the tumor as, even in the immediate postoperative period, the patient can distinguish between the pain of surgery and the pain of the osteoid osteoma. In a small number of cases, there may be one or more recurrences.

Benign Osteoblastoma

Clinical and Radiologic Features

Osteoblastoma is a rare tumor that affects children, adolescents, and young adults, with a male predominance. In contrast to that of osteoid osteoma, the most common site is the vertebra, and the central skeleton is more commonly affected than the periphery. Pain, with or without swelling, is the usual presenting symptom, and when the tumor is located in the spine, secondary scoliosis may be the presenting problem. The tumor size is greater than 1.5 cm at the time of presentation.

On plain radiographs, the lesion classically expands the bone but is well defined and surrounded by a thin shell of bone. The amount of mineralization is variable, but the radiographic appearance may be predominantly lytic. There is usually little bone reaction, but there may be soft tissue edema and inflammation, which is well demonstrated on magnetic resonance imaging (MRI).

The clinical and radiologic differential diagnosis includes giant cell tumor and aneurysmal bone cyst. As well, in adults, lytic metastases from vascular primary sites, such as kidney and thyroid, should be considered.

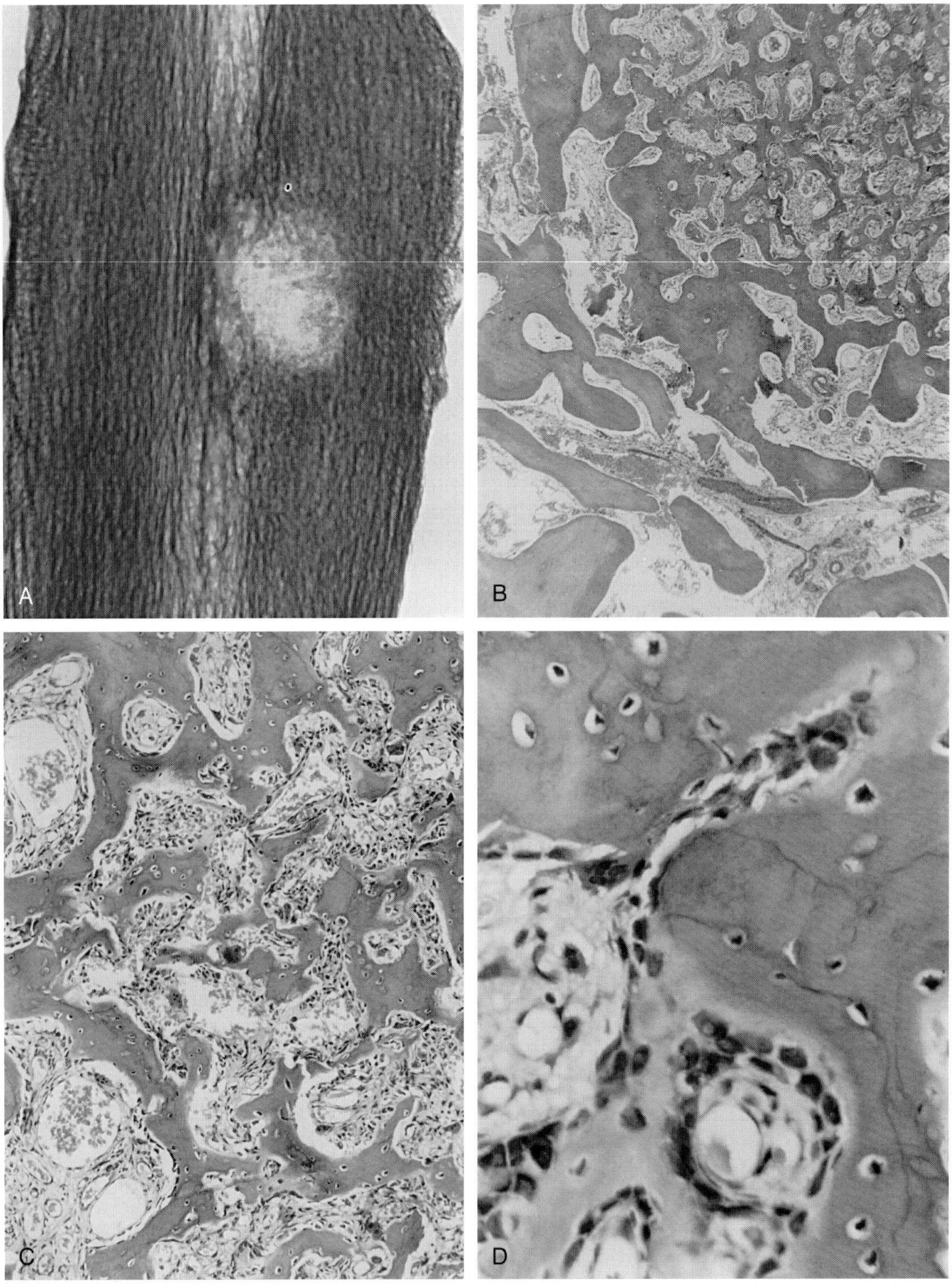

Figure 9–1. Osteoid osteoma. *A,* Fine-detail radiograph of a slice cut through an "en bloc" resection of an osteoid osteoma of the fibula showing a 1.2 cm–diameter lesion surrounded by a zone of sclerotic bone. *B,* A quadrant of the cross section of the osteoid osteoma merges with a peripheral zone of nonspecific reaction in bone and marrow. *C,* The delicate irregular bone trabeculae are covered by osteoblasts and osteoclasts, and there is prominent vascularity of the intervening tissue. *D,* At high magnification, the lesional bone has prominent cement lines and is covered by plump osteoblasts and one osteoclast.

Pathologic Features

Biopsy is usually performed prior to definitive surgery and may be troublesome as the tumor is vascular. The tissue is hemorrhagic and soft with focal gritty areas. Imprint cytology shows numerous plump and active but benign osteoblasts with many osteoclasts. Histology shows tissue with some resemblance to osteoid osteoma but with less mineralization. The trabeculae of osteoid and bone have a more open-weave appearance and a more regular configuration than in osteoid osteoma (Fig. 9–2). They are covered by plump but uniform osteoblasts, and the intertrabecular spaces are occupied by vascular tissue containing osteoclasts and spindle cells. Occasionally, sheets of poorly cellular osteoid are present. The margin is well defined but, at the periphery of the tumor, the trabeculae of tumor bone fuse imperceptibly into the adjacent mildly reactive bone. There is no permeation of pre-existing lamellar bone.

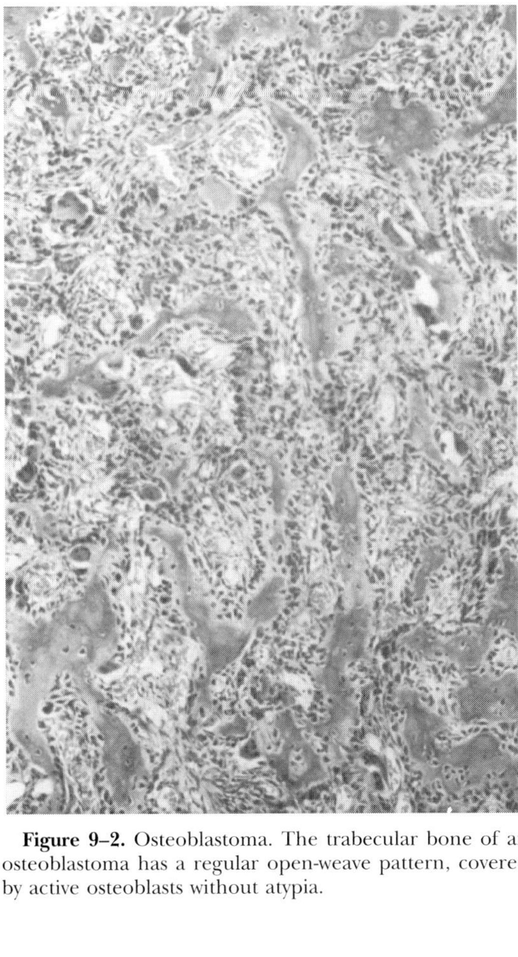

Figure 9–2. Osteoblastoma. The trabecular bone of an osteoblastoma has a regular open-weave pattern, covered by active osteoblasts without atypia.

Treatment and Prognosis

Definitive surgery is usually curettage or piecemeal removal of the tumor. This is particularly the case in the spine. Local recurrence is fairly frequent, particularly in vertebral lesions where preservation of function is at a premium. Rare cases of malignant transformation with or without radiotherapy have been reported.[3]

Differential Diagnosis

Although osteoid osteoma and benign osteoblastoma are both benign osteoblastic tumors and have similar histologic features, the differences in clinical presentation, skeletal location, biologic behavior, and radiologic appearance justify their being regarded as separate entities. The explanation for the intense pain associated with osteoid osteoma has been of interest, and published and unpublished studies using silver stains (Palmgren and Bielschowsky) to demonstrate the number of nerve fibers have shown that osteoid osteoma contains more numerous axons than does osteoblastoma in the periphery, mid-zone, and central area.[4] In addition, osteoid osteoma is associated with the production of prostaglandins, which correlates well with the pain relief afforded by aspirin and other nonsteroidal anti-inflammatory drugs.[5]

Ossifying Cementicular Fibroma

There are differing opinions among bone pathologists as to how this rare entity should be classified. The majority regard it as a variant of fibrous dysplasia, and there is no doubt that some cases of fibrous dysplasia show foci of small, rounded areas of bone resembling cementum (see Chapter 13). I have personal experience of three cases of benign tumors with extensive cementicle formation in association with areas of typical osteoblastoma (Fig. 9–3). Two of the three cases had foci of secondary aneurysmal bone cyst formation. All were solitary lesions in patients with no evidence of fibrous dysplasia in other bones and no histologic features of typical fibrous dysplasia. Two of the three lesions recurred and showed in the recurrences an identical mixture of osteoblastoma and ossifying cementicular fibroma. I therefore prefer to regard these cases as a variant of osteoblastoma. I believe that they are distinct from the original cases described by Sissons et al.[6] as ossifying fibroma, which is now regarded as osteofibrous dysplasia, and from fibrous dysplasia with foci of cementum-like bone.

Aggressive/Malignant Osteoblastoma

In 1976 Schajowicz and Lemos[7] described a series of eight cases, arising mainly in the spine and ribs, which were called *malignant osteoblastoma.* None of their cases metastasized, but the cases were associated with local recurrence and with a variety of histologic features (Fig. 9–4), including numerous mitoses, epithelioid osteoblasts, spiculated blue bone, and areas resembling giant cell tumor and aneurysmal bone cyst. No permeation of adjacent bone was present, and the lesions were often surrounded by a shell of reactive bone. Dorfman and Weiss[8] reviewed similar cases, which they preferred to call *aggressive osteoblastoma;* this seemed a more appropriate name as the tumors did not metastasize and, when they were fatal, fatality was due to local recurrence and direct extension, particularly in the spine. There remains a lack of consensus among bone pathologists as to how to define this entity. There is no doubt that osteoblastic tumors of borderline malignancy do occur, but they are rare. There is an onus on the pathologist to attempt to decide whether a tumor is benign or malignant and to place as few lesions as possible in this intermediate category. The presence of abnormal mitoses, permeation of pre-existing lamellar bone, and unequivocal malignant cells forming osteoid are the most helpful features in recognizing osteosarcoma. The confusion over this group of cases is increased by the various reports in the literature of radiotherapy associated with malignant transformation of osteoblastoma to frank osteosarcoma.

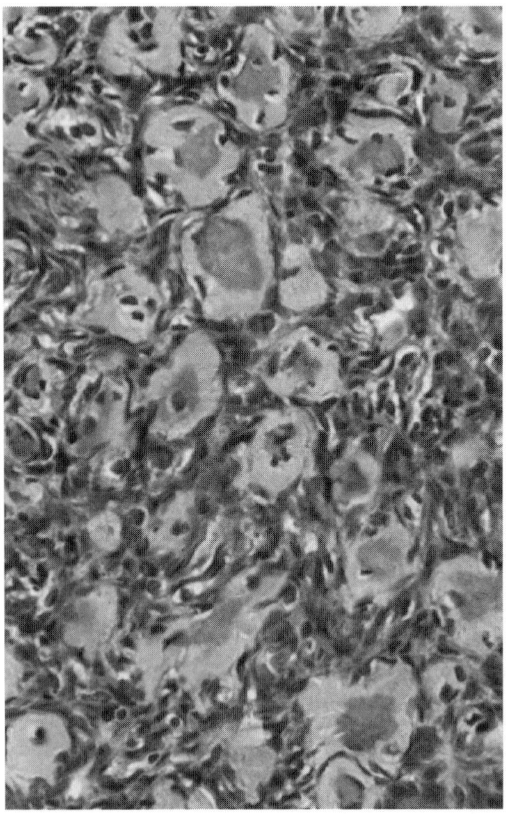

Figure 9–3. Ossifying cementicular fibroma. Distinctive rounded foci of osteoid (cementum) with central mineralization are present.

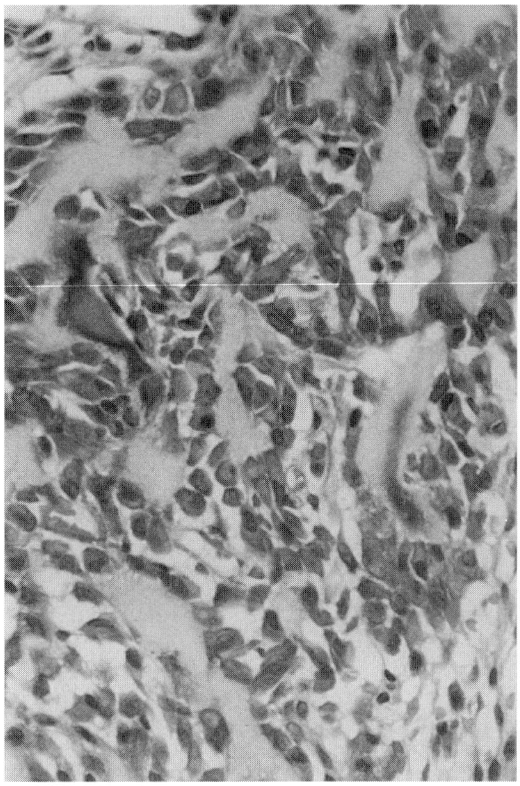

Figure 9–4. Aggressive osteoblastoma. Epithelioid osteoblasts, mitotic activity, and spiculated osteoid trabeculae are features of this tumor.

MALIGNANT BONE-FORMING TUMORS

Osteoblastoma-like Osteosarcoma

In 1985 Bertoni et al.[9] described an entity that was similar to aggressive osteoblastoma in that it resembled osteoblastoma histologically but differed by the presence of permeation of pre-existing lamellar bone. Bertoni introduced the name *osteoblastoma-like osteosarcoma* to describe this tumor. In my experience, this tumor is often diagnosed as osteoblastoma by a nonspecialist pathologist and may be curetted several times before its true nature is appreciated. It may be fairly indolent clinically but is relatively resistant to radiotherapy and chemotherapy and may prove fatal after a period of several years by distant metastases. The most helpful diagnostic feature is permeation of pre-existing bone (Fig. 9–5), which may be difficult to demonstrate in a limited biopsy sample. The permeative pattern may be reflected in a less well-defined radiologic appearance.

Low-Grade Central/Intramedullary Osteosarcoma

In 1977 Unni et al.[10] and, more recently, Kurt et al.[11] described a group of low-grade intraosseous osteosarcomas. The histologic appearance often resembled the bland features of parosteal osteosarcoma with few mitoses and minimal atypia (Fig. 9–6). Other cases resembled fibrous dysplasia with curlicue trabeculae of woven bone. This group of tumors, however, showed permeation of pre-existing bone. Mirra[12] described five patterns of low-grade intramedullary osteosarcoma. All are exceedingly rare, apart from the pattern resembling parosteal osteosarcoma or fibrous dysplasia. In my experience of 17 cases, the majority have occurred in the long bones, including the fibula and the humerus, and two have affected the foot—one in the first metatarsal and one in the proximal phalanx of the second toe. All have been fibrous dysplasia–like in histologic appearance.

If these types of osteosarcoma are diagnosed correctly and excised completely, the prognosis is excellent, being similar to that of parosteal osteosarcoma. I have seen several cases initially diagnosed as fibrous dysplasia with recurrence following curettage. As with parosteal osteosarcoma, late dedifferentiation to high-grade osteosarcoma may occur. Chemotherapy is not indicated unless dedifferentiation has occurred.

High-Grade Central Osteosarcoma

Clinical Features

High-grade central osteosarcoma is the most common primary malignant bone tumor and is commonly referred to as *osteosarcoma.* It has an estimated incidence of 2.5 per million annually, so that around 750–1000 cases will occur each year in the United States. Males are more commonly affected than females, and the tumor occurs most frequently in the period of active skeletal growth, being rare under the age of 5 years and over the age of 30 years. The fact that males are more commonly affected may be related to the earlier age of skeletal maturity in females.

The metaphysis is the most common location within bone, and the bones most frequently affected are the distal femur followed by the proximal tibia and the proximal humerus. All other sites are rare. A small number affect unusual sites such as the jaw and the spine—in these locations they may occur at any age.

In the vast majority of cases no predisposing cause is identified. There is an association with hereditary bilateral retinoblastoma, with Li-Fraumeni syndrome, and with Rothmund-Thomson syndrome. Other predisposing factors include previous irradiation and Paget's disease. Osteosarcoma is one of the patterns seen in differentiated chondrosarcoma.

In the past, fibrous dysplasia was included as one of the bone conditions in which osteosarcoma might arise. However, the recognition of low-grade (fibrous dysplasia-like) osteosarcoma, which may over time dedifferentiate into high-grade osteosarcoma, suggests that, in at least some cases, the predisposing condition had been wrongly diagnosed as fibrous dysplasia. A small number of osteosarcomas arise in middle-aged and elderly patients who have no evidence of a predisposing factor.

The majority of cases arise close to the knee joint, and the presenting symptoms include pain, swelling, and limitation of movement. Because of the age group affected, the symptoms and signs may be attributed to trauma, and there may be a considerable delay in diagnosis. Occasionally the patient presents with a pathologic fracture, having had no previous symptoms. Night pain and failure to respond to conservative treatment are indications for a plain radiograph, but a small number of patients with osteosarcoma undergo arthroscopy

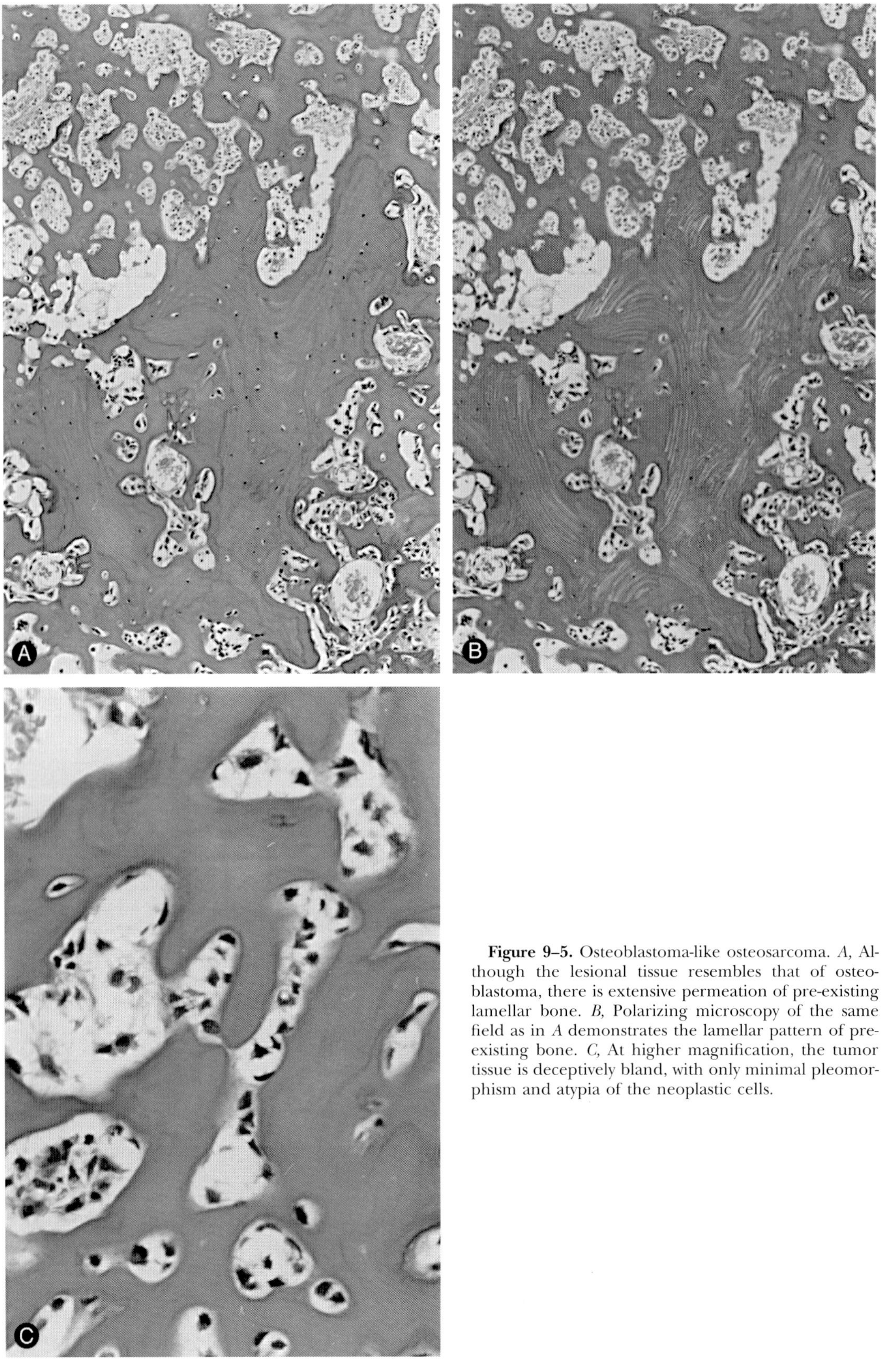

Figure 9–5. Osteoblastoma-like osteosarcoma. *A,* Although the lesional tissue resembles that of osteoblastoma, there is extensive permeation of pre-existing lamellar bone. *B,* Polarizing microscopy of the same field as in *A* demonstrates the lamellar pattern of pre-existing bone. *C,* At higher magnification, the tumor tissue is deceptively bland, with only minimal pleomorphism and atypia of the neoplastic cells.

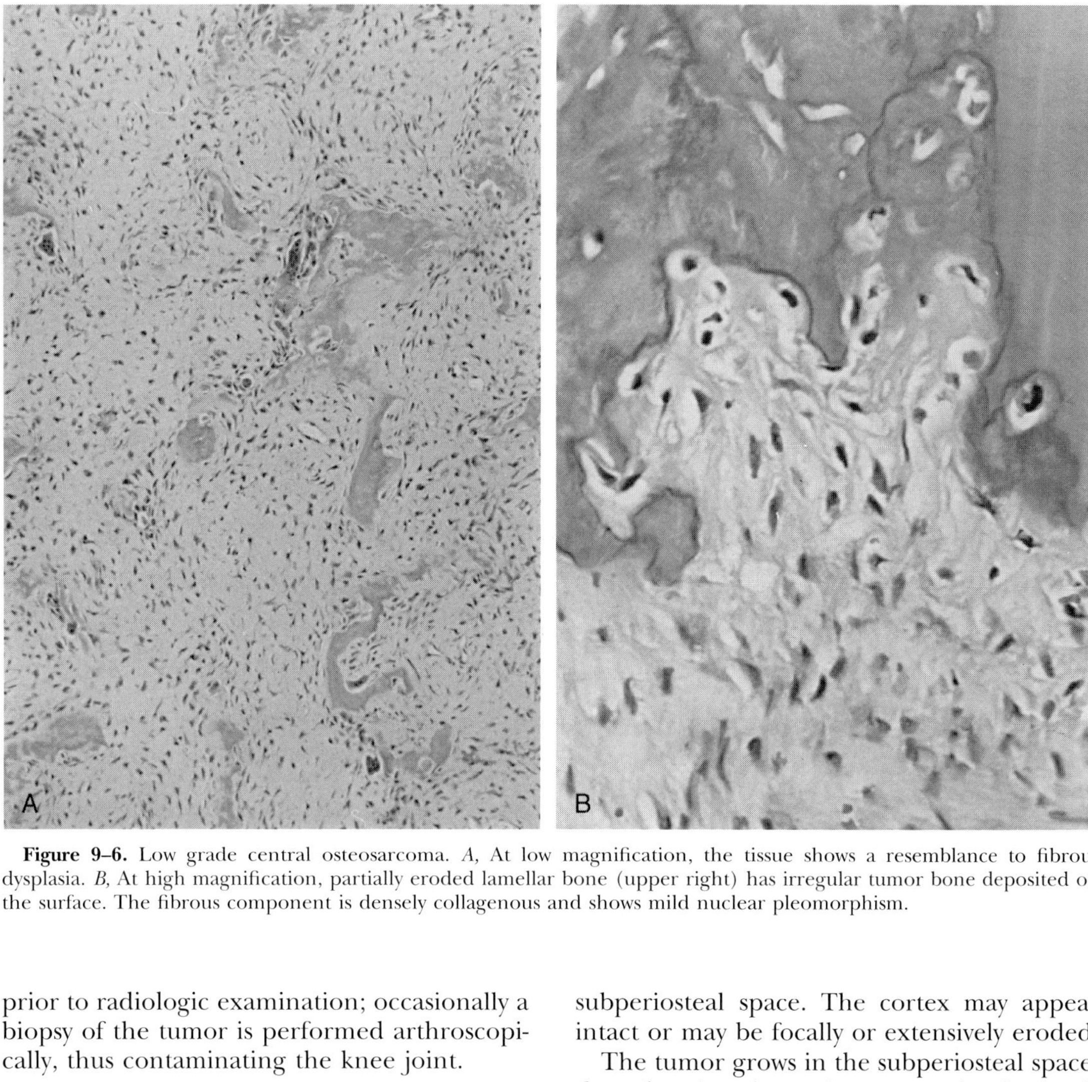

Figure 9–6. Low grade central osteosarcoma. *A,* At low magnification, the tissue shows a resemblance to fibrous dysplasia. *B,* At high magnification, partially eroded lamellar bone (upper right) has irregular tumor bone deposited on the surface. The fibrous component is densely collagenous and shows mild nuclear pleomorphism.

prior to radiologic examination; occasionally a biopsy of the tumor is performed arthroscopically, thus contaminating the knee joint.

Radiologic Features

A typical osteosarcoma arises in the metaphysis of a long bone (Fig. 9–7*A* [see also color figure]). In the immature skeleton, the majority of osteosarcomas extend to the adjacent growth plate, and a small number cross the plate into the epiphysis. This is more common in young children, in whom the growth plate is very vascular, and also in people in their late teens, in whom the growth plate is closing and there is no longer a substantial layer of cartilage. In the adult skeleton the tumor usually extends into the subarticular zone, where the articular cartilage is the barrier to extension into the adjacent joint. At the time of presentation, the majority of osteosarcomas have extended through the cortex into the subperiosteal space. The cortex may appear intact or may be focally or extensively eroded.

The tumor grows in the subperiosteal space, thus elevating the periosteum and stripping it off the cortical surface beyond the margin of the tumor mass. Periosteal reactive bone develops in this space beyond the tumor margin and appears on plain radiographs as a triangle of reactive bone, referred to as Codman's triangle (Fig. 9–7*B*). At this stage, the tumor is enclosed and constrained within the tough periosteum and is lying in the subperiosteal space it has created by stripping the periosteum off the cortex. Unfortunately, this fact is not appreciated by those with limited experience of examining resected osteosarcomas, and clinicians and radiologists loosely refer to "the soft-tissue extension of the tumor." The distinction between soft-tissue extension and subperiosteal extension is important in deciding whether soft tissue should be resected with the tumor and in considering postoperative

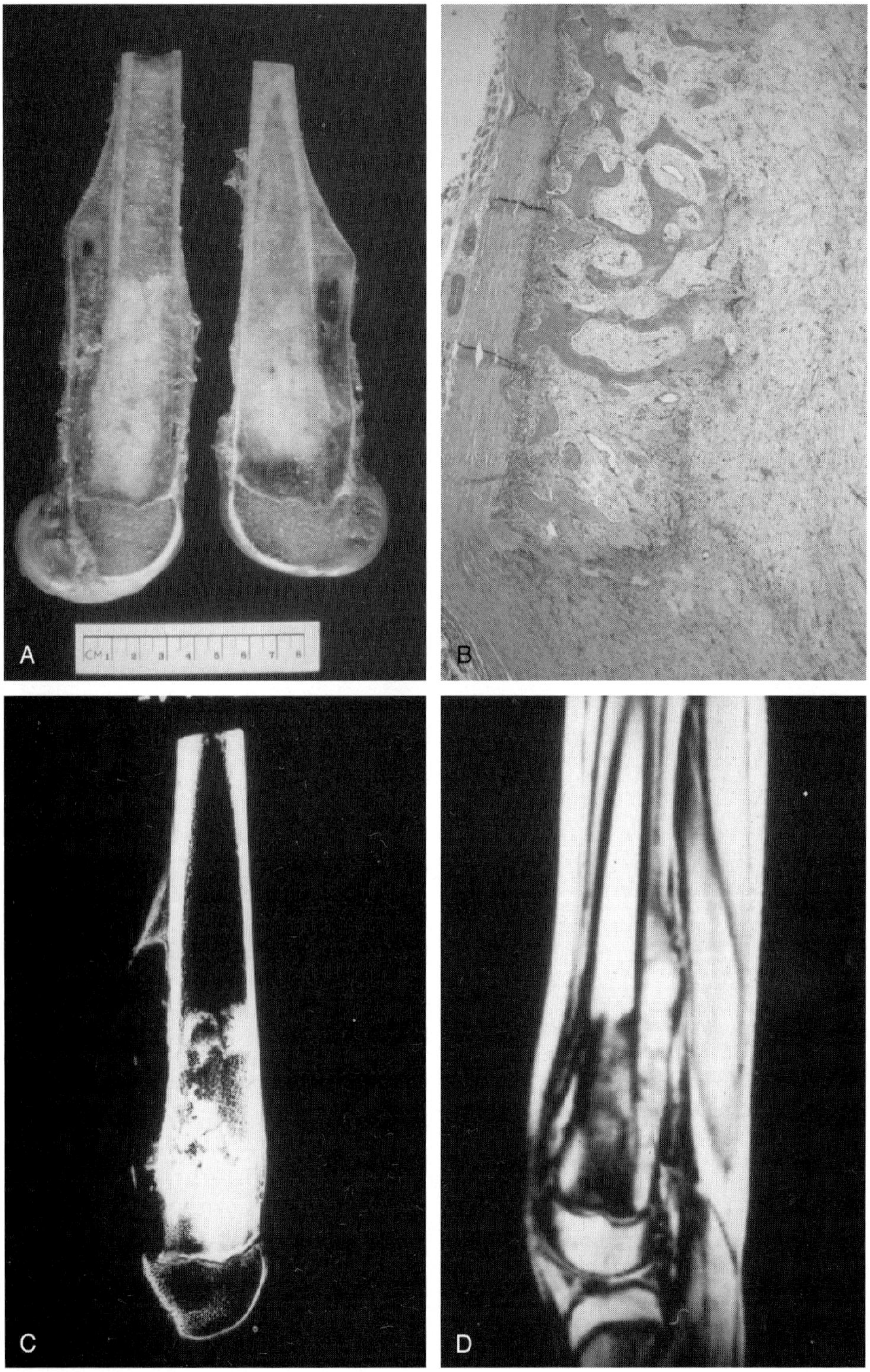

Figure 9–7. Osteosarcoma. *A,* Resected osteosarcoma of distal femur has been divided longitudinally. The tumor shows extensive necrosis after chemotherapy. The Codman's triangle is easily identified, as is the periosteal capsule surrounding and containing the tumor (see also color figure). *B,* Periosteum with a zone of reactive, new, subperiosteal bone formation covering an area of necrotic tumor. *C,* Fine-detail specimen radiograph of the osteosarcoma shows the extent of tumor in the medullary cavity and the Codman's triangle. This radiograph also shows the incomplete shell of periosteal reactive bone formed over the tumor in response to chemotherapy. *D,* Magnetic resonance imaging of the osteosarcoma clearly demonstrates the extent of the tumor including the subperiosteal extension and the Codman's triangle.

radiotherapy. Unfortunately, the standard method described by Enneking,[13] which is used for staging bone tumors, uses the cortex rather than the periosteum as the compartmental boundary of bone so that the majority of osteosarcomas are classified as stage IIB (extracompartmental) on initial staging when they are actually intracompartmental. When amputation was the standard treatment of osteosarcoma, the precise anatomy of the tumor was of no consequence. The introduction of limb-salvage surgery is a powerful reason for attempting to preserve the intact periosteum. Several factors are associated with disruption of the periosteum. Those patients who present with pathologic fracture constitute a small group in which this cannot be avoided, as do those patients who present at a late stage or who have a biologically aggressive tumor. Finally, open biopsy causes a significant defect in the periosteum and, if wrongly sited, may occasionally render conservative surgery inadvisable.[14]

A small number of osteosarcomas are sufficiently diaphyseal to permit sparing of the growth plate during tumor resection. In a series of 200 consecutive osteosarcomas affecting the long bones in an immature skeleton, the author[15] found that less than 10% were 3 cm or more from the adjacent physis.

The plain radiograph reflects the changes described above and correlates well with the different histologic subtypes, reflecting the variation in the amount of tumor bone formation (Fig. 9–7*C*). MRI has proved to be reliable in mapping the extent of the tumor (Fig. 9–7*D*) and is helpful in planning the transection plane for surgery. Radioisotope scanning is useful in demonstrating skip lesions and distant bony metastases. The most common site of distant metastasis in osteosarcoma is the lungs, and CT scanning of the chest is part of the routine staging. Lymph node involvement is rare except in the terminal stages of the disease. Metastases may occur in a variety of unusual sites in the late stage of the disease. In my experience of several hundred cases, these sites include skin and intra-abdominal and intracranial locations.

The rare multicentric osteosarcoma is now thought more likely to represent multiple bone metastases from one primary site.

A very small number of osteosarcomas arise in an intracortical location. It is possible that this is more common, but the tumor is of a size at presentation that obscures the precise site of origin. I have diagnosed only one osteosarcoma of intracortical origin in a male aged 30 years who suffered from psoriatic arthritis. An isotope scan performed to assess the activity of the arthritis identified an area of increased uptake in the distal femoral cortex. Biopsy confirmed an intracortical osteosarcoma, fortuitously diagnosed early.

Pathologic Features

In the London Bone and Soft Tissue Tumour Service, needle biopsy is the standard biopsy technique used and, combined with imprint cytology, is associated with a 97% accurate diagnosis.[16] In the last 10 years, there has been a steady trend to referral of patients with osteosarcoma prior to biopsy. A small proportion are referred following open biopsy at another hospital.

High-grade central osteosarcoma has a wide spectrum of histologic appearance and is divided into several subtypes (Table 9–2). The most common is the *common mixed* type, which can be regarded as the malignant counterpart of fracture callus, including undifferentiated areas and areas showing osteoblastic, chondroblastic, and fibroblastic differentiation. This, together with the osteoblastic category, usually contains tumor bone or osteoid even in a needle biopsy sample. Other types, such as *chondroblastic, fibroblastic, osteoclast-rich* and *telangiectatic,* may contain little or no tumor bone or osteoid. This poses a problem in establishing a definite diagnosis, which is traditionally overcome by combining the histologic appearance with the clinical and radiologic features of the case. Although the tumor cells in osteosarcoma may not be actively producing osteoid and bone, they have the potential to do so. This is often reflected in increasing bone production on radiographs associated with a response to chemotherapy. This potential can be confirmed in imprint preparations of tumor cells by demonstrating the presence of alkaline phosphatase. All osteoblasts,

Table 9–2. Histological Subtypes of High-Grade Central Osteosarcoma

Common/mixed	Telangiectatic
Fibroblastic	Small cell
Chondroblastic	Epithelioid
Osteoblastic	Anaplastic
Osteoclast-rich	

whether normal, reactive, benign, or malignant, contain alkaline phosphatase. The combination of malignant morphology with the presence of alkaline phosphatase (Fig. 9–8 [see also color figure]) is sufficient to confirm osteosarcoma where this diagnosis is consistent with other features of the case. Other cells that may contain alkaline phosphatase include endothelial cells, polymorphs, and chondrocytes associated with areas of calcification and endochondral ossification. Taking only 10–15 minutes, it is useful intraoperatively to assess tumor clearance. At present, there is no antibody for bone alkaline phosphatase that can be used in paraffin-embedded sections, and this constraint also applies to other markers of bone such as osteocalcin, osteopontin, and osteonectin. Where only paraffin-embedded material is available, the distinction between collagen and osteoid may be assisted by a reticulin stain or by immunohistochemical staining for vimentin (Fig. 9–9*A* and *B* [see also color figure]). These stains demonstrate a branching pattern typical of osteoid in contrast to a more featureless arrangement of collagen. Viewing the sections with polarized light may also help confirm the branching trabecular pattern of osteoid in contrast to the more parallel arrangement of collagen (Fig. 9–9*C*). The demonstration of matrix vesicles by transmission electron microscopy was described by Mirra[17] as the most reliable method of confirming osteoid as they are absent in collagen. However, this technique is inappropriate in a situation where the urgent diagnosis of a malignant tumor is required.

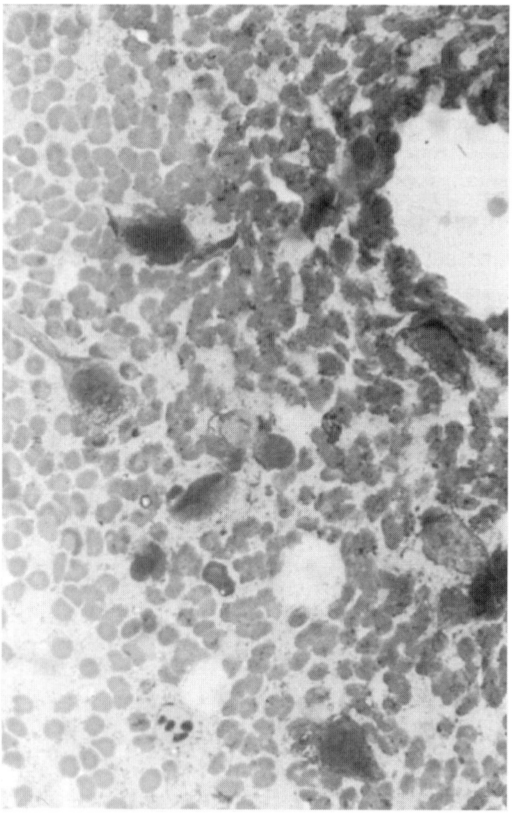

Figure 9–8. Osteosarcoma. An imprint preparation shows red blood cells, a polymorph, and several tumor cells with a high nuclear cytoplasmic ratio. The tumor cells contain many red granules of alkaline phosphatase (see also color figure).

AREAS OF DIAGNOSTIC DIFFICULTY IN THE DIAGNOSIS OF OSTEOSARCOMA

Common Mixed Osteosarcoma Versus Reactive Bone and Fracture Callus

Probably the most difficult distinction a pathologist has to make is between reactive bone and malignant bone. Assistance may be available from the history and from clinical and radiologic features, but in many cases it is determined by the pathologist's assessment of microscopic appearances. In an intraosseous setting, the most common cause of reactive bone is a fracture, including stress fracture or infraction that may not be identified easily on plain radiographs. Although fracture callus is cellular and active with quite numerous mitoses, the atypia (pleomorphism and abnormal mitoses) seen in osteosarcoma is not present. In contrast to the delicate, lace-like, spiculated blue bone associated with osteosarcoma (Fig. 9–10), reactive bone and osteoid have a more regular trabecular pattern, and the surfaces are covered by plump but uniform reactive osteoblasts (Fig. 9–11). Some progressive maturation/zoning may be seen in reactive tissue/callus, but this is of less help in an intraosseous location than in soft-tissue and surface lesions. Necrosis is not seen in reactive tissue, but focal necrosis is common in high-grade osteosarcoma. Reactive cartilage can also appear worrying (see Chapters 10 and 11) but, although cellular and active, is usually lacking in significant pleomorphism (Fig. 9–12 [see also color figure]). Areas of endochondral ossification are a reassuringly benign feature.

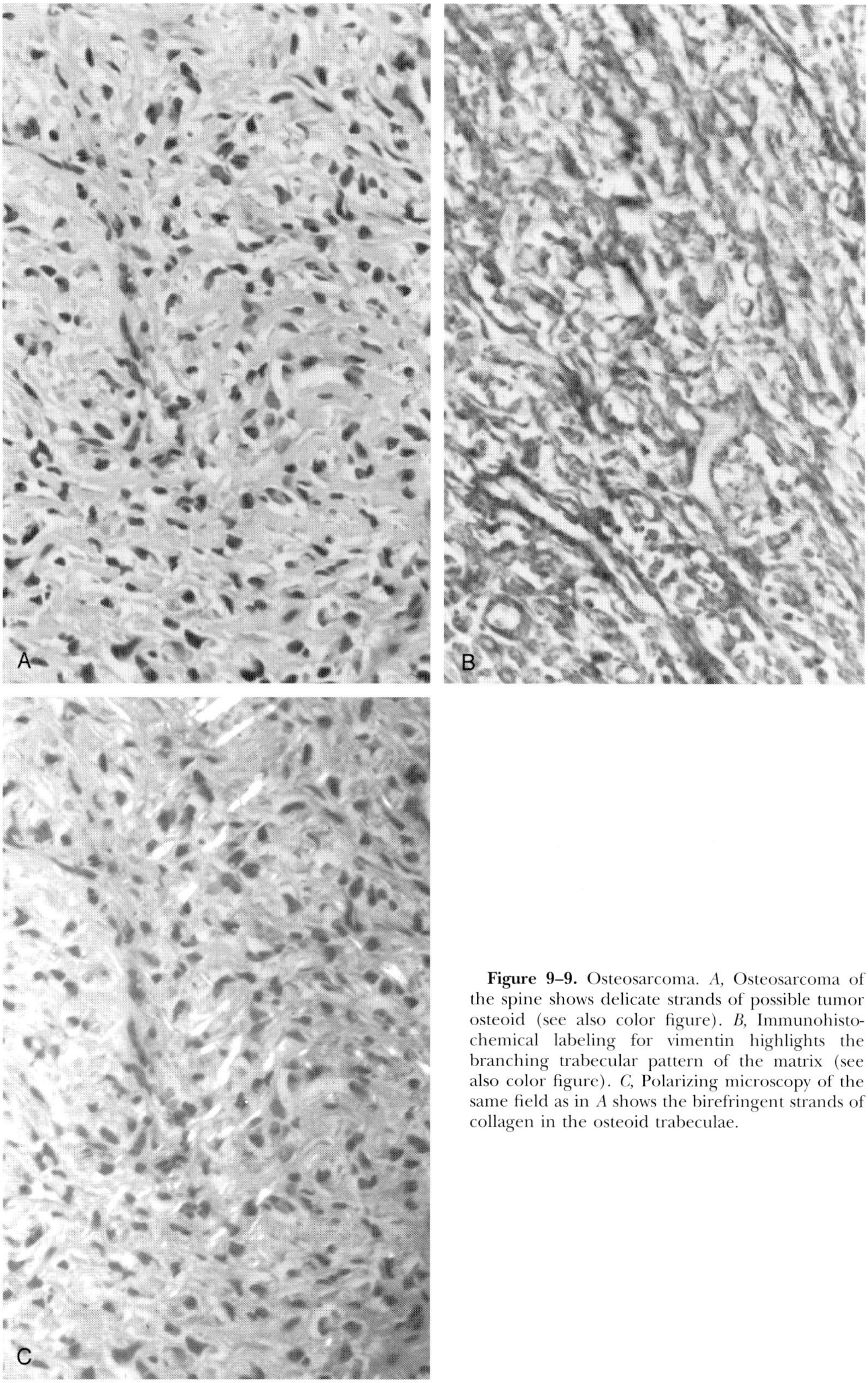

Figure 9–9. Osteosarcoma. *A,* Osteosarcoma of the spine shows delicate strands of possible tumor osteoid (see also color figure). *B,* Immunohistochemical labeling for vimentin highlights the branching trabecular pattern of the matrix (see also color figure). *C,* Polarizing microscopy of the same field as in *A* shows the birefringent strands of collagen in the osteoid trabeculae.

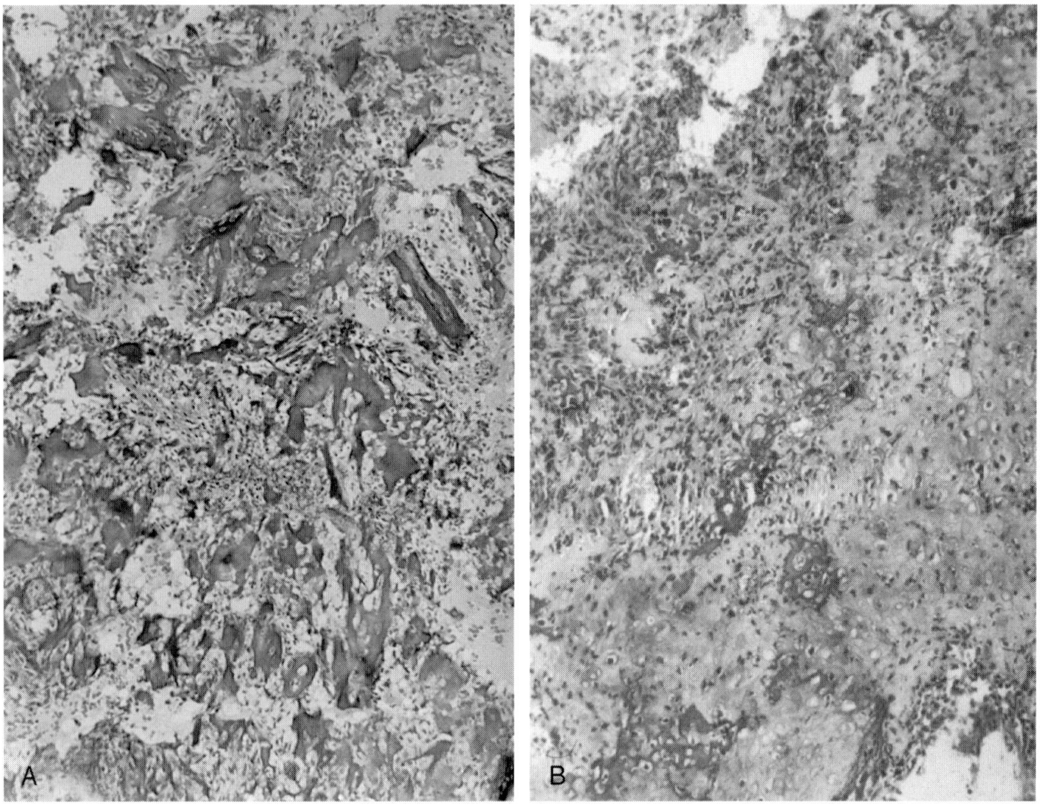

Figure 9–10. Osteosarcoma. *A,* Typical appearance of spiculated/lace-like malignant tumor bone formation. *B,* In this area, both osteoblastic and chondroblastic differentiation is present.

Chondroblastic Osteosarcoma Versus Chondrosarcoma, Mesenchymal Chondrosarcoma, and Chondroblastoma

Chondrosarcoma rarely occurs in the age group commonly affected by osteosarcoma. It usually presents with a long history and less severe pain, and it has a more centripetal skeletal distribution. Chondrosarcomas developing in patients with multiple enchondromas or diaphyseal aclasis may occur at a younger age, but their predisposing condition will be obvious clinically or radiologically. The radiographic appearance of chondrosarcoma is distinctive (see Chapters 6 and 10) with expansion of the affected bone, scalloped erosion of the endosteal surface of the cortex, and associated periosteal buttressing. The majority show delicate spotty calcification of the matrix, and a pre-existing enchondroma may be identified. This contrasts with chondroblastic osteosarcoma, which may show little evidence of bone formation (Fig. 9–13*A* and *B*) but has the features of a rapidly growing malignant tumor. Mesenchymal chondrosarcoma is very rare but may occur in the osteosarcoma age range. It is most common in the ribs, pelvis, and maxilla, and the radiograph shows distinctive "popcorn" calcification that is denser than the delicate speckled calcification seen in most chondroid tumors.

The histology may pose problems in differential diagnosis especially if clinical and radiologic features are not available. Chondroblastic osteosarcoma consists of pleomorphic cartilage that is clearly malignant (Fig. 9–13*C*). It usually lacks the distinctive lobulation of true chondrosarcoma. Careful search will usually reveal areas of pale pink osteoid matrix, but malignant bone is often completely absent. Despite the chondroid differentiation, the tumor cells of chondroblastic osteosarcoma contain alkaline phosphatase confirming their osteoblastic potential (Fig. 9–13*D* [see also color figure]).

Mesenchymal chondrosarcoma has a distinctive histological appearance (see Chapters 10 and 14), with islands of chondroid tissue of varying size surrounded by small mesenchymal cells with scanty cytoplasm often with a pericytomatoid pattern of vascular channels (Fig. 9–14*A* and *B*). Where ossification occurs, it is confined to the islands of chondroid tissue and usually centrally located within them.

Occasionally a very cellular *chondroblastoma* may be difficult to distinguish from osteosarcoma of chondroblastic or even osteoclast-rich type. Chondroblastoma usually has a typical radiographic appearance with a well defined lucency centered on the growth plate, often with spotty calcification. The histologic features may include chicken-wire calcification that may be confused with malignant spiculated blue bone (see Fig. 9–10*A*). However, the chicken-wire calcification surrounds individual cells in an orderly fashion. Although cellular, the cells have a fairly uniform rounded or polygonal configuration, and the islands of chondroid differentiation are well demarcated (see Chapter 16). Immunohistochemical labeling for S-100 protein is of no value in the differential diagnosis as there is strong expression of this antigen in the chondroblastic areas of osteosarcoma.

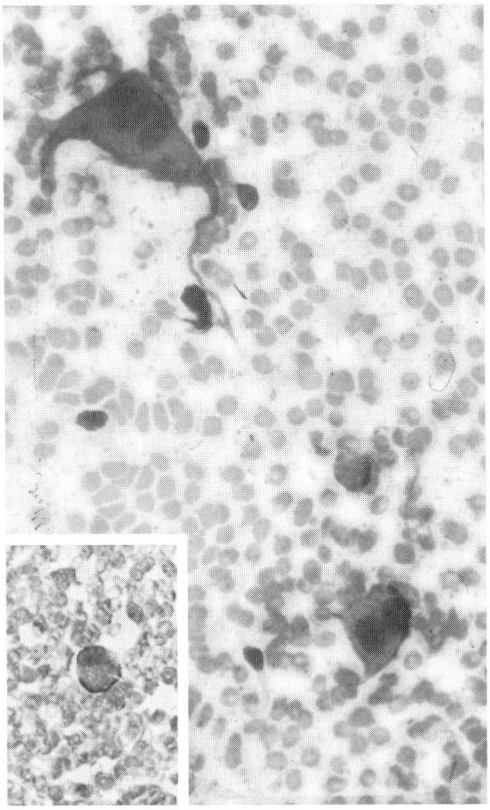

Figure 9–12. Alkaline phosphatase in osteoblastic cells. The main field shows two malignant osteoblasts that are binucleate and contain copious alkaline phosphatase (red). The insert shows a reactive osteoblast with a compact eccentric nucleus and cytoplasmic alkaline phosphatase staining (red) (see also color figure).

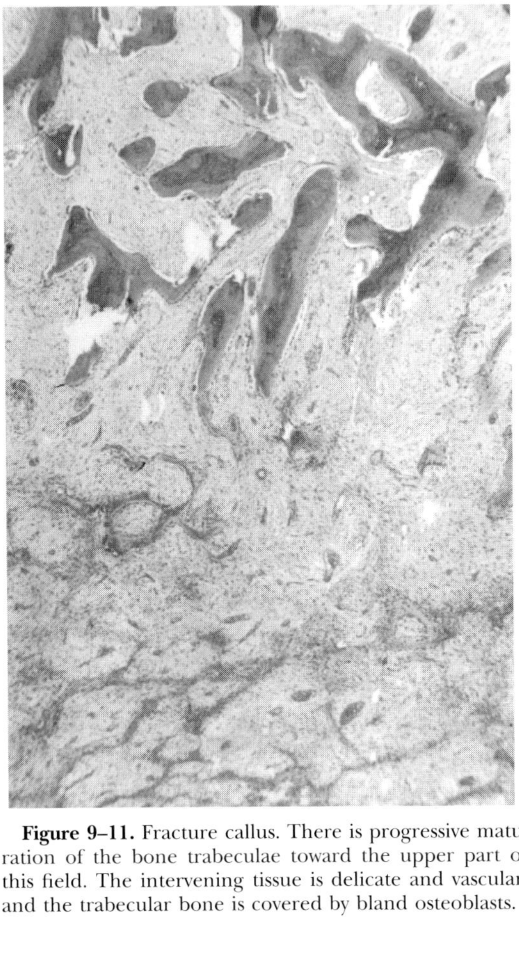

Figure 9–11. Fracture callus. There is progressive maturation of the bone trabeculae toward the upper part of this field. The intervening tissue is delicate and vascular, and the trabecular bone is covered by bland osteoblasts.

Fibroblastic Osteosarcoma Versus Fibrosarcoma/Malignant Fibrous Histiocytoma

Fibroblastic osteosarcoma is associated with a lytic destructive lesion on plain radiographs and a histological appearance that is often indistinguishable from fibrosarcoma/malignant fibrous histiocytoma (MFH) because of the paucity or complete absence of tumor bone and osteoid formation (see Figure 12–9). If imprint preparations or tissue for frozen sections is available, there is no problem as the cells of fibroblastic osteosarcoma contain alkaline phosphatase, whereas fibrosarcoma and MFH are negative. If paraffin-embedded

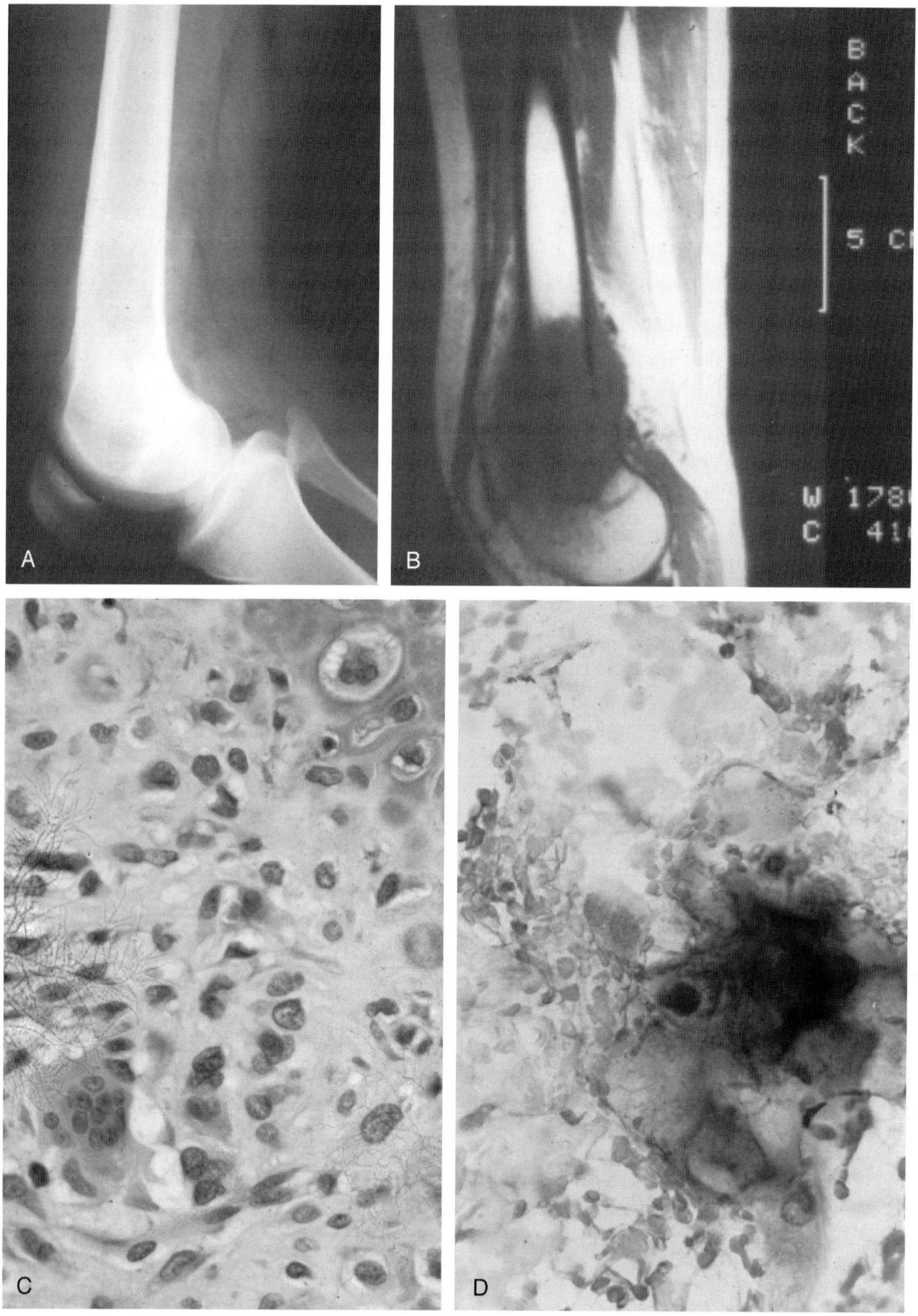

Figure 9–13. Chondroblastic osteosarcoma. *A,* Lateral plain radiograph of distal femur shows no distinct abnormality. *B,* Magnetic resonance imaging of the same bone clearly outlines a tumor of the distal metaphysis. *C,* Histology shows osteosarcoma with focal chondroblastic differentiation (top right). *D,* Imprint cytology of this case shows blue chondroid matrix with red granules of alkaline phosphatase in the tumor cells (see also color figure).

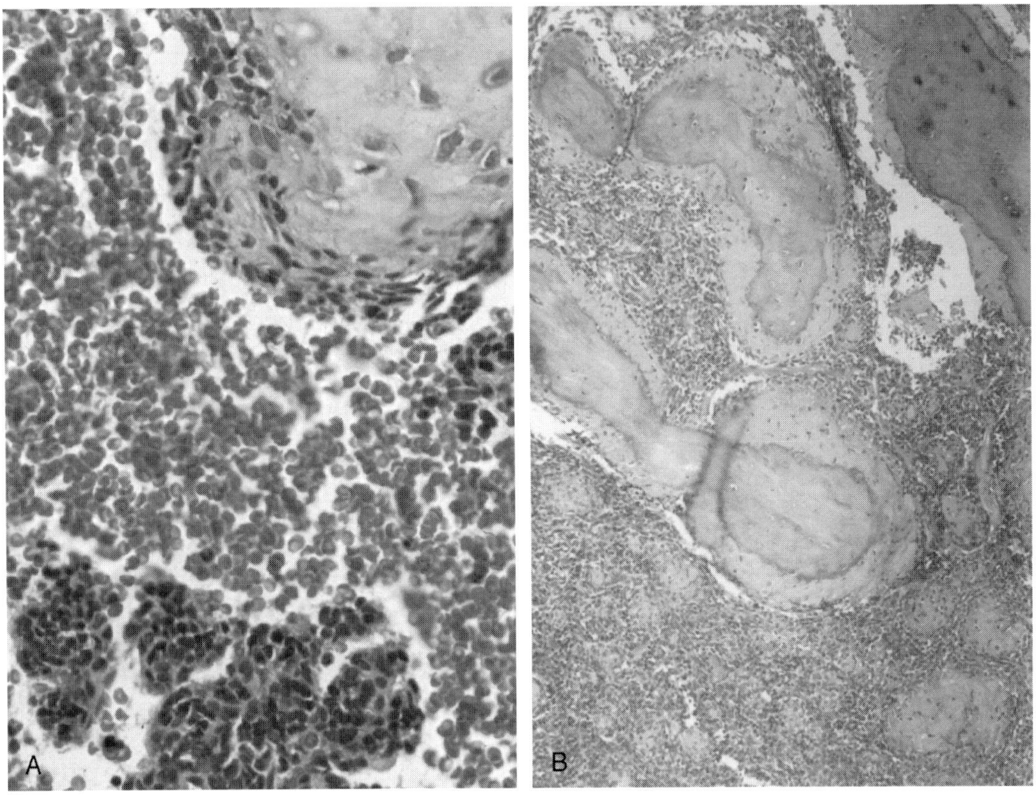

Figure 9–14. Mesenchymal chondrosarcoma. *A,* This part of a needle biopsy shows both the hemangiopericytomatous-like arrangement of the mesenchymal cells and a zone of mesenchymal cells surrounding a focus of chondroid tissue. *B,* At low magnification, the distinctive architecture of focal central ossification of large chondroid islands is seen, with small chondroid islands surrounded by mesenchymal cells.

material is all that is available, the differential diagnosis relies heavily on the age of the patient, the anatomic site of the tumor, and the radiologic features. Fibrosarcoma or MFH arising in bone is a tumor of the mature skeleton, but there is an overlap in the third decade. The most common site is the distal femur but in a more diaphyseal location than is typical for osteosarcoma. MFH may arise in association with a pre-existing bone infarct that may be detectable on plain radiographs. MFH may arise in fibrous dysplasia and may account for the dedifferentiated component in dedifferentiated chondrosarcoma. Metaplastic bone formation may occur in MFH but has a bland quality and substantial trabeculae quite different from those of malignant bone and osteoid.

Osteoblastic Osteosarcoma Versus Osteoblastoma

Osteoblastic osteosarcoma is a well differentiated bone-forming tumor that may be difficult to distinguish from osteoblastoma. Its density may cause technical difficulty and artefact in the biopsy. Permeation of pre-existing lamellar bone is the most reliable feature in diagnosing this rare type of osteosarcoma (Fig. 9–15).

Telangiectatic Osteosarcoma Versus Aneurysmal Bone Cyst

Aneurysmal bone cyst (see also Chapter 16) affects a similar age group as that of patients with telangiectatic osteosarcoma and may grow at a faster rate than does a high-grade osteosarcoma. The radiologic appearance may also give cause for concern as there may be worrying periosteal reaction, again due to the rapid expansion of the lesion (Fig. 9–16*A*). In contrast to the pattern of periosteal reaction of high-grade osteosarcoma, the outer layer of the periosteal reaction in aneurysmal bone cyst is in continuity with the expanded shell of thinned cortex that contains the lesion. On

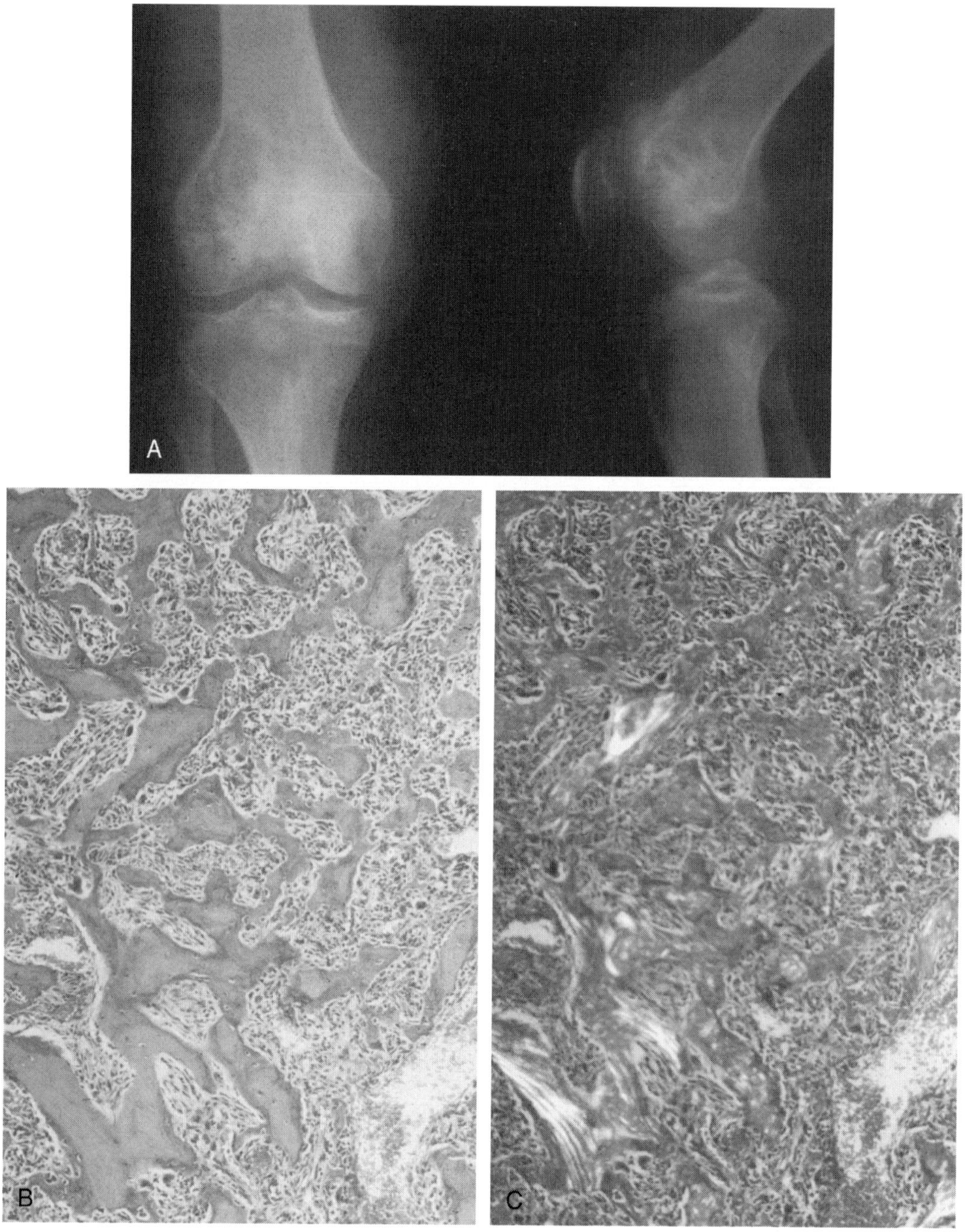

Figure 9–15. Osteoblastic osteosarcoma of the distal femur. *A*, The anteroposterior plain radiograph shows a tumor that appears to be affecting mainly the lateral condyle. The layer of periosteal reactive bone proximal to the medial femoral condyle indicates that the tumor is more extensive. The lateral view shows tumor tissue extending into the suprapatellar pouch of the knee joint. *B*, By transmitted light, it is difficult to distinguish between tumor bone and pre-existing bone trabeculae. *C*, The same field as in *B* viewed by polarized light confirms that there is permeation by tumor of pre-existing lamellar bone.

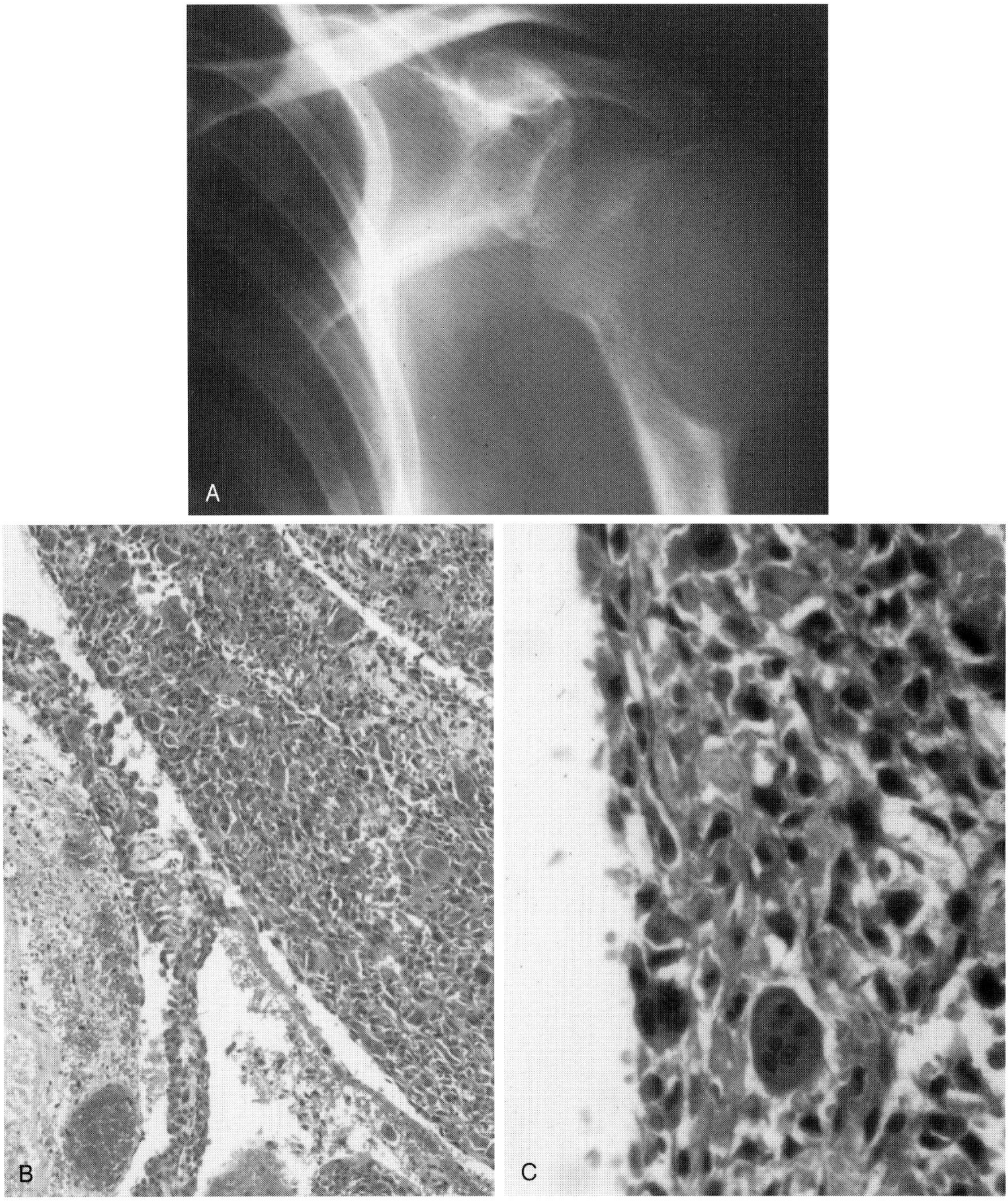

Figure 9–16. Telangiectatic osteosarcoma of the proximal humerus. *A,* The plain radiograph shows an expansile lesion with a periosteal rim. *B,* Typical histologic appearance of blood-filled spaces surrounded by thin and thicker "septal" structures. *C,* At high magnification, the pleomorphic appearance of the tumor cells is apparent. An osteoclast giant cell is included. There is no tumor bone or osteoid formation in this field.

MRI, fluid/fluid levels are a feature shared with telangiectatic osteosarcoma.

At low magnification, the histologic architecture of both lesions is similar. Alkaline phosphatase is positive in many cells of aneurysmal bone cyst, and osteoclast giant cells are present in both entities. Examination at high power will confirm the bland cytology in an aneurysmal bone cyst, and moderate numbers of normal mitoses may be present. The septa may contain significant amounts of woven trabecular bone, but the appearances are bland and the bone surface is covered by uniform osteoblasts. Occasionally there are foci of matrix calcification staining deep blue/purple that may mimic spiculated blue bone. The outer margin of an aneurysmal bone cyst is well defined and often delineated by a shell comprising attenuated cortex and reactive bone. Necrosis is not seen. In contrast, telangiectatic osteosarcoma is a high-grade malignant tumor containing lakes of blood and strands of tissue that, at high magnification, contain pleomorphic and overtly malignant cells (see Fig. 9–16*B*). Abnormal mitoses may be seen, and there may be focal or extensive necrosis. There may be no evidence of tumor bone or osteoid formation (see Fig. 9–16*C*). In a few cases the distinction may be difficult but can usually be resolved by correlation of the clinical and radiologic features with the histology.

Osteoclast-Rich Osteosarcoma Versus Giant Cell Tumor of Bone

Giant cell tumor (see Chapter 15) very rarely affects the immature skeleton, and it is more helpful in this instance to know if the skeleton is mature than to know the age of the patient. Giant cell tumor is rarer, accounting for only 5% of bone tumors, and the age group affected is older but with an overlap with osteosarcoma in the third decade. The distal femur and proximal tibia are the most common sites for both tumors, and the radiologic appearance of a lytic lesion may be similar in both lesions.

The giant cell tumor occurs at the site of a fused epiphysis (or apophysis) and classically extends to the subarticular zone of the adjacent joint. Typically, a giant cell tumor has a better-defined margin, and although the cortex may be expanded and thinned, except in the case of fracture, the tumor is usually contained within the thinned cortex at presentation and is not associated with periosteal reaction. Osteoclast-rich osteosarcoma is usually metaphyseal (Fig. 9–17*A*), but large tumors may approach the joint. There is usually some cortical destruction and a Codman's triangle may be present.

The histology of the two entities bears some similarity. Both are vascular and contain large numbers of osteoclast giant cells. The mononuclear population of a giant cell tumor consists of rounded and spindle cells with moderate numbers of normal mitoses. There is no significant pleomorphism. In contrast to this, an osteoclast-rich osteosarcoma has mononuclear cells that are very pleomorphic, and many mitoses are present, including atypical forms (Fig. 9–17*B*). Giant cell tumor is usually associated with some peripheral reactive bone and about one third contain some foci of stromal osteoid. Osteoclast-rich osteosarcoma rarely contains tumor bone or osteoid, but where it is present, it shows the malignant characteristics described earlier. Vascular invasion by tumor cells is very commonly seen in giant cell tumor, and small vascular spaces may contain single osteoclasts. This feature should not be regarded as indicative of malignancy in an otherwise typical giant cell tumor. Where imprint preparations are available, scattered mononuclear cells in giant cell tumor contain alkaline phosphatase. In contrast, the majority of the overtly malignant mononuclear cells of osteoclast-rich osteosarcoma contain alkaline phosphatase. Areas of hemorrhage and necrosis may be seen in both entities. Following chemotherapy, the osteoclast-rich osteosarcoma often develops the features of a telangiectatic osteosarcoma with strands of tumor surrounding large blood-filled spaces.

Small Cell Osteosarcoma Versus Ewing's Sarcoma

Small cell osteosarcoma is a rare histological subtype and is often associated with little tumor bone formation. Imaging studies may be of little help in distinguishing small cell osteosarcoma from Ewing's sarcoma. Glycogen may be present in the tumor cells in both entities. The cell membrane antigen detected by the *MIC2* antibody, which initially was thought to be fairly specific for Ewing's sarcoma, has been shown to be present in a number of malignant tumors of bone and soft tissue (see Chapter 14) and may be present in osteosarcoma (Fig.

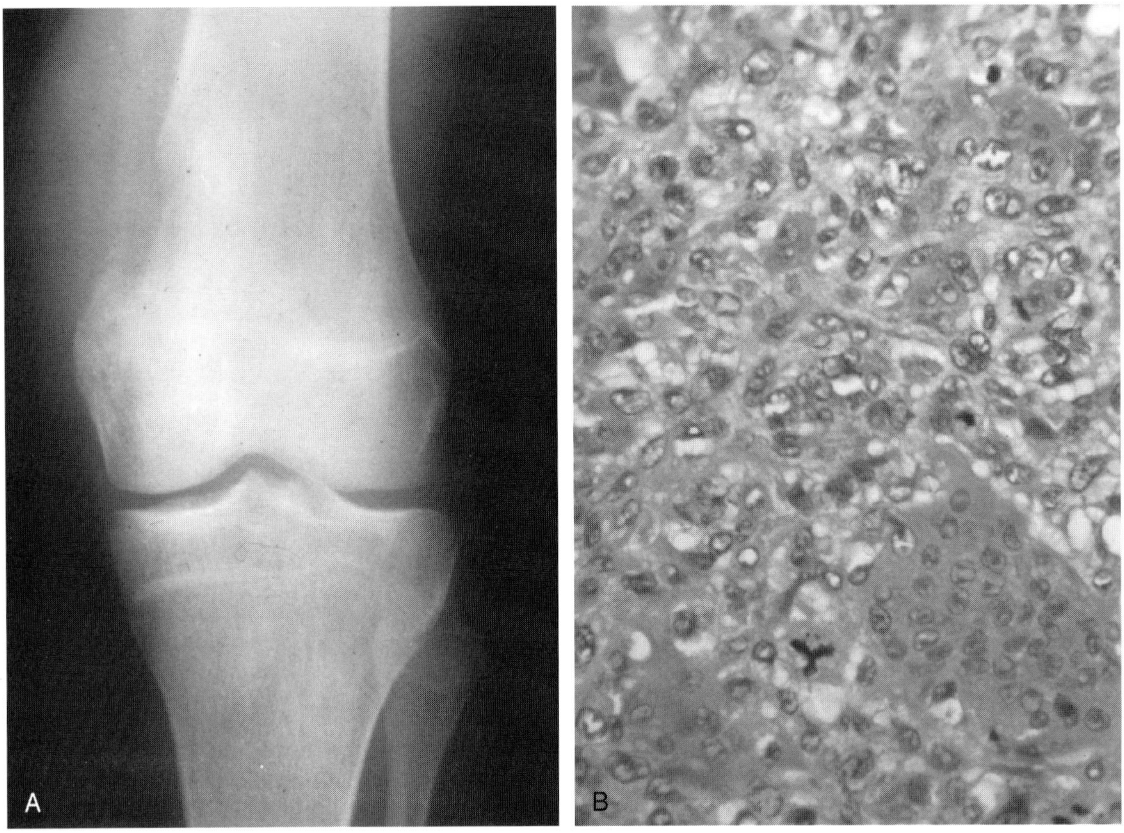

Figure 9–17. Osteoclast-rich osteosarcoma of the distal femur. *A*, Plain radiograph shows a destructive lesion of the medial aspect of the distal femoral metaphysis. *B*, At high magnification, large, multinucleate, osteoclast-like giant cells are present, together with pleomorphic mononuclear cells. A tripolar mitosis is included. No tumor bone or osteoid is present in this area.

9–18*A* [see also color figure]). The most helpful stain is the alkaline phosphatase which is negative in Ewing's sarcoma (Fig. 9–18*B* [see also color figure]). The demonstration of a reciprocal translocation between the long arms of chromosomes 11 and 22 (occasionally 21 and 22) that was thought to be specific for tumors of the Ewing's sarcoma and primitive neuroectodermal tumor (PNET) group has been described in small cell osteosarcoma (see Chapter 14), but this needs to be further tested.

Epithelioid Osteosarcoma Versus Osteoblastic Metastatic Carcinoma

Metastases to bone almost always present at an older age than does osteosarcoma, but they rarely overlap. Antibodies to cytokeratins and, in males, prostatic markers should be used to exclude osteoblastic metastases (see Chapter 17). In this instance, alkaline phosphatase is not helpful as the osteoblasts, reactive or malignant, will be positive.

Anaplastic Osteosarcoma Versus Other Poorly Differentiated High-Grade Tumors

In this instance, differentiation may be impossible and may depend mainly on the patient's age, skeletal site, and radiologic appearance. Highly anaplastic osteosarcoma (Fig. 9–19*A* and *B*) may cease to produce alkaline phosphatase, whereas other undifferentiated tumors may fail to express helpful antigens.

THE APPLICATION OF NEW TECHNIQUES TO THE DIAGNOSIS OF OSTEOSARCOMA

Osteosarcoma is traditionally defined as a primary malignant bone tumor in which the

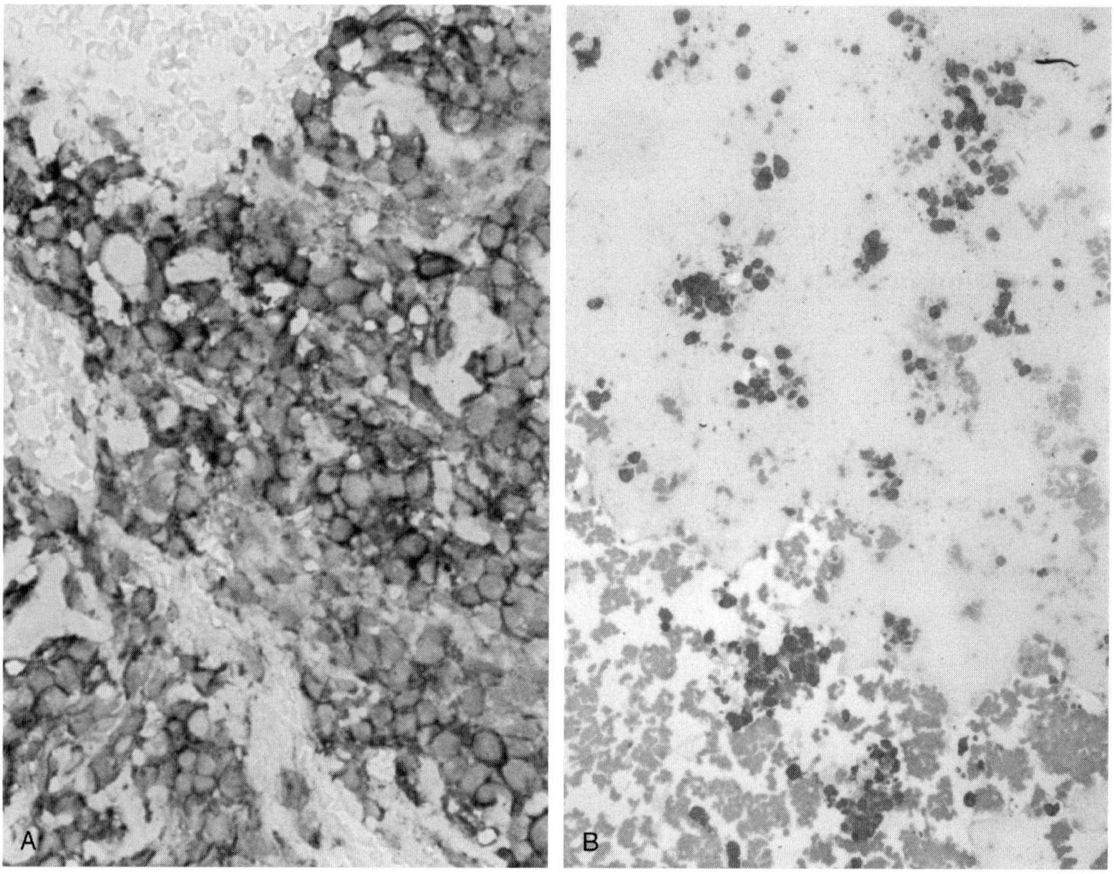

Figure 9–18. Small cell osteosarcoma (see also color figure). *A,* The neoplastic cells show intense membrane labeling for CD99 (*MIC2* antibody). *B,* Imprint preparation shows the small malignant cells contain copious alkaline phosphatase.

tumor cells are associated with the production of tumor bone and osteoid. In practice, this definition is no longer appropriate as many needle biopsy samples from cases in which all other features favor a diagnosis of osteosarcoma contain no tumor bone or osteoid. The diagnosis can be made in those cases by demonstrating alkaline phosphatase in the malignant cells. Greater experience of the very wide radiologic and histologic spectrum of osteosarcoma suggests that osteosarcoma should be regarded as a sarcoma derived from skeletal mesenchyme, which is actively producing tumor bone and osteoid or which has the potential to do so, as evidenced by the presence of alkaline phosphatase.[18] It is often said that decalcification renders immunohistochemistry difficult or impossible. In a specialist laboratory where the method of decalcification is carefully selected for each sample and the endpoint of decalcification is judged by frequent radiographic assessments, the sections will react with any antibodies that are used for undecalcified paraffin-embedded tissue. This is assisted by modern techniques for antigen retrieval.

Immunohistochemistry has a limited role in the diagnosis of osteosarcoma. The value of vimentin has already been alluded to. Bone pathologists do not routinely subject cases of osteosarcoma to a panel of immunostains. Occasionally an osteosarcoma will metastasize to an unusual site, and the histology is carried out at a hospital not involved in the biopsy and resection of the tumor. In these circumstances, the pathologist often carries out immunohistochemistry with confusing rather than helpful results, and the metastasis is then regarded as a second primary malignancy. I have subjected a small number of osteosarcomas to a panel of immunohistochemical stains; in some cases this includes the biopsy, the post-chemotherapy resection, and soft-tissue recurrence or pulmonary metastases. The pre-

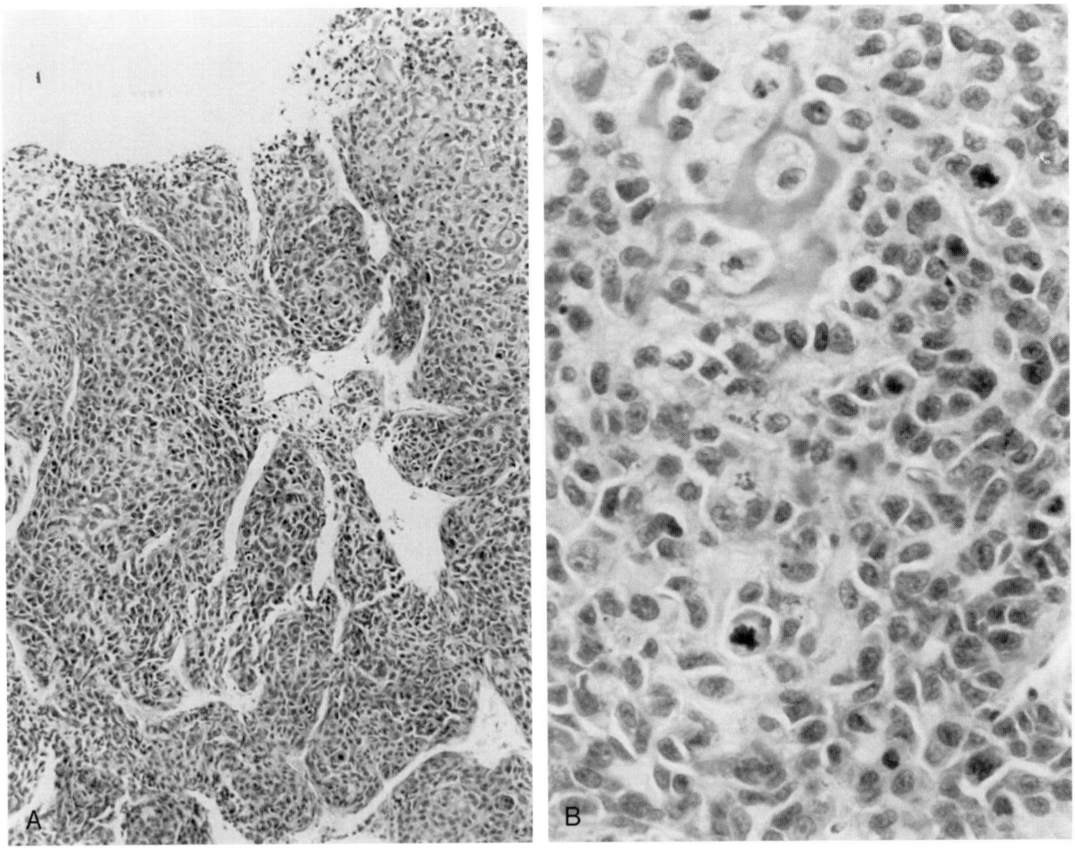

Figure 9–19. Undifferentiated/anaplastic osteosarcoma. *A*, Undifferentiated, pleomorphic tumor cells are arranged in a hemangiopericytomatous pattern. A tiny focus of bone formation is present (top right). *B*, At high magnification, the small wisps of tumor osteoid can be seen, together with the pleomorphic nature of the tumor, including mitotic figures.

liminary findings indicate that smooth muscle actin is frequently expressed in osteosarcoma, vimentin is uniformly positive in all cases, and S-100 protein is positive in areas of chondroblastic differentiation. The *MIC2* antibody may show crisp membrane staining in osteosarcoma, and this is not restricted to the small cell type.

In contrast to the findings in the Ewing's/PNET group, no consistent chromosome abnormalities have been identified in high-grade central osteosarcoma, although the presence of a ring chromosome has been described in low-grade central osteosarcomas and the closely related surface parosteal osteosarcoma. All these features support the concept of osteosarcoma representing a heterologous group of sarcomas derived from skeletal mesenchyme (malignant mesenchymomas), which have the ability to produce tumor bone and osteoid. The widely disparate histologic features seen in response to preoperative chemotherapy within the same tumor and between different tumors also reflects the polymorphic nature of osteosarcoma. Further research into the cytogenetics and molecular biology may improve understanding and classification of this challenging protean tumor.

NON-NEOPLASTIC CONDITIONS SIMULATING BONE-FORMING NEOPLASMS

Bone island, osteopoikilosis, bone infarct, fibrous dysplasia, osteofibrous dysplasia, sclerosing osteomyelitis, and Paget's disease may simulate bone-forming neoplasms on plain radiographs, and a biopsy may be required to establish an accurate diagnosis.

Bone Island

This consists of an ectopic focus of cortical bone in an intramedullary location. It is often seen as an incidental finding on plain radiographs. Typically, the trabeculae of bone merge into the trabecular structure of the adjacent cancellous bone. Occasionally these lesions show increased uptake on radioisotope scans and may very occasionally be biopsied. The histology shows a well-circumscribed area of bone, with the architecture of mature cortical bone with a peripheral zone of trabeculae merging with surrounding cancellous bone. Typically, there is little surface activity.

Osteopoikilosis

In this rare condition, the appearance on radiographs of multiple densities within bone may raise the possibility of multiple osteoblastic metastases or even multicentric osteosarcoma. These lesions are asymptomatic and are located in the epiphysis and metaphysis of long bones. The pelvis may be involved, but the skull, mandible, spine, and ribs are not affected. The lesions measure up to 5 cm in diameter. The radiologic and histologic features are similar to those of bone island. The condition may be inherited as an autosomal dominant trait, but sporadic cases occur.[19]

Bone Infarct

Bone infarct may present as a symptomatic lesion, particularly when it is near a major weightbearing joint such as in avascular necrosis of the femoral head. Many smaller areas of infarction may appear as the incidental finding of areas of increased density within the medulla on radiographs. In contrast to the rounded or ring-shaped densities of long-standing enchondromas, infarcts often have an irregular triangular or saber-shaped outline. Infarction may occur in areas of fibrous dysplasia and in metabolic diseases, such as Gaucher's disease. Those working in hyperbaric conditions, including deep-sea divers and workers on oil rigs, may develop infarcts. Multiple infarcts are common in sickle cell anemia. In the mature skeleton, an area of infarction that is symptomatic and that on radiographs is associated with a peripheral area of lucency and bone destruction should raise the possibility of malignant fibrous histiocytoma. A significant proportion of cases of this rare primary bone tumor is associated with a focus of bone infarction.

Sclerosing Osteomyelitis

This low-grade form of osteomyelitis has many names including *sclerosing osteomyelitis of Garré*[20] and, more recently, *pagetoid osteomyelitis*. It is a rare disease, but quite a large proportion of cases affect the clavicle in young females. The manubrium sterni and upper ribs are other fairly common sites. The bone is expanded irregularly and sclerotic due to extensive reactive bone formation. On radiographs it may be mistaken for a low-grade osteoblastic malignancy, and in the middle-aged and elderly an osteoblastic metastasis may be favored.

It is rare to culture a causal organism from this type of osteomyelitis, and the sclerotic nature of the bone means that biopsy is technically difficult, and any soft tissue areas will probably have significant crush artefact. The histology shows extensive areas of bone and marrow showing non-specific reactive changes. The bone surfaces are covered by plump, uniform, reactive osteoblasts, a feature that dis-

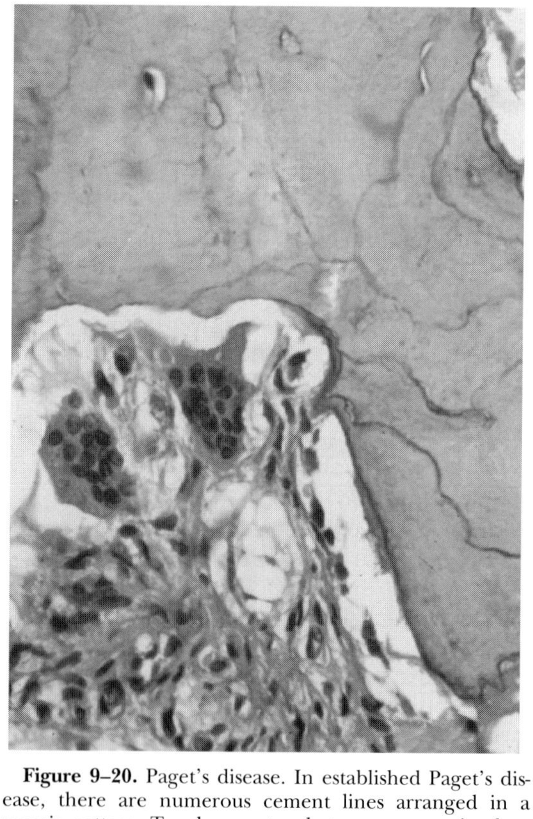

Figure 9–20. Paget's disease. In established Paget's disease, there are numerous cement lines arranged in a mosaic pattern. Two large osteoclasts are present in close apposition to active osteoblasts.

tinguishes the lesion from low-grade central osteosarcoma and parosteal osteosarcoma. Careful examination of the marrow spaces shows delicate vascular fibrous tissue and a light infiltrate of lymphocytes and occasional plasma cells. Scattered foci of more intense inflammation may be identified, and occasionally small collections of polymorphs may be seen.

Paget's Disease

Where Paget's disease is widespread in the skeleton and associated with a classic radiologic appearance, there is usually no diagnostic difficulty. However, an isolated focus of Paget's disease presenting in a younger-than-usual age group may raise the possibility of a bone-forming neoplasm.

If the lesion is sclerotic, then the Paget's disease should be well established and should not cause a diagnostic difficulty on histologic examination (Fig. 9–20). Examination with polarized light will confirm a disorderly mixture of lamellar and woven bone. The bone surfaces will contain both active osteoblasts and osteoclasts in close proximity, and the size and number of nuclei in the osteoclasts is much greater than those seen in normal bone turnover. The normal marrow tissue is replaced to a varying degree by delicate vascular fibrous tissue. Prominent irregular cement lines can be seen ramifying through the bone in a mosaic or interlocking jigsaw pattern. During preparation, the bone often separates slightly along the mosaic cement lines as the collagen fibers do not bridge them. The cement lines contain deep scallops reflecting the large size of the osteoclasts that have created the Howship's lacunae.

REFERENCES

1. McLeod RA, Dahlin DC, Beabout JWW: The spectrum of osteoblastoma. Am J Roentgenol 126:321, 1976.
2. Mazoyer JF, Kohler R, Bossard D: Osteoid osteoma: CT-guided percutaneous treatment. Radiology 181: 269, 1991.
3. Merryweather R, Middlemiss JH, Sannerkin NG: Malignant transformation of osteoblastoma. J Bone Joint Surg 62B:381, 1980.
4. Schulman L, Dorfman H: Nerve fibres in osteoid osteoma. J Bone Joint Surg 52:1351, 1970.
5. Makely J: Prostaglandins: A mechanism for pain mediation in osteoid osteoma. Orthop Trans 6:72, 1982.
6. Sissons H, Kancheria P, Wallace B: Ossifying fibroma of bone: Report of two cases. Bull Hosp Jt Dis 43:1, 1983.
7. Schajowicz F, Lemos C: Malignant osteoblastoma. J Bone Joint Surg 58B:202, 1976.
8. Dorfman HD, Weiss SW: Borderline osteoblastic tumours: Problems in the differential diagnosis of aggressive osteoblastoma and low-grade osteosarcoma. Semin Diagn Pathol 1:215, 1984.
9. Bertoni F, Unni KK, McLeod RA, et al: Osteosarcoma resembling osteoblastoma. Cancer 55:416, 1985.
10. Unni KK, Dahlin DC, McLeod RA, et al: Intraosseous well-differentiated osteosarcoma. Cancer 40:1337, 1977.
11. Kurt AM, Unni KK, McLeod RA, et al: Low-grade intraosseous osteosarcoma. Cancer 65:1418, 1990.
12. Mirra JM: Bone Tumors. Philadelphia, Lea & Febiger, 1989, p 360.
13. Enneking WF: A system of staging musculoskeletal neoplasms. Clin Orthop Rel Res 204:9, 1986.
14. Mankin HJ, Lange TA, Spanier SS: The hazards of biopsy in patients with malignant primary bone and soft tissue tumors. J Bone Joint Surg 64:1121, 1982.
15. Pringle JAS: The relationship of tumor margin to the epiphysis in 200 limb bone osteosarcomas analysed using fine detail x-ray and histopathology. J Bone Joint Surg 74B (Suppl. 3 Orthop. Proc.):277, 1992.
16. Stoker DJ, Cobb JP, Pringle JAS: Needle biopsy of musculoskeletal lesions: A review of 208 procedures. J Bone Joint Surg 73B:498, 1991.
17. Mirra JM: Bone Tumors. Philadelphia, Lea & Febiger, 1989, p 146.
18. Pringle JAS: Osteosarcoma: The experiences of a specialist unit. Curr Diagn Pathol 3:127, 1996.
19. Revell PA: Pathology of Bone. Berlin, Springer-Verlag, 1986, p 176.
20. Harris NH: Postgraduate Textbook of Clinical Orthopaedics. Oxford, Blackwell Science, 1995, p 404.

Chapter

10

CENTRAL CARTILAGINOUS NEOPLASMS OF BONE

TIMOTHY R. HELLIWELL

The diagnosis of hyaline cartilaginous lesions may be difficult for the nonspecialist pathologist, because criteria based entirely on the cytologic features of the neoplastic cells are not consistently useful in separating benign from malignant conditions. An assessment of the likely biologic behavior based on architectural features of the tissue and on imaging studies is of great value in determining the most appropriate management strategy, and the statistical approach of knowing the likely behavior of lesions presenting in a particular clinical-radiologic-pathologic context is helpful. Generalizations such as malignant lesions tend to be more than 10 cm in diameter, occur in the more proximal parts of the skeleton, and rarely occur in children[1] are of limited value; and no diagnosis should be made without integrating clinical, radiologic, and histologic appearances.

The problems surrounding the histologic diagnosis of suspected cartilaginous lesions[2] are summarized in Table 10–1. It is important for the pathologist to realize that no single radiologic or histologic criterion is sufficient to resolve all these issues. The radiologic features of the lesion are a good guide as to the reactive or neoplastic nature of the lesion and are helpful in suggesting the diagnosis of a chondroblastic osteosarcoma, particularly in younger patients.

Small fragmented biopsy specimens and fine-needle aspiration specimens are often difficult to interpret, unless a high-grade chondrosarcoma is present.[3] Given the appropriate radiologic appearances, needle core biopsy specimens can provide useful data if taken with a noncrushing needle from several sites within a lesion; they will confirm the chondroid nature and provide a general guide as to cellularity. Open biopsy including tissue from the edge of the lesion may eventually be required if other methods do not provide sufficient material on which to base a definitive diagnosis and treatment plan. The site for biopsy should be guided by the radiologic appearances because the more heavily calcified areas of chondroid tumors tend to be the more benign, whereas relatively lytic foci are the most likely areas to show features of malignancy. Artifactual changes in biopsy material may cause difficulties. Fixation of the tissues often causes shrinkage of chondrocytes, leaving a clear space between the edge of the

Table 10–1. Problems in the Diagnosis of Cartilaginous Lesions of Bone

- Is the lesion reactive or neoplastic?
- If neoplastic, is the tumor benign or malignant?
  - Is the biopsy adequate to determine the tumor architecture and cellularity?
  - How do cytologic features vary with the site and clinical syndrome?
- If it is a chondrosarcoma, how should it be graded and how likely is it to metastasize?
- If the cartilage is malignant, is the diagnosis really chondroblastic osteosarcoma?

Adapted from Reid R: New developments in the diagnosis of chondrosarcoma (editorial). J Pathol 163:93, 1991.

lacuna and the cell wall. Fortunately, the nuclear characteristics that are the key to diagnosis in some circumstances are not affected by such shrinkage.

The focus in this chapter is on the diagnosis of enchondromas and classic chondrosarcomas of bone. Consideration is also given to the special types of clear cell and dedifferentiated chondrosarcoma that may cause problems in biopsy material. Because there is a continuous spectrum of pathologic features from benign to malignant hyaline cartilaginous neoplasms, chondromas and typical chondrosarcomas are discussed together so that the similarities and differences can be emphasized. The diagnosis of cartilaginous lesions arising on the surface of the bone is discussed in detail in Chapter 11.

ENCHONDROMA AND TYPICAL CHONDROSARCOMA OF BONE

Historical Considerations

The existence of benign cartilaginous neoplasms was recognized in the 19th century, with cases of solitary or multiple enchondromas described by Sir James Paget,[4] the hereditary form of multiple enchondromas clearly defined by Ollier,[5, 6] and their association with soft tissue angiomas noted by Maffucci.[7]

Although Sir Astley Cooper described the essential characteristics of what we now know as osteosarcoma and chondrosarcoma in his essay "Exostosis" in 1818,[8] the classification of bone sarcomas devised by the Bone Sarcoma Registry of the American College of Surgeons did not recognize a separate category of chondrosarcoma until 1939,[9] after the detailed studies of Phemister.[10] The cytologic criteria that help to distinguish benign from malignant cartilaginous neoplasms were clearly defined by Lichtenstein and Jaffe,[11] and the relevance of these criteria to the diagnosis and management of cartilaginous tumors was reinforced by the observations of Barnes and Catto.[12] The description of special types of chondrosarcoma such as mesenchymal chondrosarcoma and dedifferentiated chondrosarcoma followed.[13, 14]

Clinical Presentation

Enchondroma

The true incidence of enchondromas is difficult to ascertain, because they are often asymptomatic. In the Mayo Clinic series, chondromas accounted for 13% of benign bone tumors,[15] with a slight female predominance, except that patients with multiple chondromas are more frequently male. Chondromas may present at any age, being most common in the 10- to 40-year age range. The most common sites are the small bones of the hands and feet, with relatively common sites being the proximal humerus, proximal and distal femur, tibia and fibula, and the ribs. Benign cartilaginous neoplasms of the sternum and skull are exceptionally rare. Most chondromas do not produce symptoms and are incidental findings on radiographs or radioisotope bone scans. Pain in association with a chondroma is uncommon in the absence of a fracture and should suggest continued growth and possible malignant change.[16]

Chondrosarcoma

Chondrosarcomas account for 21 to 26% of primary sarcomas of bone,[17, 18] and most occur without an obvious predisposing lesion. They are slightly more common in males. Classic chondrosarcomas present most frequently in the 30- to 60-year age range, with very few presenting in childhood.[19] Chondroid tumors in adolescents are usually chondroblastic osteosarcomas. Chondrosarcomas arise most commonly in the bones of the trunk (ribs, sternum, vertebrae, and pelvis) and in the upper ends of the femur and humerus. They are uncommon primary tumors in the hands and feet.

The clinical presentation of chondrosarcoma is usually with pain (implying active growth) and swelling. These tumors generally grow slowly, and symptoms may have been present for years before coming to medical attention. Pain is not usually severe except in rapidly growing, destructive lesions.

Multicentric chondrosarcomas are extremely rare but may present as two tumors within one bone or as tumors occurring in different bones after an interval of several years.[20] Distinction of the metachronous sarcomas from osseous metastases of the primary is often impossible. Mesenchymal chondrosarcomas are more often multifocal (7% cases) and/or have a greater tendency than conventional chondrosarcomas for osseous metastasis.[21]

Etiology

Solitary Chondromas

Enchondromas are hamartomatous lesions (dyschondroplasia) arising from chondrocytes of the epiphyseal growth plate that do not progress through the usual sequence of hypertrophy and cell death. As a consequence, a column of uncalcified cartilage extends from the growth plate into the adjacent bone, where it may become isolated and walled off by normal lamellar bone. This tissue may undergo calcification and osseous remodeling or may continue to grow as a chondroma.[22] A similar process gives rise to surface osteochondromas and may be involved in the genesis of fibrous dysplasia.

The possibility of malignant change in solitary enchondromas remains controversial, owing to differences in the interpretation of relatively mature cartilaginous elements in parts of some chondrosarcomas. Some authors regard these areas as a low-grade component of the malignancy,[17, 23] whereas others consider them to be evidence of a pre-existing chondroma.[1, 11, 16] Given the continuous spectrum of histologic appearances seen within chondroid neoplasms (see later), this debate may be resolved only when the critical genetic changes associated with these lesions are defined and can be identified in tissue sections.

Multiple Chondromas and Malignancy in Ollier's Disease

Multiple enchondromatosis or Ollier's disease is a rare, nonhereditary, nonfamilial disorder in which cartilaginous masses occur in the diaphyseal and metaphyseal regions of several bones, predominantly or exclusively on one side of the body. Enchondromatosis most commonly affects the short tubular bones of the hands and feet, with the scapulae and iliac bones being the most commonly affected flat bones. The extensive bone involvement results in skeletal deformity with swelling, shortening, angulation, and fracture contributing to the clinical presentation. Chondrosarcomas develop in about 25% of patients with Ollier's disease, most frequently in the larger long bones or the pelvis, and occasionally other malignancies including chordoma and osteosarcoma may occur.[24]

Multiple Chondromas and Malignancy in Maffucci's Syndrome

Maffucci described the association between dyschondroplasia with multiple enchondromas and soft tissue hemangiomas in 1881,[7] and many cases have since been reported. The syndrome is not familial but often presents in early childhood with cutaneous hemangiomas that histologically have a complex pattern of mixed sizes of vessels or spindle cell hemangiomas.[25] The hemangiomas are usually more extensive on one side of the body and can occur in the meninges, lungs, and gastrointestinal tract as well as in the skin.[26]

Multiple enchondromas interfere with normal bone growth, resulting in deformity, short stature, scoliosis, or fracture (see Fig. 16–6).

The incidence of malignancy in Maffucci's syndrome varies with the published series but is of a similar order to that of Ollier's disease at 25 to 30% of patients. Many benign and malignant neoplasms have been described in these patients,[26] with chondrosarcomas arising in about 15% of patients. Chondrosarcomas present at an average age of 40 years (range, 13–69 years) and are usually of low histologic grade. Other malignancies such as leukemias, soft tissue sarcomas, and astrocytomas may lead to death.

In both Ollier's disease and Maffucci's syndrome, masses of hyaline cartilage may involve the endosteal marrow and the cortex. This appears to be associated with a failure of development of the cortex and should not be taken as evidence of invasion.[1]

Other Diseases in Which Chondrosarcomas May Arise

Paget's disease of bone is complicated by the development of sarcoma in approximately 1% of patients.[27] Although the vast majority of these sarcomas are osteosarcomas or fibrosarcomas, occasional cases of chondrosarcoma have been described.[28, 29]

Malignancies rarely arise in areas of fibrous dysplasia but may affect approximately 0.5% of patients with monostotic disease and 4% of patients with polyostotic disease.[30] The most common malignancy is osteosarcoma, with occasional cases of chondrosarcoma and malignant fibrous histiocytoma or fibrosarcoma described.[30] Sarcomas may arise with or without a history of irradiation and are recognized by a combination of rapidly developing swelling and pain, appropriate imaging studies, and biopsy.

Synovial chondromatosis may rarely transform to synovial chondrosarcoma (see Chapter 18).

Chondrosarcomas may occasionally arise in the field of previous radiation[31] or after repetitive trauma to a bone over a period of many years.[32]

Molecular Biology

Cytogenetic Studies

There have been few cytogenetic studies of chondrosarcomas, and very few of chondromas, owing to the difficulty of obtaining mitotic cells from these lesions. Conventional cytogenetic analyses have found a normal karyotype in most chondromas, with chondrosarcomas showing complex karyotypes and variation in karyotype both within individual tumors and between tumors.[33, 34] Overall, structural aberrations of chromosomes 1, 12, and 15 and numerical anomalies of chromosomes 5, 7, 8, and 18 appear to be the most frequent in classic chondrosarcoma (see Chapter 4 for more details).

Comparative genomic hybridization studies of chondrosarcomas have revealed extensive chromosomal aberrations, with a mean of six changes per tumor (range, 1–24) in 72% of the tumors analyzed. More changes occur in higher-grade sarcomas. Gains of whole chromosomes or chromosomal arms occur more frequently than deletions, particularly at 1q, 8q, 12q, 14q, 16q, 17p, 20, and 21.[35] These findings may lead to the discovery of genes with important roles in the initiation and progression of chondrosarcomas. It is of interest that loss of heterozygosity for alleles at 13q and 17p is more prevalent in high-grade chondrosarcomas than in low-grade sarcomas and that in low-grade sarcomas recurrence is more frequent in tumors with loss of heterozygosity on 13q (possibly associated with the retinoblastoma gene).[36] Forty-four per cent of sporadic chondrosarcomas show loss of heterozygosity for markers linked to the loci associated with hereditary multiple exostosis, EXT1 and EXT2 on 8q and in the pericentromeric region of chromosome 11, suggesting that tumor-suppressor genes in these regions may play a role in the development of sporadic chondrosarcomas.[37]

DNA Ploidy

Aneuploidy is common particularly in Grade 2/3 chondrosarcomas, but grade and the prevalence of aneuploidy are not correlated in all series.[38–42] Aneuploid chondrosarcomas show a higher incidence of local recurrence[39] and a significantly worse 10-year survival rate.[38] In a static cytometric study, enchondromas, synovial chondromatosis, and low-grade (Grades 1 and 2) chondrosarcomas were found to be diploid, whereas Grade 3 chondrosarcomas were aneuploid.[40]

Cell Proliferation

Expression of the cell cycle–related protein, proliferating cell nuclear antigen, occurs particularly at the edges of cartilaginous nodules in chondrosarcomas, and the proportion of cells showing proliferating cell nuclear antigen immunolabeling is greater in chondrosarcomas than chondromas (which rarely show proliferating cell nuclear antigen–positive nuclei) and in the more poorly differentiated sarcomas.[43, 44] Studies of another cell cycle–associated marker detected by the Ki67 and MIB1 antibodies suggest that labeling indices are greater in high-grade chondrosarcomas than in low-grade sarcomas[45, 46] and that the MIB1 labeling index may identify prognostic groups within those patients with Grade 2 chondrosarcomas.[45]

The degree of differentiation of chondroid tumors is associated with an increased number of argyrophilic nuclear organizer regions, which are loops of DNA situated in the nucleoli that contain the genes for ribosomal RNA. Proteins associated with these genes are argyrophilic; and although the number of argyrophilic nuclear organizer regions is related to nucleolar activity, the relationship to cell proliferation is not clearly defined. In a study of two chondromas and seven chondrosarcomas, higher counts were found in sarcomas than in chondromas.[47] Whether this could help in diagnosis has not been determined.

Oncogenes and Tumor Suppressor Genes

Expression of the mutant form of the *p53* tumor suppressor gene has been studied in chondrosarcomas. Although the normal protein product of the *p53* gene cannot usually be detected in cells, missense mutations of the *p53* gene lead to an accumulation of the mutated protein that can be detected by immunocytochemistry. Such studies are complicated by the use of different antibodies by different groups and because nonsense mutations and deletions of the *p53* gene lead to a lack of p53 protein, indistinguishable on immunocytochemical preparations from normal tissue. Thus, the presence of immunocytochemically detectable p53 protein is highly predictive of a mutation but the lack of detectable protein does not exclude a mutation. Most studies have found strong immunocytochemical labeling for p53 in high-grade (Grade 3 and/or 2) chondrosarcomas, with absent or weak labeling in low-grade chondrosarcomas and in enchondromas.[40, 45, 48, 49] Mutational analysis of the *p53* gene has only been performed on a few chondrosarcomas, most showing missense mutations, although one case with a nonsense mutation has been described.[48, 49] In a patient with the Li-Fraumeni syndrome, in which there is germ-line mutation of the *p53* gene, immunohistochemical labeling for p53 was observed in the more cellular areas of a chondrosarcoma.[50]

The nm23 gene product is a nucleoside diphosphate kinase, expression of which is inversely related to metastasis in several human tumors.[51] One of 14 chondromas and 21 of 22 chondrosarcomas showed immunohistochemical reactivity for nm23, with more expression occurring in Grade 2 and 3 chondrosarcomas than in Grade 1 sarcomas.[51] The relationship between nm23 expression and prognosis in these cases remains to be determined.

Unlike in osteosarcomas, where expression of the *met* proto-oncogene product (hepatocyte growth factor) is high, in chondrosarcomas, expression of *met* appears to be low.[52] No alterations in the genes coding for a range of oncogenes (c-*myc*, N-*myc*, c-*fos*, H-*ras*, Ki-*ras*, and N-*ras*) were found in one study,[53] although others found evidence for c-*myc* amplification in two chondrosarcomas.[54] A potential role for the early response oncogene, *c-fos*, is suggested by the finding that mice that develop from embryonic stem cell chimeras selected for high exogenous *c-fos* expression show a high frequency of cartilaginous tumors after the age of 3 to 4 weeks.[55]

Immunohistochemical labeling for c-*erb*-B2, a transmembrane receptor protein with tyrosine kinase activity, has been described as being present in most chondrosarcomas but absent in most benign cartilaginous proliferations[56, 57]; others have not confirmed this observation,[58] and its potential diagnostic or prognostic use remains uncertain.

Biochemistry

A detailed study of the biochemistry of chondroid neoplasms showed an increased water content and changes in proteoglycan molecules with increased malignancy, but because there is great variability in the composition of cartilaginous tumors, these features do not appear to be of prognostic value.[59, 60]

Other Immunocytochemical Studies

The S-100 proteins are a family of acidic, calcium-binding proteins that may be involved in mineralization and that can be detected by immunocytochemistry in normal and neoplastic cartilage.[61–63] Although confirming the cartilaginous nature of an area of tissue, the detection of S-100 protein is of limited diagnostic value because expression is also found in osteoblastic areas of osteosarcomas and in other bone neoplasms.[62]

Studies of noncollagenous proteins derived from osteoblasts have been undertaken to examine whether their expression may discriminate between chondroblastic osteosarcoma and chondrosarcoma. Immunocytochemical expression for bone GLA protein occurs in most osteosarcomas and in approximately 50% of chondrosarcomas, particularly the higher-grade chondrosarcomas.[64] Osteonectin expression can be detected by immunocytochemistry in osteosarcomas, whereas chondrosarcomas are described as showing either no expression[65] or consistent positive labeling.[66] The discrepancy may be due to different experimental methods, but this suggests that immunocytochemical labeling for osteonectin should only be used with caution diagnostically. In situ hybridization for osteonectin messenger RNA may provide a more specific marker for osteogenic neoplasms.[66]

An immunocytochemical study of the expression of a range of matrix metalloproteinases (MMP) and their inhibitors suggests that when compared with benign chondroid lesions, chondrosarcomas are associated with decreased expression of MMP-3 and increased expression of MMP-1 and MMP-9.[67]

Radiologic Features

Enchondromas are typically well-defined, centrally located, geographic lesions that arise within the metaphysis, metadiaphysis, or distal diaphysis of a tubular bone (see Fig. 6–10*B*). Isolated epiphyseal involvement is uncommon and may mimic a clear cell chondrosarcoma.[68] As a chondroma expands it tends to cause endosteal scalloping and cortical remodeling of the host bone. The extent of matrix mineralization varies. The most characteristic pattern is that of "rings and arcs," which results from the formation of endochondral and reactive bone formation around cartilaginous nodules. In the more mature parts of an enchondroma where there are fewer cells, patchy mineralization of the matrix leads to a stippled and flocculent pattern of mineralization, which may eventually form a solid mass of calcified cartilage. On T2-weighted magnetic resonance imaging (MRI), calcified cartilage usually displays low signal intensity whereas uncalcified cartilage has a high signal intensity.

The majority of central chondrosarcomas are low grade and have a moderately aggressive radiographic appearance. Typically, there is a geographic pattern of bone destruction with ill-defined margins and endosteal scalloping or thickening (Fig. 10–1). More aggressive lesions penetrate the cortex and infiltrate adjacent soft tissues. Areas of stippled or "ring and arc" mineralization may be apparent in the less malignant areas, but high-grade areas are relatively radiolucent. MRI shows the lobulated pattern of growth of chondrosarcomas, particularly in low-grade sarcomas, and the fibrovascular septa between lobules are emphasized on gadolinium-enhanced T1-weighted sequences.[69] High-grade chondrosarcomas show a heterogeneous and nonspecific appearance with variable high signal intensity on T2-weighted MRI and low signal intensity foci due to mineralization.[68]

Macroscopic Pathology

Most cartilaginous lesions have a light blue, lobulated appearance macroscopically (Fig. 10–2 [see also color Figure 10–2]). Calcification and ossification appear as small, white or yellow foci within the cartilaginous lobules. Enchondromas tend to be small and well circumscribed and may be heavily calcified. In chondrosarcomas, the bone is expanded and the cortex is eventually destroyed by coalescing nodules of cartilaginous tissue ranging in size from a few millimeters to 2 to 3 cm in diameter. Myxoid (gelatinous) change in the matrix tends to liquefy the tumor tissue and tends to be associated with malignancy.

Microscopic Pathology

After consideration of the radiologic features, the most useful guide to the diagnosis is the architecture of the lesion at low magnification, although this may be difficult to appreciate in a fragmented biopsy specimen.[16] The typical patterns of enchondroma are (1) islands of cartilage separated from one an-

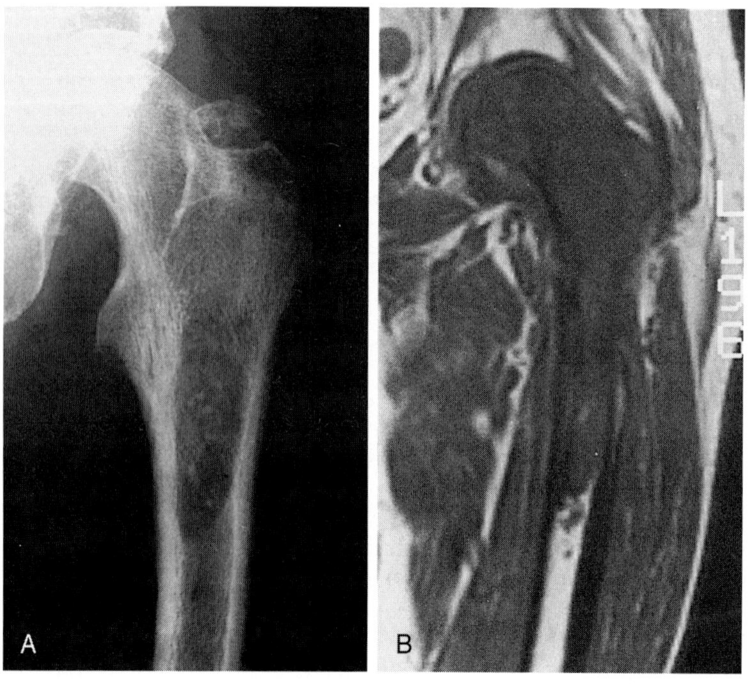

Figure 10–1. Imaging of chondrosarcoma. *A*, Plain radiograph of upper femur showing a geographic area of bone destruction in the metaphysis, with cortical erosion and small foci of mineralization within the lytic area. *B*, T1-weighted MR image shows low signal intensity for the unmineralized cartilage. More extensive changes are apparent in the femoral head as a result of avascular necrosis of the tissue secondary to the presence of chondrosarcoma.

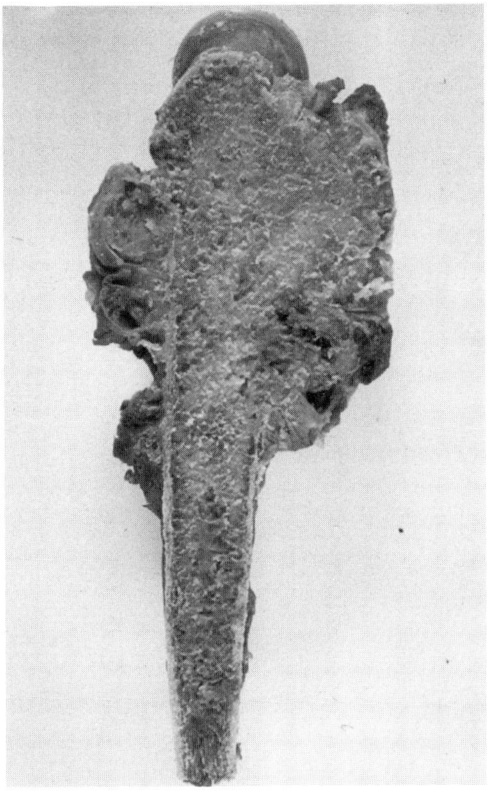

Figure 10–2. Macroscopic appearance of chondrosarcoma. Blue-gray nodules of cartilage, with yellow specks of calcification, are present centrally and extend out of the bone into soft tissues. (See also color figure.)

other by normal host bone and marrow fat and (2) the encasement of the cartilaginous islands by partial or complete shells of host lamellar or woven-lamellar bone (Fig. 10–3). Careful interpretation is required, because cartilaginous islands can occur in 40% of chondrosarcomas and the encasement (surrounding) of benign chondroid nodules by reactive bone should not be confused with the permeative pattern of chondrosarcoma between lamellar bone trabeculae. Molecular studies demonstrate that cartilaginous lobules showing the enchondroma-encasement pattern also have rims of type 1 and type 5 collagen,[70] a feature that is lost in chondrosarcomas. Dense calcification and a lack of necrosis are benign features.

In chondrosarcomas, the diagnostic appearance is one of permeation of the malignant cartilage between pre-existing lamellar bone trabeculae with obliteration of the marrow fat (Fig. 10–4*A*). This pattern may also occur in fracture callus and in chondroblastic osteosarcoma, which should be excluded on clinical and radiologic criteria. Permeation of the haversian systems of cortical bone is an analogous process to that described in the medullary cavity. Extension of chondroid tissue through the periosteum and into soft tissues is pathognomonic of malignancy but may not be apparent on biopsy material. The pattern of nodules of cartilaginous tissue separated by fibrous bands (Fig. 10–4*B*) is highly suggestive of malignancy.

The cytologic features that may help to distinguish benign from malignant cartilaginous neoplasms were first described in detail by Lichtenstein and Jaffe.[11] They found that on close inspection of viable areas of a benign tumor that the cartilage cells were consistently small, the vast majority contained one nucleus that was small in relation to the size of the cell, binucleate cells were few in number and had small nuclei, and there were no large or bizarre cells. Chondrosarcomas tended to be more cellular, with cells containing plump nuclei, many binucleate forms, and some giant cartilage cells with single or multiple nuclei. Calcified and necrotic areas of the tumor should not be used for evaluation because the nuclei of cells in these areas may show degenerative changes. High cellularity and the presence of a myxoid matrix are not by themselves important distinguishing criteria.[12]

The relevance of these criteria has been discussed by several authors[12, 16, 23, 59, 71, 72] and used to place chondrosarcomas in one of three histologic grades. Unfortunately, the precise criteria used for grading are not always clearly specified, and different authors appear to use subtly different criteria, reflecting the difficulty of dividing a continuous spectrum of appearances into discrete groups. The range of features that may generally be encountered in central cartilaginous tumors is as follows (Fig. 10–5):

- Enchondromas have abundant intercellular matrix with relatively few chondrocytes showing uniform, small, darkly stained nuclei and few binucleate forms.
- Grade 1 chondrosarcomas are more cellular with an uneven distribution of cells showing mild nuclear pleomorphism and small nucleoli, with binucleate cells easily identified.
- Grade 2 chondrosarcomas are more cellular than Grade 1 tumors and show marked nuclear pleomorphism with large cells and oc-

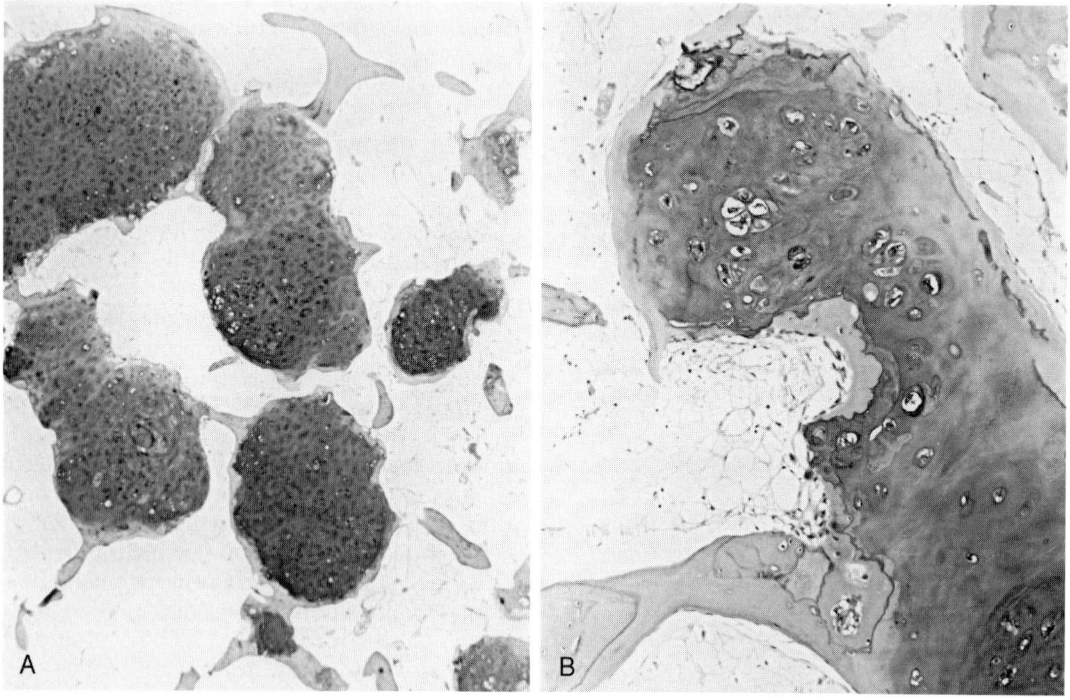

Figure 10–3. Enchondroma of the upper femur. *A,* Nodules of cartilaginous tissue are scattered through the medullary bone ("islands of cartilage" pattern). *B,* At higher magnification, the nodules are surrounded by mature, lamellar bone ("bone encasement" pattern).

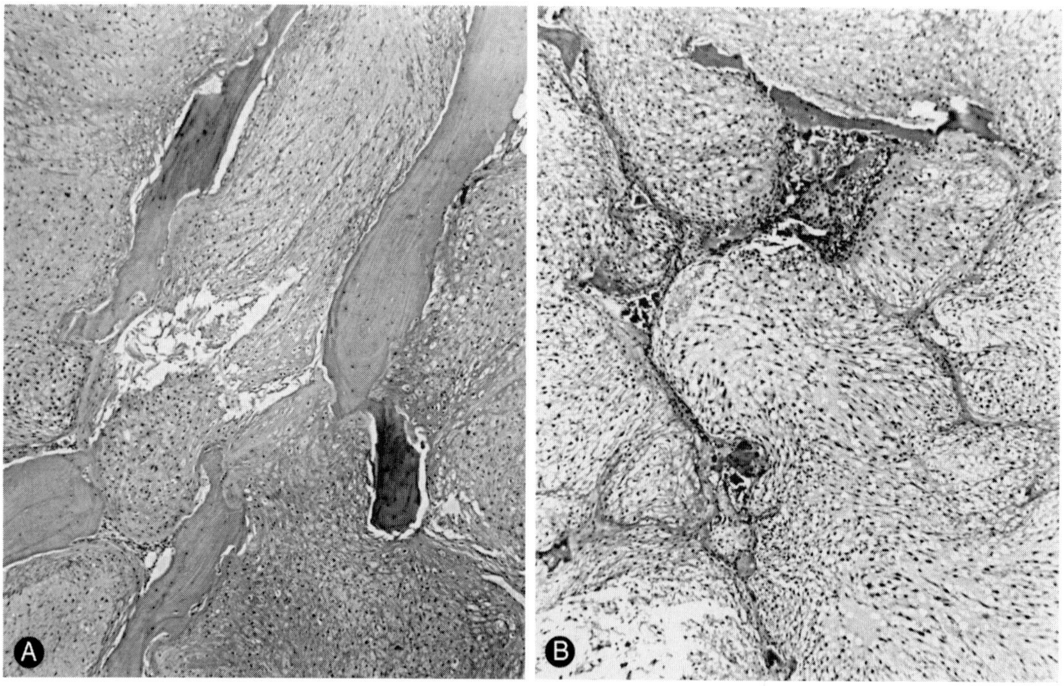

Figure 10–4. Chondrosarcoma. *A,* Sheets of malignant cartilage permeate between pre-existing bone trabeculae. *B,* Nodules of cartilage in chondrosarcoma are often separated by fibrous bands. In this area, ossification is also present between the nodules.

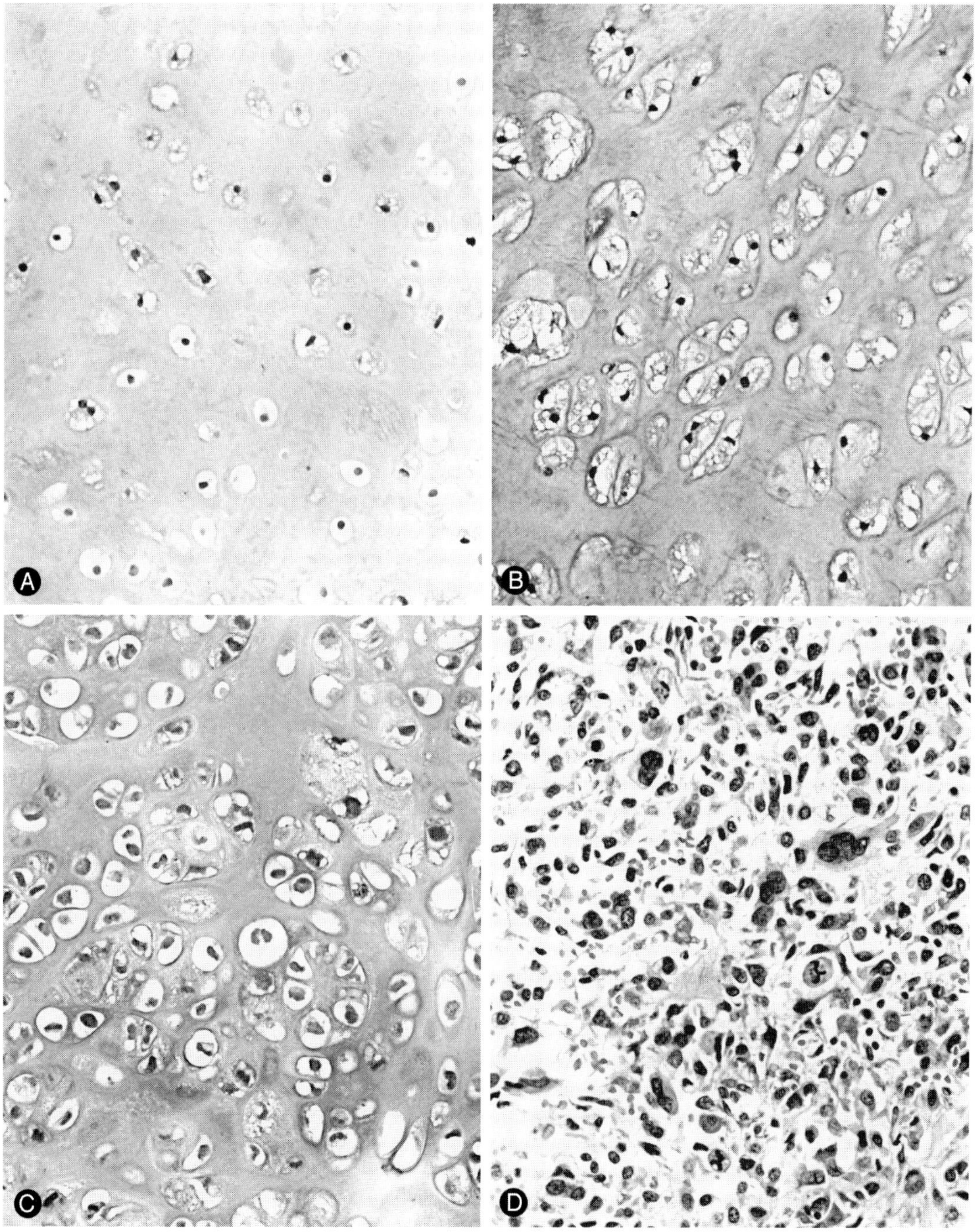

Figure 10–5. Spectrum of cytologic appearances of chondroid neoplasms. *A,* Enchondroma of the finger shows hyaline cartilage of low cellularity, chondrocytes with small nuclei, and occasional binucleate cells. *B,* Grade 1 chondrosarcoma of the femur shows hyaline cartilage of low cellularity, chondrocytes with nuclei slightly larger than those in *A,* and more frequent binucleate cells. The distinction from enchondroma can be made only on the basis of a permeative pattern of invasion seen in other areas. *C,* Grade 2 chondrosarcoma is more cellular than that in *B,* with chondrocytes having plump nuclei and several binucleate forms. *D,* Grade 3 chondrosarcoma is highly cellular with pleomorphic atypical chondrocyte nuclei, mitotic figures, and minimal matrix production. Elsewhere this tumor showed more extensive matrix production.

Table 10–2. Assessment of Malignancy of Cartilaginous Neoplasms

Tumor Type	Clinical Presentation	Radiologic Appearances	Pattern of Growth	Grade	Cellularity	Nuclear Features	Binucleate Cells	Mitotic Activity
Enchondroma	Small, often painless	Well-demarcated, heavily calcified lesion. No cortical erosion.	Nodules of cartilage encased by reactive bone	0	Low	Uniform Small Dark No nucleoli	Rare	Absent
Low-grade chondrosarcoma	Larger lesion May be painful	Poorly demarcated lesion with expansion and destruction of adjacent cortical bone. Soft tissue extension may occur. Calcification variable.	Permeation of cartilage between pre-existing bone trabeculae	1	Moderate	Slight pleomorphism Small nucleoli may be present	Common	Very rare
High-grade chondrosarcoma	Large, painful lesion	Poor demarcation with cortical destruction and soft tissue mass. Little calcification.	Permeation of cartilage between pre-existing bone trabeculae	2	High	Marked pleomorphism Large cells Occasional bizarre nuclei	Common	Occasional mitoses present
				3	High	Marked pleomorphism. Large cells. Many bizarre nuclei	Common	Many mitoses

After Mankin HJ, Cantley KP, Lippiello L, et al.: The biology of human chondrosarcomas: I. Description of the cases, grading and biochemical analyses. J Bone Joint Surg 62A:160, 1980; and Mirra JM, Gold R, Downs J, et al.: A new histologic approach to the differentiation of enchondroma and chondrosarcoma of the bones. Clin Orthop Rel Res 201:214, 1985.

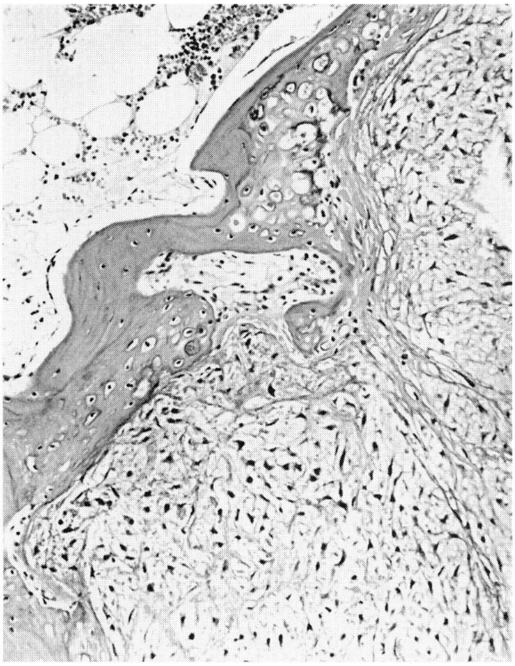

Figure 10–6. Chondrosarcoma in a case of Ollier's disease. Myxoid change is evident in the matrix.

casional bizarre forms. Binucleate cells are plentiful, and occasional mitoses may be seen.

- Grade 3 chondrosarcomas are highly cellular with little matrix. The cells show marked nuclear pleomorphism with bizarre forms and giant cells and many mitotic figures.

Morphometric analysis of nuclear size, cellularity, numbers of binucleate chondrocytes, and mitotic activity indicate that more than 25% of Grade 1 chondrosarcomas show complete cytologic overlap with enchondromas, the distinction being made on clinical and radiologic considerations.[16] For binucleate chondrocytes, only when there were more than 26 such cells in 3.2 mm^2 was there a greater than 90% probability that the diagnosis would be chondrosarcoma. Mitotic figures are very rarely seen in Grade 1 chondrosarcomas; and, therefore, although the presence of mitoses is a good indicator of malignancy, the absence of mitoses does not exclude that diagnosis.

The principles of these cytologic criteria are accepted as helpful in diagnosis, although their interpretation is necessarily subjective unless detailed morphometric studies are undertaken. Used in conjunction with the architectural pattern and clinical and radiologic features, the cytologic features are an invaluable support for most diagnoses (Table 10–2). Enchondromas are usually Grade 0. Chondrosarcomas that are clinically of low grade are usually of histologic Grade 1 but may be Grade 0. High-grade chondrosarcomas are always of histologic Grade 2 or 3 and do not usually present difficulties in diagnosis.

The same criteria can be used for the diagnosis of malignancy in Ollier's disease, with a permeative pattern of growth leading to "wall-to-wall" cartilage between lamellar bone trabeculae, and a change in character of the matrix from hyaline to myxoid (Fig. 10–6) being particularly helpful criteria.[24]

The difficulty in standardizing a grading system is reflected in the proportion of lesions placed in the different grades in series of patients from different institutions (Table 10–3), although these data may be skewed by different patterns of referral of cases or differences in the proportion of tumors from particular sites.

Variation in grade in different parts of the same tumor is well recognized[17, 73] and may lead to discrepancies in grading between biopsy and resection specimens. Approximately 10% of recurrent chondrosarcomas may have a higher histologic grade than the original tumor, either as a conventional chondrosarcoma or with areas of malignant spindle cell tissue as a dedifferentiated chondrosarcoma (see later).

The practical importance of histologic grading has been demonstrated by most groups (see Table 10–3 and the later discussion).[73]

Borderline Chondrosarcoma and Cartilaginous Lesions of Uncertain Malignant Potential

Borderline chondrosarcoma is diagnosed when the histologic features are those of an

Table 10–3. Summary of Some Studies of Grading and Prognosis in Chondrosarcomas

	Sanerkin[72]	Evans[71]	Pritchard[23]
% No. cases			
Grade 1	63	45	57
Grade 2	23	30	34
Grade 3	14	25	9
% Cases with metastases			
Grade 1	5	0	
Grade 2	14	10	
Grade 3	75	71	
% Five-year survival			
Grade 1	89	90	86
Grade 2	71	81	80
Grade 3	38	43	40

enchondroma but the radiographs show more aggressive features, including ill-defined or changing margins, and the patient complains of vague pain unrelated to athletic activity.[17, 74] Treatment by thorough curettage and bone grafting is usually successful, and recurrence is very rare. Whether these lesions should be clinically regarded as chondrosarcomas is debated. The loss of type 1 and type 5 collagen deposition around tumor nodules in these borderline lesions suggests that they show molecular features more in keeping with sarcoma than with enchondroma.[74]

The term *cartilaginous lesions of uncertain malignant potential* may be used for those lesions presenting as intermittent pain that are radiologically well marginated without cortical erosion and histologically benign. The presence of pain is the only atypical feature for an enchondroma.[16] Although such lesions may be excised *en bloc*, or by curettage, to definitively exclude a malignant histologic pattern,[75] careful radiologic follow-up to detect cortical erosion as an early sign of malignancy may be an alternative to surgery in the short term.

Chondrosarcomas of the Jaw and Facial Skeleton

Chondrosarcoma of the jaw and facial bones is a rare entity, comprising less than 3% of the Mayo Clinic series.[76] Nevertheless, any clinically significant chondroid lesion in this area should be regarded as malignant because chondromas are exceedingly rare, except as small incidental findings. Forty-one per cent of chondrosarcomas arise in the nasal septum, ethmoid, and sphenoid; 25% arise in the maxillary sinus; 20% occur in the alveolar portion of the maxilla; and 11% are found in the mandible. Clinical, radiologic, and histologic features are similar to those of chondrosarcoma of long bones. The important differential diagnostic consideration is with osteosarcoma of the jaw, which tends to be chondroblastic in 50% of cases,[77] because chondrosarcomas have a better prognosis in general than osteosarcomas at this site.[76] Although chondrosarcomas are generally regarded as resistant to radiotherapy and chemotherapy, it is interesting to note the good long-term survival of two high-grade chondrosarcomas of the jaw treated with surgery and adjunctive radiation therapy and chemotherapy because of the difficulties of achieving radical surgical margins.[78]

Cartilaginous Neoplasms of the Small Bones of the Hands

Chondromas of the digits are common, and most are cured by curettage. Chondrosarcomas are much less common than chondromas at this site, with only about 50 cases described in the literature,[79] and are often only diagnosed after recurrences follow apparently complete removal or in a tumor with rapid growth. Chondrosarcomas of the digits present most frequently in the seventh decade, rather older than typical chondrosarcomas,[80] with an enlarging, sometimes painful osseous swelling. Radiographs show bone destruction and soft tissue invasion. Histologically, enchondromas may be quite cellular but still grow in an expansile fashion. The diagnosis of chondrosarcoma is best confirmed by a permeative pattern of invasion of the adjacent bone or soft tissue. Most chondrosarcomas of the hand behave as low-grade lesions, and distant metastasis is exceptional.

Prognosis

Enchondromas are benign tumors that are usually treated by curettage and bone grafting. Recurrence is unusual, although some tumors do recur and may show greater cellular atypia than the original lesion.

Cartilage cells have low requirements for growth, and soft tissue implantation at the time of biopsy or definitive surgery may lead to recurrence. Local recurrence is more common in high-grade sarcomas,[71] although the prevalence of local recurrence is largely determined by the accessibility of the tumor to radical surgery.[72, 73]

Metastatic disease via regional veins is most commonly to the lungs, with less common sites including skin and soft tissues, and occasionally to other bones.[71, 81, 82] Chondrosarcomas of the chest wall may metastasize to the epidural space by intercostal and vertebral veins, and intravenous extension of sarcoma from the lower limb to the heart may occur without metastasis.[12] Lymph node metastasis is extremely rare.[12]

The optimal treatment of chondrosarcoma is early radical surgical resection with a wide margin of uninvolved tissue.[83] Limb-salvage surgery is now possible even for bulky tumors, although amputation may still be required for extensive tumors. Chondrosarcomas of the pelvis and thoracic regions have a relatively poor prognosis, owing to the problems of achieving total surgical excision at these sites.[73, 84]

The overall 5-year survival for chondrosarcomas is 72 to 77%, and 10-year survival is 67%, with disease-specific survival continuing to decline after 10 years because of late recurrence and metastasis.[18, 71] Survival is related to the histologic grade of the chondrosarcoma (see Table 10–3). The curability of patients who have metastatic disease is low. However, if the metastatic lesions can be surgically excised, survival is better than if surgery is not performed.[81]

CLEAR CELL CHONDROSARCOMA

Clear cell chondrosarcoma was defined as a clinicopathologic entity because of its unusual histologic appearance and epiphyseal location,[85] and subsequent reports have supported the view that this is a low-grade malignant lesion that should be distinguished both from the benign chondroblastoma that occurs at similar locations and from conventional chondrosarcomas.[86, 87]

Clinical Features

Clear cell chondrosarcomas present most commonly in the third to fifth decades of life with pain or disability, often of several years' duration. Symptoms may be referred to the adjacent joint. One third of patients develop a pathologic fracture. One case subjected to cytogenetic study showed a predominant clone with a near-haploid chromosomal content of 30 chromosomes but no structural abnormalities.[88]

Radiologic Features

These lesions are similar to chondroblastoma, except that they occur in an older age group and are usually located in the epiphyseal regions of the upper humerus or upper femur (either the femoral head or the greater trochanter),[85, 86] although other sites may occasionally be involved.[89] On plain radiographs, they are expansile, lytic lesions with a sharp line of demarcation with adjacent bone. Calcification occurs in 30% of cases. Extracortical spread is uncommon but may occur with larger lesions.

Pathologic Features

Macroscopically, these tumors are soft and gray or red; they do not usually show the glistening blue color of cartilage. Areas of high vascularity may lead to problems with hemostasis at operation. Cystic spaces may be present.

Microscopically,[85, 86] the tumor tends to have a lobulated architecture, with increased cellularity toward the edges of the lobules. The neoplastic cells have clear cytoplasm and centrally placed, monomorphic nuclei (Fig. 10–7*A*) with very few mitotic figures. Benign, osteoclast-like giant cells are often present, and about half of the tumors show areas of conventional chondrosarcoma. Generally, there is little matrix production, but some tumors show pericellular calcification as seen in chondroblastomas and frequently there are trabeculae of osteoid or bone within or between the tumor lobules (Fig. 10–7*B* and *C*). Sometimes microscopic foci of tumor can be found in the marrow space of the adjacent bone away from the main mass of tumor.[90]

Ultrastructural studies show that the clear cytoplasm of the neoplastic cells is due to glycogen accumulation, with the presence of surface microvilli being consistent with the cartilaginous nature of the cells.[91, 92]

Immunohistochemical studies show positivity for S-100 protein in the clear cells, with expression of cartilage-type collagens (collagen II and X) supporting the cartilaginous nature of the tumor.[93] The expression of osteonectin by the tumor cells[94] is consistent with the formation of reactive bone within the tumor and is not necessarily an indication of an osteoblastic origin.

Differential Diagnosis

The differential diagnosis of a locally aggressive lesion in bone containing clear cells and showing chondroid or osteoid formation includes osteoblastoma, chondroblastoma, metastatic renal adenocarcinoma and metastatic malignant melanoma, and the rare form of osteosarcoma that contains clear cells.[95, 96]

Prognosis

Clear cell chondrosarcoma is a neoplasm of low-grade malignancy. Curettage inevitably

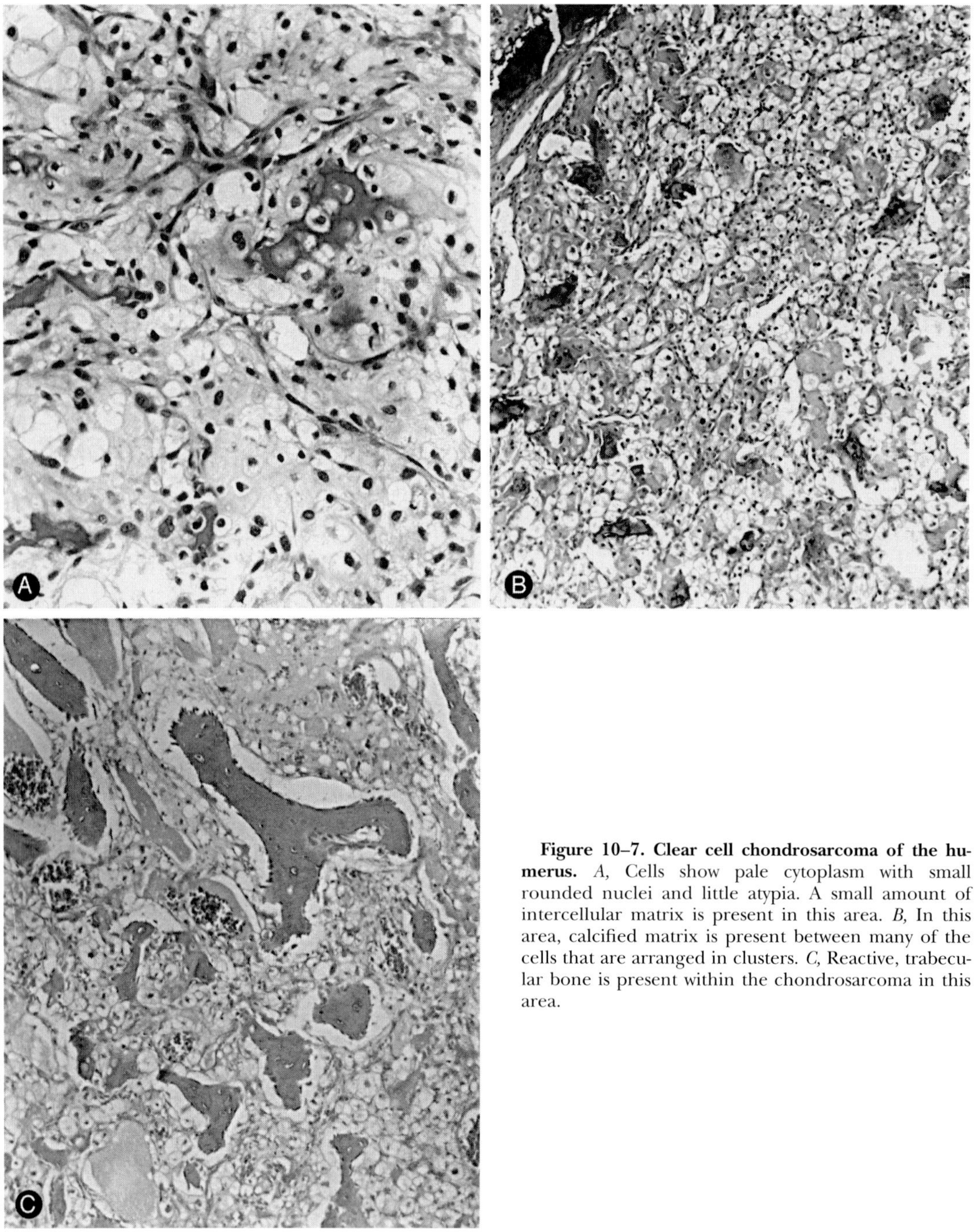

Figure 10–7. Clear cell chondrosarcoma of the humerus. *A,* Cells show pale cytoplasm with small rounded nuclei and little atypia. A small amount of intercellular matrix is present in this area. *B,* In this area, calcified matrix is present between many of the cells that are arranged in clusters. *C,* Reactive, trabecular bone is present within the chondrosarcoma in this area.

leads to local recurrence, and the optimal treatment is radical en bloc resection.[85, 86]

Metastases occur in about 25% patients, but these are not necessarily rapidly fatal. Metastases are usually to the lungs, but the involvement of multiple bones in some patients is suggestive of osseous metastasis.[85]

DEDIFFERENTIATED CHONDROSARCOMA

The term dedifferentiated chondrosarcoma was introduced by Dahlin and Beabout[13] to refer to lesions in which there are both low-grade or borderline chondrosarcomatous areas juxtaposed to areas of high-grade spindle cell tissue. The term *dedifferentiated* has been considered to be inexact by several authors, because it is unlikely that the well-differentiated cartilaginous elements undergo a failure of differentiation. Biologically, it is more likely that a daughter clone of cells with spindle cell features develops from a common progenitor cell alongside the cartilaginous tissue. Although the label of "chondrosarcoma with additional mesenchymal component" may be biologically more correct,[97] the term dedifferentiated chondrosarcoma continues to be accepted as a clinicopathologic, diagnostic entity. Some authors include tumors with Grade 2 or Grade 3 cartilaginous components,[98] although this is not generally accepted.

Clinical Features

Dedifferentiated chondrosarcomas account for about 10% of all chondrosarcomas and present at similar ages and sites to conventional chondrosarcomas.

Molecular Genetics and Molecular Biology

Cytogenetic investigation of one case of dedifferentiated chondrosarcoma with a rhabdomyosarcomatous component showed similar chromosomal anomalies in each component, supporting the theory of a common mesenchymal progenitor cell that differentiates or expresses features of more than one line of differentiation.[99] Cytogenetic studies of two other cases showed a variety of changes, but both showed breaks and rearrangements involving 1p36[100]; whether this is of pathogenetic significance is uncertain.

Overexpression of p53 protein and a high labeling index with Ki67 and PCNA were described in the spindle-cell component of two cases of dedifferentiated chondrosarcoma.[101]

Radiologic Features

Dedifferentiated chondrosarcomas usually develop centrally within a bone but may rarely develop on the surface of bone.[102] The radiologic features reflect the biphasic morphology with a combination of indolent cortical thickening and endosteal scalloping adjacent to more aggressive cortical destruction and soft tissue infiltration. As the disease progresses, the more aggressive component may overwhelm and destroy the low-grade tissue. Extracompartmental spread is best assessed by MRI.

Pathologic Features

The typical dedifferentiated chondrosarcoma shows a biphasic pattern of irregular areas of cartilaginous tissue corresponding to a borderline or low-grade chondrosarcoma, adjacent to areas of high-grade spindle cell tissue that extensively permeates the adjacent bone and extends into soft tissues (Fig. 10–8). The spindle cell (mesenchymal) component may show features of fibrosarcoma, malignant fibrous histiocytoma, osteosarcoma, angiosarcoma, or rhabdomyosarcoma.[13, 97, 103–106] Some tumors also show many osteoclast-like giant cells in parts of the spindle cell tissue.[107, 108] Immunocytochemical studies confirm the features of the specific cell types. The expression of plasminogen activators and plasminogen activation inhibitor-1 in the high-grade component of dedifferentiated chondrosarcomas may be related to the capacity of these cells to proliferate and invade adjacent tissues.[109]

The diagnosis of dedifferentiated chondrosarcomas may be difficult if the pathologist is faced with small biopsy fragments of borderline or low-grade malignant cartilage and spindle cells, but review of the radiographs and recognition of an aggressive, partly calcified, partly lytic lesion should suggest the diagnosis.

Prognosis

Dedifferentiated chondrosarcoma is an aggressive neoplasm with a median survival of 6 months and a 5-year survival of about 10%.[17, 97, 106] Metastases are usually of the spindle-cell component and occur most commonly in the lungs, but other sites including bone, thyroid, and adrenal gland have been described.[97] Radical surgery is the main treatment option, and adjuvant radiation therapy or chemotherapy, although often used, appears to have little effect on prognosis.[97, 106]

DIFFERENTIAL DIAGNOSIS OF CHONDROSARCOMA

Fracture Callus

The reactive proliferation of cartilaginous tissue in fracture callus may simulate chondro-

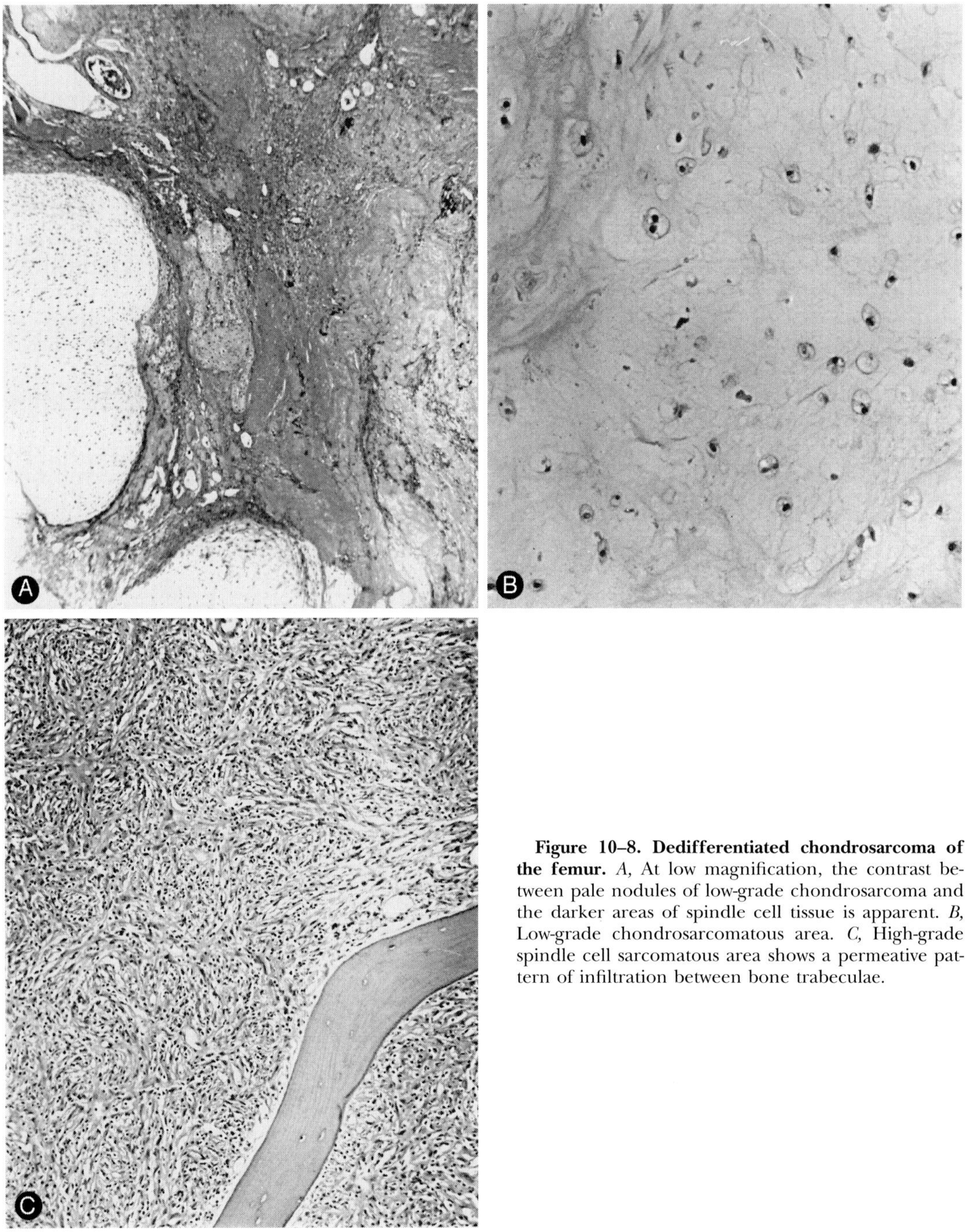

Figure 10–8. Dedifferentiated chondrosarcoma of the femur. *A,* At low magnification, the contrast between pale nodules of low-grade chondrosarcoma and the darker areas of spindle cell tissue is apparent. *B,* Low-grade chondrosarcomatous area. *C,* High-grade spindle cell sarcomatous area shows a permeative pattern of infiltration between bone trabeculae.

sarcoma through its high cellularity and the number of binucleate cells with plump nuclei (Fig. 10–9). A transition to areas of reactive, woven bone is often found but may not be present in small tissue samples. The pathologist should be provided with, or seek information on, the presence or absence of a pathologic fracture before attempting a diagnosis.

Costochondral Abnormalities

Prominence of the costochondral cartilage may lead to removal of tissue that is submitted for histologic opinion. Examination of such material shows hyaline cartilage of low cellularity with a clear line of demarcation from the underlying bone or evidence of a normal

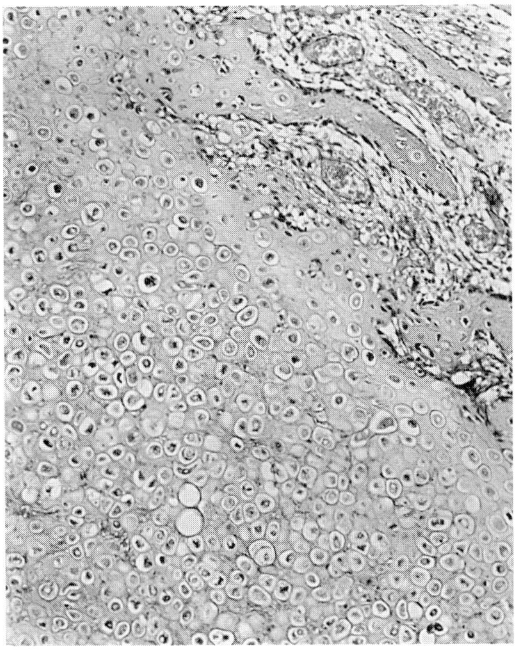

Figure 10–9. Fracture callus. Highly cellular cartilaginous tissue is present. The chondrocytes do not show cytologic atypia, and, at one edge, there is ossification with the formation of trabecular woven bone.

pattern of endochondral ossification. A normal radiologic appearance is reassuring.

Fracture of the costochondral junction of the ribs follows trauma and may produce a mass over the costochondral junction. Radiographs may be normal or may demonstrate a mass without destruction of the surrounding tissue. On biopsy, the fracture gap is surrounded by nodules of hyaline cartilage showing endochondral ossification and the adjacent rib is normal.[1]

Hamartoma (Mesenchymoma) of the Chest Wall

This lesion always presents on the chest wall of infants, leading to a mass that may interfere with breathing.[110, 111] Ribs at the center of the lesion are destroyed, and adjacent ribs may be deformed. Histologically, these lesions contain hypercellular cartilaginous areas that show endochondral ossification, trabeculae of spindle cells and bone, and aneurysmal vascular spaces. These hamartomatous lesions should not be overtreated, because they usually regress and the prognosis is good.

Fibrous Dysplasia

Cartilaginous nodules may occur within areas of monostotic and polyostotic fibrous dysplasia.[112, 113] This is most commonly observed in the proximal femur, where the ground-glass radiographic appearance of fibrous dysplasia has superimposed areas of "rim and arc" mineralization. Rarely, the cartilaginous tissue may be the dominant component of fibrous dysplasia (sometimes referred to as fibrocartilaginous dysplasia).[114, 115] The distinction from typical chondrosarcoma is made by the lack of atypia of the cartilaginous tissue and the architecture of the fibro-osseous areas, whereas dedifferentiated chondrosarcoma is excluded by the lack of cytologic atypia of the spindle cell component. Fibrous dysplasia is discussed in Chapter 13.

Fibrocartilaginous Mesenchymoma

Fibrocartilaginous mesenchymoma of bone is an extremely rare lesion that tends to affect the metaphyseal region of bones, particularly the proximal fibula. The lesion contains fibrous areas and islands of cartilage that show a pattern of organization reminiscent of epiphyseal growth plates.[116, 117] These are regarded as true neoplasms with locally aggressive behavior but that do not metastasize.

Polymorphic Fibro-osseous Lesion of the Femur

The polymorphic fibro-osseous lesion or liposclerosing myxofibrous tumor[118, 119] presents as a lucent area in the proximal femur associated with patchy central radiodensity and peripheral sclerosis. Biopsy specimens contain a complex and variable mixture of fibrous tissue and curvilinear bone trabeculae (as in fibrous dysplasia), but with mature and immature fat cells, cementum-like foci of bone, myxofibrous areas with cystic change, and cartilaginous nodules. The prognosis for these lesions is not determined; some appear to remain stable, whereas others may expand and cause pathologic fractures.

Chondroblastoma

Chondroblastoma is discussed in detail in Chapter 15. The presence of cartilaginous nodules in a cellular stroma composed of rounded or polygonal cells with scattered giant cells is a characteristic accompaniment to the typical radiologic appearance of a well-demarcated epiphyseal lesion. The overall picture is distinct from that of an enchondroma or clear cell chondrosarcoma, and the main differential diagnosis is with giant cell tumor of bone.

Chondromyxoid Fibroma

Chondromyxoid fibroma is discussed in detail in Chapter 15. This is an important histologic differential diagnosis with chondrosarcoma, owing to the presence of a lobular (zonal) growth pattern, of areas of high cellularity, and of cells with pleomorphic and hyperchromatic nuclei at the periphery of the nodules. The relatively young age of presentation (children and young adults) and the radiologic appearance of a sharply defined, purely lytic, metaphyseal lesion are most helpful in ensuring that the correct diagnosis is reached. In addition, chondromyxoid fibromas do not show the well-formed hyaline cartilage with lacunar chondrocytes seen in chondrosarcomas.[12]

Mesenchymal Chondrosarcoma

Mesenchymal chondrosarcoma is an uncommon form of chondrosarcoma, first described by Lichtenstein and Bernstein,[14] that occurs over a wide age range, most commonly in the second to fourth decades of life. The most common skeletal sites are the mandible, vertebra, ribs, pelvic bones, and femur,[21, 120] and it is rare in the extremities.[121] Radiologic features are of a lytic and destructive process that may contain stippled calcification. Cortical destruction and soft tissue extension are often present. The histologic features are those of sheets of undifferentiated small cells with small or large foci of differentiated cartilage (Fig. 10–10). The small cells have oval nuclei, are separated by a pericellular reticulin network, and are arranged in a vaguely alveolar or herringbone pattern, or with a hemangiopericytomatous pattern of cells separated by large vascular spaces. The cartilage is usually of low-grade malignancy cytologically, and reactive osteoid and bone formation may be present.

Immunocytochemical studies show labeling for S-100 protein in the cartilaginous nodules

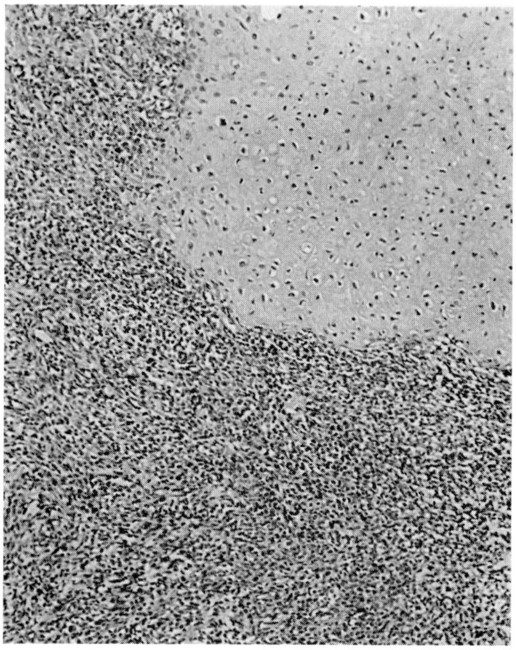

Figure 10–10. Mesenchymal chondrosarcoma. The diagnosis is made by the presence of pale nodules of low-grade chondrosarcoma surrounded by sheets of malignant small ovoid cells.

but usually in very few of the small cells; neuron-specific enolase is also present in both small cell and cartilaginous areas.[122] The *MIC2* gene product, CD99, is expressed in the small cells of mesenchymal chondrosarcomas.[123] Immunocytochemical studies therefore have only a limited role in the differential diagnosis of mesenchymal chondrosarcoma from other lesions, such as Ewing's sarcoma, peripheral neuroectodermal tumor, hemangiopericytoma, or rhabdomyosarcoma. The morphologic identification of cartilaginous nodules in adequate biopsy material remains the basis for diagnosis (see Chapter 14).

These are aggressive sarcomas, with metastases occurring in 60% of patients. The 5-year survival is about 60% and the 10-year survival rate is about 28%, but recurrent and metastatic tumors may be fatal up to 20 years after diagnosis. Radical surgery is the main treatment, although radiation therapy and chemotherapy may also have a role.[21, 120]

Myxoid Chondrosarcoma

Skeletal neoplasms that resemble histologically the myxoid chondrosarcoma (chordoid sarcoma) of soft tissues are extremely rare. The very few well-documented cases appear to be aggressive neoplasms that recur locally and develop distant metastases.[124] Immunocytochemical studies showed focal labeling for S-100 protein with no labeling for cytokeratin (AE1/AE3), factor VIII, or CD31.

Chondroblastic Osteosarcoma

The distinction of chondroblastic osteosarcoma from chondrosarcoma is important for the selection of the appropriate treatment regimen. On paraffin-embedded tissues, the presence of even a small amount of osteoid around malignant cells is sufficient to make the diagnosis of osteosarcoma. Biopsy samples from some osteosarcomas may show malignant cartilaginous tissue with no evidence of tumor bone formation. Because chondrosarcoma is rare in children and adolescents, the age and imaging appearances are important in establishing a diagnosis. The cartilage of a chondroblastic osteosarcoma is easily identified by virtue of the septal enhancement seen on Gd-DPTA–enhanced MRI.[125] If fresh tissue is available from the biopsy, histochemical staining for alkaline phosphatase may suggest the presence of osteoblastic differentiation of the malignant cells.

Some osteosarcomas contain foci of cells with clear cytoplasm resulting from glycogen accumulation.[95] The presence of an osteolytic, destructive, diaphyseal, or metaphyseal lesion radiologically, the presence of atypical osteoblastic tissue, and the lack of immunolabeling for S-100 protein should suggest the diagnosis of osteosarcoma. Clear cell chondrosarcoma can be associated with a high serum level of alkaline phosphatase, which should not be taken as suggestive of osteosarcoma.[96]

Malignant Mesenchymoma

Malignant mesenchymoma is a very rare neoplasm of bone that is defined as a sarcoma containing two or more unrelated lines of cellular differentiation, with the exclusion of fibrosarcoma. Tumors arising in bone may show osteosarcomatous, liposarcomatous, or rhabdomyosarcomatous areas and occasionally include areas of atypical cartilage that are usually regarded as a chondroblastic part of the osteosarcomatous element.[126]

Chordoma

The potential for chondroid differentiation within chordomas of the axial skeleton may lead to confusion with chondrosarcomas (see Chapter 17). The identification of more typical chordomatous tissue and the presence of immunocytochemical labeling for cytokeratins (and in some cases for epithelial membrane antigen) support the diagnosis of chordoma.[127–129] Immunocytochemical labeling for vimentin and for S-100 protein may occur in both chordomas and chondrosarcomas. The clinical relevance of making this pathologic distinction remains uncertain, because both lesions have similar long-term survival.[130]

REFERENCES

1. Schiller AL: Diagnosis of borderline cartilage lesions of bone. Semin Diagn Pathol 2:42, 1985.
2. Reid R: New developments in the diagnosis of chondrosarcoma [editorial]. J Pathol 163:93, 1991.
3. Ayala AG, Ro JY, Fanning CV, et al: Core needle biopsy and fine-needle aspiration in the diagnosis of bone and soft-tissue lesions. Hematol Oncol Clin North Am 9:633, 1995.
4. Paget J: Tumours. *In* Lectures on Surgical Pathology. London, Longman, Brown, Green & Longmans, 1853, p 171.
5. Ollier M: Exostoses osteogeniques multiples. Lyon Med 88:484, 1889.
6. Ollier M: Dyschondroplasie. Lyon Med 93:23, 1900.
7. Maffucci A: Di un caso di encondroma ed angioma multiple: Contribuzione alla genesi embrionale dei tumori. Mov Med Chir 13:399, 1881.
8. Cooper A: Exostosis. *In* Cooper A, Travers B (eds): Surgical essays. 3rd ed. London, Cox & Son, 1818, p 155.
9. Ewing J: A review of the classification of bone tumors. Surg Gynecol Obstet 68:971, 1939.
10. Phemister DB: Chondrosarcoma of bone. Surg Gynecol Obstet 50:216, 1930.
11. Lichtenstein L, Jaffe HL: Chondrosarcoma of bone. Am J Pathol 19:553, 1943.
12. Barnes R, Catto M: Chondrosarcoma of bone. J Bone Joint Surg 48B:729, 1966.
13. Dahlin DC, Beabout JW: Dedifferentiation of low-grade chondrosarcomas. Cancer 28:461, 1971.
14. Lichtenstein L, Bernstein D: Unusual benign and malignant chondroid tumours of bone. Cancer 12:1142, 1959.
15. Unni KK: Chondroma. *In* Dahlin's Bone Tumors: General Aspects and Data on 11,087 Cases. 5th ed. Philadelphia, Lippincott-Raven, 1996, p 25.
16. Mirra JM, Gold R, Downs J, et al: A new histologic approach to the differentiation of enchondroma and chondrosarcoma of the bones. Clin Orthop Rel Res 201:214, 1985.
17. Unni KK: Chondrosarcoma. *In* Dahlin's Bone Tumors: General Aspects and Data on 11,087 Cases. 5th ed. Philadelphia, Lippincott-Raven, 1996, p 71.

18. Dorfman HD, Czerniak B: Bone cancers. Cancer 75(Suppl 1):203, 1995.
19. Young CL, Sim FH, Unni KK, et al: Chondrosarcoma of bone in children. Cancer 66:1641, 1990.
20. Damron TA, Sim FH, Unni KK: Multicentric chondrosarcomas. Clin Orthop Rel Res 328:211, 1996.
21. Nakashima Y, Unni KK, Shives TC, et al: Mesenchymal chondrosarcoma of bone and soft tissue: A review of 111 cases. Cancer 57:2444, 1986.
22. Milgram JW: The origins of osteochondromas and enchondromas: A histopathologic study. Clin Orthop Rel Res 174:264, 1983.
23. Pritchard DJ, Lunke RJ, Taylor WF, et al: Chondrosarcoma: A clinicopathologic and statistical analysis. Cancer 45:149, 1980.
24. Liu J, Hudkins PG, Swee RG, et al: Bone sarcomas associated with Ollier's disease. Cancer 59:1376, 1987.
25. Suringa DWR, Ackerman AB: Cutaneous lymphangiomas with dyschondroplasia (Maffucci's syndrome). Arch Dermatol 101:472, 1970.
26. Albreghts AE, Rapini RP: Malignancy in Maffucci's syndrome. Dermatol Clin North Am 13:73, 1995.
27. Wick MR, Siegal GP, Unni KK, et al: Sarcomas of bone complicating osteitis deformans (Paget's disease): Fifty years' experience. Am J Surg Pathol 5:47, 1981.
28. Schajowicz F, Santini Araujo E, Berenstein M: Sarcoma complicating Paget's disease of bone: A clinicopathological study of 62 cases. J Bone Joint Surg 65B:299, 1983.
29. Haibach H, Farrell C, Dittrich FJ: Neoplasms arising in Paget's disease of bone: A study of 82 cases. Am J Clin Pathol 83:594, 1985.
30. Ruggieri P, Sim FH, Bond JR, et al: Malignancies in fibrous dysplasia. Cancer 73:1411, 1994.
31. Schwarz RE, Burt M: Radiation-associated malignant tumors of the chest wall. Ann Surg Oncol 3:387, 1996.
32. Ron IG, Amir G, Inbar MJ, et al: Clear cell chondrosarcoma of rib following repetitive low-impact trauma. Am J Clin Oncol 18:87, 1995.
33. Mandahl N, Heim S, Arheden K, et al: Chromosomal rearrangements in chondromatous tumors. Cancer 65:242, 1990.
34. Orndal C, Mandahl N, Rydholm A, et al: Chromosome alterations and cytogenetic intratumor heterogeneity in chondrosarcomas. J Cancer Res Clin Oncol 120:51, 1993.
35. Larramendy ML, Tarkkanen M, Valle J, et al: Gains, losses, and amplifications of DNA sequences evaluated by comparative genomic hybridization in chondrosarcomas. Am J Pathol 150:685, 1997.
36. Yamaguchi T, Toguchida J, Wadayama B, et al: Loss of heterozygosity and tumor suppressor gene mutations in chondrosarcomas. Anticancer Res 16:2009, 1996.
37. Raskind WH, Conrad EU, Chansky H, et al: Loss of heterozygosity in chondrosarcomas for markers linked to hereditary multiple exostosis loci on chromosomes 8 and 11. Am J Hum Genet 56:1132, 1995.
38. Kreicbergs A, Boquist L, Borssen B, et al: Prognostic factors in chondrosarcoma: A comparative study of cellular DNA content and clinicopathologic features. Cancer 50:577, 1982.
39. Helio H, Karaharju E, Bohling T, et al: Chondrosarcoma of bone: A clinical and DNA flow cytometric study. Eur J Surg Oncol 21:408, 1995.
40. Coughlin B, Feliz A, Ishida T, et al: p53 expression and DNA ploidy of cartilage lesions. Hum Pathol 26:620, 1995.
41. Adler CP, Herget GW, Neuburger M: Cartilaginous tumors: Prognostic applications of cytophotometric DNA analysis. Cancer 76:1176, 1995.
42. Mankin HJ, Connor JF, Schiller AL, et al: Grading of bone tumors by analysis of nuclear DNA content using flow cytometry. J Bone Joint Surg 67A:404, 1985.
43. Hasegawa T, Seki K, Yang P, et al: Differentiation and proliferative activity in benign and malignant cartilage tumors of bone. Hum Pathol 26:838, 1995.
44. Chano T, Ishizawa M, Matsumoto K, et al: The identity of proliferating cells in bone tumors with cartilaginous components: Evaluation by double-immunohistochemical staining using proliferating cell nuclear antigen and S-100 protein. Eur J Histochem 39:21, 1995.
45. Nawa G, Ueda T, Mori S, et al: Prognostic significance of Ki67 (MIB1) proliferation index and p53 over-expression in chondrosarcomas. Int J Cancer 69:86, 1996.
46. Scotlandi K, Serra M, Manara MC, et al: Clinical relevance of Ki-67 expression in bone tumors. Cancer 75:806, 1995.
47. Clohisy JC, Schajowicz F, Vaziri DM, et al: Assessment of argyrophilic nucleolar organizer region quantification in benign and malignant bone tumors. Clin Orthop Rel Res 310:229, 1995.
48. Dobashi Y, Sugimura H, Sato A, et al: Possible association of p53 overexpression and mutation with high-grade chondrosarcoma. Diagn Mol Pathol 2:257, 1993.
49. Wadayama B, Toguchida T, Yamaguchi T, et al: p53 expression and its relationship to DNA alterations in bone and soft tissue sarcomas. Br J Cancer 68:1134, 1993.
50. King P, Craft AW, Malcolm AJ: p53 expression in three separate tumours from a patient with Li-Fraumeni's syndrome. J Clin Pathol 46:676, 1993.
51. Oda Y, Walter H, Radig K, et al: Immunohistochemical analysis of nm23 protein expression in malignant bone tumors. J Cancer Res Clin Oncol 121:667, 1995.
52. Scotlandi K, Baldini N, Oliviero M, et al: Expression of Met/hepatocyte growth factor receptor gene and malignant behavior of musculoskeletal tumors. Am J Pathol 149:1209, 1996.
53. Pompetti F, Rizzo P, Simon RM, et al: Oncogene alterations in primary, recurrent, and metastatic human bone tumors. J Cell Biochem 63:37, 1996.
54. Barrios C, Castresana JS, Falkmer UG, et al: *C-myc* oncogene amplification and cytometric DNA ploidy pattern as prognostic factors in musculoskeletal neoplasms. Int J Cancer 58:781, 1994.
55. Wang ZQ, Grigoriadis AE, Mohle Steinlein U, et al: A novel target cell for c-*fos*-induced oncogenesis: Development of chondrogenic tumours in embryonic stem cell chimeras. EMBO J 10:2437, 1991.
56. Wrba F, Gullick WJ, Fertl H, et al: Immunohistochemical detection of the c-*erb*B-2 proto-oncogene product in normal, benign and malignant cartilage tissues. Histopathology 15:71, 1989.
57. Davis RI, Foster H, Biggart DJ: C-*erb* B-2 staining in primary synovial chondromatosis: A comparison with other cartilaginous tumours. J Pathol 179:392, 1996.
58. Battifora H: c-*erb*B-2 proto-oncogene product. Histopathology 16:105, 1990.

59. Mankin HJ, Cantley KP, Schiller AL, et al: The biology of human chondrosarcoma: II. Variation in chemical composition among types and subtypes of benign and malignant cartilage tumors. J Bone Joint Surg 62A:176, 1980.
60. Mankin HJ, Cantley KP, Lippiello L, et al: The biology of human chondrosarcomas: I. Description of the cases, grading and biochemical analyses. J Bone Joint Surg 62A:160, 1980.
61. Monda L, Wick MR: S-100 protein immunostaining in the differential diagnosis of chondroblastoma. Hum Pathol 16:287, 1985.
62. Okajima K, Honda I, Kitagawa T: Immunohistochemical distribution of S-100 protein in tumors and tumor-like lesions of bone and cartilage. Cancer 61:792, 1988.
63. Weiss A-PC, Dorfman HD: S-100 protein in human cartilage lesions. J Bone Joint Surg 68A:521, 1986.
64. Iwasaki R, Yamamuro T, Kotourar Y, et al: Immunohistochemical study of bone GLA protein in primary bone tumours. Cancer 70:619, 1992.
65. Serra M, Morini MC, Scotlandi K, et al: Evaluation of osteonectin as a diagnostic marker of osteogenic bone tumors. Hum Pathol 23:1326, 1992.
66. Park YK, Yang MH, Park HR: The impact of osteonectin for differential diagnosis of osteogenic bone tumors: An immunohistochemical and in situ hybridization approach. Skeletal Radiol 25:13, 1996.
67. Kawashima A, Okada Y, Nakanishi I, et al: Immunolocalization of matrix metalloproteinases and tissue inhibitors of metalloproteinases in human chondrosarcomas. Gen Diagn Pathol 142:129, 1997.
68. Ragsdale BD, Sweet DE, Vinh TN: Radiology as gross pathology in evaluating chondroid lesions. Hum Pathol 20:930, 1989.
69. Geirnaerdt MJA, Bloem JL, Eulderink F, et al: Cartilaginous tumors: Correlation of gadolinium-enhanced MR imaging and histopathologic findings. Radiology 186:813, 1993.
70. Ueda Y, Oda Y, Tsuchiya H, et al: Immunohistological study on collagenous proteins of benign and malignant human cartilaginous tumours of bone. Virchows Arch (A) 417:291, 1990.
71. Evans HL, Ayala AG, Romsdahl MM: Prognostic factors in chondrosarcoma of bone: A clinicopathologic analysis with emphasis on histologic grading. Cancer 40:818, 1977.
72. Sanerkin NG, Gallagher P: A review of the behaviour of chondrosarcoma of bone. J Bone Joint Surg 61B:395, 1979.
73. Meachim G: Histological grading of chondrosarcomata. J Bone Joint Surg 61B:393, 1979.
74. Tsuchiya H, Ueda Y, Morishita H, et al: Borderline chondrosarcoma of long and flat bones. J Cancer Res Clin Oncol 119:363, 1993.
75. Feaux de Lacroix W, Dietlein M, Schmidt J, et al: Histological investigation for comparison of cartilaginous tumors of unknown biological course with unequivocal chondrosarcomas. Zentralbl Pathol 138:339, 1992.
76. Saito K, Unni KK, Wollan PC, et al: Chondrosarcoma of the jaw and facial bones. Cancer 76:1550, 1995.
77. Clark JL, Unni KK, Dahlin DC, et al: Osteosarcoma of the jaw. Cancer 51:2311, 1983.
78. Molla MR, Ijuhin N, Sugata T, et al: Chondrosarcoma of the jaw: Report of two cases. J Oral Maxillofac Surg 45:453, 1987.
79. Damron TA, Rock MG, Unni KK: Subcutaneous involvement after a metacarpal chondrosarcoma. Clin Orthop Rel Res 316:189, 1995.
80. Roberts PH, Price CHG: Chondrosarcoma of the bones of the hand. J Bone Joint Surg 59B:213, 1977.
81. Ozaki T, Hillmann A, Linder N, et al: Metastasis of chondrosarcoma. J Cancer Res Clin Oncol 122:629, 1996.
82. Disler DG, Rosenberg AE, Springfield D, et al: Extensive skeletal metastases from chondrosarcoma without pulmonary involvement. Skeletal Radiol 22:595, 1993.
83. Ozaki T, Lindner N, Hillmann A, et al: Influence of intralesional surgery on treatment outcome of chondrosarcoma. Cancer 77:1292, 1996.
84. Sheth DS, Yasko AW, Johnson ME, et al: Chondrosarcoma of the pelvis: Prognostic factors for 67 patients treated with definitive surgery. Cancer 78:745, 1996.
85. Unni KK, Dahlin DC, Beabout JW, et al: Chondrosarcoma: Clear-cell variant: A report of sixteen cases. J Bone Joint Surg 58A:676, 1976.
86. Le Charpentier Y, Forest M, Postel M, et al: Clear-cell chondrosarcoma: A report of five cases including ultrastructural study. Cancer 44:622, 1979.
87. Bjornsson J, Unni KK, Dahlin DC, et al: Clear cell chondrosarcoma of bone: Observations in 47 cases. Am J Surg Pathol 8:223, 1984.
88. Sreekantaiah C, Leong SP, Davis JR, et al: Cytogenetic and flow cytometric analysis of a clear cell chondrosarcoma. Cancer Genet Cytogenet 52:193, 1991.
89. Ogose A, Motoyama T, Hotta T, et al: Clear cell chondrosarcomas arising from rare sites. Pathol Int 45:684, 1995.
90. Present DA, Bonar SF, Greenspan A, et al: Clear-cell chondrosarcoma: An unusual case complicated by a microinfiltrative pattern of bone marrow involvement and postsurgical myositis ossificans. Clin Orthop Rel Res 237:164, 1988.
91. Faraggiana T, Sender B, Glicksman P: Light- and electron-microscopic study of clear cell chondrosarcoma. Am J Clin Pathol 75:117, 1981.
92. Ohno T, Park P, Oguro K, et al: Ultrastructural study of a clear cell chondrosarcoma. Ultrastruct Pathol 10:321, 1986.
93. Aigner T, Dertinger S, Belke J, et al: Chondrocytic cell differentiation in clear cell chondrosarcoma. Hum Pathol 27:1301, 1996.
94. Bosse A, Ueda Y, Wuisman P, et al: Histogenesis of clear cell chondrosarcoma: An immunohistochemical study with osteonectin, a non-collagenous structure protein. J Cancer Res Clin Oncol 117:43, 1991.
95. Povysil C, Matejovsky Z, Zidkova H: Osteosarcoma with a clear-cell component. Virchows Arch (A) 412:273, 1988.
96. Brien EW, Mirra JM, Ippolito V, et al: Clear-cell chondrosarcoma with elevated alkaline phosphatase, mistaken for osteosarcoma on biopsy. Skeletal Radiol 25:770, 1996.
97. Johnson S, Tetu B, Ayala AG, et al: Chondrosarcoma with additional mesenchymal component (dedifferentiated chondrosarcoma): I. A clinicopathologic study of 26 cases. Cancer 58:278, 1986.
98. Capanna R, Bertoni F, Bettelli G, et al: Dedifferentiated chondrosarcoma. J Bone Joint Surg 70A:60, 1988.
99. Bridge JA, DeBoer J, Travis J, et al: Simultaneous interphase cytogenetic analysis and fluorescence immunophenotyping of dedifferentiated chondrosar-

coma: Implications for histopathogenesis. Am J Pathol 144:215, 1994.
100. Zalupski MM, Ensley JF, Ryan J, et al: A common cytogenetic abnormality and DNA content alterations in dedifferentiated chondrosarcoma. Cancer 66:1176, 1990.
101. Simms WW, Ordonez NG, Johnston D, et al: p53 expression in dedifferentiated chondrosarcoma. Cancer 76:223, 1995.
102. Bertoni F, Present D, Bacchini P, et al: Dedifferentiated peripheral chondrosarcoma. Cancer 63:2054, 1989.
103. Dervan PA, O'Loughlin J, Hurson BJ: Dedifferentiated chondrosarcoma with muscle and cytokeratin differentiation in the anaplastic component. Histopathology 12:517, 1988.
104. Reith JD, Bauer TW, Fischler DF, et al: Dedifferentiated chondrosarcoma with rhabdomyosarcomatous differentiation. Am J Surg Pathol 20:293, 1996.
105. Tetu B, Ordonez NG, Ayala AG, et al: Chondrosarcoma with additional mesenchymal component (dedifferentiated chondrosarcoma): II. An immunohistochemical and electron microscopic study. Cancer 58:287, 1986.
106. Mercuri M, Picci P, Campanacci L, et al: Dedifferentiated chondrosarcoma. Skeletal Radiol 24:409, 1995.
107. Sissons HA, Matlen JA, Lewis MM: Dedifferentiated chondrosarcoma: Report of an unusual case. J Bone Joint Surg 73A:294, 1991.
108. Ishida T, Dorfman HD, Habermann ET: Dedifferentiated chondrosarcoma of humerus with giant cell tumor-like features. Skeletal Radiol 24:76, 1995.
109. Hackel C, Czerniak B, Ayala AG, et al: Expression of plasminogen activators and plasminogen activator inhibitor 1 in dedifferentiated chondrosarcoma. Cancer 79:53, 1997.
110. Mcleod RA, Dahlin DC: Hamartoma (mesenchymoma) of the chest wall in infancy. Radiology 131:657, 1979.
111. Baretton G, Stehr M, Nerlich A, et al: Chest wall hamartoma in infancy: A case report with immunohistochemical analysis of various interstitial collagen types. Pediatr Pathol 14:3, 1994.
112. Lichtenstein L, Jaffe HL: Fibrous dysplasia of bone. Arch Pathol 33:777, 1942.
113. Harris WH, Dudley HR, Barry RJ: The natural history of fibrous dysplasia—an orthopaedic, pathological, and roentgenographic study. J Bone Joint Surg 44A:207, 1962.
114. Ishida T, Dorfman HD: Massive chondroid differentiation in fibrous dysplasia of bone (fibrocartilaginous dysplasia). Am J Surg Pathol 17:924, 1993.
115. Hermann G, Klein M, Abdelwahab IF, et al: Fibrocartilaginous dysplasia. Skeletal Radiol 25:509, 1996.
116. Bulychova IV, Unni KK, Bertoni F, et al: Fibrocartilaginous mesenchymoma of bone. Am J Surg Pathol 17:830, 1993.
117. Dahlin DC, Bertoni F, Beabout JW, et al: Fibrocartilaginous mesenchymoma with low-grade malignancy. Skeletal Radiol 12:263, 1984.
118. Gilkey FW: Liposclerosing myxofibrous tumor of bone. Hum Pathol 24:1264, 1993.
119. Ragsdale BD: Polymorphic fibro-osseous lesions of bone: An almost site-specific diagnostic problem of the proximal femur. Hum Pathol 24:505, 1993.
120. Takahashi K, Sato K, Kanazawa H, et al: Mesenchymal chondrosarcoma of the jaw—report of a case and review of 41 cases in the literature. Head & Neck 15:459, 1993.
121. Sans M, Nubiola D, Alejo M, et al: Mesenchymal chondrosarcoma of the foot, an unusual location: Case report and review of the literature. Med Pediatr Oncol 26:139, 1996.
122. Swanson PE, Lillemoe TJ, Manivel JC: Mesenchymal chondrosarcoma: An immunohistochemical study. Arch Pathol Lab Med 114:943, 1990.
123. Granter SR, Renshaw AA, Fletcher CD, et al: CD99 reactivity in mesenchymal chondrosarcoma. Hum Pathol 27:1273, 1996.
124. Kilpatrick SE, Inwards CY, Fletcher CD, et al: Myxoid chondrosarcoma (chordoid sarcoma) of bone: A report of two cases and review of the literature. Cancer 79:1903, 1997.
125. Bloem JL, Reisre M, Vanel D: MRI contrast agents in the evaluation of the musculo-skeletal system. Magn Res Q 6:136, 1990.
126. Kessler S, Mirra JM, Ishii T, et al: Primary malignant mesenchymoma of bone: Case report, literature review, and distinction of this entity from mesenchymal and dedifferentiated chondrosarcoma. Skeletal Radiol 24:291, 1995.
127. Nabeshima K, Sato S, Sameshima T, et al: Intraoperative squash and touch cytology of chondroid chordoma of the skull base: Report of a case with immunocytochemical and immunohistochemical studies. Acta Cytol 41:913, 1997.
128. Rosenberg AE, Brown GA, Bhan AK, et al: Chondroid chordoma—a variant of chordoma: A morphologic and immunohistochemical study. Am J Clin Pathol 101:36, 1994.
129. Wojno KJ, Hruban RH, Garin-Chesa P, et al: Chondroid chordomas and low-grade chondrosarcomas of the craniospinal axis. Am J Surg Pathol 16:1144, 1992.
130. Mitchell A, Scheithauer BW, Unni KK, et al: Chordoma and chondroid neoplasms of the spheno-occiput: An immunohistochemical study of 41 cases with prognostic and nosologic implications. Cancer 72:2943, 1993.

Chapter

11

BONE NEOPLASMS AND TUMOR-LIKE LESIONS ON THE BONE SURFACE

ROBIN P. REID

Whereas most bone tumors and tumor-like lesions arise within the medullary canal, a variety of tumors can occur on the bone surface,[1] including the most common primary bone "tumor," osteocartilaginous exostosis. In addition, reactive conditions are common at this site, rendering it an area rich in diagnostic pitfalls. It must be emphasized that the pathologist confronted with a biopsy sample from the surface of a bone is no less dependent on full clinical and radiologic information than when examining material derived from the medullary canal. In this chapter, the discussion will concentrate mainly on those tumors and reactive conditions that typically arise in relation to the periosteum and adjacent soft tissue. Those that are rare on the bone surface but occur more commonly at other sites will receive only brief mention here and are discussed fully in the appropriate chapters.

The nomenclature of surface lesions is confusing, and definition of terms is required.[1] Lesions can be found in any of the anatomic planes and may give rise to different reactions from the surrounding normal tissues, depending on the precise location and the rate of growth of the lesion. From within outwards, there are four planes:

- **Cortical** lesions arise in the bone cortex and often extend beneath or through the periosteum. These are not discussed in this chapter.
- **Subperiosteal** lesions form in the potential space between the cortex and the periosteum. They lift the periosteum, which responds by laying down bone in a variety of patterns depending on the speed of the process.
- **Periosteal** lesions arise from the deep layer of the periosteum and also provoke periosteal bone formation.
- **Parosteal** lesions are believed to arise from the outer part of the periosteum outside the cambium layer of the periosteum and do not stimulate an overlying periosteal reaction.

The term *juxtacortical* is a useful generic term for lesions on the surface of bone when a more specific anatomic origin cannot be determined. The tendency of tumors arising on the bone surface to invade the underlying medulla gives rise to another conceptual difficulty. It could be argued that any such tumor should be regarded as a central tumor with soft-tissue extension, but in general it is agreed that if the epicenter of the tumor lies outside the cortex, then a juxtacortical origin can be accepted.

REACTIVE TUMOR-LIKE LESIONS

Reactive Subperiosteal New Bone Formation

It may seem strange to start this section with such a nonspecific topic, but the distinction of reactive from tumor bone is of critical importance. Active subperiosteal new bone formation, whatever the cause, can be confused with a bone-forming neoplasm because the osteoblasts are large and the matrix is primitive. The reassuring development of an oriented trabecular architecture with osteoblastic rimming and foci of more mature bone is more apparent on low-power examination. Not infrequently a biopsy of a suspected tumor is too superficial and shows reactive new bone only: the pathologist must not overinterpret this but rather ask for a deeper biopsy sample. The radiologic appearances of a periosteal reaction to an underlying bone neoplasm are shown in Chapter 6, Figure 6–11.

Fracture Callus

External fracture callus may give rise to diagnostic difficulty, especially if it is presented to the pathologist in the early days after injury as a soft tissue mass and without the relevant history. Under these circumstances, it is too easy to overdiagnose the lesion as a sarcoma. The appearances are of a "tissue culture" of unoriented plump spindle and stellate cells with prominent nucleoli, rich in normal mitoses, lying in a pale-staining myxoid matrix and infiltrating between skeletal muscle fibers. In places the spindle cells may be plumper, aggregated in small clusters around short, branching stands of faintly eosinophilic primitive osteoid matrix. Small lobules of cartilage with plump and sometimes binucleate cells may also be present. These features may suggest an osteosarcoma or, before matrix forms, a myxoid soft-tissue sarcoma. Later, the mitotic activity lessens, recognizable woven bone trabeculae rimmed by osteoblasts appear, and orientation may develop in a parallel stranded or arcade pattern. Diagnostic difficulty then tends to center around the islands of cartilage, the cells of which have plump, open nuclei, sometimes two to a cell (Fig. 11–1). Reassuringly, however, the cartilage typically merges with the maturing woven bone. The presence of foci of hemorrhage, hemosiderin, fibrin, and fragments of dead bone from the fracture site may alert the pathologist to the possibility of callus; once considered, the differential diagnosis is not difficult. As always, review of the clinical history and radiologic images further diminishes the chance of a potentially catastrophic histopathologic error.

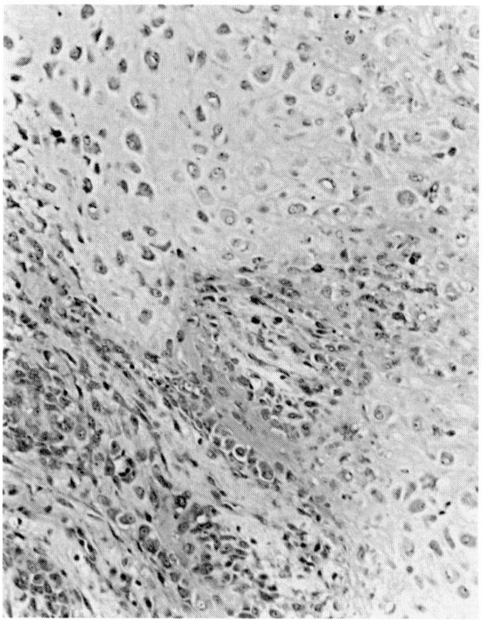

Figure 11–1. Fracture callus. Abundant cartilage may form at a fracture site, particularly when there is excessive movement. The cartilage in this callus shows significant cytologic atypia, but the pattern in which the cartilage merges with reactive bone is a clue that the tissue is reactive.

Stress Fracture

Stress fractures typically affect the metatarsals (march fracture) or the junction between the upper and middle thirds of the tibia and occur in individuals who have taken unaccustomed or excessive exercise.[2] Stress fractures of the femoral shaft, particularly in children, are less well recognized.[3] Clinically recognized stress fractures are seldom subject to biopsy, so when the pathologist receives tissue from one, it is usually because the surgeon suspects or wishes to exclude a malignant bone tumor. The concern is evoked by the patient's complaint of pain and, in the absence of a recognizable fracture line, the radiologic appearance of a periosteal reaction with multiple parallel lamellae (onion skinning) or a Codman's reactive triangle. Sometimes there is an ill-defined zone of sclerosis in the adjacent medulla and an extensive area of abnormal intramedullary signal on magnetic resonance imaging (MRI), appearances that raise the possibility of an osteosarcoma or Ewing's sarcoma. The biopsy material may consist only of reactive new bone, perhaps with cartilage, and a specific histologic diagnosis cannot be reached. If the biopsy material contains the stress fracture itself, it can be identified as a crack in the cortex that may extend into the periosteal new bone; the presence of fibrin within the defect and a surrounding callus reaction distinguish the stress fracture from an artifactual crack in the section.

Myositis Ossificans (Pseudomalignant Osseous Tumor of Soft Tissues; Periostitis Ossificans; Florid Reactive Periostitis; Fibro-Osseous Pseudotumor of Digits)

This section discusses a group of pseudomalignant reactive lesions with similar histologic features of proliferating fibroblastic tissue with focal formation of bone and sometimes cartilage. The nomenclature of these lesions is confusing, reflecting the different anatomic sites, but the basic process appears to be the same in each. In its classic form, myositis ossificans occurs deep within skeletal muscle, particularly of the buttock and thigh, where it simulates a soft-tissue sarcoma.[4] It is often close enough to the underlying bone to induce a periosteal reaction, and in a proportion of cases particularly of long bones, the lesion itself lies close to the periosteum and may be confused with bone surface tumors, especially parosteal osteosarcoma. The term *periostitis ossificans* has been applied to such cases. Similar lesions within the hands and feet have been referred to as florid reactive periostitis[5] and fibro-osseous pseudotumor of digits.[6]

Myositis ossificans typically affects young adults; around one-half give a definite history of trauma to the area 1 to 4 weeks before the mass appears, but the cause of the lesion in the remaining patients is unknown. The short history and rapid growth of the lesion raise clinical suspicion of malignancy and, like those of other reactive conditions, the histologic appearance may be equally alarming, particularly in the early stages of the lesion. In one-third of patients an infective origin is considered and antibiotics are prescribed on the basis of local heat and tenderness with elevation of the erythrocyte sedimentation rate, neutrophil leukocytosis, and, occasionally, mild fever.

Radiologic Appearances

Early in the evolution of the lesion, plain radiographs are normal or show a soft-tissue mass, better demonstrated by computed tomography (CT) or MRI.[7] Within a few weeks, focal ossification develops in soft tissue or close to the periosteum. Lesions in deep soft tissue form a round or oval mass, with ossification most marked at the periphery, although a linear periosteal reaction may be present on the adjacent bone. Progressive maturation occurs in a few weeks to a benign-looking lesion in which a pattern of bony trabeculae can be seen.[8] In lesions close to bone (periostitis ossificans) this regular linear ossification has been described as a "dotted veil" (see Chapter 6, Fig. 6–13).

Pathologic Appearances

The histology of myositis ossificans reflects the changing radiologic appearances. In the early stage, proliferating fibroblasts are seen in a loose myxoid background. The cells have the "tissue culture" appearance associated with other reactive conditions such as fracture callus and nodular fasciitis. Although mitotic figures are numerous, they are normal in form, and the cells show little atypia. In areas, the cells "round up" to assume an osteoblastic phenotype and are associated with a primitive osteoid matrix, which is often present in linear strands well demonstrated by viewing in plane-polarized light.[9] Only tiny foci of more mature, often lightly calcified, woven bone may be present. It is at this early stage, when the clinical and radiologic appearances are most worrying, that the risk of an erroneous diagnosis of malignancy is highest, especially when the appearances occur at an unusual age or site.[10] Later, the zoning phenomenon, beautifully described by Ackerman,[4] becomes more apparent. Three concentric zones are seen: an innermost actively proliferating fibroblastic area, an intermediate zone of active osteoblasts and primitive osteoid, and an outer shell of fairly mature woven bone sometimes with nodules of cartilage (Fig. 11–2). Recognition of this zoning pattern with peripheral maturation is one of the keys to the diagnosis; in parosteal osteosarcoma, in contrast, the most mature bone lies in the depths of the lesion, with the spindle cell areas at the periphery. It must be remembered that zoning is poorly defined in early lesions and in lesions in the hands. In addition, even when well developed, the zoning need not be complete, so that proliferating spindle-celled areas may, focally, lie at the margin of the lesion and infiltrate skeletal muscle.

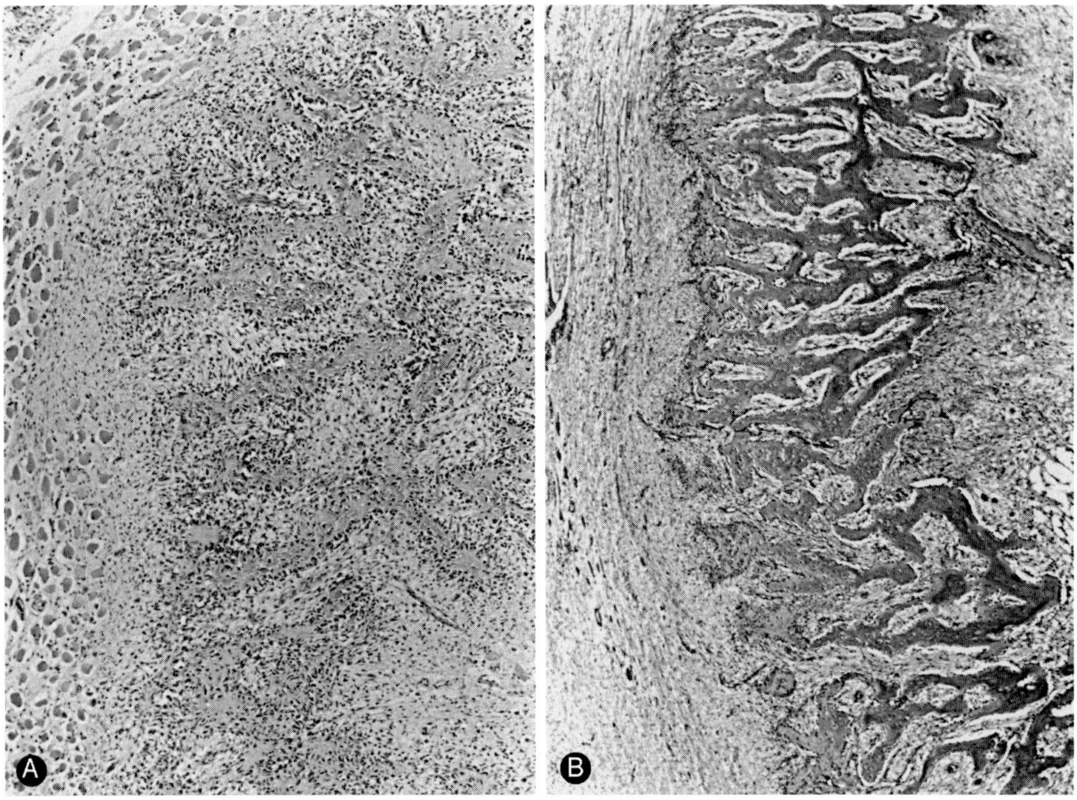

Figure 11–2. Myositis ossificans. *A,* In an early lesion, the outer zone of tissue consists of ill-defined trabeculae of woven bone. *B,* In later lesions, the bone progressively matures into well-defined arcades.

On needle biopsies, the lack of significant atypia should suggest a reactive diagnosis. The diagnosis of soft-tissue osteosarcoma in the young or of parosteal osteosarcoma should never be made without first considering myositis ossificans.

Prognosis and Treatment

Myositis ossificans is a benign, self-limiting condition that progressively matures to a bony mass, sometimes becoming attached to the underlying cortex. Local excision may be necessary to remove a symptomatic large lump. It has been suggested that malignant transformation of myositis ossificans occurs occasionally.[11]

Parosteal Fasciitis and Cranial Fasciitis

Nodular fasciitis usually occurs in a superficial location, in superficial fascia, in subcutis, or within skeletal muscle. Rarely, histologically similar lesions consisting of proliferating fibroblasts with a tissue culture pattern are found close to bone, and the term *parosteal fasciitis* is applied.[12, 13] *Cranial fasciitis* is a variant of nodular fasciitis that chiefly but not exclusively affects infants and involves the deep layers of the scalp.[14] Erosion of the outer table of the skull is common, and penetration of the inner table with meningeal involvement can occur.

Subungual Exostosis

This reactive lesion is found under or beside the nail, especially of the hallux, usually of adolescents and young adults.[15] Local trauma, infection, and tight footwear are implicated in its pathogenesis. Occasional examples are seen in the hand, particularly the thumb and index finger. The lesion is painful and may lift the nail, whereas secondary infection or hemorrhage may cause the lesion to appear black or brown and simulate a malignant melanoma. This clinical problem has been complicated by the description of subungual osteoblastic melanoma, a rare variant of melanoma that contains reactive bone.[16]

Radiologic and Pathologic Appearances

Frequently, no radiograph is taken preoperatively. The lesion is a well-defined calcified spur attached to the distal phalanx of the toe, but unlike an osteochondroma it lacks continuity with the cortex and spongiosa of the underlying bone (Fig. 11–3*A*). On gross inspection, if removed intact, the lesion has a rough-surfaced, irregular fibrocartilaginous cap and a bony base. On microscopy,[15, 17] there is a superficial zone of proliferating fibrous tissue that can contain many, but normal, mitotic figures. The fibrous tissue undergoes cartilaginous metaplasia to form the chondroid cap of the lesion (Fig. 11–3*B*). The cartilage can be cellular with binucleate cells and plump nuclei. In turn, the cartilage undergoes endochondral ossification, often with an irregular pattern. The intertrabecular spaces contain fat or proliferating fibrous tissue. Subungual exostosis is entirely benign, although recurrence may follow incomplete excision.

Bizarre Parosteal Osteochondromatous Proliferation

This lesion, first described by Nora et al.,[18] is closely related to subungual exostosis but, by definition, occurs in sites other than the distal phalanges. Most occur on the surface of the tubular bones of the hands and feet, with occasional examples on long bones. In fact, one-quarter of cases in one series[19] arose from

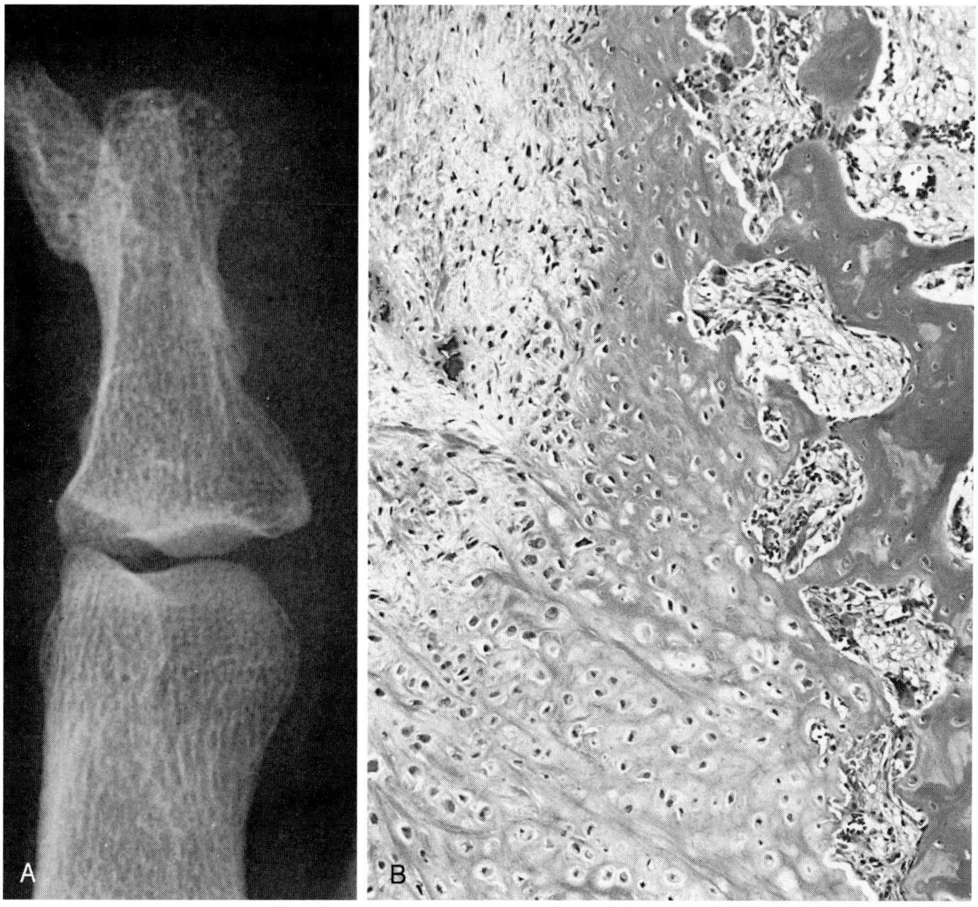

Figure 11–3. Subungual exostosis. *A,* This bony spur stuck on the surface of the terminal phalanx has the typical radiologic appearance of subungual exostosis. *B,* The surface of the exostosis consists of cellular fibrous tissue and reactive cartilage that undergoes endochondral ossification.

long bones, but it is likely that referral of unusual cases accounts for this high proportion. There is a history of trauma in one-third of patients.

Radiologic and Pathologic Appearances

Radiographs show a well-defined mass with stippled calcification, stuck on the surface of the bone (Fig. 11–4*A*). Histologic appearance shows a cap of cellular cartilage, arising by metaplasia from fibrous tissue and undergoing irregular endochondral ossification to distinctive, coarse hematoxyphilic woven bone with crenated cement lines (Fig. 11–4*B* and *C*). Adipose tissue and spindle-celled fibrous tissue sometimes mixed with cartilage fill the intertrabecular spaces. Recurrence is seen in one-third of patients, but because no metastases have been reported, the lesion is generally regarded as reactive rather than neoplastic in nature, although Schajowicz[20] suggests that some are periosteal chondrosarcomas. It has been proposed, on radiologic evidence, that bizarre parosteal osteochondromatous proliferation is related to the group of myositis ossificans–like lesions in the hand,[21] but the dissimilar histologic appearances militate against this view.

Cortical Irregularity Syndrome (Periosteal Desmoid)

This lesion commonly occurs in young children on the flare of the posteromedial aspect of the distal femoral metaphysis[22, 23] and is believed to result from traction at or avulsion of the insertion of adductor magnus. The child may complain of pain, or the lesion may be noted incidentally on plain radiographs. Small, well-defined lucencies are seen that may resemble a fibrous cortical defect, and there may be a spiculated periosteal reaction (Fig. 11–5*A*). If the radiologist recognizes the lesion, there is no need for biopsy. On histologic appearance, cellular fibrous tissue with occasional mitoses is seen (Fig. 11–5*B*), in keeping with the erroneous name "periosteal desmoid." The underlying bone shows active osteoclasis and formation of callus-like new bone and cartilage. Awareness of the entity and the lack of significant atypia will prevent overdiagnosis of a sarcoma.[24] It should not be confused with true periosteal fibromatosis, an aggressive lesion (see Chapter 12).

Aneurysmal Bone Cyst

Aneurysmal bone cysts (see Chapter 16) are usually eccentrically located in the bone, but about 7% arise beneath the periosteum.[25]

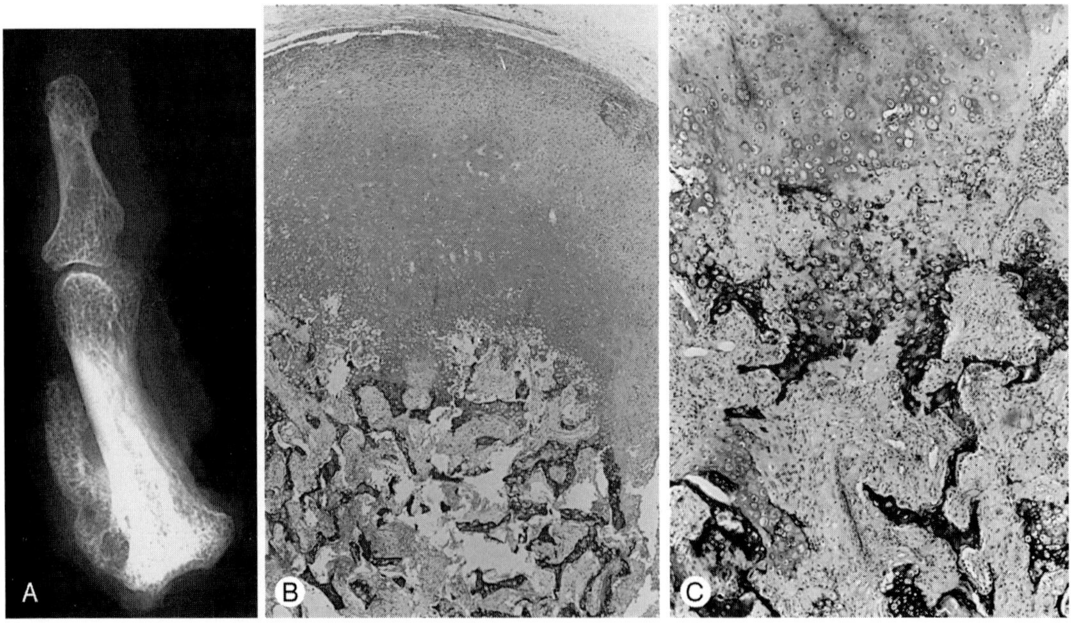

Figure 11–4. Bizarre parosteal osteochondromatous proliferation. *A,* Plain radiograph shows a well-defined bony mass stuck on the surface of the phalanx. *B,* The surface of the lesion shows irregular areas of cellular fibrous tissue, cartilage, and bone. *C,* Endochondral ossification proceeds in an irregular fashion.

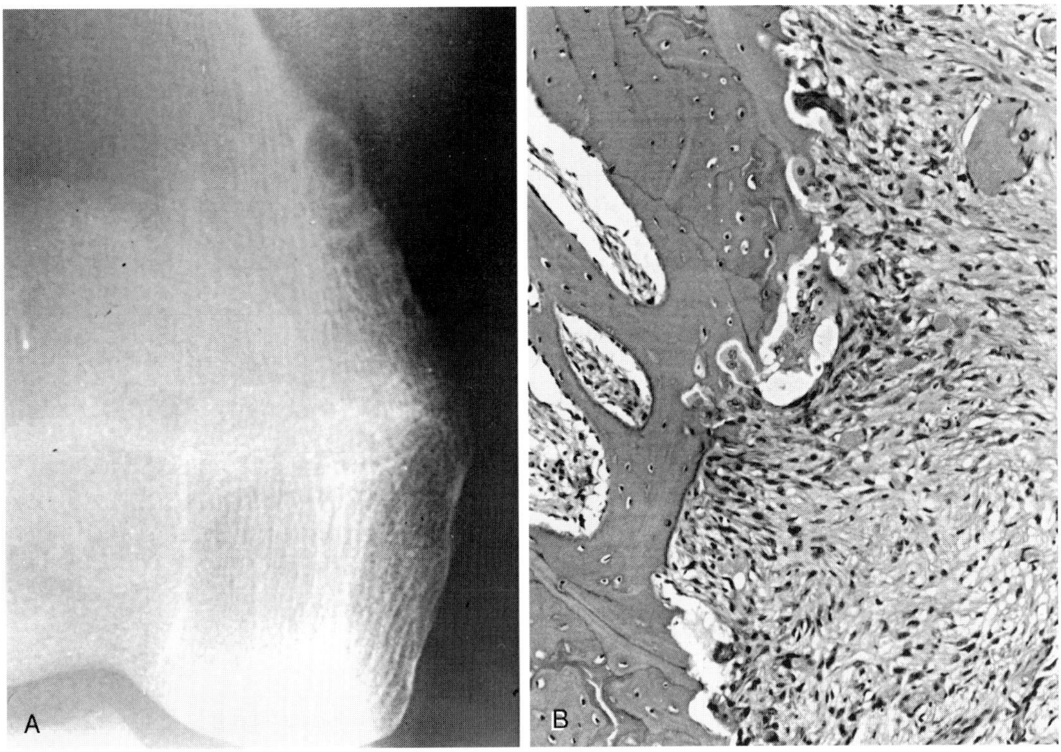

Figure 11–5. Cortical irregularity syndrome. *A*, Plain radiograph shows a small, well-defined area of lucency on the medial femoral condyle. *B*, The lesion is composed of cellular fibrous tissue with bone formation and active osteoclasis.

OSTEOSARCOMAS ON THE BONE SURFACE

The variants of surface osteosarcoma are by far the most important of the bone-forming tumors that arise on the bone surfaces. The 7% of osteosarcomas that arise at this site are divided into three main categories.[20, 26, 27] They form a spectrum from low-grade tumors with a small risk of metastasis to high-grade sarcomas whose behavior is similar to that of conventional central osteosarcoma. The low-grade *parosteal osteosarcoma* was first described by Geschickter and Copeland in 1951 as parosteal osteoma,[28] this erroneous name reflecting the low grade of the tumor. The malignant nature of the lesion was soon recognized, and the entity was subsequently separated from *periosteal osteosarcoma,* which differs in radiologic and pathologic appearances and has a significantly worse prognosis.[29, 30] The self-explanatory term, *high-grade surface osteosarcoma,* was introduced in 1984,[31] although the concept that otherwise typical osteosarcomas could occasionally arise on the bone surface was not new. In each type of surface osteosarcoma, cortical erosion and penetration may lead to medullary involvement, but in general this should be slight, because by convention a tumor with extensive intraosseous and extraosseous components is regarded as a primary central tumor with subperiosteal or soft-tissue extension. The extremely uncommon *intracortical osteosarcoma*[32, 33] is discussed in Chapter 9.

Parosteal (Juxtacortical) Osteosarcoma

Parosteal osteosarcoma is the most common surface osteosarcoma, representing 4 to 5% of all osteosarcomas, and is usually a slow-growing tumor with a relatively good prognosis. Perhaps partly because of this slow growth, it affects a much wider age range than conventional intramedullary osteosarcoma, with 80% of patients presenting between 20 and 50 years of age. Some series[34, 35] have a slight female preponderance. Parosteal osteosarcoma typically arises at the metaphysis of long bones. By far the most common site is the posterior aspect of the distal femur, where around 70% of examples are found, with the proximal humerus, tibia, and femur next in frequency. Occasionally the tumor may arise in other sites,[35] including the skull[36, 37] and the hand[38]; it must be remembered that reactive lesions simulating sarcoma are far more common than sarcomas in the extremities. Most patients present with a slowly growing mass; some tumors are painful, and up to one-third interfere with the function of the neighboring joint.[35] A tumor arising following therapeutic irradiation has been reported.[39]

Radiologic Appearances

Typically, the tumor is a lobulated and heavily ossified mass stuck onto the underlying cortex, often by a broad base, and occasionally encircles much of the remainder of the bone.[40] In most cases a translucent line may be seen between part of the lesion and the underlying cortex in some projections; this may cause confusion with myositis ossificans unless the attachment of lesion to bone is demonstrated by other views, CT, or MRI. In one-quarter of cases, CT and MRI will show that the tumor erodes the cortex and extends into the medulla.[35, 41] While some authors have taken an extreme view and have regarded any tumor with an intraosseous component as being, by definition, a central osteosarcoma, others acknowledge that intramedullary extension is part of the natural history of these tumors and accept as a parosteal osteosarcoma any tumor with typical histology involving less than 25% of the medulla,[35] especially if there is a long history of a palpable mass. Although the tumor is often less heavily mineralized toward the periphery, the outer border of the tumor is usually smooth. A tumor with an ill-defined margin and poorly mineralized deep areas is likely to be of higher than average grade.[42] A biopsy should be directed toward these areas to avoid underestimating the grade of the tumor.

Pathologic Appearances

In keeping with the radiologic appearance, the tumor is usually a white, heavily ossified mass (Fig. 11–6*A*), but toward the periphery there are softer, more fibrous areas that may infiltrate surrounding soft tissue or muscle. Islands of cartilage are seen in one-half of the lesions and in one-quarter form a cap at the periphery, thus simulating the appearance of an osteochondroma.[35] Unlike an osteochondroma, whose cortex and spongiosa are in continuity with that of the bone of origin, a parosteal osteosarcoma is attached to the underlying cortex, although erosion or even penetration may be seen.

At first sight the histologic features of a low-grade parosteal osteosarcoma do not look like those of a sarcoma. They consist of arrays of parallel, ribbon-like trabeculae of woven bone that are separated by a poorly cellular fibroblastic stroma (Fig. 11–6*B* and *C*). The bony trabeculae lack a covering of osteoblasts (osteoblastic rimming) and show progressive maturation toward the base of the lesion. Irregular "pagetoid" cement lines may be seen in these thick trabeculae. The fibroblastic component shows only mild cytologic atypia with occasional mitotic figures, features that are most evident at the periphery, where there may be infiltration of skeletal muscle, sometimes in a manner reminiscent of a fibromatosis. The cartilage, present in nodules or as a cap, is usually well differentiated, with some cells having plump nuclei and with occasional binucleate cells; it usually lacks the ordered arrays of cells of a growing exostosis. In the depths of the 15% or so of particularly well differentiated tumors, the mature bony trabeculae (sometimes described as "normalized") may be separated by fatty or hemopoietic marrow. In a few tumors, foci of giant cells are seen, leading to the description of a giant cell-rich parosteal osteosarcoma.[43]

Grading, Treatment, and Prognosis

All authors agree that parosteal osteosarcomas vary in grade, from extremely well-differentiated tumors showing minimal atypia to more mitotically active and cytologically atypical tumors, and that histologic grade is of major prognostic importance.[34, 44] The criteria for each grade differ, and the number of patients in each grade in most series is small so that it is difficult to compare figures for clinical outcome. The following are guidelines for grading parosteal osteosarcoma:

- **Grade 1** tumors have a fibroblastic component that is only moderately cellular and contains much collagen. The fibroblastic cells are uniform and show little pleomorphism or hyperchromasia. Mitotic figures are rare, averaging around 1 per 10 high-power fields. The bony trabeculae are mature and often, particularly in the depths of the le-

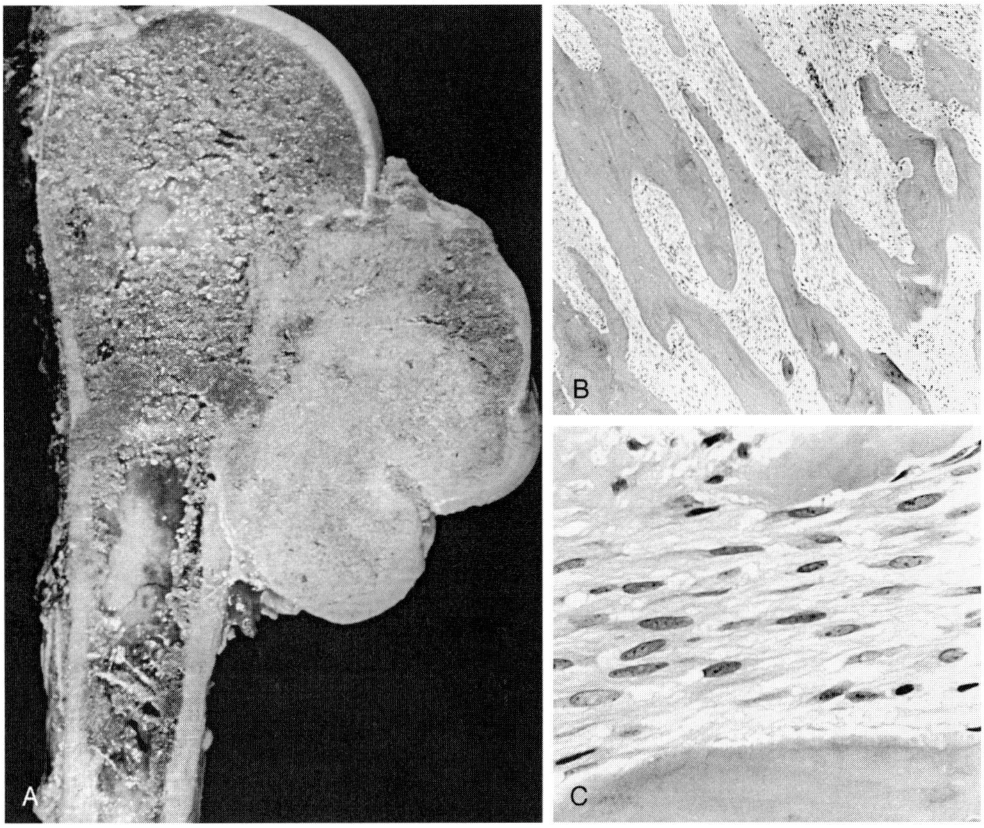

Figure 11–6. Parosteal osteosarcoma. *A,* This tumor lies on the proximal humeral metaphysis and shows early invasion of the underlying medulla. *B,* The surface of the tumor has a smooth cartilaginous cap. The tumor consists of parallel arrays of mature bone separated by a spindle-cell stroma. *C,* At high magnification, the spindle cells show little cytologic atypia.

sion, contain lamellar bone. Any cartilage present is bland cytologically, at worst resembling a grade 1 chondrosarcoma.

- **Grade 2** tumors have a more cellular stroma, in small or large areas. The spindle cells have plumper nuclei showing some pleomorphism and hyperchromasia. Mitoses are more common, averaging around 5 per 10 high-power fields. Irregular foci of osteoid or bone may be seen in the fibrous component between mature trabeculae. Cartilage, if present, corresponds to that in grade 2 chondrosarcoma.
- **Grade 3** tumors show frankly malignant fibroblastic, cartilaginous, or osteoblastic tissue.

Parosteal osteosarcoma almost invariably recurs after intralesional excision (see Chapter 6, Fig. 6–21) and commonly after marginal excision[45, 46]; accordingly, wide surgical excision is the treatment of choice.[47] Local recurrences are often of higher grade. Grade 1 tumors metastasize uncommonly, perhaps in 5 to 10% of cases, in contrast to 20 to 40% of grade 2 tumors.[29, 30, 34, 35, 40, 48] Around 50% of grade 3 tumors metastasize, and for this reason some authors regard them as high-grade surface osteosarcomas.[49] Chemotherapy is usually given to these patients. Some studies[34] have shown that tumors with intramedullary extension are more likely to metastasize, but this may be explained by the positive correlation between medullary involvement and increasing tumor grade rather than as an independent variable. Around 80 to 90% of patients with parosteal osteosarcoma should survive for a long time.

Dedifferentiated Parosteal Osteosarcoma

This term describes the combination of a low-grade parosteal osteosarcoma and a high-grade sarcoma, usually an osteosarcoma or malignant fibrous histiocytoma (Fig. 11–7). The

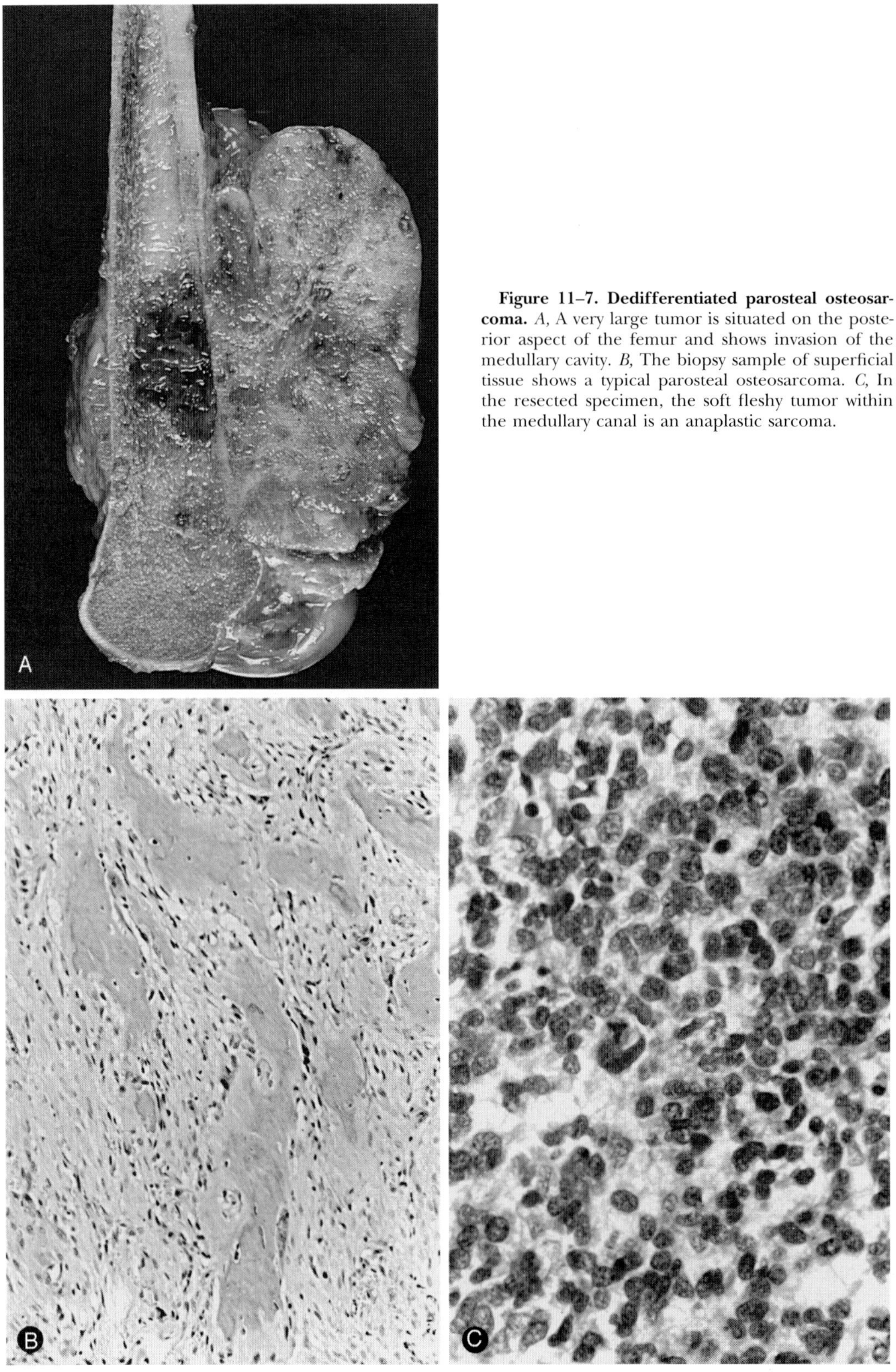

Figure 11–7. Dedifferentiated parosteal osteosarcoma. *A,* A very large tumor is situated on the posterior aspect of the femur and shows invasion of the medullary cavity. *B,* The biopsy sample of superficial tissue shows a typical parosteal osteosarcoma. *C,* In the resected specimen, the soft fleshy tumor within the medullary canal is an anaplastic sarcoma.

high-grade component may be present at initial diagnosis or after repeated local recurrences and may be found in a parosteal or intramedullary location.[50] These tumors represent approximately 20% of all parosteal osteosarcomas in most series[51] and as many as 43% in one study.[52] The identification of focal hypervascularity on angiography appears to correlate better with dedifferentiation[52] than the presence of deeply placed lytic areas on plain film or CT images.[42] These tumors have a poor prognosis, comparable to that of high-grade osteosarcomas, and require similar treatment with chemotherapy.

Cytogenetic Analysis

The small number of parosteal osteosarcomas examined cytogenetically have shown ring chromosomes,[53] a finding seen in other low-grade tumors such as dermatofibrosarcoma protuberans, in contrast to the complex abnormalities seen in conventional osteosarcoma. Similarly, most parosteal osteosarcomas are diploid, whereas conventional osteosarcomas are usually aneuploid. Perhaps unsurprisingly, the high-grade component of one dedifferentiated tumor has been shown to be aneuploid.[54]

Differential Diagnosis

The cartilage cap of a parosteal osteosarcoma may suggest the diagnosis *of "atypical osteocartilaginous exostosis,"* but this common error can be avoided if the spindle-celled component is identified and the radiographs and imaging are carefully examined to determine the relationship of the lesion to the cortex. The pattern of mature but irregular woven bone trabeculae in a fairly bland fibrous stroma may be reminiscent of *fibrous dysplasia*, but this diagnosis is untenable if the lesion is confined to the bone surface. The term *fibrous dysplasia protuberans* has been proposed for a very rare variant of fibrous dysplasia presenting as an exophytic mass.[55] The bony trabeculae of this lesion are more randomly arranged than those of parosteal osteosarcoma, and the stromal cells show no atypia. In addition, the adjacent medullary canal is also affected. The differential diagnosis between fibrous dysplasia and low-grade central osteosarcoma, the intramedullary equivalent of parosteal osteosarcoma, is discussed in Chapters 9 and 13. The distinction from myositis ossificans and bizarre parosteal osteochondromatous proliferation was discussed earlier in this chapter.

Periosteal Osteosarcoma

Periosteal osteosarcoma[30, 56, 57] is a chondroblastic osteosarcoma of intermediate grade with a prognosis between those of parosteal osteosarcoma and conventional osteosarcoma. Fewer than 2% of osteosarcomas are in this category. The age distribution is similar to that of conventional osteosarcoma and younger than that of parosteal osteosarcoma. Most examples arise on the diaphyses of long bones, especially the tibia, femur, and humerus, and the majority of patients present with swelling and pain.

Radiologic Appearances

The appearance on plain radiographs is distinctive.[58] The lesion consists of an ill-defined and lightly calcified mass lying in a saucerized defect in the cortex, which may be thickened (Fig. 11–8*A*). Within the lesion, there are usually spicules of reactive bone perpendicular to the long axis of the bone. Although erosion of the cortex is common, only very superficial medullary involvement is allowable; if spread within the bone is extensive, the tumor is best regarded as a central osteosarcoma with extraosseous extension.

Pathologic Appearances

Grossly, the tumor is composed of lobules of cartilage in which white bony spicules may be seen. On microscopy, the lesion is rich in malignant-appearing cartilage, corresponding to a grade 2 to 3 central chondrosarcoma. At the periphery of the lobules there are atypical spindle-shaped cells between which osteoid may be seen (Fig. 11–8*B*). In some cases it can be extremely difficult to find the convincing "tumor bone" that is, by definition, required to make this diagnosis. Trabeculae of bone are often seen at the center of the lobules, but it can be difficult to distinguish these from foci of reactive new bone. Trabeculae arranged perpendicular to the bone surface, corresponding to the spiculation seen radiologically, are usually reactive in nature.

Differential Diagnosis

The overtly malignant nature of the cartilage exceeds that permissible in a periosteal

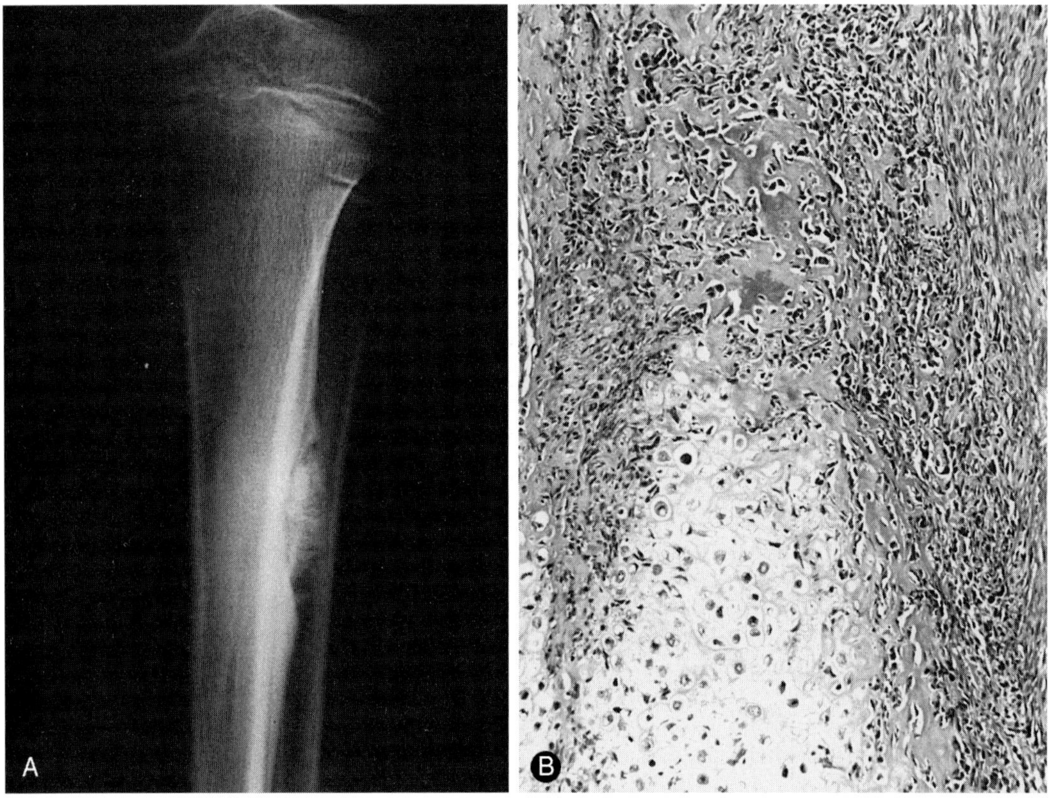

Figure 11–8. Periosteal osteosarcoma. *A,* The tumor consists of a calcified mass lying in a saucerized depression on the underlying cortex of the tibial metaphysis. *B,* Microscopic examination shows cellular cartilage with cytologic atypia, spindle cells, and areas where tumor cells form osteoid, some lightly calcified.

chondroma but is less than is seen in a high-grade (grade 4) *chondroblastic osteosarcoma,* which is usually larger, has a worse prognosis, and should not be included in this category. In general, *periosteal chondrosarcoma* has a more lobulated architecture, and spindle-celled areas are found only at the margin of the lobules in the uncommon high-grade examples; it lacks the spiculated intralesional bone of periosteal osteosarcoma. Crucially, it does not contain areas of osteoid formation.

Treatment and Prognosis

The prognosis of periosteal osteosarcoma lies between that of parosteal osteosarcoma and conventional osteosarcoma, and around 15% of patients develop lung metastases. Local control requires wide or radical excision.[27]

High-Grade Surface Osteosarcoma

This, the least common surface osteosarcoma, represents less than 1% of all osteosarcomas.[31] Most tumors occur on the diaphysis or diaphyso-metaphysis of long bones, especially the femur and humerus, in young patients who present with swelling or pain.

The tumor is typically large; the extent of mineralization varies from minimal to densely sclerotic. It is attached to or erodes the cortex but, by definition, shows no or only slight medullary involvement. Histologic examination shows a high-grade osteosarcoma with any of the patterns seen in conventional central osteosarcoma[49] (see also Chapter 9).

This tumor has the same prognosis as conventional osteosarcoma, and the same principles of treatment apply.

PERIOSTEAL OSTEOID OSTEOMA AND OSTEOBLASTOMA

Osteoid osteoma (see Chapter 9) most commonly occurs within the cortex, stimulating dense reactive sclerosis, or in the medullary cavity, where there is little reaction. It occurs least commonly on the surface of bone,[59] where it may induce subperiosteal new bone formation, giving an appearance similar to a cortical lesion. A juxta-articular osteoid osteoma arising on the bone surface tends to cause little new bone formation, and the diagnosis is often delayed because the pain may suggest arthritis. A typical site is the neck of the talus. A few *multifocal periosteal osteoid osteomas* have been described with several nidi, each less than 1 cm in diameter and embedded in reactive bone.[60] *Periosteal osteoblastoma* is very rare[61, 62]; the tumor is usually covered by a thin shell of reactive bone and is histologically identical to its more common intramedullary form.

PAROSTEAL OSTEOMA

Osteomas (see Chapter 9) are predominantly tumors of the craniofacial skeleton. Osteomas on the surface of long bones are extremely rare. Only four cases were found in the files of the Mayo Clinic, and a further 10 cases among the consultation cases, from more than 40,000 cases of bone tumors.[63] Parosteal osteomas are heavily ossified masses on the surface, principally of long bones, in adults. Some patients have tuberous sclerosis or Gardner's syndrome. Most patients complain of a swelling, sometimes painful, but on occasion the lesion is an incidental radiologic finding. Radiographs show a densely sclerotic mass, varying from 2 to 20 cm, with a lobulated or smooth surface and without intralesional areas of lucency (Fig. 11–9*A*).

Histologically, the tumor consists of compact lamellar bone with haversian systems (Fig. 11–9*B*). Irregular cement lines resembling those of Paget's disease are common. On the surface of the lesion is a thin layer of fibrous tissue with no cytologic atypia. No cartilage is present, and the presence of a spindle-cell stroma within the tumor, no matter how bland, should suggest the diagnosis of low-grade parosteal osteosarcoma.

The lesion can closely resemble a parosteal osteosarcoma radiologically and therefore requires to be excised or at least subjected generously to biopsy.

CARTILAGINOUS NEOPLASMS

Osteochondroma (Osteocartilaginous Exostosis)

Osteochondroma is regarded as the most common benign tumor of bone. It accounts for more than one-third of benign bone tumors,[27] although it is a developmental abnormality rather than a true neoplasm. An osteochondroma is believed to derive from a displaced section of physeal growth plate herniating through a defect in the periosteum.[64] Proliferation of cartilage followed by endochondral ossification results in a cartilage-capped bony mass attached to the metaphysis. The osteochondroma may be sessile or pedunculated with a slender stalk. Due to continuing physeal growth, the point of attachment of the osteochondroma seems to move toward the diaphysis (although, in reality, the physis grows away from the osteochondroma). Occasionally, growth of the osteochondroma may continue for a few years after closure of the physis from which it is derived.[65] Half of all osteochondromas are found at the lower femur, upper tibia, and proximal humerus, but any bone, except those formed by membranous ossification (principally the craniofacial skeleton), may be affected. Solitary osteochondromas rarely affect the hands and feet.

Whereas many small osteochondromas are asymptomatic, patients with larger lesions usually present in adolescence or early adult life complaining of swelling. Pain may be due to fracture of the stalk, due to pressure on an artery causing claudication or formation of a false aneurysm,[66] or due to inflammation of an overlying bursa[67] that may show synovial chondrometaplasia.[68] Peripheral nerves or the spinal cord may be compressed. In the absence of such a cause, pain, particularly in adult life and especially when associated with resumption of growth, is suspicious of malignant transformation. Approximately 12% of children who receive therapeutic irradiation for childhood malignancy may develop osteochondromas.[69, 70]

Multiple exostoses are a part of the autosomal dominant syndrome of diaphyseal aclasis,[71–73] in which there is failure of remodeling of the metaphysis into the diaphysis. Diaphyseal aclasis appears to be a result of a mutation in one of at least three genes, EXT1, EXT2, and EXT3, located on chromosomes 8q24, 11p13, and 19q.[74] Most patients have many osteochondromas (Fig. 11–10) and are usually of mildly shortened stature, and many have skeletal deformity, particularly of the forearm bones. The individual osteochondromas are similar to solitary lesions but are more commonly sessile.[75]

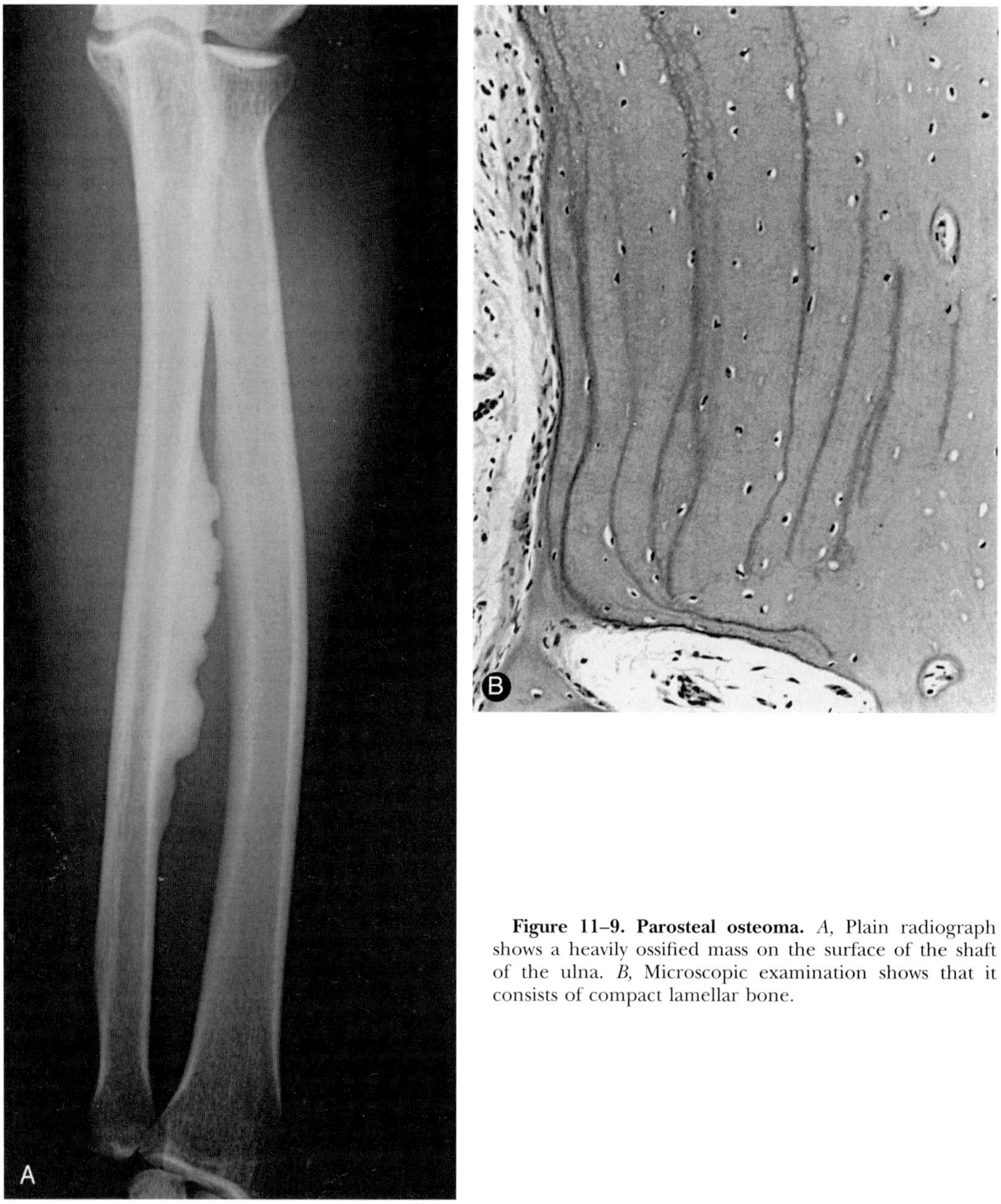

Figure 11–9. Parosteal osteoma. *A*, Plain radiograph shows a heavily ossified mass on the surface of the shaft of the ulna. *B*, Microscopic examination shows that it consists of compact lamellar bone.

Radiologic and Pathologic Appearances

Radiographs show a pedunculated or sessile projection from the metaphysis of the bone, which usually points away from the adjacent joint (see Fig. 11–10). The cortex and the medulla of the exostosis are continuous with those of the parent bone. In contrast, a parosteal osteosarcoma is separated from the medullary canal by an intact or partially eroded cortex. The bony stalk has a trabecular pattern and is usually well defined; however, the cartilage cap is difficult to see on plain radiographs. The cartilage cap is normally thin, usually no more than 1 cm in adults (Fig. 11–11*A*), but thicker in children, and occasionally there are large areas of heavily calcified and necrotic cartilage in "ancient" exostoses. The surface, although often lobulated, is smooth, and there is a covering of

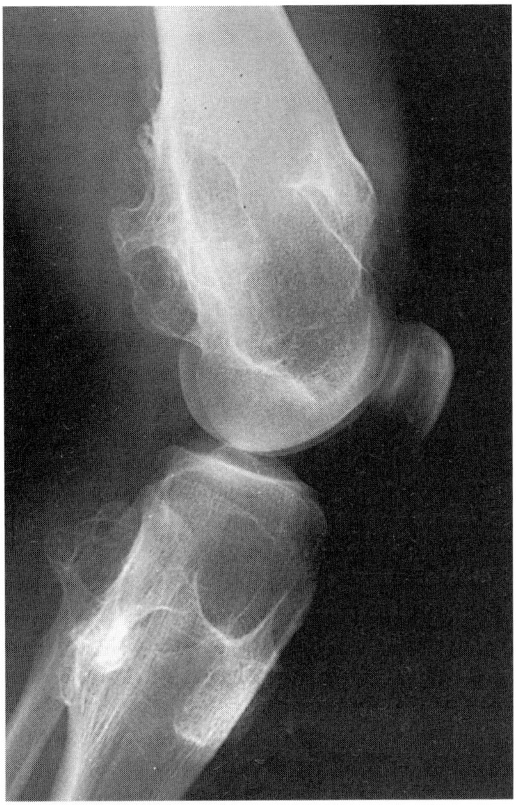

Figure 11–10. Diaphyseal aclasis. Plain radiograph shows multiple osteochondromas around the knee joint. The metaphyses are widened as a result of a failure of remodeling.

fibrous perichondrium. Histologically, the cap consists of hyaline cartilage that is replaced by endochondral ossification at its base (Fig. 11–11*B*). The cartilage of growing exostoses mimics that of the growth plate, with its chondrocytes arranged in columns. Once skeletal growth has finished, the cartilage cap is progressively replaced by bone, and the lesion becomes covered by a layer of fibrous tissue in which a few chondroid nodules may remain. Occasionally, histologically benign osteochondromas with very thin cartilage caps are found in adults who report clinical growth.

Very rarely, an eccentrically placed enchondroma, usually of the humerus, bulges out to form an exophytic mass that may simulate an exostosis; the term *enchondroma protuberans* has been applied to this phenomenon.[76, 77] Curettage has been curative in the few reported cases.

Prognosis and Treatment

Osteochondroma is almost always cured by complete excision, but occasionally recurrence follows incomplete removal, perhaps due to growth of small satellite nodules remaining in the perichondrium. Malignant change, almost always to low-grade chondrosarcoma, occurs in less than 1% of clinically apparent exostoses, and the true risk is even lower if small asymptomatic lesions are included. The risk of chondrosarcoma in diaphyseal aclasis is higher and in many series is between 5 and 25% in hospital patients, although population studies suggest that the true incidence is much smaller, probably around 1%.[78, 79]

Peripheral "Secondary" Chondrosarcoma

In contrast to central chondrosarcomas, most of which arise in apparently normal bone, the majority of peripheral chondrosarcomas complicate osteocartilaginous exostoses and are therefore described as "secondary." The small number of remaining chondrosarcomas on the bone surface are discussed in the following section on subperiosteal cartilage tumors.

In general, patients with chondrosarcomas complicating exostoses, whether solitary or in diaphyseal aclasis, are around a decade younger than those with "primary" chondrosarcomas. Most tumors arise in relation to long bones and the pelvis.[27, 80] Because many are low-grade and well differentiated, histologic diagnosis can be difficult, so that knowledge of the clinical and radiologic features is essential; resumption of growth of an exostosis in an adult should raise a strong suspicion of malignancy, particularly if the lesion is painful. A higher proportion of middle- or high-grade chondrosarcomas arise in diaphyseal aclasis than in solitary exostoses.

Radiologic and Pathologic Appearances

On radiographs, a chondrosarcoma has an irregular and thickened cartilage cap, more than 1 to 2 cm in depth, with ill-defined borders and often containing flocculent calcification.[75] CT and MRI demonstrate the extent of the cartilaginous component and any soft-tissue extension better than plain radiographs. The thickened cartilage cap is also the most important pathologic evidence of malignancy (Fig. 11–12); often the cartilage is poorly cellular, and its cytology is unimpressive, with only an occasional binucleate cell or cell with a

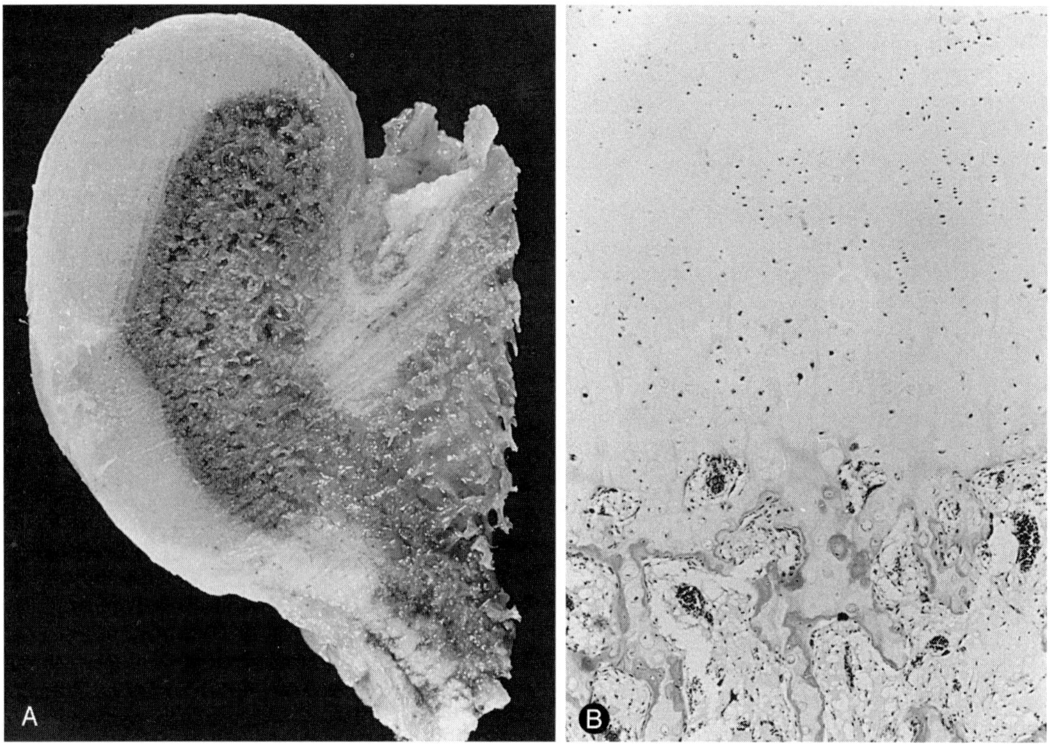

Figure 11–11. Osteochondroma. *A,* This osteochondroma consists of a central core of cancellous bone covered by a smooth cartilage cap. *B,* Chondrocytes are arranged in columns resembling those of the growth plate; at the base, the cartilage undergoes endochondral ossification.

plump nucleus.[80] The entire biopsy material should be processed and thoroughly sectioned to search for any foci showing more atypia. Some tumors are more obviously malignant, although still usually grade 1 or occasionally grade 2; there is often an increase in grade with local recurrence. Very occasionally, peripheral chondrosarcomas show dedifferentiation (see Chapter 10), with an associated high-grade nonchondroid sarcoma.[81]

Prognosis and Treatment

Because the majority of peripheral chondrosarcomas are low-grade, morbidity is more often related to local extension and recurrence than to distant metastases. The major determinant of local recurrence is the completeness of excision, which depends on the skill of the surgeon and the anatomic site of the tumor. Pelvic, chest wall, and spinal tumors are particularly difficult to eradicate completely. Chondrosarcomas should be treated by wide or radical excision, taking care to avoid any breach of the "capsule" around the tumor because chondrocytes seeded into the operation site are prone to form recurrent nodules. It is important to remove the tumor by surgery; chemotherapy and radiotherapy have little effect in the treatment of low-grade chondrosarcomas.

Subperiosteal Cartilage Tumors

Subperiosteal cartilage tumors are rare, representing less than 1% of bone tumors; most are benign (periosteal chondroma); about one-quarter are malignant (periosteal chondrosarcoma). The distinction between these is not always easy as they form a spectrum of pathologic appearances, and sometimes it is necessary to report a periosteal cartilage tumor as "borderline."

Periosteal Chondroma

Periosteal chondroma, the periosteal equivalent of enchondroma, occurs over a wide age range but especially in the second and third decades of life; two-thirds of patients are male.[82–84] It is a slow-growing, usually painless tumor that most commonly affects the proximal humerus and the femur and the tubular bones of the hands and feet. The tumor is commonly 1 to 3 cm and rarely more than 5 cm in size and lies in the long axis of the bone, more commonly in the metaphysis than in the diaphysis and rarely in the epiphysis (Fig. 11–13). It erodes the underlying cortex, giving a well-defined oval defect with a sclerotic base.[85] Half of the lesions show punctate calcification, and in one-third there is a complete or partial shell of subperiosteal new bone on the outer surface. Histologically, periosteal chondromas consist of lobules of cartilage, usually hyaline but occasionally focally myxoid. Some examples are highly cellular and show a degree of cytologic atypia that at other sites, e.g., in a central cartilage tumor of the pelvis, would indicate low-grade malignancy (see Chapter 10). In a few tumors, nodules of cartilage are seen pushing into the underlying medullary canal, but there is no evidence of a permeative growth pattern, and the innermost margin is usually surrounded by a rim of lamellar bone.[82] As local recurrence sometimes follows curettage, block excision with a margin of normal tissue is the recommended treatment.

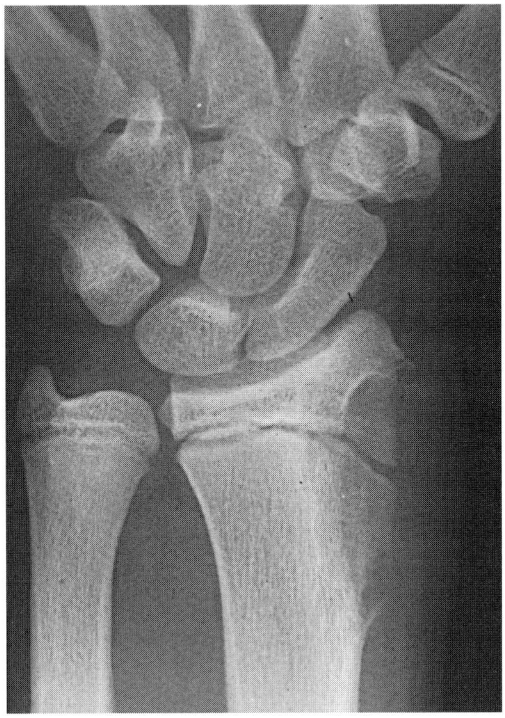

Figure 11–13. Periosteal chondroma. Plain radiograph shows the tumor lies on the surface of the distal radius in a scalloped defect. The adjacent periosteum is elevated with the formation of a Codman's triangle.

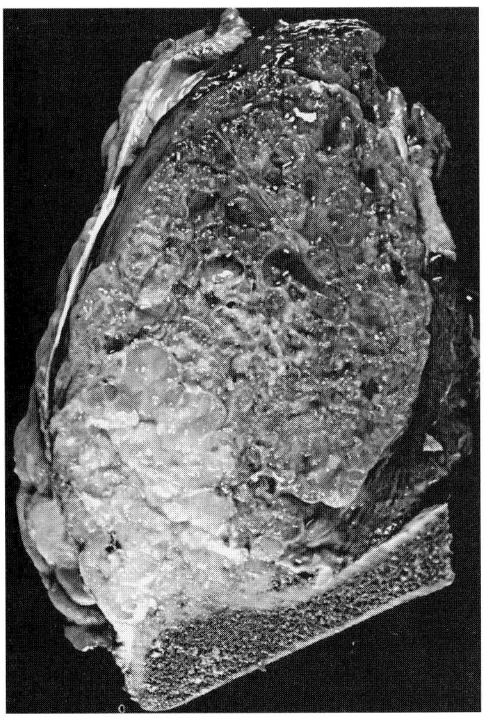

Figure 11–12. Peripheral chondrosarcoma. This large chondrosarcoma arising from the iliac crest is composed entirely of lobules of cartilage that on histologic examination were of low-grade malignancy.

Periosteal Chondrosarcoma

The tumors in this small group are usually of low- to middle-grade malignancy and account for less than 4% of all chondrosarcomas. Most are large, lobulated masses (usually greater than 5 cm) that lie on the metaphyses of long bones of adults of a wide age range.[86, 87] The distinction from periosteal chondroma may be difficult. In general, periosteal chondrosarcoma tends to be larger and usually shows more cytologic atypia. The architectural and radiologic features are often most helpful. A cartilage tumor whose cytology is equivalent to a grade 2 central chondrosarcoma or worse, which permeates rather than erodes the underlying cortex (Fig. 11–14) or infiltrates adjacent soft tissue, should be regarded as malignant.[88] Excision with a wide or radical margin is the appropriate treatment for periosteal chondrosarcoma, but a small proportion of patients develop lung metastases, the histo-

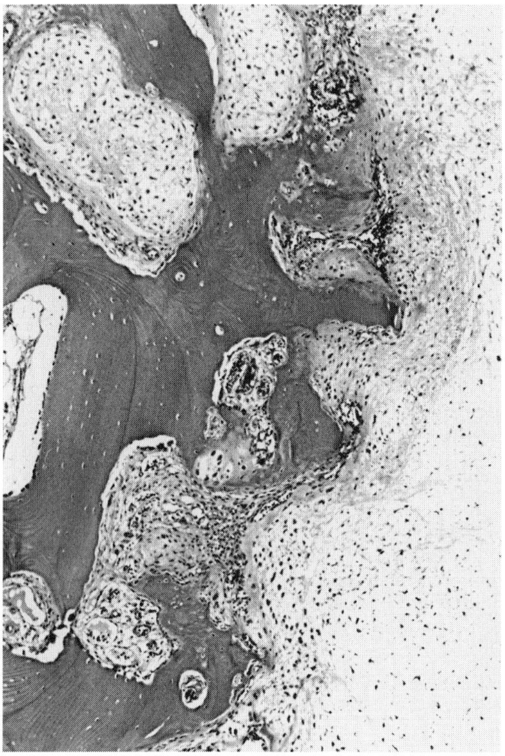

Figure 11–14. Periosteal chondrosarcoma. This cartilaginous tumor is moderately cellular, shows myxoid change, and has invaded the underlying cortex *(top left)*.

logic grade being an important prognostic indicator.

Periosteal Chondromyxoid Fibroma

Whereas chondromyxoid fibroma usually arises within the medullary cavity, there are occasional case reports of tumors arising on the surface of bone[27]; a study of 14 such tumors has been published in abstract form.[89] These tumors are described as showing more marked calcification than is usually seen. The rare phenomenon of a surface origin for chondromyxoid fibroma should be distinguished from the much more common soft-tissue implantation that may follow curettage of an intramedullary tumor.

SUBPERIOSTEAL FIBROUS TUMORS

Fibrosarcomas of bone arise predominantly in the medullary cavity. Most authors[20, 27, 90] take the view that the majority of spindle-cell sarcomas lying adjacent to the cortex are of soft-tissue origin. In contrast, Huvos and Higinbotham[91] found that almost one-third of their large series of fibrosarcomas were periosteal in origin. Cases regarded as malignant fibrous histiocytoma have also been described in a periosteal site.[92]

Occasionally, otherwise typical musculoaponeurotic fibromatoses arise in deep soft tissue and erode adjacent bone. These should not be confused with so-called "periosteal desmoid."

OTHER TUMORS

Almost all tumors that usually arise within bone have on occasion been described on the bone surface. In general, the histologic appearances are identical to those of the intramedullary counterpart. Only a brief comment will be made on these entities.

A small proportion of *Ewing's tumors* arise on the bone surface.[93, 94] Typically, there is elevation of the periosteum, with saucerization of the underlying cortex. There may be microscopic evidence of invasion of the superficial cortex, but by definition the medullary cavity is not involved. MRI is the best modality to exclude medullary involvement preoperatively.

Adamantinoma of long bones typically arises in the cortex (see Chapter 17) but frequently extends into the medullary canal and not uncommonly beneath the periosteum and into soft tissue. In contrast, primary periosteal adamantinoma is very rare. A few cases, including a "Ewing-like adamantinoma,"[95] have been described at this site.

Periosteal hemangioma most often occurs in adolescents and young adults and affects the diaphysis of long bones, especially the tibia and fibula.[96] Most patients complain of pain. Radiographs show a lytic lesion on the bone surface, usually accompanied by periosteal reaction and cortical thickening. The radiologic appearances are often suggestive of an osteoid osteoma. The histologic features are the same as those of hemangiomas within bone (see Chapter 16).

Solitary fibrous tumor, originally described in the pleura, has been reported in an increasing variety of sites, including the periosteum of the tibia in a woman 35 years of age.[97] The histologic appearance—that of a fibroblastic tumor of varying cellularity containing hypocellular collagenous areas—is in keeping with that seen at other sites where CD34 expression is common.

Parosteal lipoma is a slow-growing mass found in middle-aged adults.[98] Radiographs show a well-defined lesion attached to the bone surface. The cortex is often depressed, and there is a shell of subperiosteal new bone. Ossification within the lesion may be marked.[99]

Periosteal ganglion causes a scalloped area of cortical erosion with an adjacent soft-tissue mass. The tibia and femur appear to be affected most often. The histologic appearances are identical to those of the common soft-tissue ganglion.[100] MRI shows a low signal on both T1- and T2-weighted images.[1]

REFERENCES

1. Kenan S, Abdelwahab IF, Klein MJ, et al: Lesions of juxtacortical origin (surface lesions of bone). Skeletal Radiol 22:337, 1993.
2. Ihmeidan I, Tehranzadeh J, Oldham SA, et al: Case Report 443: Florid cortical and periosteal reactions due to stress fractures of the right femur and left calcaneus in a "break dancer." Skeletal Radiol 16:581, 1987.
3. Meaney JEM, Carty H: Femoral stress fractures in children. Skeletal Radiol 21:173, 1992.
4. Ackerman LV: Extraosseous localised non-neoplastic bone and cartilage formation (so-called myositis ossificans). J Bone Joint Surg Am 40A:279, 1958.
5. Spjut HJ, Dorfman HD: Florid reactive periostitis of the tubular bones of the hands and feet: A benign lesion which may simulate osteosarcoma. Am J Surg Pathol 5:423, 1981.
6. Dupree WB, Enzinger FM: Fibro-osseous pseudotumor of the digits. Cancer 58:2103, 1986.
7. De Smet AA, Norris MA, Fisher DR: Magnetic resonance imaging of myositis ossificans: Analysis of seven cases. Skeletal Radiol 21:503, 1992.
8. Norman A, Dorfman HD: Juxtacortical circumscribed myositis ossificans: Evolution and radiographic features. Radiology 96:301, 1970.
9. Lagier R, Cox JN: Pseudomalignant myositis ossificans. Hum Pathol 6:653, 1975.
10. Nuovo MA, Norman A, Chumas AJ, et al: Myositis ossificans with atypical clinical, radiographic or pathological findings: A review of 23 cases. Skeletal Radiol 21:87, 1992.
11. Huvos AG: The spontaneous transformation of benign into malignant soft tissue tumors (with emphasis on extraskeletal osseous, lipomatous and schwannian lesions). Am J Surg Pathol 9(Suppl):7, 1985.
12. Hutter RV, Foote FW, Francis KC, et al: Parosteal fasciitis: A self-limiting benign process that simulates a malignant neoplasm. Am J Surg 104:800, 1962.
13. McCarthy EF, Ireland DCR, Sprague BL, et al: Parosteal (nodular) fasciitis of the hand. J Bone Joint Surg Am 58A:714, 1976.
14. Lauer DH, Enzinger FM: Cranial fasciitis of children. Cancer 45:401, 1980.
15. Landon GC, Johnson KA, Dahlin DC: Subungual exostosis. J Bone Joint Surg Am 61A:256, 1979.
16. Lucas DR, Tazelaar HD, Unni KK, et al: Osteogenic melanoma: A rare variant of malignant melanoma. Am J Surg Pathol 17:400, 1993.
17. Miller-Breslow A, Dorfman HD: Dupuytren's (subungual) exostosis. Am J Surg Pathol 12:368, 1988.
18. Nora FE, Dahlin DC, Beabout JW: Bizarre parosteal osteochondromatous proliferations of the tubular bones of the hands and feet. Am J Surg Pathol 7:245, 1983.
19. Meneses MF, Unni KK, Sweet RG: Bizarre parosteal osteochondromatous proliferation of bone (Nora's lesion). Am J Surg Pathol 17:691, 1993.
20. Schajowicz F: Tumors and Tumorlike Lesions of Bone: Pathology, Radiology and Treatment. 2nd ed. Berlin, Springer-Verlag, 1994.
21. Yuen M, Friedman L, Orr W, et al: Proliferative periosteal processes of the phalanges: A unitary hypothesis. Skeletal Radiol 21:301, 1992.
22. Dunham WK, Marcus NW, Enneking WF, et al: Developmental defects of the distal femoral metaphysis. J Bone Joint Surg Am 62A:801, 1980.
23. Resnick D, Greenway G: Distal femoral cortical defects, irregularities and excavations. Diagn Radiol 143:345, 1982.
24. Craigen MAC, Bennet GC, MacKenzie JR, et al: Symptomatic cortical irregularities of the distal femur simulating malignancy. J Bone Joint Surg Br 76B:814, 1994.
25. Vergel De Dios AM, Bone JR, Shives TC, et al: Aneurysmal bone cyst: A clinicopathologic study of 238 cases. Cancer 69:2921, 1992.
26. Raymond AK: Surface osteosarcoma. Clin Orthop Rel Res 270:140, 1991.
27. Unni KK: *In* Unni KK (ed): Dahlin's Bone Tumors: General Aspects and Data on 11,807 Cases. 5th ed. Philadelphia, Lippincott-Raven, 1996.
28. Geschickter CF, Copeland MM: Parosteal osteoma of bone: A new entity. Ann Surg 133:790, 1951.
29. Unni KK, Dahlin DC, Beabout JW, et al: Parosteal osteogenic sarcoma. Cancer 37:2466, 1976.
30. Unni KK, Dahlin DC, Beabout JW: Periosteal osteogenic sarcoma. Cancer 37:2476, 1976.
31. Wold LE, Unni KK, Beabout JW, et al: High-grade surface osteosarcomas. Am J Surg Pathol 8:181, 1984.
32. Kyriakos M: Intracortical osteosarcoma. Cancer 46:2525, 1980.
33. Vigorita VJ, Jones JK, Ghelman B, et al: Intracortical osteosarcoma. Am J Surg Pathol 8:65, 1984.
34. Campanacci M, Picci P, Gherlinzoni F, et al: Parosteal osteosarcoma. J Bone Joint Surg Br 66B:313, 1984.
35. Okada K, Frassica FJ, Sim FH, et al: Parosteal osteosarcoma: A clinicopathological study. J Bone Joint Surg Am 76A:366, 1994.
36. Hinton CE, Turnbull AE, O'Donnell HDT, et al: Parosteal osteosarcoma of the skull. Histopathology 14:322, 1989.
37. Kumar R, Moser RP Jr, Madewell JE, et al: Parosteal osteogenic sarcomas arising in cranial bones: Clinical and radiologic features in eight patients. Am J Roentgenol 155:113, 1990.
38. Van der Walt JD, Ryan JF: Parosteal osteogenic sarcoma of the hand. Histopathology 16:75, 1990.
39. Masuda S, Murakawa Y: Postirradiation parosteal osteosarcoma: A case report. Clin Orthop Rel Res 184:204, 1984.
40. Levine E, De Smet AA, Huntrakoon M: Juxtacortical osteosarcoma: A radiologic and histologic spectrum. Skeletal Radiol 14:38, 1985.

41. Lindell MM, Shirkhoda A, Raymond AK, et al: Parosteal osteosarcoma: Radiologic-pathologic correlation with emphasis on CT. Am J Roentgenol 148:323, 1987.
42. Bertoni F, Present D, Hudson T, et al: The meaning of radiolucencies in parosteal osteosarcoma. J Bone Joint Surg Am 67A:901, 1985.
43. Sciot R, Samson I, Dal Cin P, et al: Giant cell-rich parosteal osteosarcoma. Histopathology 27:51, 1995.
44. Ahuja SC, Villacin AB, Smith J, et al: Juxtacortical (parosteal) osteogenic sarcoma: Histological grading and prognosis. J Bone Joint Surg Am 59A:632, 1977.
45. Luck JV Jr, Luck JV, Schwinn CP: Parosteal osteosarcoma: A treatment-orientated study. Clin Orthop Rel Res 153:92, 1980.
46. Enneking WF, Springfield D, Gross M: The surgical treatment of parosteal osteosarcoma in long bones. J Bone Joint Surg Am 67A:125, 1985.
47. Kavanagh TG, Cannon SR, Pringle J, et al: Parosteal osteosarcoma: Treatment by wide resection and prosthetic replacement. J Bone Joint Surg Br 72B:959, 1990.
48. Ritschl P, Wurnig C, Lechner G, et al: Parosteal osteosarcoma: 2–23 year follow-up of 33 patients. Acta Orthop Scand 62:195, 1991.
49. Schajowicz F, McGuire MH, Santini Araujo E, et al: Osteosarcomas arising on the surfaces of long bones. J Bone Joint Surg Am 70A:555, 1988.
50. Pintado SO, Lane J, Huvos AG: Parosteal osteogenic sarcoma of bone with co-existent low- and high-grade sarcomatous components. Hum Pathol 20:488, 1989.
51. Wold LE, Unni KK, Beabout JW, et al: Dedifferentiated parosteal osteosarcoma. J Bone Joint Surg Am 66A:53, 1984.
52. Sheth DS, Yasko AW, Raymond AK, et al: Conventional and dedifferentiated parosteal osteosarcoma: Diagnosis, treatment and outcome. Cancer 78:2136, 1996.
53. Sinovic JF, Bridge JA, Neff JR: Ring chromosome in parosteal osteosarcoma: Clinical and diagnostic significance. Cancer Genet Cytogenet 50:125, 1990.
54. Van Oven MW, Molenaar WM, Freling NJ, et al: Dedifferentiated parosteal osteosarcoma of the femur with aneuploidy and metastases. Cancer 63:807, 1989.
55. Dorfman HD, Ishida T, Tsuneyoshi M: Exophytic variant of fibrous dysplasia (fibrous dysplasia protuberans). Hum Pathol 25:2434, 1994.
56. Hall RB, Robinson LH, Malawar MM, et al: Periosteal osteosarcoma. Cancer 55:165, 1985.
57. Ritts GD, Pritchard DJ, Unni KK, et al: Periosteal osteosarcoma. Clin Orthop Rel Res 219:299, 1987.
58. de Santos LA, Murray JA, Finklestein JB, et al: The radiographic spectrum of periosteal osteosarcoma. Radiology 127:123, 1978.
59. Tanaka C, Fujiwara Y, Yamamuro T: Intraperiosteal osteoid osteoma: A case report. Clin Orthop Rel Res 175:190, 1983.
60. Glynn JJ, Lichtenstein L: Osteoid osteoma with multicentric nidus: A report of two cases. J Bone Joint Surg Am 55A:855, 1973.
61. Goldman R: The periosteal counterpart of benign osteoblastoma. Am J Clin Pathol 56:73, 1971.
62. Gentry JF, Schechter JJ, Mirra JM: Case report 574: Periosteal osteoblastoma of rib. Skeletal Radiol 18:551, 1989.
63. Bertoni F, Unni KK, Beabout JW, et al: Parosteal osteoma of bones other than of the skull and face. Cancer 75:2466, 1995.
64. Milgram JW: The origins of osteochondromas and enchondromas. Clin Orthop Rel Res 174:264, 1983.
65. Krieg JC, Buckwalter JA, Peterson KK, et al: Extensive growth of an osteochondroma in a skeletally mature patient. J Bone Joint Surg Am 77A:269, 1995.
66. Vallance R, Hamblen DL, Kelly IG: Vascular complications of osteochondroma. Clin Radiol 36:639, 1985.
67. El Khoury GY, Bassett GS: Symptomatic bursa formation with osteochondromas. Am J Roentgenol 133:895, 1979.
68. Borges AM, Huvos AG, Smith J: Bursa formation and synovial chondrometaplasia associated with osteochondromas. Am J Clin Pathol 75:648, 1981.
69. Libschitz HI, Cohen MA: Radiation-induced osteochondromas. Radiology 142:643, 1982.
70. Herman TE, McAlister WH, Rosenthal D, et al: Case report 691: Radiation-induced osteochondromas (RIO) arising from the neural arch and producing compression of the spinal cord. Skeletal Radiol 20:472, 1991.
71. Solomon L: Hereditary multiple exostosis. J Bone Joint Surg Br 45B:292, 1963.
72. Shapiro F, Simon S, Glimcher MJ: Hereditary multiple exostoses: Anthropometric, roentgenographic and clinical aspects. J Bone Joint Surg Am 61A:815, 1979.
73. Schmale GA, Conrad EU, Raskind WH: The natural history of hereditary multiple exostoses. J Bone Joint Surg Am 76A:986, 1994.
74. Hecht JT, Hogue D, Wang Y, et al: Hereditary multiple exostoses (EXT): Mutational studies of familial EXT1 cases and EXT-associated malignancies. Am J Hum Genet 60:80, 1997.
75. Norman A, Sissons HA: Radiographic hallmarks of peripheral chondrosarcoma. Radiology 151:589, 1984.
76. Caballes RL: Enchondroma protuberans masquerading as osteochondroma. Hum Pathol 13:734, 1982.
77. Crim JR, Mirra JM: Enchondroma protuberans: Report of a case and its distinction from chondrosarcoma and osteochondroma adjacent to an enchondroma. Skeletal Radiol 19:431, 1990.
78. Voutsinas S, Wynne-Davies R: The infrequency of malignant disease in diaphyseal aclasis and neurofibromatosis. J Med Genet 20:345, 1983.
79. Peterson HA: Multiple hereditary osteochondromata. Clin Orthop Rel Res 239:22, 1989.
80. Garrison RC, Unni KK, McLeod RA, et al: Chondrosarcoma arising in osteochondroma. Cancer 49:1890, 1982.
81. Bertoni F, Present D, Bacchini P, et al: Dedifferentiated peripheral chondrosarcomas: A report of seven cases. Cancer 63:2054, 1989.
82. Bauer TW, Dorfman HD, Latham JTJ: Periosteal chondroma: A clinicopathologic study of 23 cases. Am J Surg Pathol 6:631, 1982.
83. Boriani S, Bacchini P, Bertoni F, et al: Periosteal chondroma: A review of twenty cases. J Bone Joint Surg Am 65A:205, 1983.
84. Lewis MM, Kenan S, Yabut SM, et al: Periosteal chondroma: A report of ten cases and review of the literature. Clin Orthop Rel Res 256:185, 1990.
85. de Santos LA, Spjut HJ: Periosteal chondroma: A radiographic spectrum. Skeletal Radiol 6:15, 1981.
86. Schajowicz F: Juxtacortical chondrosarcoma. J Bone Joint Surg Br 59B:473, 1977.
87. Bertoni F, Boriani S, Laus M, et al: Periosteal chon-

drosarcoma and periosteal osteosarcoma: Two distinct entities. J Bone Joint Surg Br 64B:370, 1982.
88. Nojima T, Unni KK, McLeod RA, et al: Periosteal chondroma and periosteal chondrosarcoma. Am J Surg Pathol 9:666, 1985.
89. Robinson LH, Unni KK, O'Laughlin S, et al: Surface chondromyxoid fibroma of bone. Mod Pathol 7:10A, 1994.
90. Taconis WK, Van Rijssel TG: Fibrosarcoma of long bones: A study of the significance of areas of malignant fibrous histiocytoma. J Bone Joint Surg Br 67B:111, 1985.
91. Huvos AG, Higinbotham NL: Primary fibrosarcoma of bone: A clinicopathologic study of 130 patients. Cancer 35:837, 1975.
92. Kemp HBS, Byers PD: Case report 444: Subperiosteal malignant fibrous histiocytoma (MFH) of thigh with involvement of femur. Skeletal Radiol 16:584, 1987.
93. Bator SM, Bauer TW, Marks KE, et al: Periosteal Ewing's sarcoma. Cancer 58:1781, 1986.
94. Shapeero LG, Vanel D, Sundaram M, et al: Periosteal Ewing sarcoma. Radiology 191:825, 1994.
95. Ishida T, Kikuchi F, Oka T, et al: Case report 727: Juxtacortical adamantinoma of humerus. Skeletal Radiol 21:205, 1992.
96. Devaney K, Vinh TN, Sweet DE: Surface-based hemangiomas of bone: A review of 11 cases. Clin Orthop Rel Res 300:233, 1994.
97. O'Connell JX, Logan M, Beauchamp CP: Solitary fibrous tumor of the periosteum. Hum Pathol 26:460, 1995.
98. Fleming RJ, Alpert M, Garcia A: Parosteal lipoma. Am J Roentgenol 87:1075, 1962.
99. Jones JG, Haberman ET, Dorfman HD: Case report 553: Parosteal ossifying lipoma of femur. Skeletal Radiol 18:537, 1989.
100. McCarthy EF, Matz S, Steiner GC, et al: Periosteal ganglion: A cause of cortical bone erosion. Skeletal Radiol 10:243, 1983.

Chapter

12

SPINDLE CELL LESIONS OF BONE

SCOTT E. KILPATRICK and K. KRISHNAN UNNI

Spindle cell lesions of bone can be divided into neoplasm simulators and true neoplasms. The true neoplasms are divided into four subgroups—fibrous neoplasms, fibrohistiocytic neoplasms, myogenic neoplasms, and neurogenic neoplasms (Table 12–1). Tumors with spindle cell features exhibiting osseous or cartilaginous production (e.g., fibrous dysplasia) are discussed as part of the differential diagnosis but are considered in detail in other chapters. We consider fibrous neoplasms to include desmoplastic fibroma, fibrosarcoma, and congenital fibromatosis. Although avulsive cortical irregularity and metaphyseal fibrous defect are fibrous lesions, they do not represent "true" neoplasms and hence are included under the designation of neoplasm simulators. Fibrohistiocytic neoplasms of bone comprise benign or atypical fibrous histiocytoma and malignant fibrous histiocytoma. Metastatic "spindle cell" carcinomas may mimic both fibrosarcoma and malignant fibrous histiocytoma and are discussed within the differential diagnosis of these tumors. Myogenic neoplasms include only leiomyosarcoma of bone. To our knowledge, leiomyoma of bone does not exist. Similarly, neurogenic neoplasms of bone include only neurilemoma (schwannoma). We have not encountered any examples of neurofibroma or neurofibrosarcoma of bone.

Table 12–1. Spindle Cell Lesions of Bone

Neoplastic simulators
Metaphyseal fibrous defect
Avulsive cortical irregularity
Fibrous neoplasms of bone
Desmoplastic fibroma
Congenital fibromatosis
Fibrosarcoma
Fibrohistiocytic neoplasms of bone
Benign fibrous histiocytoma
Malignant fibrous histiocytoma
Myogenic neoplasms of bone
Leiomyosarcoma
Neurogenic neoplasms of bone
Schwannoma

Spindle cell lesions of bone, like other bone lesions, may pose significant problems for pathologists, radiologists, and orthopedic surgeons because they are uncommon conditions, and the diagnosis of malignancy often results in drastic consequences (surgical amputation and/or chemotherapy) frequently affecting young children. The wide variety of lesions that may mimic malignancy causes further apprehension for the surgical pathologist involved with a diagnosis of a bone tumor.

One aspect of the surgical pathologic diagnosis of bone lesions that cannot be overemphasized is the importance of radiographic interpretation. Firstly, the radiograph is important in the recognition of certain benign tumors or tumor-like conditions that do not require further analysis or treatment. One such example is metaphyseal fibrous defect. A radiologist experienced with bone lesions will readily identify its classic features and, unless the lesion is complicated by fracture or associated with atypical features, surgical intervention is not warranted, as the majority of these lesions will resolve on their own. Secondly, when necessary, the radiographs aid the surgeon in choosing the optimal site for tissue biopsy. Third, for the surgical pathologist, accurate assessment of features such as location, size and shape, pattern of bone destruction, matrix, margins, periosteal reaction, and concomitant soft tissue abnormalities usually relate to the aggressiveness of the lesion and, therefore, allow for a more specific diagnosis. In this manner, radiographs serve as the "gross bone specimen" for the pathologist.

Unfortunately, the interpretation of radiographs has its limitations, and, in some cases, the radiographic appearance can be quite misleading. An aneurysmal bone cyst may show very aggressive and even "malignant" features on radiographs. In contrast, intraosseous osteosarcomas may sometimes appear innocuous. For these reasons, radiographic features should not supplant histologic interpretation in establishing a diagnosis. Nevertheless, we believe the pathologic diagnosis of a bone tumor should be a multidisciplinary one comprising clinical data, radiographic features, and optimal histology. Using this approach, the surgical pathologist can avoid potential misdiagnoses.

Regarding classification of bone tumors, we employ the one first proposed by Lichtenstein,[1] which is based predominately on the cytologic features of the individual cells and specific matrix production by the lesion. Our grading system of bone tumors follows that proposed by Broders[2] and Unni and Dahlin.[3] Although Broders's original report involved squamous cell carcinoma of the lip, the same criteria may be applied to bone tumors. Importantly, histologic grade applies only to malignant tumors and is based on the resemblance of the neoplastic cells to their normal counterparts. Our grading scale encompasses four levels of histologic differentiation (i.e., I–IV). Thus, neoplasms that closely resemble normal cells should receive the lowest grade (i.e. grade I or II), whereas less differentiated tumors, which least resemble normal cells, would receive the highest grade (grade III–IV). Grading is only applicable to those tumors showing cytologic variation, and some tumors, such as Ewing's sarcoma, are considered by nature poorly differentiated, and hence are not further graded.

NEOPLASM SIMULATORS

Metaphyseal Fibrous Defect (Nonossifying Fibroma)

Metaphyseal fibrous defects typically involve the metaphysis of a long bone and probably do not represent true neoplastic change. Terms such as nonossifying fibroma, fibroma, and fibrous cortical defect are considered synonymous.

Clinical Features

In general, metaphyseal fibrous defects are incidental findings presenting between 10 and 20 years of age and affecting males and females equally. Physical examination rarely reveals any significant swelling or overlying skin changes. Occasional patients may present with pathologic fracture. The most common anatomic locations in decreasing order of frequency are distal femur, distal tibia, proximal tibia, proximal fibula, and proximal humerus. Rarely, the defect may involve the clavicle or the ribs. Although usually solitary, multiple lesions sometimes occur and, rarely, may be associated with extraosseous features (Jaffe-Campanacci syndrome).[4, 5] These stigmata may include café-au-lait-like skin patches (in the absence of neurofibromas), cryptorchidism, and mental retardation. We have never encountered malignant transformation in a metaphyseal fibrous defect; however, Kyriakos and Murphy[6] reported a case of concurrent osteosarcoma and metaphyseal fibrous defect.

Radiologic Features

Almost without exception, metaphyseal fibrous defects are eccentrically located along the long axis of the metaphyseal portion of bone. Size is variable and may range from small, intracortical lesions to those involving virtually the entire diameter of the bone. In young to middle-aged adults, the lesions may be diaphyseally centered and show mineralization (healing). The lesion may be expansile but is sharply marginated with a sclerotic ("scalloped") margin (Fig. 12–1). Rarely, multiple lesions may be present. The radiographic differential diagnosis includes chondromyxoid fibroma, fibrous dysplasia, and Langerhans' cell histiocytosis.

Pathologic Features

On gross inspection, the curettage specimen consists of firm red-tan to gray tissue with varying amounts of yellow coloration, depending upon the amount of lipid-laden macrophages. Microscopically, metaphyseal fibrous defects are hypercellular lesions composed of a uniform population of spindle cells characteristi-

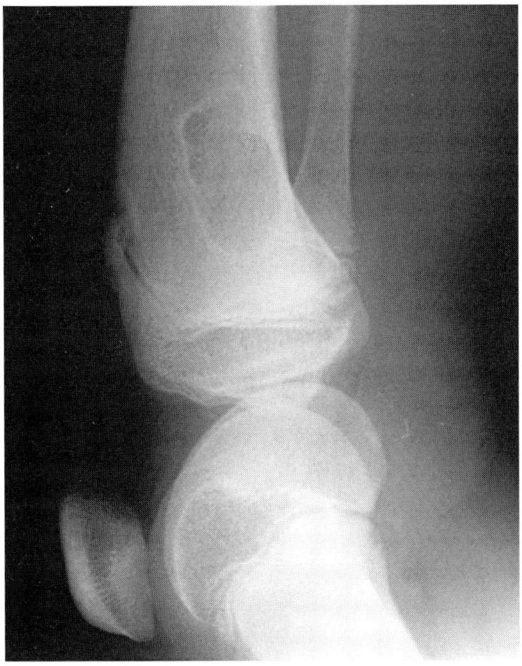

Figure 12–1. Classic metaphyseal fibrous defect involving the proximal tibia in a 13-year-old boy. Note the sharp margination and rim of sclerosis.

cally arranged in a storiform pattern (Fig. 12–2*A*). The spindle cells may show numerous mitoses, especially in the early proliferative phase of the lesion; however, atypical mitoses are absent. The nuclei of the spindle cells may display prominent nucleoli but remain regular and monotonous. Scattered throughout the lesion are often numerous osteoclast-type giant cells, foamy macrophages, and even hemosiderin-laden macrophages (Fig. 12–2*B*). Reactive new bone formation rimmed by a thin layer of osteoblasts may also be present, especially in the presence of pathologic fracture. Older lesions may also show a considerable amount of mature trabecular bone. For these reasons, we avoid using the term *nonossifying fibroma,* since this suggests a total absence of bone.

Differential Diagnosis

The differential diagnosis of metaphyseal fibrous defect includes benign fibrous histiocytoma and giant cell tumor. Both entities generally pose little diagnostic difficulty if correlation with radiographic and clinical features is obtained.

The term *benign fibrous histiocytoma* describes lesions with the histologic features of a metaphyseal fibrous defect but that do not have the characteristic clinical or radiographic findings. Benign fibrous histiocytomas tend to occur in nonmetaphyseal locations such as the epiphyses of a long bone or the pelvic bones (see later discussion).

Giant cell tumors are generally seen in skeletally mature (≥18 years of age) individuals and usually involve the epiphysis of a long bone (see Chapter 15). The background stromal cells in giant cell tumors are oval and only slightly elongated in contrast to the slender, more elongated cells in metaphyseal fibrous defect. Furthermore, a well-developed storiform pattern is rarely seen in giant cell tumor. In our opinion, the number of osteoclast-type giant cells or the number of nuclei present within the giant cells is not useful in this distinction.

Prognosis and Treatment

In those cases in which the integrity of the bone is not compromised, simple observation is adequate treatment. The vast majority of cases ultimately "heal," probably by cortical remodeling and reparative ossification. Lesions occupying more than 50% of the bone diameter represent a significant risk for fracture.[7] In these cases, bone curettage with grafting is curative.

Avulsive Cortical Irregularity (Periosteal Desmoid)

Synonyms for avulsive cortical irregularity include periosteal desmoid, cortical desmoid, distal metaphyseal femoral defect, distal femoral cortical defect, and cortical irregularity syndrome.

Clinical Features

Avulsive cortical irregularity is almost exclusively found on the posterior medial distal femur at or near the insertion of the adductor magnus muscle.[8, 9] Similar lesions have been described involving the humerus at the insertion of the pectoralis major muscle.[10] The majority of patients are younger than 20 years of age; boys are affected more often than girls (3:1). Interestingly, some of these lesions are bilateral.[11] Most often, they present as incidental findings following minor trauma.

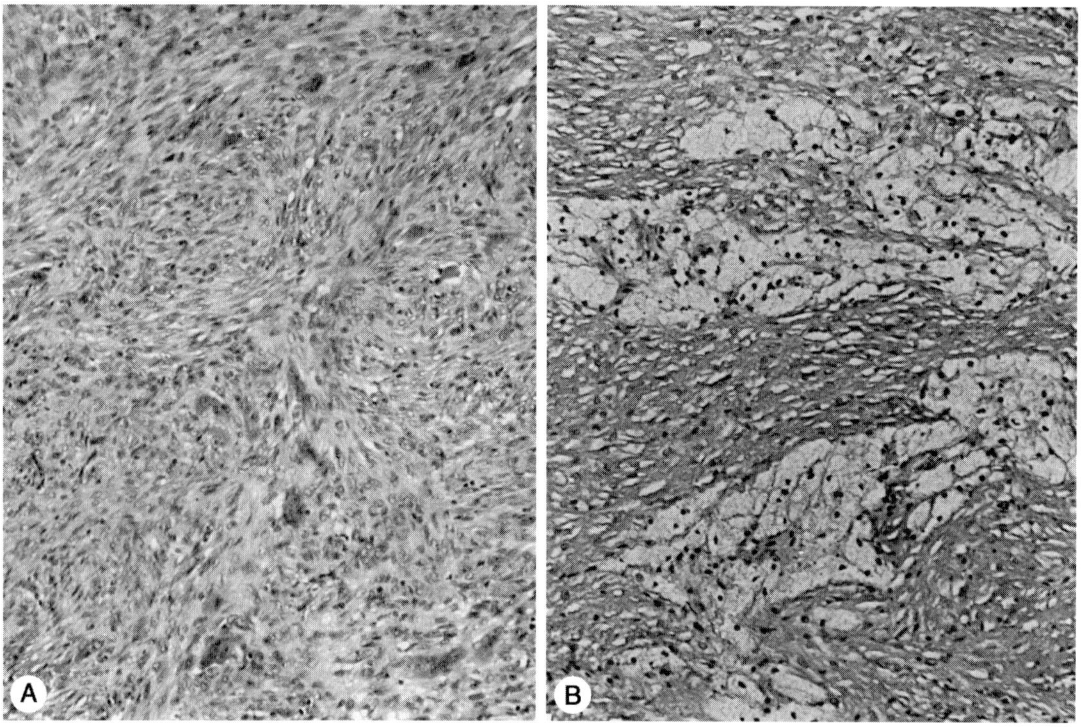

Figure 12–2. Metaphyseal fibrous defect. *A*, Classic storiform pattern of hypercellular metaphyseal fibrous defect. Individual cells are remarkably uniform despite the fact that numerous mitoses may be present. Scattered osteoclast-type giant cells are also evident. *B*, Occasional areas within metaphyseal fibrous defects may show aggregates of "foamy" lipid-laden macrophages.

Radiologic Features

Avulsive cortical irregularities in the femur typically present as radiolucent areas located along the medial posterior subcondylar ridges superior to the epiphyseal plate (Fig. 12–3*A*). Frequently, cortical "fuzziness" is also present. A soft tissue mass is never seen.

Pathologic Features

The lesion is composed of abundant stromal collagen reminiscent of tendon-like fibrous tissue and is distinctly hypocellular. Cytologically, individual cells are uniformly spindled and lack significant atypia (Fig. 12–3*B*). A few benign-appearing giant cells may be scattered throughout the lesion. Rarely, reactive bone or cartilage resembling callus may also be present.

Prognosis and Treatment

In most cases with classic radiographic features, no therapy is needed. Biopsy or curettage may be indicated in those patients in whom the radiologic features are atypical. Treated or untreated, the prognosis is excellent and recurrences do not occur following biopsy.[12]

FIBROUS NEOPLASMS OF BONE

Desmoplastic Fibroma

Clinical Features

Desmoplastic fibroma of bone is an extraordinarily rare tumor that represents the intraosseous equivalent of aggressive fibromatosis (desmoid tumor) of soft tissues. Excluding consultation cases, there are only nine examples of desmoplastic fibroma of bone in the Mayo Clinic files. Age at diagnosis ranges from 1 to 70 years; however, the majority of patients are diagnosed in the first three decades of life. In our experience, there is a slight male predominance. Desmoplastic fibromas commonly arise from the metaphysis or metadiaphysis of the long bones (femur, tibia, humerus, and radius); nevertheless, the single

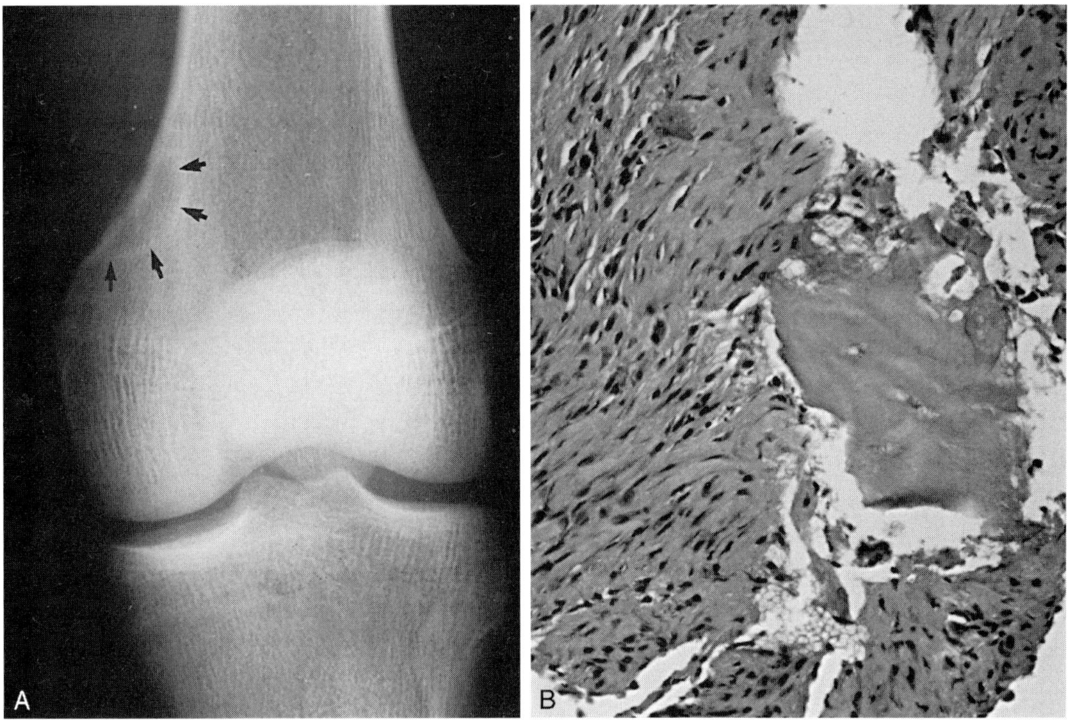

Figure 12–3. Avulsive cortical irregularity. *A*, Radiolucent defect *(arrows)* with a sclerotic margin on the posterior-medial distal femoral metaphysis. *B*, Tendon-like fibrous tissue and uniform, banal-appearing spindle cells. A fragment of cortical bone is also present.

most common skeletal site is the mandible.[13, 14] The most common presenting complaint is localized pain. Desmoplastic fibroma has been reported associated with Paget's disease and fibrous dysplasia.[15, 16]

Radiologic Features

Desmoplastic fibromas usually present as expansile, lytic, and lobulated lesions often described as having a "soap bubble" appearance and void of matrix production (Fig. 12–4*A*). Periosteal reaction is generally lacking, and the margin is sharply defined. Sclerosis is occasionally present. The radiographic differential diagnosis includes simple bone cyst, metaphyseal fibrous defect, chondromyxoid fibroma, and fibrous dysplasia. Rarely, more obvious bone destruction associated with a soft tissue mass may simulate malignancy (i.e., fibrosarcoma or osteosarcoma).

Pathologic Features

Grossly, desmoplastic fibroma is gray-white and fibrous in appearance, with scattered small cystic spaces (Fig. 12–4*B*). The microscopic morphology of desmoplastic fibroma is identical to that of aggressive fibromatosis of soft tissues. Characteristic features include sweeping fascicles of uniform-appearing spindle cells within a variably collagenized stroma (Fig. 12–4*C*). Although usually hypocellular in appearance, occasional foci of hypercellularity may also be present. The collagen within the stroma may range from thin wavy fibers to thick keloid-like bundles (Fig. 12–4*D*). In areas of absent or sparse collagen production, myxoid changes may be apparent. Cytologically, individual cells contain slender to elongated monotonous nuclei and inconspicuous nucleoli, lacking significant nuclear pleomorphism or hyperchromasia. Mitotic activity is rare. Sections from the periphery of the tumor may show permeation of existing bony trabeculae and even surrounding soft tissues.

Differential Diagnosis

Clinically, the most important distinction is separating desmoplastic fibroma from fibrosarcoma. Generally, fibrosarcomas are more hypercellular than desmoplastic fibromas, and the characteristic herring-bone pattern of fi-

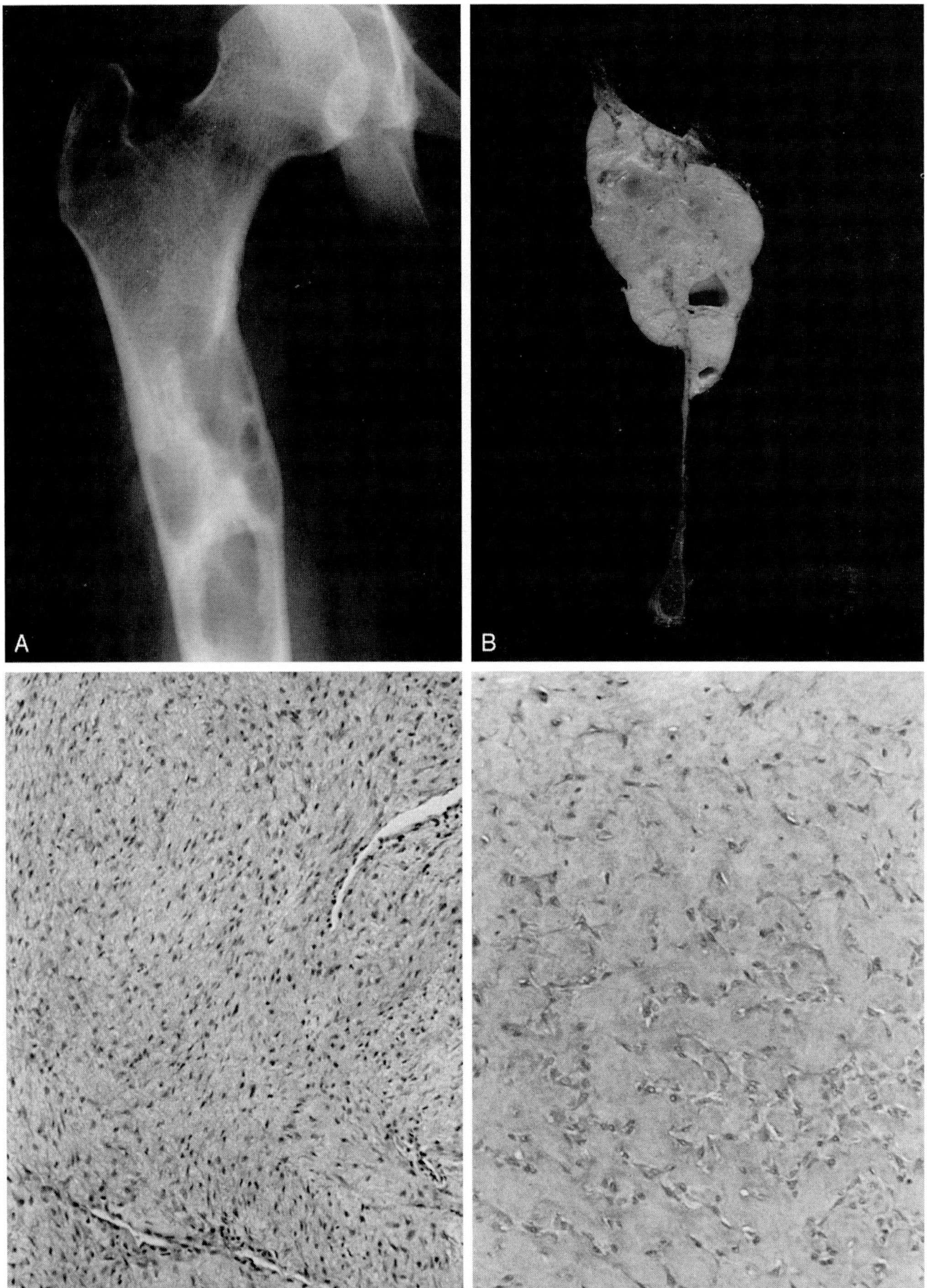

Figure 12–4. Desmoplastic fibroma of bone. *A*, Radiograph of the metadiaphysis of the proximal femur in an 18-year-old woman. The bone is expanded and shows lytic areas transversed by irregular trabeculations. *B*, Specimen from the scapula in a 36-year-old woman showing homogenous fibrous appearance and cystic spaces. *C*, Classic case with "sweeping" fascicles of uniform spindle cells and a collagenous background. Note the close resemblance to desmoid tumor of soft tissue. *D*, Occasional examples demonstrate keloid-like bundles of collagen fibers.

brosarcoma is never seen in desmoplastic fibroma. Cytologically, more nuclear atypia is observed in fibrosarcoma. In most cases, separation of fibrosarcoma from desmoplastic fibroma will not pose a diagnostic problem. However, in low-grade fibrosarcomas, this distinction may be very difficult. Of comfort to the pathologist faced with this dilemma is the fact that the behavior of low-grade fibrosarcoma (i.e., frequent recurrences but metastasis less likely) is not appreciably different from that of desmoplastic fibroma. Bone tumors focally resembling desmoplastic fibroma of bone but cytologically displaying hyperchromasia, anaplasia, and significant mitotic activity should be regarded as fibrosarcoma.

Perhaps a more common scenario is the differential diagnosis of fibrous dysplasia and desmoplastic fibroma. In those cases of fibrous dysplasia in which bone is not readily identified, the distinction of its stroma from that seen in desmoplastic fibroma may also prove difficult. However, the nuclei in the stromal cells of fibrous dysplasia are shorter and usually more compact in appearance when compared to the elongated slender nuclei typically seen in desmoplastic fibroma.

Prognosis and Treatment

Desmoplastic fibroma of bone should be regarded as a low-grade "borderline" malignancy because of its tendency toward locally aggressive behavior but absence of metastatic potential. Recurrence rates following surgical treatment range up to 47%. For this reason, en bloc resection of the lesion with a wide margin is recommended.[13, 14] At the present time, there appears to be no role for radiation therapy or chemotherapy in the treatment of desmoplastic fibroma.

Congenital Fibromatosis (Infantile Myofibromatosis)

Clinical Features

Congenital fibromatosis is a rare disease most commonly seen in infancy and childhood. Age at diagnosis ranges from birth to 16 years; however, the majority of patients are less than 2 years of age at presentation. It may present as a solitary subcutaneous nodule, multiple masses involving the skeleton and soft tissues, or involvement of visceral organs. The craniofacial skeleton, specifically the skull followed by the mandible, represents the most frequent site of osseous involvement.[17] Those cases involving soft tissue usually involve the head and neck region, followed in frequency by the trunk and proximal extremities. Distal extremity involvement (i.e., hands or feet) does not usually occur.[18]

Radiologic Features

Regardless of whether the lesion is solitary or multicentric, congenital fibromatosis typically presents as a lucent lesion with a sclerotic rim (Fig. 12–5*A*).[19, 20] Lesions in the mandible are lucent and sharply marginated but lack marginal sclerosis. In the multicentric form, multiple, bilateral, and symmetrical lesions are frequently seen in the metaphyses of the long bones. Usually, as the patients mature, the lesions spontaneously heal. Whether some such lesions in the long bones represent concomitant metaphyseal fibrous defects is unclear. Radiographic differential diagnosis includes metaphyseal fibrous defect, aneurysmal bone cyst, chondromyxoid fibroma, and Langerhans' cell histiocytosis. Extraskeletal tumors present on radiographs as soft tissue masses, often with foci of calcification.[18]

Pathologic Features

Grossly, submitted tissue is white-gray to tan and usually fibrous, although some areas may be firm and cartilaginoid. Microscopically, congenital fibromatosis of bone shows bundles, whorls, and nodules of smooth muscle–appearing cells alternating with fascicles of spindled fibroblast-like cells (Fig. 12–5*B* and *C*). Frequently, within the fascicular areas between the nodules are slit-like to cleft-shaped vascular spaces (Fig. 12–5*D*). In some cases, this vascular pattern may predominate, the histologic picture mimicking hemangiopericytoma. The background stroma is usually "loose" in appearance and may focally show myxoid or even chondroid changes. Occasionally, foci of necrosis or calcification are also apparent. Although mitoses are present in the majority of cases, they are generally not numerous, and atypical forms are absent. In contrast to desmoplastic fibroma, congenital fibromatosis is usually well circumscribed and only rarely exhibits infiltration of surrounding bony trabeculae. An immunohistochemical and ultrastructural study of a single skeletal

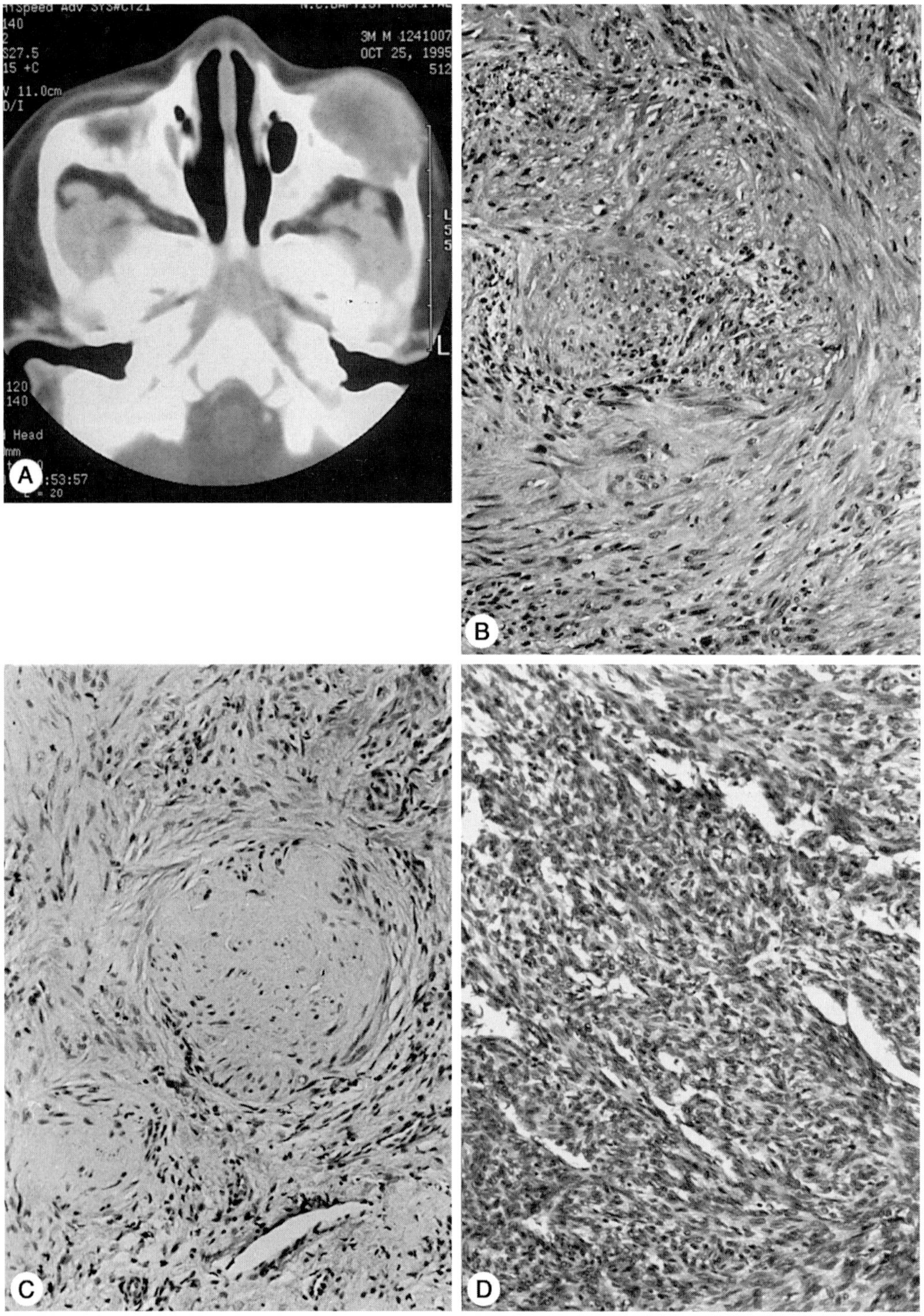

Figure 12–5. Congenital fibromatosis. *A,* Computed tomography of the skull discloses a well-circumscribed mass involving the inferior orbital and zygomatic bones in a 3-month-old boy. Biopsy showed classic features of congenital fibromatosis. *B,* Characteristic myofibroblastic fascicles of congenital fibromatosis. *C,* Characteristic myofibroblastic nodules of congenital fibromatosis. *D,* Slit-like vascular spaces within fascicular areas of congenital fibromatosis. Such areas may predominate, mimicking hemangiopericytoma.

case reported immunoreactivity for vimentin and α–smooth muscle actin.[21]

Differential Diagnosis

The differential diagnosis for congenital fibromatosis of bone includes desmoplastic fibroma, metaphyseal fibrous defect, and fibrosarcoma. Aside from the obvious clinical and radiographic differences, the most important diagnostic feature of congenital fibromatosis is the presence of a myofibroblastic nodular appearance within a hemangiopericytoma-like to chondroid-appearing stroma. The classic herring-bone pattern of fibrosarcoma is not seen in congenital fibromatosis.

Prognosis and Treatment

In the solitary osseous form of the disease, conservative surgical treatment with simple excision is recommended. Local recurrence in solitary osseous lesions is not typically seen and if present should lead to a reassessment of the diagnosis.[17] Once the diagnosis of congenital fibromatosis is established, further studies should be performed to exclude multicentric disease. Most patients do well, even in the presence of multiple bone and soft tissue lesions. Chung and Enzinger[18] reported 15 patients with multicentric involvement; 12 of these patients were alive and without active disease at last contact, and 5 of the 12 showed spontaneous regression. Patients with extensive visceral involvement have a significantly higher risk of disease progression and death; of the four patients in this study with extensive visceral involvement, three died shortly after birth.[18]

Fibrosarcoma

Clinical Features

Fibrosarcoma of bone occurs over a broad age range, and, unlike with osteosarcoma, there is no predilection for the second decade of life. Males and females appear to be affected equally. Although any portion of the skeleton may be involved, the majority of cases involve the bones around the knee and pelvis. Specifically, the most common locations in decreasing order of frequency are the distal femur, the proximal tibia, the ilium, the mandible, and the sacrum and proximal humerus. Clinical symptoms usually include pain and soft tissue swelling over the affected bone. Importantly, fibrosarcomas may arise from preexisting bone conditions, including fibrous dysplasia, Paget's disease, irradiated bone, and chronic osteomyelitis.[22, 23]

Radiologic Features

The radiographic features of fibrosarcoma are, in general, nonspecific and may be seen in any number of malignancies. Typically, the lesion is metaphyseally located, purely lytic, and lacks marginal sclerosis. The margin is poorly defined, and cortical destruction with extension into surrounding soft tissues is common. Rarely, low-grade lesions may be sharply marginated but still lack a sclerotic rim.

Pathologic Features

Well-differentiated, low-grade fibrosarcomas tend to be well-circumscribed, white-tan, and fibrous due to abundant collagen. More commonly, high-grade lesions have indistinct permeative margins and often foci of yellow-tan necrosis (Fig. 12–6*A*). Microscopically, fibrosarcomas are characteristically hypercellular high-grade lesions composed of fascicles of spindle cells frequently arranged in a herring-bone pattern (Fig. 12–6*B*). Collagen production may be abundant in less cellular, lower grade lesions, making the distinction from desmoplastic fibroma difficult (Fig. 12–6*C*). Cytologically, the cells of fibrosarcoma of bone range from typical elongated, fibroblastic-appearing nuclei to short, blunted nuclei that may focally resemble Ewing's sarcoma (Fig. 12–6*D*). Osteoclast-type giant cells may be seen but are rarely numerous.

Low-grade (grade I–II) tumors are characterized by mild to moderate cellularity and abundant collagen production. Cytologically, the individual cells resemble normal fibroblasts. High-grade (grade III–IV) tumors exhibit marked cellularity and minimal to absent collagen production and often display the characteristic herring-bone pattern. Mitotic figures are abundant.

Differential Diagnosis

The differential diagnosis of fibrosarcoma of bone includes, at the low-grade end of the spectrum, desmoplastic fibroma and congenital fibromatosis (see previous sections) and, at

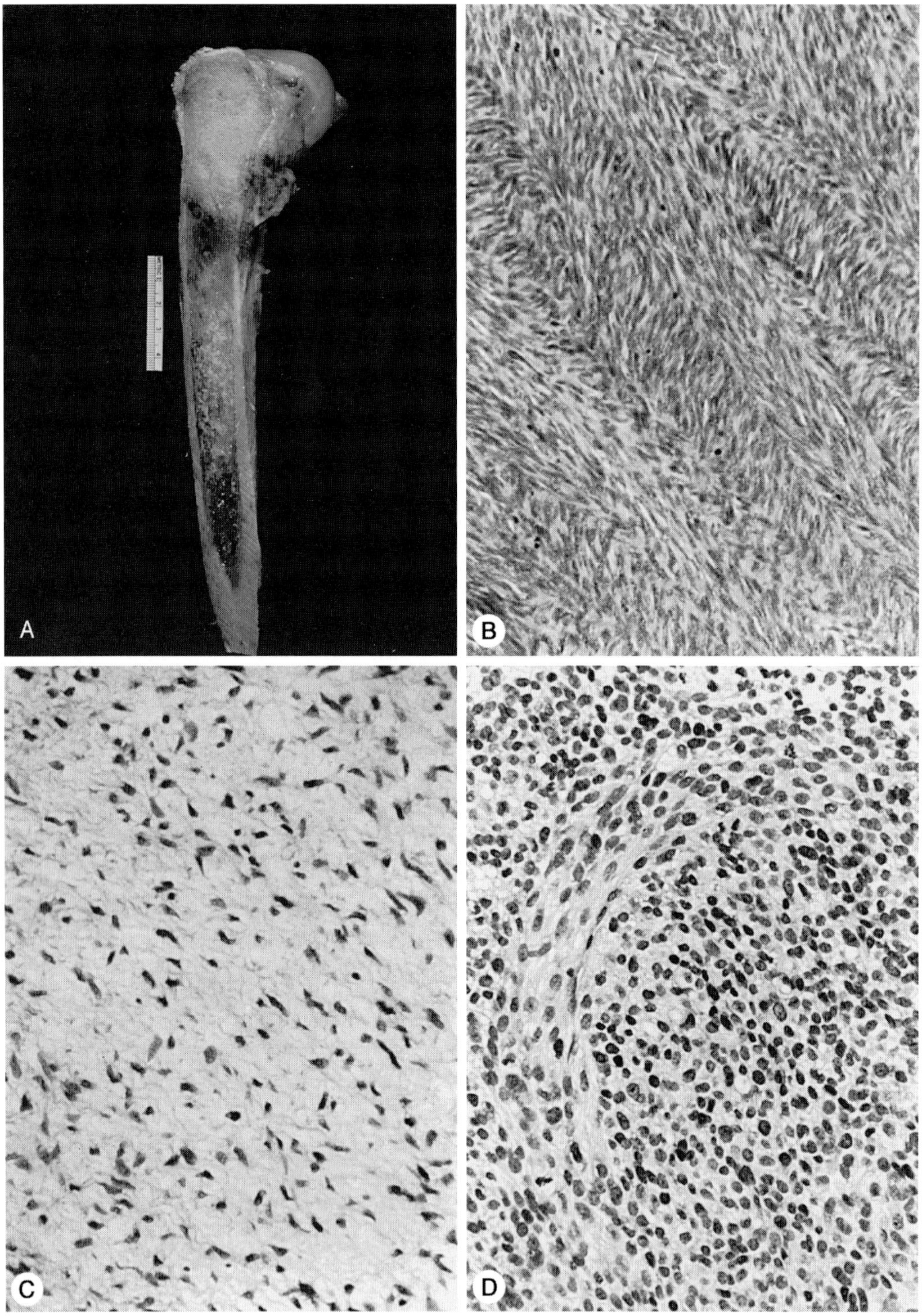

Figure 12–6. Fibrosarcoma. *A*, Lesion permeating and replacing the bone marrow of the distal femur in a 36-year-old woman. *B*, Classic herring-bone pattern of high-grade fibrosarcoma. The neoplasm is hypercellular and mitoses are frequent. *C*, Low-grade, mildly to moderately cellular fibrosarcoma with abundant background collagen resembling desmoplastic fibroma. Cytologically, individual cells show more nuclear hyperchromasia and atypia than is seen in desmoplastic fibroma. *D*, Occasional examples may contain more "rounded" cells, resembling Ewing's sarcoma. Importantly, the presence of even minor "spindling" features almost always excludes the diagnosis of Ewing's sarcoma.

the high-grade end of the spectrum, fibroblastic osteosarcoma, malignant fibrous histiocytoma, and metastatic carcinoma. Generally speaking, the collagen fibers in fibrosarcoma are thinner than those seen in desmoplastic fibroma. Depending on the degree of malignancy, mitotic activity ranges from sparse to abundant but generally exceeds that seen in desmoplastic fibroma or congenital fibromatosis.

The lack of osseous matrix production in fibrosarcoma is the only reliable feature separating it from fibroblastic osteosarcoma. By definition, fibrosarcomas lack the marked nuclear pleomorphism and atypical giant cells characteristic of malignant fibrous histiocytoma.

The presence of short, blunt-ended nuclei in fibrosarcoma may lead to confusion with Ewing's sarcoma. Importantly, the cells of Ewing's sarcoma are never spindled, so that the presence of even minor "spindled" cytomorphology excludes the diagnosis of Ewing's sarcoma. If in doubt, immunohistochemical or molecular studies may be performed (see Chapter 14).

In older adults, it is necessary to exclude metastatic carcinoma. Metastatic sarcomatoid renal cell carcinomas are especially prone to exhibit fibrosarcoma-like features. Immunohistochemical stains for epithelial markers and a good clinical examination are the best tools for establishing this diagnosis.

Prognosis and Treatment

In fibrosarcoma, the prognosis directly correlates with the histologic grade of the neoplasm.[24, 25] For low-grade lesions, conservative surgical excision is usually adequate treatment. In contrast, high-grade lesions may require preoperative chemotherapy and limb-sparing resection with reconstruction when feasible. In certain cases, amputation may be indicated. Radiation therapy may be employed for surgically inaccessible lesions.

FIBROHISTIOCYTIC NEOPLASMS

Benign (Atypical) Fibrous Histiocytoma

Clinical Features

Benign (also referred to as atypical) fibrous histiocytoma of bone is an extremely rare (somewhat controversial) tumor generally found in adults. Females are affected slightly more commonly than males (1.5:1). The most common anatomic site is the ilium; other common locations include the femur and tibia. In general, most patients are asymptomatic, and routine physical examination is unrevealing.

Radiologic Features

Radiographically, benign fibrous histiocytoma is a lytic lesion with sharp margination and focal sclerosis.[26] Matrix mineralization is distinctly absent (Fig. 12–7*A*). Expansion of the affected bone is commonly seen. The radiographic differential diagnosis includes fibrous dysplasia, giant cell tumor, and chondromyxoid fibroma.

Pathologic Features

As has already been mentioned, the morphology of benign fibrous histiocytoma and metaphyseal fibrous defect are virtually identical. On gross inspection, the curettage specimen ranges from gray-white to yellow-tan, depending on the amount of lipid present. Microscopically, the tumor is composed of uniform-appearing, spindled-shaped cells frequently arranged in a storiform pattern. Foamy macrophages are often present, and osteoclast-type giant cells are scattered throughout the lesion (Fig. 12–7*B*). Hemosiderin-laden macrophages are common. Although mitotic figures may be numerous, atypical mitoses are never present. Cytologically, individual cells lack significant nuclear pleomorphism or anaplasia.

Differential Diagnosis

The differential diagnosis of the benign fibrous histiocytoma includes metaphyseal fibrous defect, giant cell tumor, and malignant fibrous histiocytoma. Distinction morphologically from metaphyseal fibrous defect may be very difficult. We believe that painful lesions in adult patients, especially in nonmetaphyseal locations, should be regarded as benign fibrous histiocytoma. In contrast, metaphyseal fibrous defect is virtually always observed in children and, unless associated with fracture, usually is not painful.

Those cases of fibrous histiocytoma involving the epiphysis may be difficult to distinguish from giant cell tumor. Given the rarity

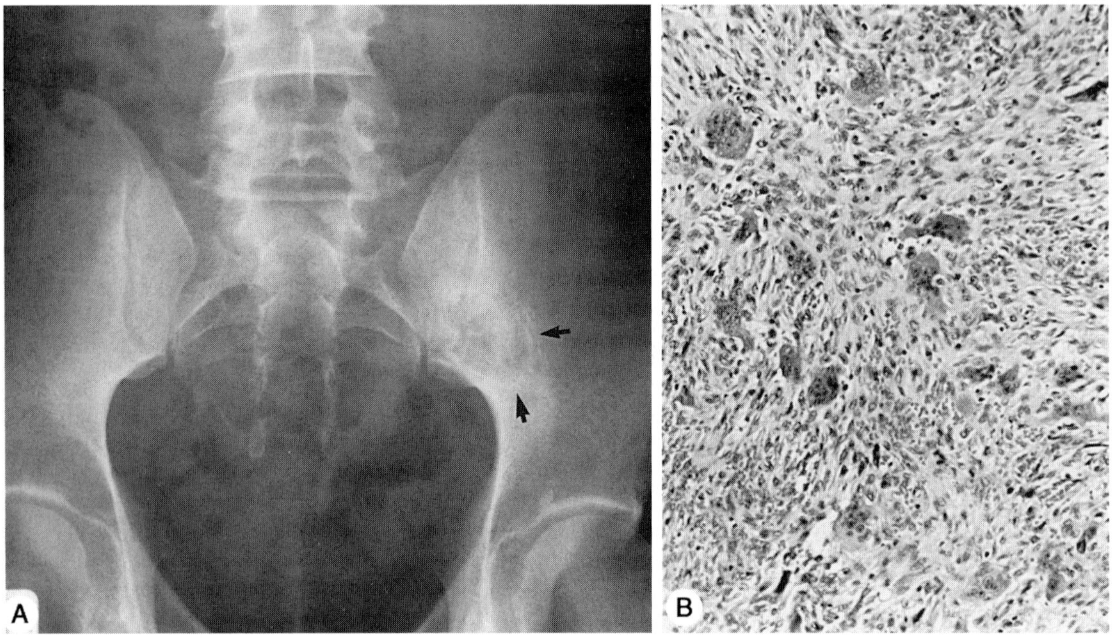

Figure 12–7. Benign fibrous histiocytoma. *A*, Radiograph from a 29-year-old man showing sharply marginated and focally sclerotic, lytic lesion in the left ilium *(arrows)*. *B*, Benign fibrous histiocytoma resembles metaphyseal fibrous defect, being composed of a uniform population of spindle cells arranged in storiform pattern and scattered osteoclast-type giant cells. Clinical and radiologic correlation is needed.

of benign fibrous histiocytoma, the vast majority of such cases will represent giant cell tumor of bone, and foci of typical giant cell tumor will be found if carefully sought.[27] In comparison to malignant fibrous histiocytoma, its benign counterpart lacks significant cytologic atypia, nuclear pleomorphism, and mitotic activity.

Prognosis and Treatment

Generally, benign fibrous histiocytoma can be treated by simple curettage and bone grafting.[28] En bloc resection may be necessary for lesions located in the ilium. Aggressive behavior overall is uncommon; however, unlike metaphyseal fibrous defect, local recurrence may occur.[26]

Malignant Fibrous Histiocytoma

In contrast to those originating in soft tissue, malignant fibrous histiocytoma of bone is an uncommon tumor. This may be, in part, related to its considerable histologic overlap with fibrosarcoma and fibroblastic osteosarcoma. In the literature, its true incidence varies depending on intraobserver criteria.

Clinical Features

Although malignant fibrous histiocytoma is seen in patients over a broad age range, it clearly predominates in adults. Males and females are involved with equal frequency. Like fibrosarcoma and osteosarcoma, the bones around the knee are most commonly afflicted. The most common anatomic sites in decreasing order of frequency are the distal femur, proximal femur, proximal tibia, ilium, and skull (calvarium). Most patients present with complaints of a soft tissue mass, which may be associated with pain. As with fibrosarcoma, malignant fibrous histiocytoma may arise from pre-existing conditions such as prior irradiation, bone infarcts, or Paget's disease.[29, 30]

Radiologic Features

Malignant fibrous histiocytoma of bone most often displays a lytic pattern within the metaphysis of a long bone. Cortical destruction associated with a soft tissue mass is commonly seen (Fig. 12–8*A*). The radiographic differential diagnosis includes other obvious malignant bone tumors, including osteosarcoma, fibrosarcoma, malignant lymphoma, and metastatic carcinoma.

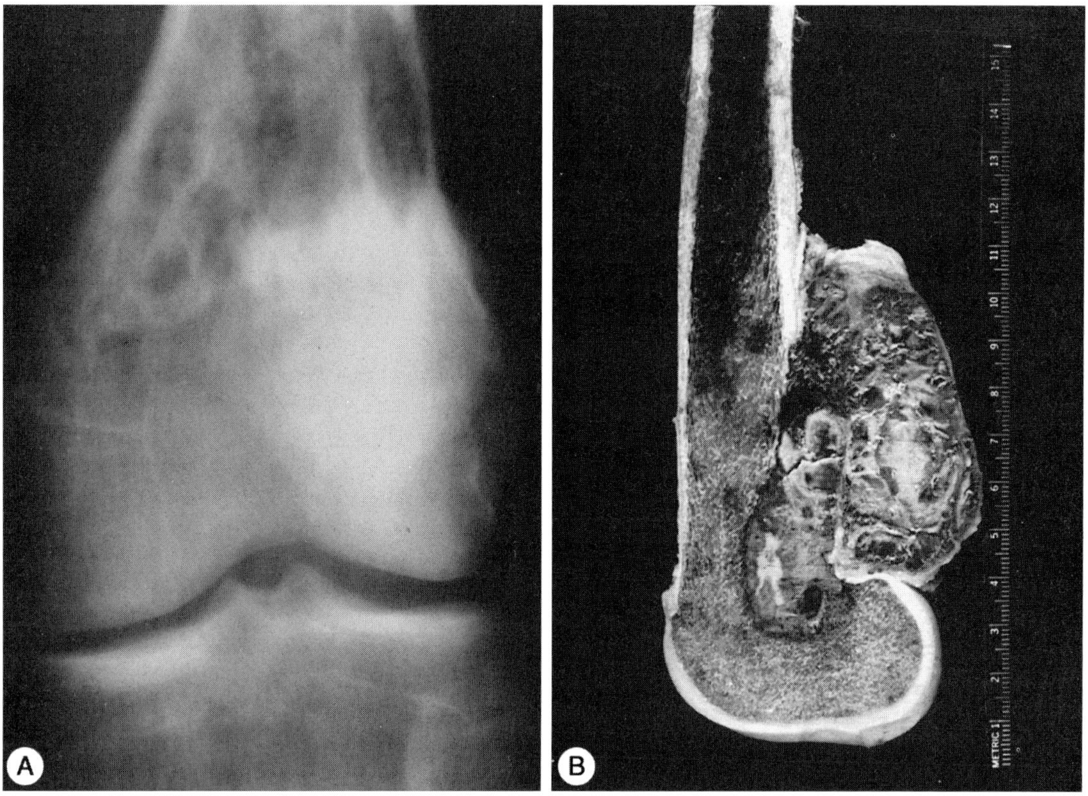

Figure 12–8. Malignant fibrous histiocytoma of bone. *A*, Case involving the metaphysis of the distal femur. Note the ill-defined permeative appearance. *B*, Case involving the distal femur of a 45-year-old woman. Note the large soft tissue mass.

Pathologic Features

Resected specimens are tan-brown, hemorrhagic, and focally necrotic with permeative, ill-defined margins. A soft tissue mass is commonly present (Fig. 12–8*B*). Microscopically, the lesion is composed of a spindle cell proliferation frequently arranged in a storiform pattern. By definition, malignant fibrous histiocytoma contains anaplastic giant cells and marked nuclear pleomorphism (Fig. 12–9*A* [see also color Figure 12–9]). Benign osteoclast-type giant cells are often admixed with the atypical malignant giant cells. Osteoid and cartilage production by the malignant cells is never seen and its presence excludes the diagnosis of malignant fibrous histiocytoma.

Differential Diagnosis

The differential diagnosis of malignant fibrous histiocytoma includes fibrosarcoma, fibroblastic osteosarcoma, and metastatic carcinoma. Generally, the degree of nuclear pleomorphism and anaplasia in malignant fibrous histiocytoma far exceeds that seen in fibrosarcoma. The presence of even minor foci of osteoid matrix production by the tumor cells confirms the diagnosis of osteosarcoma and effectively excludes the diagnosis of malignant fibrous histiocytoma (Fig. 12–9*B*). For the latter reason, we rarely make the diagnosis of malignant fibrous histiocytoma.

The possibility of malignant lymphoma and metastatic sarcomatoid carcinoma in the differential diagnosis of malignant fibrous histiocytoma should be considered in any older adult patient. The presence of extensive lymphocytic infiltrates and background sclerosis strongly suggests malignant lymphoma. Immunohistochemical stains for lymphocytic markers are invaluable in this setting. As in fibrosarcoma of bone, metastatic sarcomatoid carcinomas, especially those originating from the kidney, may pose an especially difficult problem (Fig. 12–10). Although immunohistochemistry (i.e., epithelial membrane antigen and cytokeratin) may be helpful in this setting, in our experience, a thorough clinical exami-

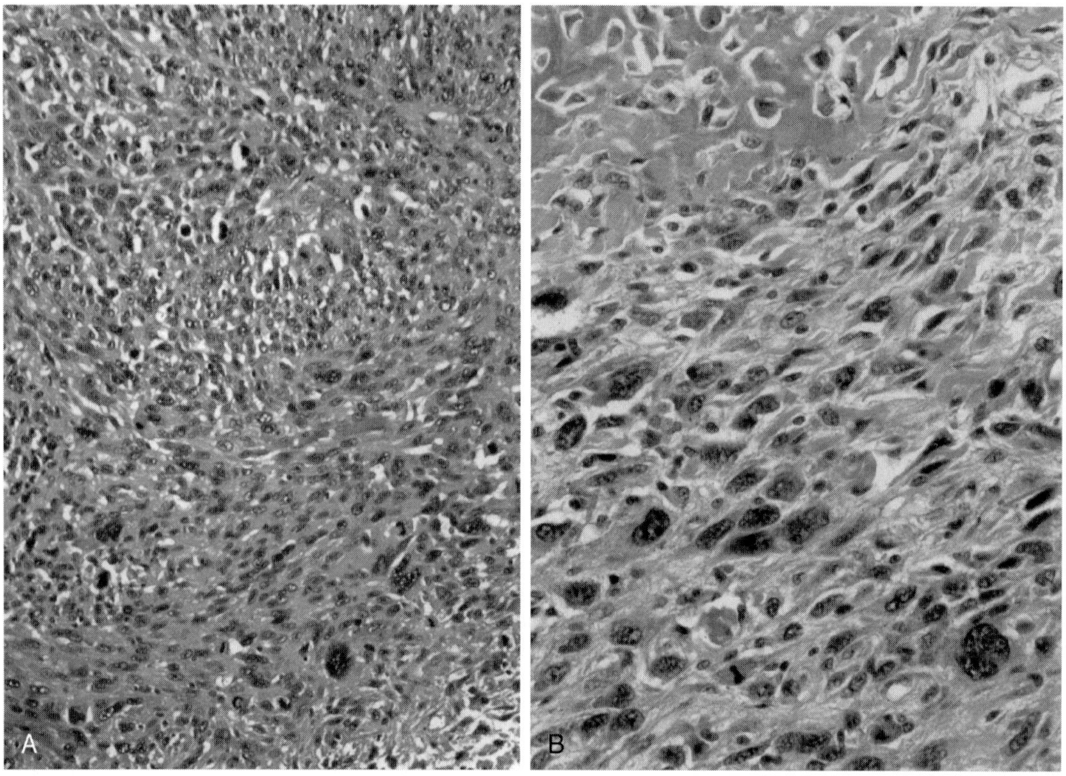

Figure 12–9. Malignant fibrous histiocytoma of bone. *A*, Classic case with markedly anaplastic spindle cells. *B*, Malignant fibrous histiocytoma–like osteosarcoma. The presence of osteoid production by the tumor cells *(upper left)* excludes the diagnosis of malignant fibrous histiocytoma. (See also color figure.)

nation is most beneficial in avoiding a misdiagnosis.

Prognosis and Treatment

In general, the clinical behavior of malignant fibrous histiocytoma of bone parallels that seen in high-grade fibrosarcoma and fibroblastic osteosarcoma.[30–32] Preoperative chemotherapy and limb salvage resection are used when possible. In certain cases, amputation may be necessary. Similar to high-grade fibrosarcoma, radiation therapy may be effective in those cases in which the tumors are surgically inaccessible.

MYOGENIC NEOPLASMS OF BONE

Leiomyosarcoma of Bone

Clinical Features

To our knowledge, leiomyoma of bone does not exist. Leiomyosarcoma of bone is a rare entity with fewer than 50 cases reported in the literature. Our experience includes five cases at the Mayo Clinic. Although leiomyosarcoma of bone may be found in patients over a broad age range, it is most commonly seen in patients older than 20 years of age. Males and females are affected equally. The most common anatomic site is the distal femur; other common locations include the proximal humerus and the proximal tibia. Pain is the most common presenting complaint.

Radiologic Features

The radiographic features for leiomyosarcoma of bone are those of a lytic, poorly marginated defect usually within the metaphysis (Fig. 12–11). Most cases also show cortical destruction, periosteal reaction, and frequently a soft tissue mass.[33] Mineralization within the tumor is distinctly absent. The radiographic differential diagnosis includes fibrosarcoma, malignant fibrous histiocytoma, metastatic carcinoma, and, less likely, malignant lymphoma.

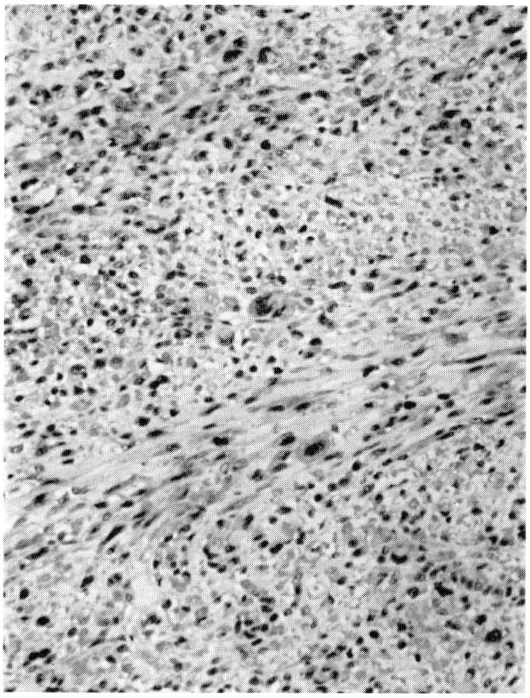

Figure 12–10. Metastatic "sarcomatoid" carcinomas may resemble malignant fibrous histiocytoma. This example represents metastasis from the kidney. Immunohistochemically, the neoplastic cells expressed keratin.

Pathologic Features

On gross inspection, the tumor is tan-white, often exhibiting a whorled appearance, and may show foci of necrosis. Microscopically, leiomyosarcoma of bone is composed of intersecting fascicles of spindle cells containing cigar-shaped nuclei and tapering eosinophilic cytoplasm (Fig. 12–12*A* [see also color Figure 12–12]). Although nuclear pleomorphism typically ranges from mild to moderate, occasional high-grade cases will show a pattern reminiscent of malignant fibrous histiocytoma (Fig. 12–12*B* [see color Figure 12–12]).[34] Likewise, mitotic activity is variable. All cases show obvious permeation of surrounding bone. Osteoclast-type giant cells may be prominent and should not deter one from the diagnosis of leiomyosarcoma if classic morphologic features are present.

In our experience and that of others, immunohistochemical studies show strong expression of α–smooth muscle actin and muscle specific actin (HHF-35) in virtually all cases, with up to 50% of cases showing desmin expression.[34]

Differential Diagnosis

The most important diagnostic consideration is metastatic leiomyosarcoma, especially from the uterus, which may rarely present as a skeletal metastasis. A thorough clinical examination is thus recommended to exclude this possibility.

High-grade leiomyosarcoma may be indistinguishable morphologically from malignant fibrous histiocytoma, and immunohistochemical stains are necessary to establish a definitive diagnosis. This distinction is probably of academic but not prognostic importance.

Prognosis and Treatment

The prognosis for primary leiomyosarcoma of bone is poor.[34–36] Although fewer than 50 cases have been reported in the literature, wide resection (i.e., limb salvage or amputation) appears to be the treatment of choice. The role of chemotherapy at this time has not been well established.

NEUROGENIC NEOPLASMS OF BONE

Although cases of intraosseous neurofibroma and even neurofibrosarcoma (malignant peripheral nerve sheath tumor) have been reported,[37–39] we have not encountered either of these entities. Histologically acceptable examples of malignant peripheral nerve

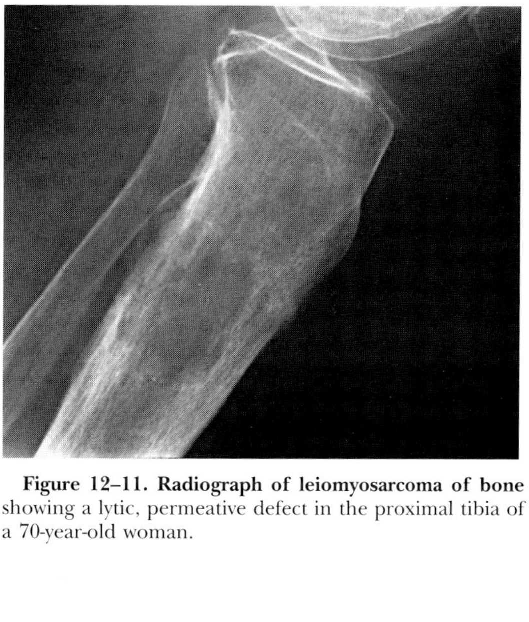

Figure 12–11. Radiograph of leiomyosarcoma of bone showing a lytic, permeative defect in the proximal tibia of a 70-year-old woman.

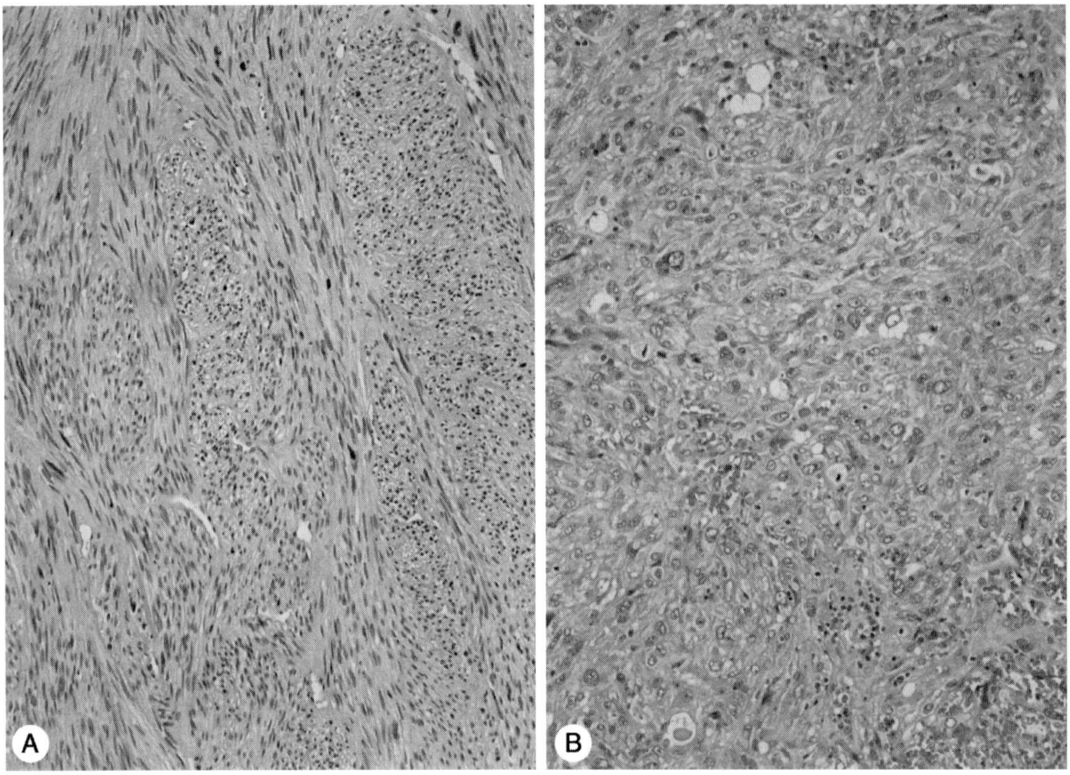

Figure 12–12. Leiomyosarcoma. *A*, Case with intersecting fascicles of spindle cells containing cigar-shaped nuclei and tapering eosinophilic cytoplasm. *B*, Occasional cases may show more obvious nuclear anaplasia resembling malignant fibrous histiocytoma. Immunohistochemical staining for α–smooth muscle actin is needed to make this distinction. (See also color figure.)

sheath tumors are difficult to establish, since most are rather nondescript spindle cell sarcomas. There are three examples in the Mayo Clinic files of intraosseous sarcomas associated with neurofibromatosis; however, all three were classified as fibrosarcomas and not malignant peripheral nerve sheath tumors.[40] We should also point out that S-100 immunopositivity may be absent in up to 50% of malignant peripheral nerve sheath tumors, adding further difficulty in establishing this diagnosis.[41] Non-neoplastic skeletal diseases that may be associated with neurofibromatosis include congenital bowing of the tibia, predisposition to fractures and poor fracture healing, and congenital pseudoarthrosis.[42, 43]

Schwannoma (Neurilemoma)

Clinical Features

Primary neurilemoma of bone is an extraordinarily rare lesion and is found in patients over a broad age range. Females are afflicted slightly more often than males. The most common anatomic location is the mandible, possibly related to the presence of the mental nerve. Most of the reported cases of osseous neurofibroma have also occurred in this location[37]; however, in our experience, all such cases have represented neurilemomas and not neurofibromas. Other common locations include the distal femur, scapula, ribs, sacrum, and skull (calvarium).[44, 45] The majority of patients are asymptomatic at diagnosis. Association with neurofibromatosis (von Recklinghausen disease) may be evident.

Radiologic Features

In general, neurilemoma of bone has a distinctly benign lytic appearance on radiographs, with sharply defined margins and focal sclerosis (Fig. 12–13*A*). In the long bones, a metaphyseal localization is common. The radiologic differential diagnosis includes mainly metaphyseal fibrous defect. Nonosseous neuri-

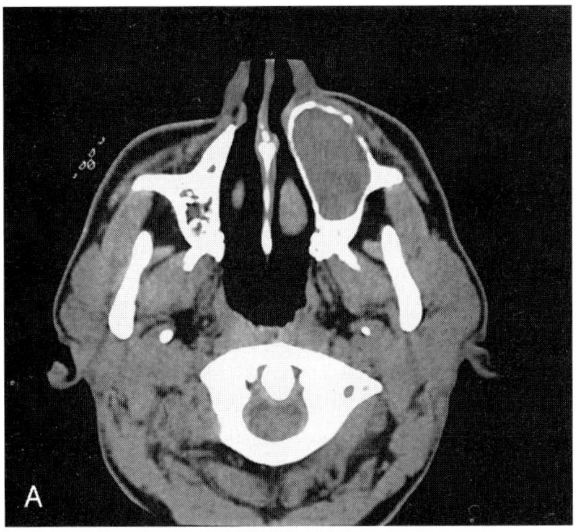

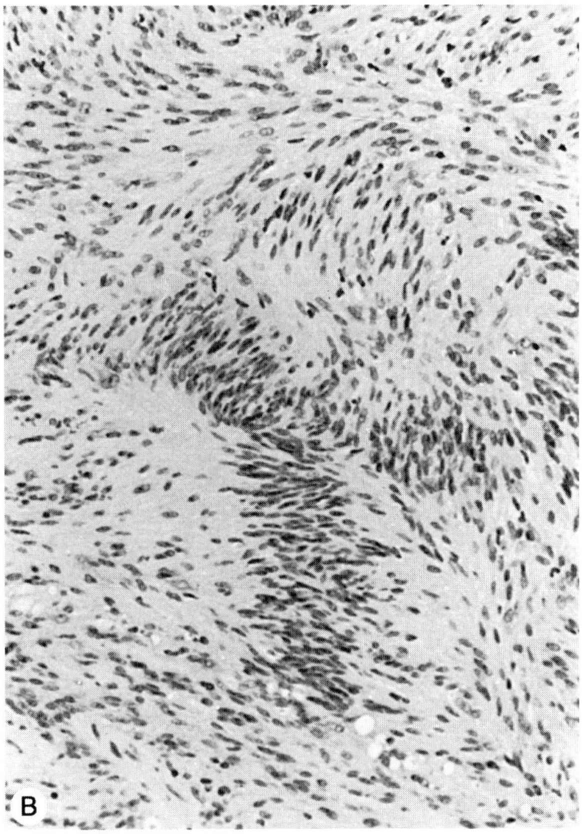

Figure 12–13. Neurilemoma. *A*, Computed tomography of neurilemoma involving the maxillary sinus of a 37-year-old man. Note the well-circumscribed outline and rim of bone surrounding the tumor indicative of slow growth. (Courtesy of Dr. Samuel Dachs, Great Falls, Montana.) *B*, Nuclear palisading characteristic of neurilemoma.

lemomas secondarily involving bone, especially when originating from spinal nerve roots, are far more common than their skeletal counterpart.

Pathologic Features

The morphologic appearance of neurilemoma of bone is identical to that seen in soft tissue. The submitted tissue is gray-tan to yellow and may be focally cystic. At low power, the tumor is composed of variable amounts of hypercellular Antoni type A regions alternating with loosely-packed hypocellular Antoni B regions. Frequently, in the Antoni A areas, the spindle cells will align in a linear fashion, producing the so-called Verocay bodies (Fig. 12–13*B*). Cytologically, the nuclei are generally small and hyperchromatic and have a wavy appearance. Occasionally, degenerative changes may produce more irregular and pleomorphic nuclei. Like their soft tissue counterpart, intraosseous neurilemomas often contain lipid-laden macrophages and hyalinized blood vessels. Rare cases of skeletal melanotic (psammomatous) schwannomas have also been reported.[46] Immunohistochemically, neurilemomas of bone are uniformly positive for S-100 protein.

Differential Diagnosis

The differential diagnosis of intraosseous neurilemoma includes benign fibrous histiocytoma, metaphyseal fibrous defect, and desmoplastic fibroma. The presence of alternating hypercellular Antoni A areas with hypocellular Antoni B regions easily establishes the diagnosis of neurilemoma. Although thin collagen fibers are frequently seen in intraosseous neurilemoma, collagen is more abundant and thicker in desmoplastic fibroma. The storiform pattern typical of metaphyseal fibrous defect and benign fibrous histiocytoma is virtually never seen in neurilemoma. Furthermore, the neoplastic cells of neurilemoma show strong and diffuse cytoplasmic immunoreactivity for S-100 protein.

Prognosis and Treatment

Surgical curettage is generally effective treatment, and the prognosis is excellent.

REFERENCES

1. Lichtenstein L: Classification of primary tumors of bone. Cancer 4:335, 1951.
2. Broders AC: Squamous-cell epithelioma of the lip: A study of five hundred and thirty-seven cases. JAMA 74:656, 1920.
3. Unni KK, Dahlin DC: Grading of bone tumors. Semin Diagn Pathol 1:165, 1984.
4. Campanacci M, Laus M, Boriani S: Multiple non-ossifying fibromata with extraskeletal anomalies: A new syndrome? J Bone Joint Surg 65B:627, 1983.
5. Mirra JM, Gold RH, Rand F: Disseminated non-ossifying fibromas in association with cafe-au-lait spots (Jaffe-Campanacci Syndrome). Clin Orthop 168:192, 1982.
6. Kyriakos M, Murphy WA: Concurrence of metaphyseal fibrous defect and osteosarcoma: Report of a case and review of the literature. Skeletal Radiol 6:179, 1981.
7. Arata MA, Peterson HA, Dahlin DC: Pathological fractures through non-ossifying fibromas. Review of the Mayo Clinic experience. J Bone Joint Surg 63A:980, 1981.
8. Kimmelstiel P, Rapp I: Cortical defect due to periosteal desmoids. Bull Hosp Jt Dis 12:286, 1951.
9. Barnes GR Jr, Gwinn JL: Distal irregularities of the femur simulating malignancy. Am J Roentgenol 122:180, 1974.
10. Chadwick CJ: Tendinitis of the pectoralis major insertion with humeral lesions: A report of two cases. J Bone Joint Surg 71B:816, 1989.
11. Dunham WK, Marcus NW, Enneking WF, et al: Developmental defects of the distal femoral metaphysis. J Bone Joint Surg 62A:801, 1980.
12. Resnick D, Greenway G: Distal femoral cortical defects, irregularities, and excavations: A critical review of the literature with the addition of histologic and paleopathologic data. Radiology 143:345, 1982.
13. Inwards CY, Unni KK, Beabout JW, et al: Desmoplastic fibroma of bone. Cancer 68:1978, 1991.
14. Bohm P, Krober S, Greshniok A, et al: Desmoplastic fibroma of the bone: A report of two patients, review of the literature, and therapeutic implications. Cancer 78:1011, 1996.
15. West R, Huvos AG, Lane JM: Desmoplastic fibroma of bone arising in fibrous dysplasia. Am J Clin Pathol 79:630, 1983.
16. Hillman JS, Mesgarzadeh M, Tang CK, et al: Case Report 481: Benign intraosseous fibroma (desmoplastic fibroma) associated with Paget's disease of the iliac bone. Skeletal Radiol 17:356, 1988.
17. Inwards CY, Unni KK, Beabout JW, et al: Solitary congenital fibromatosis (infantile myofibromatosis) of bone. Am J Surg Pathol 15:935, 1991.
18. Chung EB, Enzinger FM: Infantile myofibromatosis. Cancer 48:1807, 1981.
19. Condon VR, Allen RP: Congenital generalized fibromatosis: Case report, with roentgen manifestations. Radiology 76:444, 1961.
20. Heiple KG, Perrin E, Aikawa M: Congenital generalized fibromatosis: A case limited to osseous lesions. J Bone Joint Surg 54A:663, 1972.
21. Hasegawa T, Hirose T, Seki K, et al: Solitary infantile myofibromatosis of bone: An immunohistochemical and ultrastructural study. Am J Surg Pathol 17:308, 1993.
22. Campanacci M, Olmi R: Fibrosarcoma of bone: A study of 114 cases. Ital J Orthop Traumatol 3:199, 1977.
23. Morris JM, Lucas DB: Fibrosarcoma within a sinus tract of chronic draining osteomyelitis. J Bone Joint Surg 46A:853, 1964.
24. Bertoni F, Capanna R, Calderoni P, et al: Primary central (medullary) fibrosarcoma of bone. Semin Diagn Pathol 1:185, 1984.
25. Jeffree GM, Price CHG: Metastatic spread of fibrosarcoma of bone: A report of forty-nine cases and a comparison with osteosarcoma. J Bone Joint Surg 58B:418, 1976.
26. Clarke BE, Xipell JM, Thomas DP: Benign fibrous histiocytoma of bone. Am J Surg Pathol 9:806, 1985.
27. Matsuno T: Benign fibrous histiocytoma involving the ends of long bone. Skeletal Radiol 19:561, 1990.
28. Bertoni F, Calderoni P, Bacchini P, et al: Benign fibrous histiocytoma of bone. J Bone Joint Surg 68A:1225, 1986.
29. Frierson HF Jr, Fechner RE, Stallings RG, et al: Malignant fibrous histiocytoma in bone infarct: Association with sickle cell trait and alcohol abuse. Cancer 59:496, 1987.
30. Huvos AG, Heliweil M, Bretsky SS: The pathology of malignant fibrous histiocytoma of bone: A study of 130 patients. Am J Surg Pathol 9:853, 1985.
31. Capanna R, Bertoni F, Bacchini P, et al: Malignant fibrous histiocytoma of bone. The experience at the Rizzoli Institute: Report of 90 cases. Cancer 54:177, 1984.
32. Nishida J, Sim FH, Wenger DE, et al: Malignant fibrous histiocytoma of bone: A clinicopathologic study of 81 patients. Cancer 79:482, 1997.
33. Berlin O, Angervall L, Kindblom LG, et al: Primary leiomyosarcoma of bone: A clinical, radiographic, pathologic-anatomic, and prognostic study of 16 cases. Skeletal Radiol 16:364, 1987.
34. Myers JL, Arocho J, Bernreuter W, et al: Leiomyosarcoma of bone: A clinicopathologic, immunohistochemical, and ultrastructural study of five cases. Cancer 67:1051, 1991.
35. Young CL, Wold LE, McLeod RA, et al: Primary leiomyosarcoma of bone. Orthopedics 11:615, 1988.
36. Kawai T, Suzuki M, Mukai M, et al: Primary leiomyosarcoma of bone: An immunohistochemical and ultrastructural study. Arch Path Lab Med 107:433, 1983.
37. Prescott GH, White RE: Solitary central neurofibroma of the mandible: Report of a case and review of the literature. J Oral Maxil Surg 28:305, 1970.
38. Kameyama Y, Maeda H, Nakane S, et al: Malignant schwannoma of the mandible in a patient without neurofibromatosis. Histopathol 11:1205, 1987.
39. Bullock MJ, Bedard YC, Bell RS, et al: Intraosseous malignant peripheral nerve sheath tumor: Report of a case and review of the literature. Arch Path Lab Med 119:367, 1995.
40. Ducatman BS, Scheithauer BW, Dahlin DC: Malignant bone tumors associated with neurofibromatosis. Mayo Clin Proc 58:578, 1983.
41. Johnson TL, Lee MW, Meis JM, et al: Immunohistochemical characterization of malignant peripheral nerve sheath tumors. Surg Pathol 4:121, 1991.
42. Masserman RL, Peterson HA, Bianco A: Congenital pseudoarthrosis of the tibia: A review of the literature and 52 cases from the Mayo Clinic. Clin Orthop 99:140, 1974.

43. Green WT, Rudo N: Pseudoarthrosis and neurofibromatosis. Arch Surg 46:639, 1943.
44. de la Monte SM, Dorfman HD, Chandra R, et al: Intraosseous schwannoma: Histologic features, ultrastructure, and review of the literature. Hum Pathol 15:551, 1984.
45. Divertie MB, Dahlin DC: Neurilemmoma of rib: Report of a case. Dis Chest 44:635, 1963.
46. Myers JL, Bernreuter W, Dunham W: Melanotic schwannoma of bone: Clinicopathologic, immunohistochemical, and ultrastructural features of a rare primary bone tumor. Am J Clin Pathol 93:424, 1990.

Chapter

13

BENIGN FIBRO-OSSEOUS LESIONS OF BONE

KENNETH DEVANEY

There are a number of different fibro-osseous lesions that, while all benign, differ in their histologic appearances and their clinical features. It is in recognition of these differences that, rather than diagnosing a single encompassing entity (such as "benign fibro-osseous lesion of bone, not further subclassified"), pathologists attempt to arrive at a more precise diagnosis whenever possible. This process of subclassification is complicated by the need, in most instances, to involve the radiologic findings (which may be unfamiliar to general pathologists), and by the fact that some of the benign fibro-osseous lesions (particularly those arising in the head and neck area) are defined differently by different expert pathologists.

In this chapter, the well-defined benign fibro-osseous lesions of bone, as well as some of the more nebulous entities, are discussed (Table 13–1). Radiographs are not presented here, as most entities are discussed in Chapter 6. The importance of the pertinent radiographic findings and accompanying radiographic differential diagnostic considerations is emphasized in the text so as to afford the surgical pathologist an opportunity to make the best use of the information provided by his or her radiologic colleagues. This may be an appropriate point at which to insert a caveat: Plain film radiographs are sometimes obtained in private physicians' offices and subsequently interpreted by those same clinicians. It may in such instances be prudent for the surgical pathologist to request the loan of the radiographs for review by a radiologist practicing at that pathologist's hospital.

There will be instances in which the pathologist, despite having correlated the light microscopic findings with the radiographic and clinical information, is able to proffer no more precise a diagnosis than "benign fibro-osseous lesion of bone, not further subclassified." The pathologist must take comfort in the knowledge that such cases do occur and that the attending surgeon has actually been aided greatly by the histologic exclusion of malignancy or other lesions for which a different therapy might be applied.

FIBROUS DYSPLASIA

Historical and Etiologic Considerations

Several of the classic clinicopathologic descriptions of fibrous dysplasia date back to the early part of the 20th century.[1–3] It is likely, however, that fibrous dysplasia was recognized much earlier than this and considered among series of patients with osseous neoplasms and other processes. Indeed, clinicians in the late 19th and early 20th centuries seem to have confused the clinical features of fibrous dysplasia, neurofibromatosis, and the skeletal changes of hyperparathyroidism, resulting in the designation of fibrous dysplasia by such ponderous labels as "osteitis fibrosa generalisata" and "osteitis fibrosa cystica localisata et disseminata (von Recklinghausen)."[4] Le-

Table 13–1. Benign Fibro-osseous Lesions of Bone and Their Differential Diagnosis

Lesion	Differential Diagnosis
Fibrous dysplasia	Low-grade and parosteal osteosarcoma Nonossifying fibroma Osteoblastoma Fibro-osseous pseudotumor (of the rib) Liposclerosing myxofibrous tumor Chondroid tumors Paget's disease, fracture callus, hyperparathyroidism Neurofibromatosis
Cortical osteofibrous dysplasia	Adamantinoma
Fibro-osseous lesions of the facial skeleton	Chronic sclerosing osteomyelitis Paget's disease Osteoma Benign cementoblastoma Idiopathic osteosclerosis Cherubism Ossification of other intramedullary lesions of bone

sions of fibrous dysplasia are seen in animals[5, 6] as well as in ancient skeletal remains.[7–9]

Although fibrous dysplasia is sometimes considered along with the true neoplasms of bone (in recognition of its presentation as a mass lesion), it is a form of hamartoma and thus similar in behavior to the osteochondroma (see Chapter 11). Fibrous dysplasia and osteochondroma are the two most commonly encountered developmental anomalies of bone. Osteochondromas are 10 to 40 times more commonly encountered than fibrous dysplasia in surgical biopsy practice, although their relative incidence is influenced by the prevailing surgical philosophy.

Clinical Features

Fibrous dysplasia is a sporadic process that does not show an increased incidence in the family members of those affected by either monostotic or polyostotic disease. The sex incidence is equal, except for the specific subset of patients with Albright's syndrome (see later), which is more common in females.

The patient with conventional fibrous dysplasia may have a single affected bone (monostotic), or several skeletal sites may be involved (polyostotic). In clinical series that depend on clinical and radiographic features and are not necessarily biopsy driven, monostotic disease is five to 10 times more common than its polyostotic counterpart.[2, 3, 10] Polyostotic disease is either unilateral or, when bilateral, asymmetric in its distribution, favoring one side of the body over another.

Clinical presentations may include a sudden onset of pain, signaling a pathologic fracture through a previously unsuspected lesion; a more chronic pain, a limp, or limb length discrepancy; or a painless deformity or asymmetry, particularly in polyostotic disease; or the lesions may be asymptomatic.

Virtually any bone of the body may be involved by fibrous dysplasia; among the particularly common sites affected are the ribs, the long bones (particularly the femur, tibia, and humerus), the pelvis, the mandible and maxilla (discussed with the fibro-osseous lesions of the facial skeleton), and the skull. When fibrous dysplasia arises in the long bone, it may occupy either the diaphysis or the metaphysis, or both. Epiphyseal involvement is not usually seen until after closure of the growth plate.

While patient age may vary widely, the majority of cases are diagnosed between 3 and 20 years of age. It is most unusual for fibrous dysplasia to be diagnosed in the first year or two of life (in this age group, in the tibial and fibular regions in particular, cortical osteofibrous dysplasia is a more likely possibility, as discussed later) or in patients over the age of 40 years. The lesions of fibrous dysplasia typically exhibit their greatest period of growth in tandem with the growth of the skeleton as a whole, stabilizing to some extent after the epiphyses have closed. Pregnancy can produce growth of lesions in some women.[11, 12]

The size of a given lesion of fibrous dysplasia may vary from a small focus measuring a centimeter or less in greatest dimension, to massive involvement of virtually the entire length of a long bone such as the femur.

Associated Diseases. A well-established clinical association is the triad of fibrous dysplasia, patches of cutaneous pigmentation, and precocious puberty, known as the McCune-Albright syndrome, or Albright's syndrome.[1] The full-blown triad of Albright's syndrome is rarely seen, occurring in less than 5% of patients with fibrous dysplasia; but cutaneous pigmentation without precocious puberty is more common, occurring in 25 to 50% of fibrous dysplasia patients. Whether fibrous dysplasia is associated with endocrine disease other than the precocious puberty of Albright's syndrome is not clear; the concurrence of fibrous dysplasia and hyperparathyroidism and hyperthyroidism has been reported, but this may be a chance occurrence.[13–17]

Although the majority of soft tissue myxomas are isolated lesions, a minority of myxomas (usually intramuscular) are found in close proximity to a skeletal lesion of fibrous dysplasia (Mazabraud's syndrome).[18–22]

Malignant Transformation. Rarely, fibrous dysplasia may be complicated by the development of another lesion. Desmoplastic fibroma has been reported in two patients with fibrous dysplasia, for example.[23, 24] Of greater import is the association between fibrous dysplasia and the development of malignancy in the same bone. This malignant change may take the form of an osteosarcoma, fibrosarcoma, chondrosarcoma, malignant fibrous histiocytoma, or simply high-grade sarcoma, not further subclassified.[25–34]

Some investigators have suggested that the likelihood of malignant transformation is greater in polyostotic than in monostotic disease, although this may simply reflect the greater number of lesions with the potential for undergoing malignant change in the polyostotic patients, a situation similar to that seen in solitary and multiple osteochondromas (see Chapter 11). Some of these sarcomas have followed a course of radiation therapy for fibrous dysplasia; others, however, have arisen in the absence of intervening therapy (other than surgical excision or biopsy of the fibrous dysplasia). Irrespective of the precise histologic subtyping, sarcomas arising in the setting of pre-existing fibrous dysplasia are high-grade lesions with a generally poor prognosis.

Radiologic Features

Well-developed intramedullary lesions of monostotic and polyostotic fibrous dysplasia are marked by three features on plain film radiographs: relative lucency (lytic) compared with the adjacent bone; a surrounding rim of sclerosis; and expansion of the contours of the host bone (see Fig. 6–5*B*).[35] The classic radiologic description of fibrous dysplasia includes the "ground glass" character of the lytic lesion, a reference to its homogeneous density, which lies somewhere between that of fatty marrow and cortical bone and which replaces the normal trabecular bone of the medulla,[35] and a "geographic" pattern of bone destruction that suggests a slowly growing lesion (and thus likely to be benign). Except when complicated by a pathologic fracture, fibrous dysplasia does not usually show an accompanying periosteal reaction.

The three key features of lucency, sclerotic rim, and expansion are subject to variation. The lytic (cystic, or lucent) character of fibrous dysplasia may also incorporate patchy irregular calcifications with irregularly shaped sclerotic zones, particularly in the craniofacial lesions (see discussion following). The sclerotic rim may be partially or even completely lacking. Finally, the expansile character of fibrous dysplasia may not produce a significant widening of the contours of the host bone, but rather may manifest as endosteal scalloping.

Additional radiographic observations may include a significant deformity of the affected bone (as, for example, the "shepherd's crook" deformity of the proximal femur, a result of the combination of a growing mass lesion with pathologic fracture), a disparate growth of paired skeletal structures when compared from right to left, and an acceleration of osseous maturation in the vicinity of lesions of fibrous dysplasia.

One particularly rare appearance of fibrous dysplasia is that of a surface-based lesion that may mimic an osteochondroma radiologically and surgically. On histologic examination, however, the core of this exophytic lesion as well as that of the adjacent intramedullary bone is occupied by the fibro-osseous proliferation of fibrous dysplasia, an appearance referred to as *fibrous dysplasia protuberans* (analagous to a similarly rare presentation of enchondromas as exophytic lesions, a process termed *enchondroma protuberans*).[36]

The radiologic differential diagnosis of fibrous dysplasia is summarized in Table 13–2, so as to provide some "moral support" to the diagnostic surgical pathologist who is presented with a confident clinical diagnosis of fibrous dysplasia but a biopsy specimen looking nothing like a fibro-osseous proliferation. Conversely, when the problem is that the biopsy specimen is reminiscent of fibrous dysplasia but the clinical diagnosis is one of a different entity, it is comforting to know that the diagnosis being considered by the microscopist actually may enter into the radiographic differential. Although the radiologic differential diagnosis includes many diseases, the options are reduced when the age of the patient and the site are considered (see Chapters 1 and 6).

The lesions of fibrous dysplasia are "hot"

Table 13–2. Radiologic Differential Diagnosis of Fibrous Dysplasia

Radiologic Finding	Differential Diagnosis
Solitary expansile lytic lesions	Enchondroma, chondromyxoid fibroma Aneurysmal bone cyst Nonossifying fibroma Giant cell tumor of bone Osteoblastoma Plasmacytoma Chondrosarcoma Brown tumor of hyperparathyroidism Metastasis
Solitary, nonexpansile lytic lesions (with or without peripheral sclerosis)	Langerhans' cell histiocytosis Simple bone cyst Enchondroma, chondroblastoma Chronic osteomyelitis Brown tumor of hyperparathyroidism Metastasis
Multifocal skeletal disease	Langerhans' cell histiocytosis Brown tumor of hyperparathyroidism Metastasis Multiple nonossifying fibromas Enchondromatosis Paget's disease

on radionuclide scanning (i.e., exhibit markedly increased uptake). This is not a particularly specific finding but is useful in distinguishing monostotic from polyostotic disease. Computed tomographic scanning will precisely delineate the extent of disease.[35, 37] Magnetic resonance (MR) scanning reveals a lesion that is relatively dark (low or intermediate signal intensity) on T1 weighted images and variable on T2 weighted images.[38]

Pathology

The usual specimen of fibrous dysplasia provided for the surgical pathologist is a curettage, consisting of an aggregate of firm, gray-white tissue fragments that cut with a gritty sensation. In a minority of lesions, grossly recognizable nodules of cartilage may be present.

The histologic appearances of monostotic and polyostotic fibrous dysplasia are identical. The essence of fibrous dysplasia is a proliferation of thin, wavy spicules of woven bone (sometimes likened to thin, delicate "Chinese characters," or a bowl of "alphabet soup") disposed in a slightly to moderately cellular, cytologically bland fibrous background (Fig. 13–1*A&B*). Mineralization of these woven bone trabeculae lends to the lesions of fibrous dysplasia the "ground glass" radiologic appearance. The woven bone trabeculae are distinguished by an absence of rimming osteoblasts and appear instead to spring directly from the background fibrous stroma, an appearance likened by some to a process of fibro-osseous metaplasia (Fig. 13–1*C*). These osseous trabeculae are usually thinner than the normal host bone trabeculae and often appear as discrete (i.e., not interconnected) structures (see Fig. 13–1*B*). In general, osteoclastic activity is conspicuous by its absence.

Variations on this basic fibro-osseous theme include the following:

- The presence or absence of cystic degeneration (Fig. 13–1*D*)
- Scattered foci of osteoblastic rimming of the bone trabeculae
- Thickening of the bone trabeculae approaching or even exceeding that of the host cancellous bone (Fig. 13–2*A*)
- The usually discrete woven bone trabeculae may be interconnected and may produce a pattern reminiscent of the "Roman bridge" formation seen in fracture callus formation (see Fig. 13–2*A*)
- Scattered trabeculae of lamellar bone are infrequently seen, apparently a product of previous pathologic fracture of fibrous dysplasia.
- The ratio of osseous to fibrous tissue may be highly variable, ranging from a predominance of woven bone trabeculae to a predominance of fibrous tissue.

The osseous structures of fibrous dysplasia very occasionally adopt a rounded or spherical configuration; these structures have been referred to by a variety of names, including psammomatoid bodies, cementum, and cementicles (Fig. 13–2*B*).[39–45] Although some investigators have suggested that lesions containing a preponderance of these cementicles are distinct entities when they arise outside of the craniofacial bones (advocating diagnoses such as ossifying fibroma, cementoma, cemento-ossifying fibroma, or cementifying fibroma of the long bones), such lesions are probably best regarded as variants of fibrous dysplasia. This is supported by several reports in which the cementicle-containing areas have been observed to blend into regions recognizable as conventional fibrous dysplasia.[39, 44, 45] The special circumstance of such lesions aris-

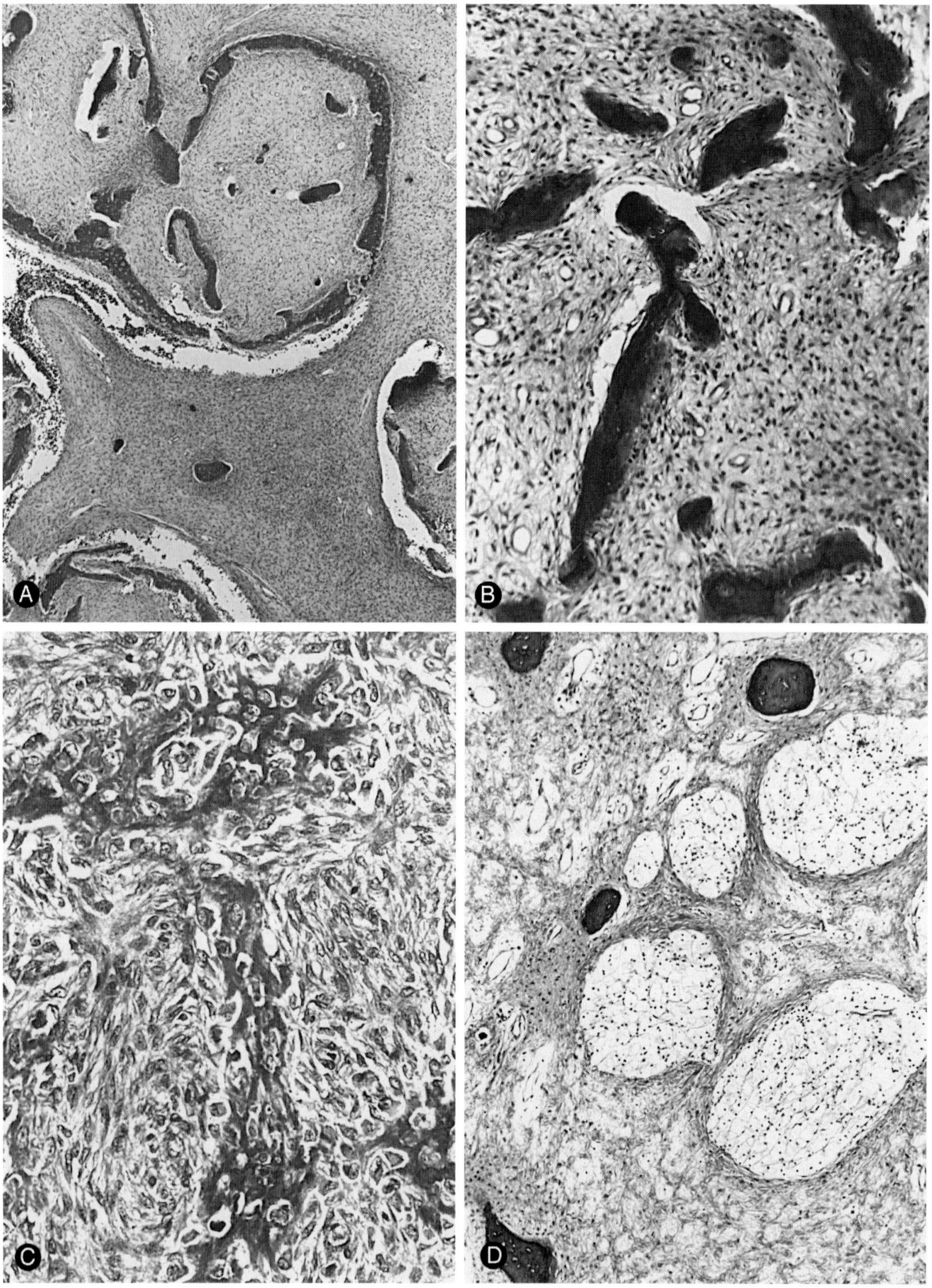

Figure 13–1. Fibrous dysplasia. *A*, The classic appearance of fibrous dysplasia combines thin, arcing trabeculae of woven bone with a moderately cellular fibrous stroma. *B*, The thin woven bone trabeculae of fibrous dysplasia are typically discrete structures, separated from one another by the intervening fibrous stroma. *C*, The transition from stroma to woven bone trabeculae is an abrupt one, without an intervening row of osteoblasts (so-called "osseous metaplasia"). *D*, Cystic change, either as a microscopic or a gross phenomenon, may occur.

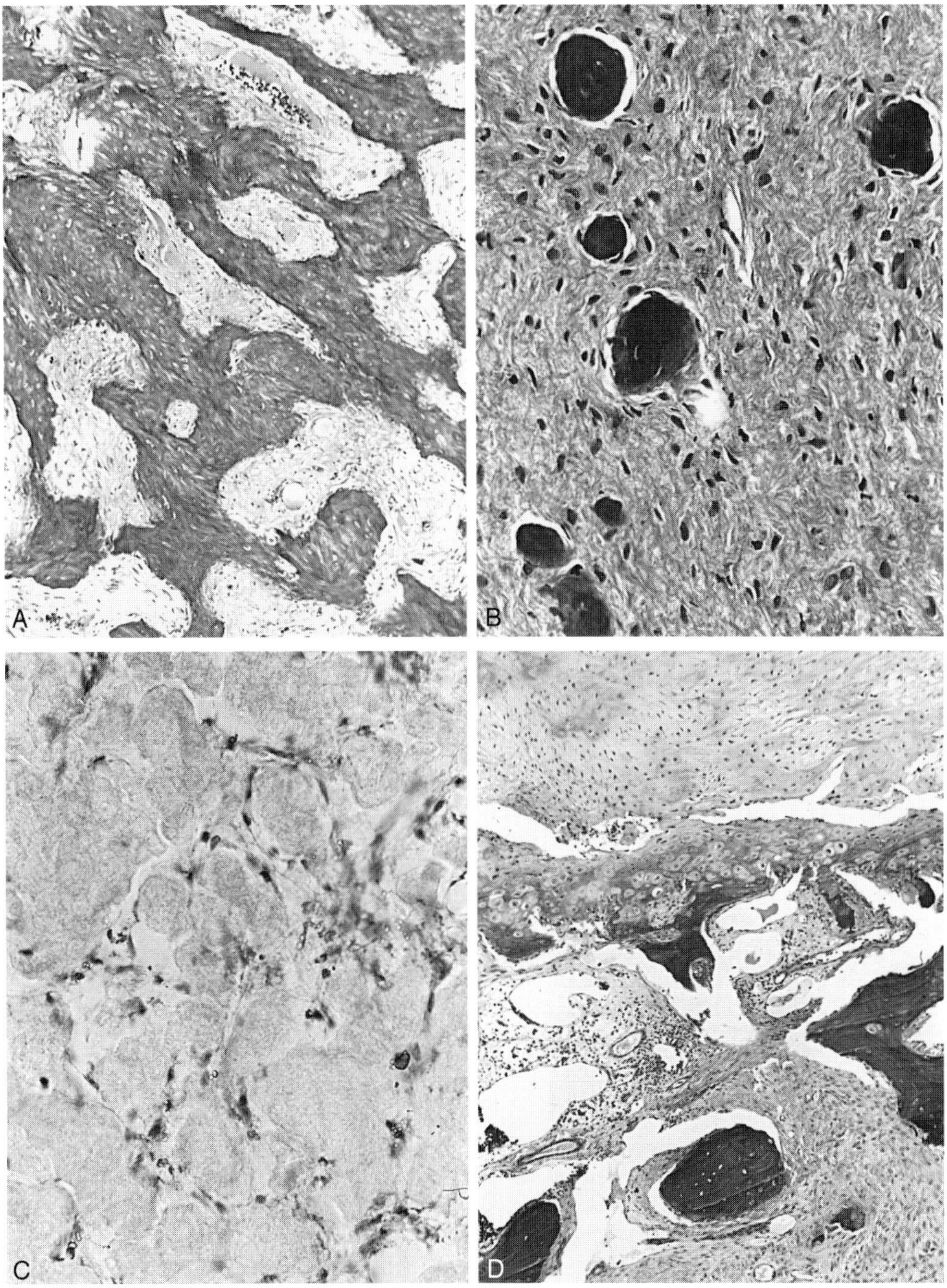

Figure 13–2. Variations of fibrous dysplasia. *A*, In some lesions of fibrous dysplasia (as in this humeral lesion) the woven bone trabeculae are broader than usual and may adopt an interconnecting configuration; the stroma, however, continues to be a moderately cellular one. *B*, Benign fibro-osseous lesions of the extragnathic bones (as in this lesion of the tibia) and the mandible and maxilla may sometimes contain small rounded mineralized structures (ossicles, cementum, or psammomatoid bodies). *C*, Simple bone cyst. Primarily cystic lesions of bone may contain small rounded amorphous masses within their walls; although these structures may resemble cementum, the lesion as a whole is probably best classified as a form of simple bone cyst (in the absence of other areas more typical of fibrous dysplasia). *D*, Uncommonly, lesions of fibrous dysplasia contain cartilaginous nodules. This mid-diaphyseal lesion of the femur shows, in the upper part of the figure, an island of cartilage, while a short transitional zone of endochondral ossification bridges the gap to the adjacent fibro-osseous proliferation.

ing in the craniofacial bones is discussed in the next section.

As a component of a very real terminological conundrum, however, this does prompt a consideration of a group of lesions of long bone that are primarily cystic but contain diffuse rounded masses of amorphous material that some have likened to what has been called cementum in jaw lesions. These long bone lesions have also been called *cementomas* or *cementifying fibromas*. However, in view of their largely cystic nature, the extensive nature of the formation of the cementum-like material (in contrast to the small, rounded cementicles seen in fibrous dysplasia), and the absence of well-defined regions reminiscent of conventional fibrous dysplasia, it seems reasonable to regard this change as an aberrant pattern of mineralization in the wall of a simple (unicameral) bone cyst and not as a variant of fibrous dysplasia (Fig. 13–2*C*).[44, 46, 47]

In adults, uncomplicated lesions of fibrous dysplasia are essentially without mitotic activity. More than a rare mitosis in this age group is cause for concern and should prompt a search for both cytologic atypia and radiographic evidence of a destructive mass lesion. In children, by contrast, a mitosis every 5 or 10 high-power fields may be encountered and should not, as an isolated finding, be taken to suggest the presence of a sarcoma.

Rarely, nodules of cartilage are identified in association with the otherwise typical fibro-osseous proliferation of fibrous dysplasia (Fig. 13–2*D*).[48–51] These cartilaginous nodules are entirely benign in their cellularity and cytologic features and probably derive from misplaced portions of growth plate.

Fibrous dysplasia may be complicated by secondary aneurysmal bone cyst formation (see Chapter 16).[12, 52, 53] This change may overshadow the underlying (minor) component of fibrous dysplasia, and so evidence of an underlying lesion should always be assiduously sought by surgical pathologists who are contemplating a diagnosis of primary aneurysmal bone cyst.

Ancillary Studies. Immunohistochemistry is rarely required in the evaluation of an otherwise uncomplicated case of fibrous dysplasia. The spindle cells of conventional fibrous dysplasia will fail to stain with antibodies to cytokeratin and epithelial membrane antigen (in contrast to cortical osteofibrous dysplasia; see later discussion), and show no labeling for S-100 protein.

Serum calcium and phosphorus levels will be normal for age in fibrous dysplasia; while some elevation of alkaline phosphatase levels may be seen, this elevation rarely reaches the level seen in Paget's disease, osteosarcoma, or hyperparathyroidism.[10]

Treatment and Prognosis

As the incidence of malignant transformation is less than 1% in monostotic fibrous dysplasia,[54] these lesions are regarded clinically as benign processes, and therapy is largely directed toward the correction of symptomatic deformities via osteotomy and the treatment of incipient or fully developed pathologic fractures. The confident clinical and radiographic diagnosis of fibrous dysplasia (particularly in polyostotic disease), means that diagnostic biopsy may not always be necessary. Following curettage and packing with bone chips, recurrences of fibrous dysplasia are common, and so these lesions are likely to present lingering problems requiring long-term follow-up and management.

Differential Diagnostic Considerations

The formation of spicules of metaplastic, woven bone in a spindle cell background is not restricted to fibrous dysplasia. A similar fibro-osseous pattern is encountered in some *low-grade intraosseous osteosarcomas* (see Chapter 9) and in *parosteal osteosarcomas* (see Chapter 11), which represent the key light microscopic differential diagnostic considerations for the surgical pathologist (Fig. 13–3*A*).[55, 56] As a light microscopic clue to differential diagnosis, osteoblastic rimming may be found in both low-grade intraosseous osteosarcoma and in parosteal osteosarcoma but is lacking in uncomplicated cases of fibrous dysplasia; this, however, can be a subjective as well as focal finding, and so may not be an entirely reliable guide in each instance. Although radiographic imaging can minimize this differential diagnostic problem in most instances (i.e., the surface location of parosteal osteosarcoma and the massive destructive nature of an intraosseous well-differentiated osteosarcoma diverge from the usual appearance of fibrous dysplasia), the fact remains that some surgical pathologists succumb to the temptation to diagnose osseous tumors without any knowledge of the accompanying imaging findings. Although

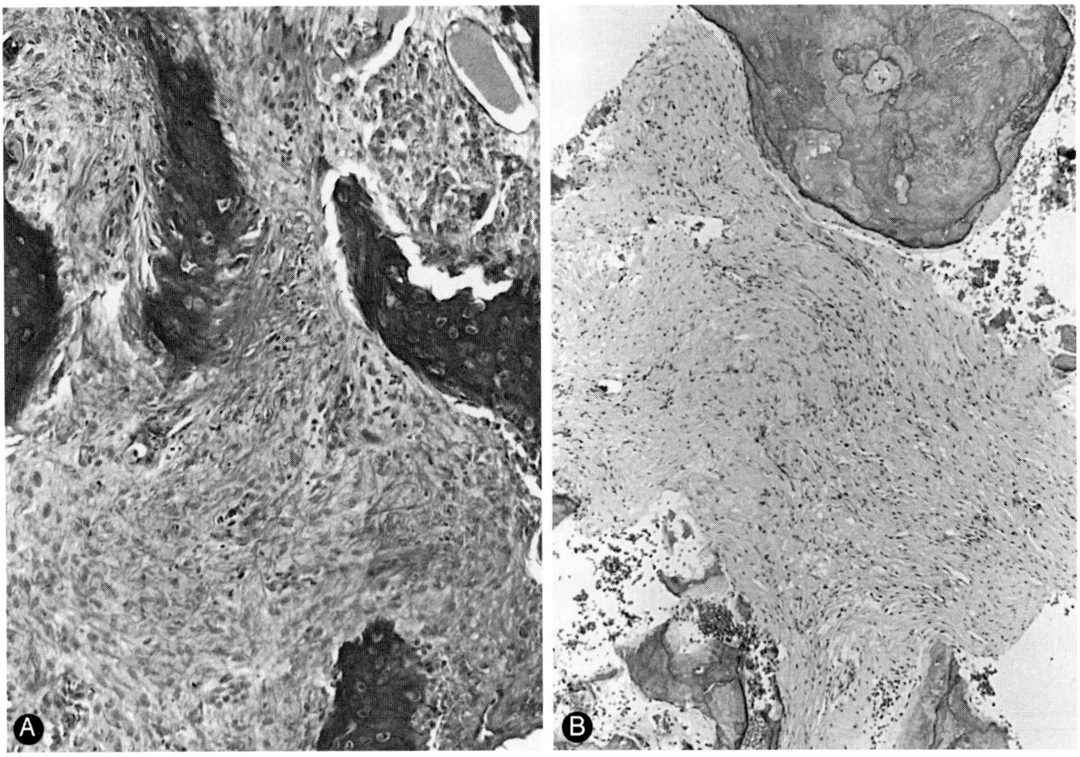

Figure 13–3. Differential diagnosis of fibrous dysplasia. *A*, Osteosarcoma. Both a low-grade intraosseous osteosarcoma (seen here) and a parosteal osteosarcoma may be confused on light microscopic grounds with fibrous dysplasia; attention to radiographic features of such lesions is essential to avoid this diagnostic pitfall. *B*, Liposclerosing myxofibrous tumor (polymorphic fibro-osseous lesion) of the femur is characterized by the presence of areas identical to fibrous dysplasia as well as large masses of lamellar and woven bone, with prominent cement lines.

this practice is to be deplored (being dangerous both for the patient and for the pathologist), the reality is that a routine, universal integration of radiologic data into pathologic interpretation has not yet been achieved. Those who feel too pressured by a busy practice to consult with orthopedic surgeons and radiologists before rendering diagnoses should be aware that, while such a practice will probably do limited harm when the issues are trivial, the surgical pathologist working in isolation will not always be able to identify those cases in which the issues are of greater magnitude, and so is at risk of making diagnostic errors.

The proportions of fibrous to osseous tissues within a given lesion are subject to great variation in fibrous dysplasia; particularly at frozen section (when less ossified tissues are preferentially selected), fibrous dysplasia may appear to be largely fibrous and so invite consideration of other fibrous lesions such as *nonossifying fibroma* or a reactive process.[57] On thorough sampling, the foci of woven bone formation will reveal the true nature of a lesion as fibrous dysplasia.

While the largely sclerotic character of osteoid osteoma usually prevents its confusion with fibrous dysplasia, *osteoblastoma* has been mistaken for fibrous dysplasia on occasion. While most osteoblastomas have a richly vascular loose stroma (unlike fibrous dysplasia), some osteoblastomas are marked by a denser, more fibrous stroma. The osteoblastic rimming of bone trabeculae and the clinical and radiographic characteristics of an osteoblastoma will aid in its recognition.

First recognized in the ribs (and almost exclusive to that site), a form of *fibro-osseous pseudotumor* has been recognized that resembles fibrous dysplasia.[58–60] This fibro-osseous pseudotumor includes areas of woven bone arising from a fibrous stroma in a fashion similar to that seen in fibrous dysplasia. In addition, however, the fibro-osseous pseudotumor also includes areas of lamellar bone formation at its periphery (yielding a "zonal" sort of architecture), which is not a typical feature of uncomplicated fibrous dysplasia.

A lesion that appears to be virtually specific to the intertrochanteric region of the proximal femur was recently reported under the heading of *polymorphic fibro-osseous lesion of bone.*[61] This same lesion has been referred to by the Armed Forces Institute of Pathology, where it was first recognized, as a *liposclerosing myxofibrous tumor.*[62] In contrast to conventional fibrous dysplasia, this lesion is characterized by, among other changes, the presence of lamellar bone, often with prominent cement lines (Fig. 13–3*B*). It is not entirely clear whether this "new entity" will prove to be nothing more than a peculiar site-specific variant of fibrous dysplasia, but experience from other centers has yet to accrue.

Although it is uncommon for lesions of fibrous dysplasia to manifest cartilaginous differentiation, such a change may invite consideration of a diagnosis of *enchondroma* (see Chapter 10). The finding of islands of hyaline cartilage in association with a fibro-osseous proliferation should suggest the correct interpretation of fibrous dysplasia, as an enchondroma does not exhibit a spindle cell component, except when a pathologic fracture is present.

The *fibrocartilaginous mesenchymoma* is also reminiscent of fibrous dysplasia with islands of cartilage, but it differs from fibrous dysplasia in two key ways: first, architecturally complex structures that resemble the formation of true epiphyseal plates are formed within the fibrocartilaginous mesenchymoma; second, its spindle cells are in areas arranged in well-formed fascicles.[63, 64] The fibrocartilaginous mesenchymoma has been regarded as a true benign neoplasm, and not as a hamartoma, with a capacity for exhibiting locally aggressive behavior but no apparent metastatic potential.

The rare occurrence of nodules of cartilage in association with otherwise typical changes of fibrous dysplasia may invite consideration of *chondrosarcomatous change* in fibrous dysplasia; however, in "fibrocartilaginous dysplasia," the chondroid islands lack both the increased cellularity and the cytologic atypia that would support a diagnosis of chondrosarcoma. Similarly, the spindle cell component lacks the pronounced cytologica atypia and mitotic activity that would support a diagnosis of dedifferentiated chondrosarcoma (see Chapter 10).

While *chondromyxoid fibroma* is not usually considered to be an ossifying lesion, both the fibrous component of chondromyxoid fibroma and the occasional ossification of the chondroid islands may cause confusion with fibrous dysplasia. Moreover, when pathologic fracture of a chondromyxoid fibroma has supervened, the reparative bone formation may further cloud this issue. Chondromyxoid fibroma can usually be distinguished from fibrous dysplasia by its distinctly lobular architecture, its absence of trabeculae of woven bone, and the presence of islands of cartilage (see Chapter 15).

Lesions of Paget's disease of bone are not usually considered to be fibro-osseous proliferations; however, *Paget's disease of bone* and *primary* or *secondary hyperparathyroidism* have on occasion been confused with fibrous dysplasia. In these entities, however, the trabeculae are usually formed by lamellar bone (not the woven bone of fibrous dysplasia), and the osteoclastic and osteoblastic activity typically far outstrip such activities in the usual lesion of fibrous dysplasia.

Other sclerosing lesions such as *fracture callus* may be confused with fibrous dysplasia. Attention to the well-developed osteoblastic rimming in callus formation will aid in making this distinction.

Adamantinoma has been confused with fibrous dysplasia on occasion and is considered under a discussion of cortical osteofibrous dysplasia (see Chapter 17).

In view of the recognized association of polyostotic fibrous dysplasia in some patients with cutaneous pigmentation (Albright's syndrome), it will come as no surprise to learn that such a presentation may be confused on clinical grounds with *neurofibromatosis* (von Recklinghausen's disease). This potential for confusion is further exacerbated by reports of fibro-osseous lesions in patients with neurofibromatosis.[65] However, although benign nerve sheath tumors may rarely occupy an intraosseous location in patients with neurofibromatosis, the fibro-osseous proliferation of fibrous dysplasia is not seen in those patients with neurofibromatosis and skeletal lesions. Should such a concurrence be found in a given patient, it is likely that the individual suffers both from fibrous dysplasia and from von Recklinghausen disease.

CORTICAL OSTEOFIBROUS DYSPLASIA

Historical and Etiologic Considerations

The lesion designated here as *cortical osteofibrous dysplasia* (COFD) was initially included in most early observers' groupings of fibrous dysplasia. Subsequently, ossifying fibroma of long bone, congenital pseudarthrosis of the tibia, congenital kyphoscoliotic tibia, infantile pseudarthrosis of the tibia, localized osteitis fibrosa, congenital fibrous defect, osteofibrous dysplasia, and Campanacci's disease have each enjoyed some favor as designations for this process.[66–76] In recognition of the fact that there already exists a substantial degree of overlap between many of the other benign fibro-osseous lesions of bone, it seems as though the designation *cortical osteofibrous dysplasia*[77] is the one most likely to clearly convey the lesion's essence.

As COFD is often first recognized as a congenital lesion, it is tempting to regard it as a developmental anomaly; however, there are some similarities between COFD and adamantinoma, which have prompted speculation about its possible neoplastic nature (see following discussion).

Clinical Features

Cortical osteofibrous dysplasia is a benign process without a familial tendency or predilection for one sex. In biopsy material, it is seen approximately 10 times less often than material from fibrous dysplasia. While fibrous dysplasia may involve virtually any bone in the body, COFD is almost always restricted to the anterior cortex of the tibia or the fibula; very rare reports of involvement of other bones such as the radius may be found.[77]

The typical COFD patient presents in the first decade of life with signs and symptoms that may include a congenital deformity, a mass lesion, bowing of the affected lower extremity, or pain attendant upon pathologic fracture.[78, 79] Very rarely, patients do not present until the second or even third decades of life.

While a potential association between COFD and the later development of a soft tissue sarcoma in the same extremity has been described, it is not clear whether this is a chance association or a true increased incidence of the two lesions occurring in the same individual.[80]

Cortical osteofibrous dysplasia follows a capricious course. In some children, the lesion may be identified only incidentally and observed over time to regress, whereas in other patients it may be the cause of gross deformity and even progress in tandem with the growth of the skeleton. Once skeletal maturation has been achieved, however, even progressive lesions of COFD may be expected to stabilize and then regress. It is for this reason that many surgeons have found that the optimal management is conservative therapy, resisting the temptation to overtreat, preferring instead to try to "wait out" the disease process.[57, 81]

While this advice has been successfully employed by some centers, there is a critical caveat that this conservative advice is only applicable if the lesion is truly one of COFD. If, on the other hand, the lesion is actually an adamantinoma with COFD-like areas (discussed later), then such a watchful, waiting approach would be unwise. In view of this concern, some have suggested that en bloc excision is the prudent course of action for both diagnosis and treatment of COFD, as this is the only method to definitively exclude the diagnosis of adamantinoma. The solution to this clinical dilemma will revolve around how certain surgeons and radiologists can be that a partially sampled lesion with a tentative diagnosis of COFD can be safely followed clinically. Those who feel confident that they are able to monitor and control such a situation will opt for biopsy and follow-up, whereas those less confident of their ability to follow such patients clinically or radiographically will favor an en bloc excision so as not to be surprised subsequently by an occult aggressive component.

Radiologic Features

Cortical osteofibrous dysplasia involves the anterior cortex of long bones (virtually always the tibia, fibula, or both), unlike fibrous dysplasia, which is not centered in the cortex. COFD is a lytic lesion, surrounded by a rim of sclerosis. The lytic interior will, at times, adopt a homogeneous appearance similar to that of the "ground glass" pattern of conventional fibrous dysplasia. The larger lesions of COFD usually are oval, with their long axes running parallel to the long axes of the host bone. The typical location within the long bone is in the diaphysis; COFD may extend into the metaphysis but usually spares the epiphysis.[78]

Variations on the basic theme include secondary expansion to encroach upon or extend into the medullary space; involvement of both the tibia and the fibula; formation of a pseudarthrosis; gross distortion of the tibia or fibula to produce a distinct bowing of the lower extremity; and, rarely, involvement of other bones (as, for example, the radius).

Radionuclide bone scanning usually reveals increased uptake in lesions of COFD.[78] Experience with MR imaging is limited, but these lesions are likely to image similarly to fibrous dysplasia.[82]

The radiologic differential diagnosis is similar to that of fibrous dysplasia and includes other cortical-based lesions such as fibrous cortical defect, nonossifying fibroma, osteoid osteoma, cortical chondroma, chronic osteomyelitis, surface-based hemangioma, adamantinoma, and metastasis.[77, 83] The radiologic differential of COFD in the newborn period includes other causes of congenital pseudarthrosis such as fracture and neurofibromatosis.

Pathology

The typical curettage specimen of COFD will take the form of several nodules of firm, rubbery, gray-white tissue that give a gritty feeling when cut with a scalpel blade. Gross cystic change is less common in COFD than in conventional fibrous dysplasia, and cartilaginous nodules are not found.

Cortical osteofibrous dysplasia is a distinctly different lesion from fibrous dysplasia on light microscopic as well as clinical grounds. The lesions of COFD show a recognizable pattern of osteoblastic rimming, with palisading of osteoblasts around the trabeculae of woven bone (Fig. 13–4*A&B*). This osteoblastic rimming pattern may be diffuse or only focal in a given lesion, but it is usually identifiable in at least some areas on close scrutiny of the whole biopsy specimen. The woven bone trabeculae do not usually achieve the long, delicate character of the "Chinese characters" seen in conventional fibrous dysplasia but are somewhat shorter.

The fibrous stroma is similar to that of fibrous dysplasia, differing only in that later-stage lesions are not usually as heavily collagenized (Fig. 13–4*C*).

Although the usual specimen from COFD is a fragmented curettage specimen, on occasion these lesions have been removed in their entirety. Study of such specimens has revealed that the architecture of COFD is a zonal one, with thin, delicate trabeculae of woven bone occupying the central region, while at the periphery a corona of radial woven bone trabeculae interdigitates with thicker trabeculae of lamellar bone, which in turn bridge the gap between the lesion and the dense cortical bone.[77]

Immunohistochemistry. The immunohistochemical features of COFD are distinctive. In over 90% of biopsies of COFD, immunohistochemical staining for cytokeratin or epithelial membrane antigen reveal scattered positive cells throughout the fibrous stroma (Fig. 13–4*D*).[77, 84] These cytokeratin-positive cells are usually inapparent on routine hematoxylin and eosin–stained sections and should not form aggregates of more than five or 10 cells (larger aggregates of cytokeratin-positive cells are features of adamantinoma).

Differential Diagnostic Considerations

While the osteoblastic rimming of the bone trabeculae is a useful differentiating point between COFD and conventional fibrous dysplasia, it must be conceded that this rimming phenomenon may be focal in COFD, and so may not be sampled. Nevertheless, the relative youth of the patient, the lesion's cortical location, and the localization of the process to the tibia or the fibula should still provide the surgical pathologist with a strong suspicion that such a lesion is best diagnosed as COFD, an impression that can usually be confirmed by immunohistochemical positivity for cytokeratin.[77] The pathologic differential of conventional fibrous dysplasia applies to COFD.

One of the most intriguing aspects of COFD is its virtual identity in location and the similarity of the histologic features with areas of tissue seen in a low-grade malignant tumor of bone, the *adamantinoma*.[84–94] This entity is considered at greater length in Chapter 17. It is difficult to imagine that such similarities are wholly coincidental, and many authors have grappled with the implications of these observations. Some, for example, have suggested that at least some lesions of COFD may represent a stage in the evolution of adamantinoma—specifically, a "burned-out" end stage form of adamantinoma whose light microscopic features presumably represent a process of maturation or regression of the neoplasm (differentiated adamantinoma).[95] Preliminary results of karyotypic analysis of COFD lesions have suggested that trisomies may be found that might be common to both COFD and adamantinoma (see Chapter 4).[96]

These theoretical considerations notwithstanding, a practical approach to the distinc-

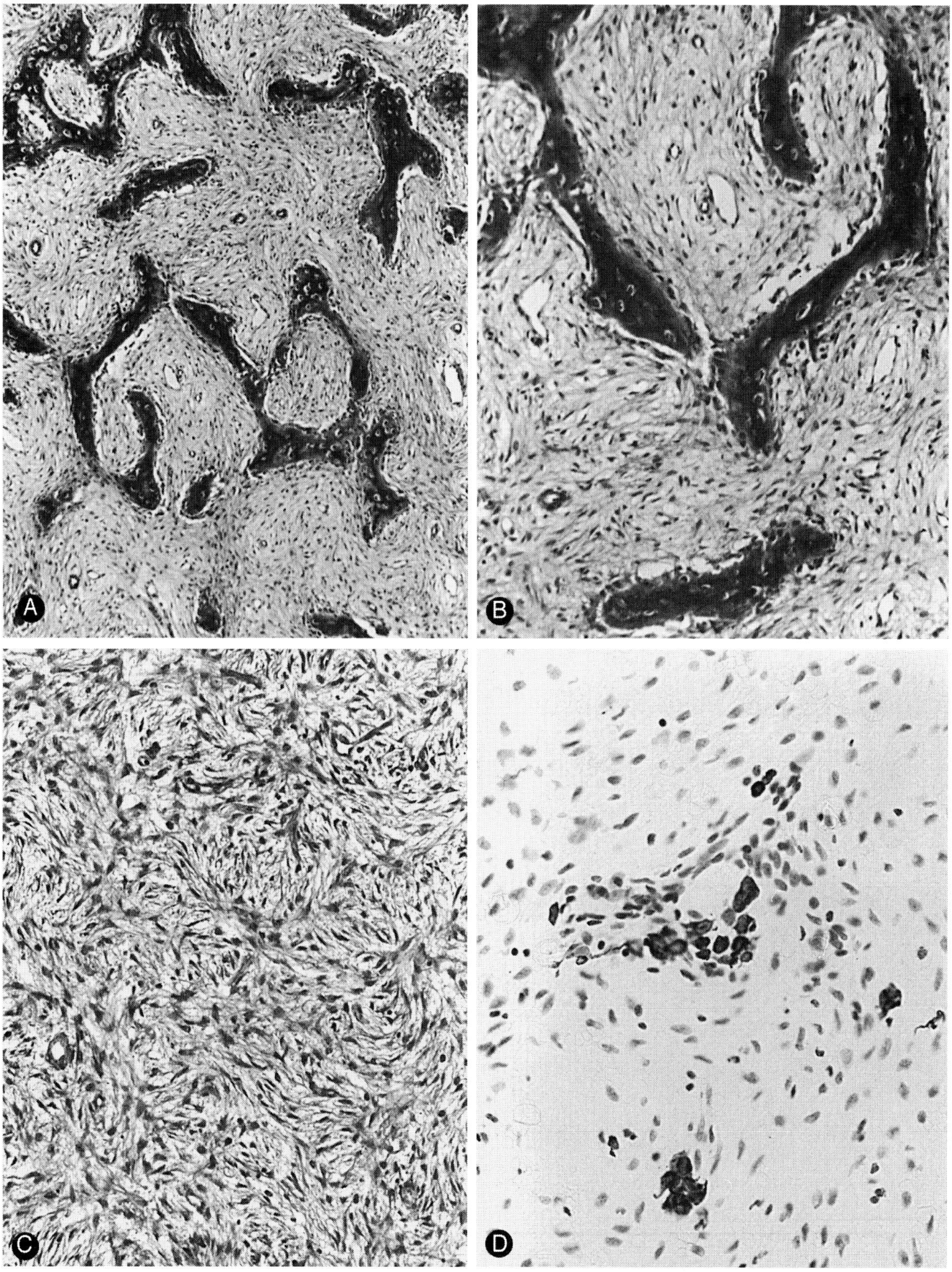

Figure 13–4. Cortical osteofibrous dysplasia. *A*, The formation of woven bone trabeculae in association with a fibrous stroma is reminiscent of that seen in fibrous dysplasia. *B*, In contrast to conventional fibrous dysplasia, osteoblastic rimming of woven bone trabeculae is a characteristic feature of cortical osteofibrous dysplasia (same lesion as shown in *A*). *C*, The stroma of cortical osteofibrous dysplasia is less heavily collagenized than in conventional fibrous dysplasia. Note that large masses of epithelioid or spindled cells that would support a diagnosis of adamantinoma are not present. *D*, While they are inapparent on routine light microscopy, scattered cytokeratin-positive cells are identifiable in the vast majority of cortical osteofibrous dysplasia lesions on immunohistochemical staining.

tion of COFD from adamantinoma, in the absence of a complete local excision of the lesion, is that any biopsy specimen with features only of COFD should be diagnosed as such, but with the caveat that adamantinoma may contain areas indistinguishable from COFD, and so clinical and radiographic follow-up of that patient is essential to monitor the course of disease. Should evidence develop suggesting aggressive disease, then repeat biopsy to exclude the possibility of an adamantinoma with COFD-like areas is warranted.

Another clinical differential diagnostic consideration for COFD is that of neurofibromatosis (von Recklinghausen disease). In the newborn, congenital pseudarthroses are a rare orthopedic problem that often triggers a search for stigmata of neurofibromatosis. The clinician should be reminded that congenital pseudarthroses may be associated with the fibro-osseous lesions of COFD as well as with those of von Recklinghausen disease, and so biopsy to better define the nature of the process may be helpful in some instances.[97–100]

FIBRO-OSSEOUS LESIONS OF THE FACIAL SKELETON

Historical and Etiologic Considerations

The group of fibro-osseous lesions arising within the facial skeleton are often treated as a discrete family of lesions for two principal reasons: firstly, they show a greater degree of variation than do the benign fibro-osseous lesions of the long bones; and secondly, the facial lesions include lesions of the jaw bones, which have most often been studied by oral pathologists and thus been treated to the application of a nosology different in some ways from that employed by orthopedic pathologists.[101–110]

Some explanation for the differing histologic patterns produced by the craniofacial fibro-osseous lesions may be drawn from both the embryology and the anatomy of the region. It should be recalled that (save for the condyle of the mandible, which has a true epiphysis) the bones of this region are formed by a process of intramembranous ossification, not by enchondral ossification. The skeletal underpinnings that define the facial structures include the upper face (devoted to the formation of the forehead), the mid-face (which includes the orbit, the nose, and the maxilla) and the lower face (mandible). The two entities that are most familiar to diagnostic surgical pathologists are fibrous dysplasia and ossifying fibroma, which may be encountered in any of these three facial regions. Fibrous dysplasia and ossifying fibroma of the facial skeleton appear more akin to developmental lesions than to true neoplasms.

The mandible and maxilla are hosts to the periodontal structures, which are responsible for supporting the teeth. These periodontal structures include the gingiva, the periodontal ligament (a thin structure lying between the cementum-covered tooth root and the bone of the adjacent socket, which contains fibroblasts, osteoblasts/cementoblasts, and osteoclasts), the bone surrounding the teeth themselves (the alveolar bone), the cementum (woven bone surrounding the dentin of the teeth), and the epithelial rests of Malassez. The tumors that arise from these odontogenic structures may be placed into three large categories: epithelial tumors (such as the ameloblastoma and the calcifying epithelial odontogenic tumor), combined epithelial and mesenchymal tumors (including the odontoma and the ameloblastic fibroma), and mesenchymal lesions. Only the benign, pure mesenchymal odontogenic family lesions with a fibro-osseous character are considered here (Table 13–3). The light microscopic appearances of these pure mesenchymal fibro-osseous odontogenic lesions may, in many areas, show little or no difference from the appearances of fibrous dysplasia or ossifying fibroma arising elsewhere in the craniofacial skeleton; the reasons for naming these jaw-related lesions separately de-

Table 13–3. Benign Fibro-osseous Lesions of the Mandible and Maxilla: A Lexicon

Conventional fibrous dysplasia (monostotic and polyostotic)
Ossifying fibroma
Aggressive psammomatoid ossifying fibroma (sinonasal)
Cementifying fibroma (synonym: ossifying fibroma)
Periapical fibrous dysplasia (synonyms: periapical cemental dysplasia, cementoma)
Florid osseous dysplasia (synonyms: cemento-osseous dysplasia, gigantiform cementoma, multiple cemento-ossifying fibromas, multiple periapical osteofibromatosis, multiple enostosis, multiple osteomas, periapical cementoblastoma, sclerotic cemental masses of the jaw, and Paget's disease of the mandible)
Benign fibro-osseous lesion, not further subclassified

rive from their location in association with dental structures and from their clinical features.

It is not clear whether the cementifying fibroma, florid osseous dysplasia, and periapical fibrous dysplasia are true neoplasms or are reactive or developmental processes. As they are often first identified later in life (thus, apparently, manifesting as acquired lesions), they are probably best regarded as lesions whose etiologies remain to be defined. The criteria presented here for distinguishing these lesions have not been universally adopted, and so areas of potential overlap between competing classification schemes are indicated where necessary.

Cementum is the layer of woven bone that bridges the gap between the dentin of the tooth and the dense collagenous tissue of the periodontal ligament. Oral pathologists list four types of cementoma: cementoblastoma (discussed only as a differential diagnostic consideration), cementifying fibroma (considered here as a variant of ossifying fibroma), florid osseous dysplasia (discussed separately), and periapical cemental dysplasia (discussed separately).[111, 112] The light microscopic features of neoplastic cementum are those of small or large amorphous masses of bony material. These bony masses are blunter or more rounded than the thin, arcing, woven bone trabeculae of conventional fibrous dysplasia, and their internal texture usually appears rather amorphous (in contrast to the linear appearance of typical woven bone trabeculae). Nevertheless, although mention is often made of the basophilia of cementum, this material is not greatly different from bone formed elsewhere and so is identified principally by its location in association with dental structures. Consequently, the further away the "cementum" is from the tooth, the more difficult it is to argue that it is actually a different substance from bone. Some observers, seeking to avoid the difficulty of distinguishing bone from cementum, have employed the descriptor *psammomatoid* to indicate the presence of small mineralized spherules within the fibro-osseous proliferation.[113–116]

The descriptor *aggressive* has been employed variously in the diagnosis of some members of this group of lesions; lesions reaching greater than 5 cm in greatest dimension have been called aggressive by some, while others have reserved the term aggressive for lesions with cytologic atypia (thus inviting consideration of such lesions as low-grade osteosarcoma as well as a benign fibro-osseous lesion). In light of these differing usages, this qualifier will not be employed here except for a subset of ossifying fibroma recently described in the sinonasal area.

Clinical Features

Several of the important discriminatory clinicopathologic features of these lesions are summarized in Table 13–4. Craniofacial fibrous dysplasia shows neither a familial nor a gender predilection. Ossifying fibroma (and its jaw-specific subtype, cementifying fibroma), periapical fibrous dysplasia, and florid osseous dysplasia are more often seen in female patients but do not show a familial predilection.

The most common presentation of *craniofacial fibrous dysplasia* is as a painless mass in the first or second decade of life.[117] Within the jaw, fibrous dysplasia is found slightly more frequently in the maxilla than in the mandible. Fibrous dysplasia involving the craniofacial bones may be monostotic or polyostotic and may be associated with cutaneous pigmentation with or without precocious puberty (Albright's syndrome). Some (small) risk of sarcomatous degeneration exists for craniofacial fibrous dysplasia.

In the craniofacial bones, the term *ossifying fibroma* designates a lesion that, in contrast to fibrous dysplasia, is radiographically rather well circumscribed. The diagnosis is most often initially made when affected individuals present with painless masses in the third or fourth decade of life. Ossifying fibroma is more often found in the mandible than in the maxilla. A variant of ossifying fibroma, variously named aggressive active ossifying fibroma, juvenile active ossifying fibroma, juvenile ossifying fibroma, and trabecular desmo-osteoblastoma, has been segregated by some authors, in consideration of its more aggressive course and the younger age at presentation of some patients.[108, 118] While rather well circumscribed radiographically, these lesions appear to be more likely to recur locally than other lesions of ossifying fibroma, particularly when arising in sites other than the mandible and maxilla. They are grouped here with the other lesions of ossifying fibroma, as it is not entirely clear whether these lesions diverge so significantly from ossifying fibroma as to warrant the creation of a separate diagnostic category (particularly in the mandible

Table 13–4. Benign Fibro-osseous Lesions of the Craniofacial Skeleton: Key Diagnostic Features

Type	Clinical Features	Radiologic Features	Histopathologic Features
Fibrous dysplasia	Male = female 1st and 2nd decades Painless mass Maxillary predominance	Lytic, may be "ground glass" Poorly marginated	Woven bone trabeculae in fibrous background No lamellar bone, no osteoblasts
Ossifying fibroma	Female predominance Age 20–40 years Painless mass Mandibular predominance	Lytic, usually not "ground glass" Well marginated	Woven and lamellar bone Spherules may occur Osteoblasts present
Cementifying fibroma	Identical to ossifying fibroma, but associated with teeth	As ossifying fibroma	As ossifying fibroma
Periapical fibrous dysplasia	Mostly black females Age 20–50 years Painless mass Mandibular predominance	Lytic lesion, may have internal densities Often multiple Associated with teeth	Early: fibrous with little bone. Later: woven bone and dense masses of cementum
Florid osseous dysplasia	Mostly black females Aged 30–50 years Painless masses, often multiple and symmetrical	Largely sclerotic May have lobulated border Associated with teeth	Woven bone in fibrovascular stroma Spherules and larger masses of cementum present Osteoblasts may be present

and maxilla), and because the differential diagnostic considerations (which include a low-grade osteosarcoma and osteoblastoma) remain prime considerations in their analysis.

A particular variant of ossifying fibroma localized to the bones of the sinonasal region is the *aggressive psammomatoid ossifying fibroma.* This is an uncommon lesion that spans a wide age range at initial diagnosis (median 33 years) and that is distinguished not so much by its radiographic image or its light microscopic appearance as by its clinical course, because these lesions are locally infiltrative and likely to recur. As a consequence, en bloc excision is recommended, instead of the less aggressive curettage or enucleation that might be employed in the treatment of the usual ossifying fibroma.[116]

The *cementifying fibroma* is probably best approached as a variant of ossifying fibroma, which is distinguished by its association with dental structures in the mandible or maxilla; otherwise, this is a lesion whose clinical features parallel those of ossifying fibroma, including female predominance and peak age of presentation in the fourth decade of life. Cementifying fibromas are particularly likely to occur in the molar or premolar regions of the mandible.

Periapical fibrous dysplasia (also known as periapical cemental dysplasia and as cementoma) is, like florid osseous dysplasia, a condition that predominantly affects black females, with a peak incidence in the third through fifth decades. Most of these lesions arise in the vicinity of the incisors of the mandible and are identified only as incidental findings.

Florid osseous dysplasia (also known as cemento-osseous dysplasia, gigantiform cementoma, multiple cemento-ossifying fibromas, multiple periapical osteofibromatosis, multiple enostosis, multiple osteomas, periapical cementoblastoma, sclerotic cemental masses of the jaw, and Paget's disease of the mandible) is seen principally in black females who are usually in their fourth or fifth decades of life at the time of diagnosis. The lesions of florid osseous dysplasia are often multiple and symmetrical in their distribution. Some investigators regard florid osseous dysplasia not as a distinct entity but rather as an exuberant variant of periapical fibrous dysplasia.

One association peculiar to the fibro-osseous lesions arising in the craniofacial bones is the development of a mucocele in the same vicinity.[119, 120]

Radiologic Features

The large family of fibro-osseous lesions of the facial bones is difficult to separate into its component parts in the absence of clinical and radiographic data.[105, 121–124] Computed tomography is particularly useful in the anatomically complicated territory of the craniofacial region in delineating the extent of fibro-osseous lesions.[125]

Fibrous dysplasia in the facial region is a lytic lesion with an ill-defined border, with or without a "ground glass" pattern of homogeneous internal density.[126, 127] One radiographic finding that is more commonly seen in fibrous dysplasia of the craniofacial bones than elsewhere in the body is a pronounced degree of sclerosis of the affected bone—a finding (particularly at the base of the skull) sometimes described by radiologists as *leontiasis ossea*.[107, 117, 121–123, 126–131]

In contrast to fibrous dysplasia, *ossifying fibroma* is a lytic lesion that is sharply demarcated from the adjacent bone, with a very narrow zone of transition. A homogeneous internal pattern of "ground glass" density is observed less frequently than in fibrous dysplasia.

The *aggressive psammomatoid ossifying fibroma* shares many similarities with ossifying fibroma and appears to be a rather well circumscribed (albeit radiodense) lesion with a sclerotic rim. Some of these lesions, however, betray their aggressive nature by a radiographic pattern of an infiltrative, ill-defined lesion that erodes bone and may extend into the intracranial space.[116, 132]

The *cementifying fibroma* is a sharply circumscribed lytic lesion that is similar to ossifying fibroma, apart from its association with dental structures.

In *periapical fibrous dysplasia*, the typical radiographic image early in the genesis of the lesion is one of a well-circumscribed lytic lesion that may or may not show internal densities or a "ground glass" appearance. As the lesion matures, it acquires an increasingly radiodense character. In the late stages of periapical fibrous dysplasia, a radiolucent periphery often surrounds the variably sclerotic central portion of the lesion.

The lesions of *florid osseous dysplasia* are usually multiple and densely sclerotic. In some instances, lytic areas may contain irregular masses of dense material (bone or cementum).

The radiologic differential of fibro-osseous lesions of the facial bones is similar to that of conventional fibrous dysplasia (see Table 13–2). Both Paget's disease of the skull and meningioma with sclerosis of the adjacent bone may mimic fibrous dysplasia radiographically. The radiologic differential considerations specific to the facial bones include sclerosing osteomyelitis and cherubism.[123, 133, 134]

Pathology

Curettages from a craniofacial benign fibro-osseous lesion are usually gray-white, with varying degrees of cystic change. However, these tissues have a gritty to a very densely sclerotic cut surface, a result of their osseous component. In contrast to fibrous dysplasia of the long bones, cartilaginous nodules do not appear to be a component of the craniofacial fibro-osseous lesions.

Fibrous dysplasia, ossifying fibroma, cementifying fibroma, periapical fibrous dysplasia, and florid osseous dysplasia may all present, in areas, a very similar histologic appearance. Here, the light microscopic features that ideally will permit distinction between these entities are described, with the qualification that clinical and radiographic information is invaluable in the classification of these lesions, as light microscopic features taken in isolation are as likely to confuse as they are to clarify a given diagnostic problem (see Table 13–4).

In *fibrous dysplasia* of the facial bones, trabeculae of woven bone appear to spring fully formed from the associated fibrous stroma by a process of "osseous metaplasia." Neither osteoblastic rimming nor the presence of lamellar bone are features of the uncomplicated lesion of fibrous dysplasia of the facial bones (Fig. 13–5*A*).

The trabeculae of an *ossifying fibroma* (and its subtypes, aggressive psammomatoid ossifying fibroma and cementifying fibroma) often show (at least in areas) rimming of the osseous trabeculae by plump osteoblasts and foci of woven bone appliquéd on the surfaces of woven bone trabeculae—neither of which are features of the typical lesion of fibrous dysplasia (Fig. 13–5*B*).[135] The bony ossicles ("cementicles") in *cementifying fibromas* often adopt a somewhat blunter, more amorphous appearance than that created by the delicately curved "Chinese characters" of conventional fibrous dysplasia (Fig. 13–6*A*).

In *periapical fibrous dysplasia*, an appearance similar to that of florid osseous dysplasia is produced, with woven bone trabeculae and oddly shaped masses of bone ("cementum") set in a fibrous background. Osteoblastic rimming may be found in areas (Fig. 13–6*B*).

The lesions of *florid osseous dysplasia* combine trabeculae of woven bone with irregularly shaped masses of bone ("cementum") (which may be large masses or smaller globular struc-

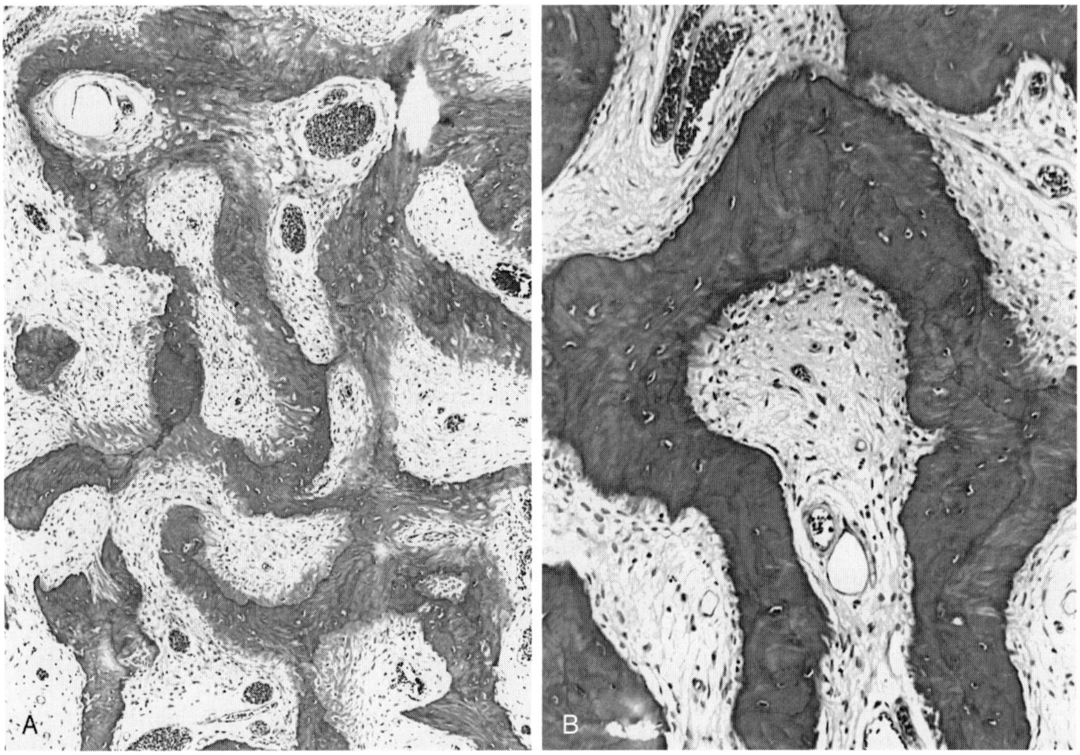

Figure 13–5. Fibro-osseous lesions of the facial bones. *A*, Fibrous dysplasia of the maxilla. This lesion shows interconnecting trabeculae of woven bone that are broader than are those in many cases of fibrous dysplasia of long bones; however, there is neither osteoblastic rimming nor lamellar bone, and as the lesion was radiographically poorly circumscribed, the features supported an interpretation of fibrous dysplasia. *B*, Ossifying fibroma of the mandible. The trabeculae often combine woven and lamellar bone with foci of osteoblastic rimming, and individual trabeculae often appear thicker than those of fibrous dysplasia. Of great import, this lesion is well circumscribed on plain radiographs.

tures) in a fibrovascular stroma. Osteoblastic rimming is usually found, at least focally (Fig. 13–6*C*).

As with conventional fibrous dysplasia arising elsewhere, fibro-osseous lesions of the facial bones may undergo secondary aneurysmal bone cyst formation.[136]

Ancillary Studies. While these lesions have not been subjected to extensive immunohistochemical analysis, it is likely that benign fibro-osseous lesions of the facial skeleton will not exhibit cytokeratin positivity. Serum calcium and phosphorus levels will be normal for age in the fibro-osseous lesions of the facial region; although an elevation of serum alkaline phosphatase levels may be seen in fibrous dysplasia, this rarely reaches the levels seen in Paget's disease, osteosarcoma, or hyperparathyroidism.

Treatment and Prognosis

The craniofacial fibro-osseous lesions are clinically benign, and treatment is directed toward relieving the cosmetic problems presented by the deforming mass lesions and the pressure effects attendant upon their growth in the confined space of the facial skeleton. Recurrences of craniofacial fibro-osseous lesions may be seen despite surgery. Malignant transformation is a highly lethal, albeit rare, complication of craniofacial fibrous dysplasia,[137] but it has not been established for other benign fibro-osseous lesions in this location.

Fibrous dysplasia may be treated surgically to achieve a more pleasing cosmetic result, but such an intervention is usually delayed until after skeletal growth has ceased. Radiation therapy does not seem to be of great use in the treatment of craniofacial fibrous dysplasia. Lesions of ossifying fibroma (and its jaw-specific subtype, cementifying fibroma) are often approached by either curettage or en bloc excision, an approach that is facilitated by the sharp circumscription of ossifying fibroma, which may permit the surgeon to ''shell out'' the lesion. When complete removal of ossi-

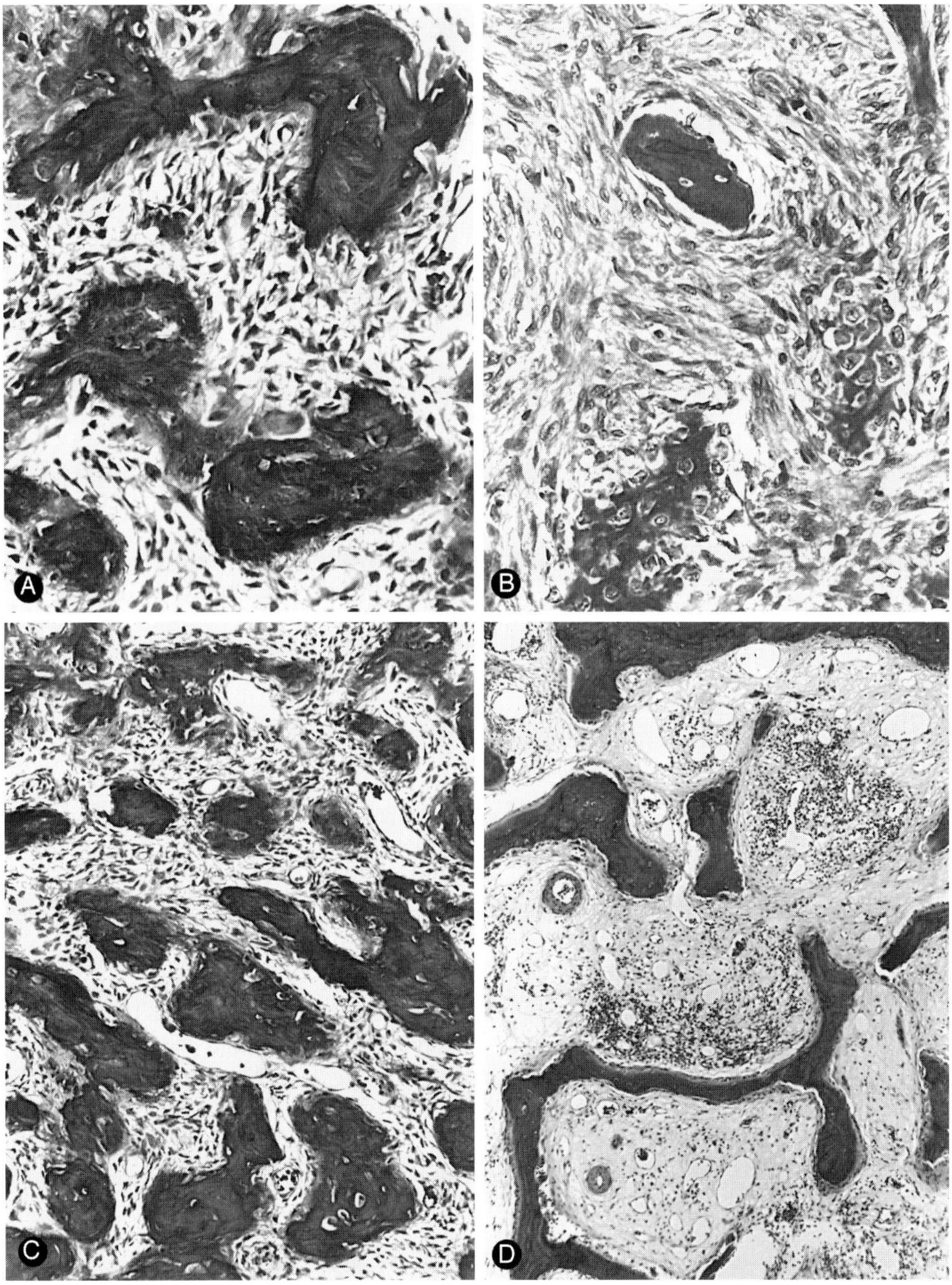

Figure 13–6. Fibro-osseous lesions of the jaw bones. *A*, Cementifying fibroma, a variant of ossifying fibroma, combines amorphous masses of bone ("cementum") with trabeculae of woven and lamellar bone, both set in a rather cellular fibrous stroma as in this mandibular lesion. *B*, Periapical fibrous dysplasia is characterized by a combination of woven and lamellar bone (with osteoblastic activity) set in a fibrous stroma. This asymptomatic mandibular lesion surrounded the apex of a tooth and, in areas, the amorphous bony material ("cementum") coalesced to form large masses. *C*, Florid osseous dysplasia. This lesion, one of several within this patient's mandible and maxilla, contained large and small masses of amorphous to trabecular bony material with osteoblasts and a fibrous stroma. *D*, Chronic sclerosing osteomyelitis. This osseous proliferation was associated with a painful tooth and clinical pulpitis. Between the trabeculae of woven bone are scattered aggregates of chronic inflammatory cells, a finding not usually seen in other benign fibro-osseous lesions of bone.

fying fibroma has been achieved by enucleation, the recurrence rate is quite low (as contrasted with fibrous dysplasia, which is difficult to extirpate surgically). Periapical fibrous dysplasia is, in general, not treated surgically. Florid osseous dysplasia is a disease process upon which oral surgeons are reluctant to operate, in view of the risk of complication by osteomyelitis.

Differential Diagnosis

The differential diagnostic considerations are similar to those for fibrous dysplasia (see Table 13–1), with some specifically craniofacial considerations.[138]

The light microscopic appearance of *chronic sclerosing osteomyelitis* (*condensing osteitis*) may overlap with that of a benign fibro-osseous lesion.[104, 134, 139–141] An important clinical clue to the correct diagnosis is the association of osteomyelitis with an inflamed tooth. The lesion presumably results from extension of a pulpitis into the adjacent alveolar bone, which shows a sclerotic reaction surrounding the apex of the involved tooth. In an ideal world, chronic sclerosing osteomyelitis would show, in addition to the bony overgrowth characteristic of a reparative reaction, a chronic inflammatory infiltrate, which is not a typical feature of the fibro-osseous lesions of bone (Fig. 13–6*D*). This is not always the case, and some observers have questioned whether chronic sclerosing osteomyelitis might actually encompass a variety of entities, including florid osseous dysplasia. It is probably wise to restrict the use of the diagnosis of chronic sclerosing osteomyelitis to those cases in which an accompanying dental lesion can be identified.

Paget's disease of bone may at times be confused with fibro-osseous lesions, particularly on radiographic grounds. In its early stages, however, Paget's disease is marked by a prominent osteoclastic or osteoblastic reaction that is not typical of the fibro-osseous lesions of bone. In the late stage lesions of Paget's disease, the dense sclerotic masses of bone may suggest a fibro-osseous lesion, but the rather cellular fibrous stromal component of such a process is lacking in Paget's disease.[142]

Osteomas of bone may prompt inclusion of fibro-osseous lesion in the differential diagnosis on biopsy material. However, while it is true that osteomas do contain a minimal amount of fibrous tissue, the bulk of the lesion is composed of lamellar or woven bone, or both, as opposed to fibro-osseous lesions, which contain a greater proportion of fibrous tissue.

The lesion known as the *benign cementoblastoma* is very like an osteoma, differing principally in that the cementoblastoma is attached to a tooth. Cementoblastomas are most often found in the mandible of males in the first three decades of life and are distinguished by an abundance of lamellar and amorphous bone; cement lines may be so prominent here as to invite consideration of Paget's disease of bone. However, cementoblastomas lack the well-developed fibrous stromal component that would support an interpretation of a benign fibro-osseous lesion. Cementoblastomas may also exhibit a looser, more richly vascular stroma and so suggest the possibility of an osteoid osteoma or an osteoblastoma.

Idiopathic osteosclerosis is a lesion not associated with a tooth and is marked by a predominance of bony material and a paucity of fibrous stroma and so diverges from the appearance of the typical fibro-osseous lesion of bone.

Cherubism may be difficult to distinguish from fibrous dysplasia, both as a result of clinical similarities between the two lesions and as a result of definitional overlap. The waters are muddied yet further by reports of concurrence of both fibrous dysplasia and cherubism in the same patient.[143] In its best developed form, cherubism is defined clinically as a process seen in children who present with bilateral swellings of the jaw. The designation "cherubism" was selected to acknowledge the physical appearance of the affected children, whose diffusely enlarged lower faces and correspondingly upwards looking eyes reminded the authors of the cherubs so frequently captured on canvas by Renaissance artists.[144] Most regrettably, however, these authors entitled their article "a familial fibrous dysplasia," which continues to produce nomenclatural confusion. Osseous proliferation is not a feature of cherubism and, when bone is found within such lesions, it is a minimal and secondary feature. Instead, the light microscopic appearance is an admixture of fibroblasts, mononucleated and multinucleated giant cells, and collagen, an appearance more reminiscent of a giant cell reparative granuloma or a brown tumor of hyperparathyroidism than of a benign fibro-osseous lesion of bone. Cherubism is inherited by an autosomal dominant pathway.[145–148]

OSSIFICATION IN OTHER INTRAMEDULLARY LESIONS OF BONE

The ability of some skeletal tumors of the sort usually *not* thought to be bone-forming lesions to develop foci of ossification may on occasion confound attempts by the surgical pathologist to construct a differential diagnosis for a given bone biopsy. By way of example, giant cell tumor, brown tumors of hyperparathyroidism, nonossifying fibroma, and giant cell reparative granuloma are all lesions that occasionally exhibit an intimate admixture of bone trabeculae with the lesional tissue. These entities are discussed in detail elsewhere in this book, but it should be noted at this time that not all bone formation within a lesion is necessarily proof that the given lesion is one of the fibro-osseous tumors. While such bone formation may, in some cases, be attributed to the occurrence of a pathologic fracture, in other instances no such fracture can be documented. As a guide, in each of the differential considerations noted earlier, the mononuclear cells usually adopt a plumper configuration than that of the rather more spindled cells that make up the fibrous tissue of fibrous dysplasia. The stroma itself in fibrous dysplasia is typically more heavily collagenized. Finally, the osseous trabeculae may show osteoblastic rimming in these differential possibilities, while such rimming is not a characteristic feature of conventional fibrous dysplasia. These are admittedly subjective distinctions in some instances, which may be clouded by regression and pathologic fracture in any of the lesions being discussed, and so there may be cases in which the best diagnosis is one of "consistent with" or "suggestive of" a given pathologic entity.

REFERENCES

1. Albright F, Butler AM, Hampton AO, et al: Syndrome characterized by osteitis fibrosa disseminata, areas of pigmentation and endocrine dysfunction, with precocious puberty in females. N Engl J Med 216:727, 1937.
2. Lichtenstein L: Polyostotic fibrous dysplasia. Arch Surg 36:874, 1938.
3. Lichtenstein L, Jaffe HL: Fibrous dysplasia of bone. Arch Pathol 33:777, 1942.
4. Thannhauser S: Neurofibromatosis (von Recklinghausen) and osteitis fibrosa cystica localisata et disseminata (von Recklinghausen). Medicine 23:105, 1944.
5. Williamson WM, Lombard LS, Firfer HS: Fibrous dysplasia in a monkey and a kudu. J Am Vet Med Assoc 147:1049, 1965.
6. Liu SK, Dorfman HD, Patnaik AK: Primary and secondary bone tumors in the cat. J Small Anim Pract 15:141, 1974.
7. Wells C: Polyostotic fibrous dysplasia in a seventh century Anglo-Saxon. Br J Radiol 36:925, 1963.
8. Canalis RF, Aragon RM, Cabieses F, et al: Fibrous dysplasia. Findings in a pre-Columbian skull. Am J Otolaryngol 1:131, 1980.
9. Gregg JB, Reed A: Monostotic fibrous dysplasia in the temporal bone: A late prehistoric occurrence. Am J Phys Anthropol 52:587, 1980.
10. Harris WH, Dudley HR, Barry RJ: The natural history of fibrous dysplasia: An orthopaedic, pathological, and roentgenographic study. J Bone Joint Surg 44A:207, 1962.
11. Henry A: Monostotic fibrous dysplasia. J Bone Joint Surg 51B:300, 1969.
12. Mintz MC, Dalinka MK, Schmidt R: Aneurysmal bone cyst arising in fibrous dysplasia during pregnancy. Radiology 165:549, 1987.
13. Ehrig V, Wilson D: Fibrous dysplasia of bone and primary hyperparathyroidism. Ann Intern Med 77:234, 1972.
14. Benjamin D, McRoberts J: Polyostotic fibrous dysplasia associated with Cushing's syndrome. Arch Path Lab Med 96:175, 1973.
15. Firat D, Stutzman L: Fibrous dysplasia associated with multiple endocrinopathy. Am J Med 44:421, 1968.
16. Danon M, Robbov S, Kim S, et al: Cushing's syndrome, sexual precocity and polyostotic fibrous dysplasia in infancy. J Pediat 87:1019, 1975.
17. Rosen IB, Palmer JA: Fibroosseous tumors of the facial skeleton in association with primary hyperparathyroidism: An endocrine syndrome or coincidence? Am J Surg 142:494, 1981.
18. Wirth WA, Leavitt D, Enzinger FM: Multiple intramuscular myxomas: Another extraskeletal manifestation of fibrous dysplasia. Cancer 27:1167, 1971.
19. Ireland DC, Soule EH, Ivins JC: Myxoma of somatic soft tissues. A report of 58 cases, 3 with multiple tumors and fibrous dysplasia of bone. Mayo Clin Proc 48:401, 1973.
20. Sundaram M, McDonald DJ, Merenda G: Intramuscular myxoma: A rare but important association with fibrous dysplasia of bone. AJR Am J Roentgenol 153:107, 1989.
21. Prayson MA, Leeson MC: Soft-tissue myxomas and fibrous dysplasia of bone: A case report and review of the literature. Clin Orthop 291:222, 1993.
22. Aoki T, Kouho H, Hisaoka M, et al: Intramuscular myxoma with fibrous dysplasia: A report of two cases with a review of the literature. Pathol Int 45:165, 1995.
23. West R, Huvos AG, Lane JM: Desmoplastic fibroma of bone arising in fibrous dysplasia. Am J Clin Pathol 79:630, 1983.
24. Bridge JA, Rosenthal H, Sanger WG, et al: Desmoplastic fibroma arising in fibrous dysplasia. Chromosomal analysis and review of the literature. Clin Orthop 247:272, 1989.
25. Huvos AG, Higinbotham NL, Miller TR: Bone sarcomas arising in fibrous dysplasia. J Bone Joint Surg 54A:1047, 1972.
26. Feintuch TA: Chondrosarcoma arising in a cartilaginous area of previously irradiated fibrous dysplasia. Cancer 31:877, 1973.

27. Milgram JW: Malignant degeneration of polyostotic fibrous dysplasia of bone. Bull Hosp Jt Dis 36:137, 1975.
28. Halawa M, Aziz AA: Chondrosarcoma in fibrous dysplasia of the pelvis. A case report and review of the literature. J Bone Joint Surg 66B:760, 1984.
29. Yabut SM, Kenal S, Sissons HA, et al: Malignant transformation of fibrous dysplasia. A case report and review of the literature. Clin Orthop 228:281, 1988.
30. Taconis WK: Osteosarcoma in fibrous dysplasia. Skeletal Radiol 17:163, 1988.
31. Mortensen A, Bojsen-Moller M, Rasmussen P, et al: Fibrous dysplasia of the skull with acromegaly and sarcomatous transformation: Two cases with a review of the literature. J Neurooncol 7:25, 1989.
32. Ishida T, Machinami R, Kojima T, et al: Malignant fibrous histiocytoma and osteosarcoma in association with fibrous dysplasia of bone. Report of three cases. Pathol Res Pract 188:757, 1992.
33. Blackwell JB: Mesenchymal chondrosarcoma arising in fibrous dysplasia of the femur. J Clin Pathol 46:961, 1993.
34. Ruggieri P, Sim FH, Bond JR, et al: Malignancies in fibrous dysplasia. Cancer 73:1411, 1994.
35. Kransdorf MJ, Moser RP, Gilkey FW: Fibrous dysplasia. Radiographics 10:519, 1990.
36. Dorfman HD, Ishida T, Tsuneyoshi M: Exophytic variant of fibrous dysplasia (fibrous dysplasia protuberans). Hum Pathol 25:1234, 1994.
37. Daffner RH, Kirks DR, Gehweiler JA, et al: Computed tomography of fibrous dysplasia. AJR Am J Roentgenol 139:943, 1982.
38. Utz JA, Kransdorf MJ, Jelinek JS, et al: MR appearance of fibrous dysplasia. J Comput Assist Tomogr 13:845, 1989.
39. van Horn PE, Dahlin PE, Bickel WH: Fibrous dysplasia: A clinical pathologic study of orthopaedic surgical cases. Mayo Clin Proc 38:175, 1963.
40. Kolar JJ, Horn V, Zidkova H, et al: Cementifying fibroma (so-called "cementoma"). Br J Radiol 54:989, 1981.
41. Horn V, Bozdech Z, Macek M, et al: Cementoma-like tumours of bone. Arch Orthop Trauma Surg 100:267, 1982.
42. Sissons HA, Kancheral PL, Lehman WB: Ossifying fibroma of bone: Report of two cases. Bull Hosp Jt Dis 43:1, 1983.
43. Povysil C, Matejovsky Z: Fibro-osseous lesion with calcified spherules (cementifying fibroma-like lesion) of the tibia. Ultrastruct Pathol 17:25, 1993.
44. Sissons HA, Steiner GC, Dorfman HD: Calcified spherules in fibro-osseous lesions of bone. Arch Path Lab Med 117:284, 1993.
45. Voytek TM, Ro JY, Edeiken J, et al: Fibrous dysplasia and cemento-ossifying fibroma. A histologic spectrum. Am J Surg Pathol 19:775, 1995.
46. Adler CP: Tumor-like lesions in the femur with cementum-like material: Does a "cementoma" of long bones exist? Skeletal Radiol 14:26, 1985.
47. Mirra JM, Bernard GW, Bullough PG, et al: Cementum-like bone production in solitary bone cysts: So-called "cementoma" of long bones. Clin Orthop 135:295, 1978.
48. Sanerkin NG, Watt I: Enchondromata with annular calcification in association with fibrous dysplasia. Br J Radiol 54:1027, 1981.
49. Drolshagen LF, Reynolds WA, Marcus NW: Fibrocartilaginous dysplasia of bone. Radiology 156:32, 1985.
50. Zayer M: Tibia vara in focal fibrocartilaginous dysplasia: A report of 2 cases. Acta Orthop Scand 63:353, 1992.
51. Ishida T, Dorfman HD: Massive chondroid differentiation in fibrous dysplasia of bone (fibrocartilaginous dysplasia). Am J Surg Pathol 17:924, 1993.
52. Buraczewski J, Dabska M: Pathogenesis of aneurysmal bone cyst. Relationship between the aneurysmal bone cyst and fibrous dysplasia of bone. Cancer 28:597, 1971.
53. Diercks RL, Sauter AJ, Mallens WM: Aneurysmal bone cyst in association with fibrous dysplasia. J Bone Joint Surg 68B:144, 1986.
54. Ruggieri P, Sim FH, Bond JR, et al: Malignancies in fibrous dysplasia. Cancer 73:1411, 1994.
55. Unni KK, Dahlin DC, Beabout JW, et al: Parosteal osteogenic sarcoma. Cancer 37:2466, 1976.
56. Bertoni F, Bacchini P, Fabbri N, et al: Osteosarcoma. Low-grade intraosseous-type osteosarcoma, histologically resembling parosteal osteosarcoma, fibrous dysplasia, and desmoplastic fibroma. Cancer 71:338, 1993.
57. Marks KE, Bauer TW: Fibrous tumors of bone. Orthop Clin North Am 20:377, 1989.
58. Kandel RA, Pritzker KP, Bedard YC: Symmetrical fibro-osseous dysplasia of rib–post-traumatic dysplasia? Histopathology 5:651, 1981.
59. McCarthy EF, Moses DC, Zibreg JW, et al: Painless fibro-osseous lesion of the rib resembling osteoid osteoma: A report of six cases. Skeletal Radiol 13:263, 1985.
60. Kessler S, Mirra JM, Gordon P: Case report 823: Fibro-osseous pseudotumor of the scapula. Skeletal Radiol 23:73, 1994.
61. Ragsdale BD: Polymorphic fibro-osseous lesions of bone: An almost site-specific diagnostic problem of the proximal femur. Hum Pathol 24:505, 1993.
62. Gilkey FW: Liposclerosing myxofibrous tumor of bone. Hum Pathol 24:1264, 1993.
63. Dahlin DC, Bertoni F, Beabout JW, et al: Fibrocartilaginous mesenchymoma with low-grade malignancy. Skeletal Radiol 12:263, 1984.
64. Bulychova IV, Unni KK, Bertoni F, et al: Fibrocartilaginous mesenchymoma of bone. Am J Surg Pathol 17:830, 1993.
65. Schotland HM, Eldridge R, Sommer SS, et al: Neurofibromatosis 1 and osseous fibrous dysplasia in a family. Am J Med Genet 43:815, 1992.
66. Frangenheim P: Angeborene Ostitis als Ursache einer intrauterinen Unterschenkelfraktur. Arch Klin Chir 117:22, 1921.
67. Compere EL: Localized osteitis fibrosa in the newborn and congenital pseudarthrosis. J Bone Joint Surg 18:513, 1936.
68. Aegerter AE: The possible relationship of neurofibromatosis, congenital pseudarthrosis, and fibrous dysplasia. J Bone Joint Surg 32A:618, 1950.
69. Badgley CE, O'Connor SJ, Kudner DF: Congenital kyphoscoliotic tibia. J Bone Joint Surg 34A:349, 1952.
70. Boyd HB, Sage FP: Congenital pseudarthrosis of the tibia. J Bone Joint Surg 40A:1245, 1958.
71. Kempson RL: Ossifying fibroma of the long bones: A light and electron microscopic study. Arch Pathol 82:218, 1966.
72. Semian DW, Willis JB, Bove KE: Congenital fibrous defect of the tibia mimicking fibrous dysplasia. J Bone Joint Surg 57A:854, 1975.
73. Goergen TG, Dickman PS, Resnick D, et al: Long bone ossifying fibromas. Cancer 39:2067, 1977.

74. Markel SF: Ossifying fibroma of long bone: Its distinction from fibrous dysplasia and its association with adamantinoma of long bone. Am J Clin Pathol 69:91, 1978.
75. Campbell CJ, Hawk T: A variant of fibrous dysplasia (osteofibrous dysplasia). J Bone Joint Surg 64A:231, 1982.
76. Castellote A, Garcia-Pena P, Lucaya J, et al: Osteofibrous dysplasia: A report of two cases. Skeletal Radiol 17:483, 1988.
77. Sweet DE, Vinh TN, Devaney K: Cortical osteofibrous dysplasia of long bones and its relationship to adamantinoma. A clinicopathologic study of 30 cases. Am J Surg Pathol 16:282, 1992.
78. Blackwell JB, McCarthy SW, Xipell JM, et al: Osteofibrous dysplasia of the tibia and fibula. Pathology 20:227, 1988.
79. Park YK, Unni KK, McLeod RA, et al: Osteofibrous dysplasia: Clinicopathologic study of 80 cases. Hum Pathol 24:1339, 1993.
80. Ben Arush MW, Ben Arieh Y, Bialik V, et al: Synovial sarcoma associated with osteofibrous dysplasia: A case report and review of the literature. Am J Pediat Hematol 14:261, 1992.
81. Campanacci M, Laus M: Osteofibrous dysplasia of the tibia and fibula. J Bone Joint Surg 63A:367, 1981.
82. Dominguez R, Saucede J, Fenstermacher M: MRI findings in osteofibrous dysplasia. Magnet Reson Imag 7:567, 1989.
83. Bloem JL, van der Heul RO, Schuttavaer HM, et al: Fibrous dysplasia vs adamantinoma of the tibia: Differentiation based on discriminant analysis of clinical and plain film reading. AJR Am J Roentgenol 156:1017, 1991.
84. Benassi MS, Campanacci L, Gamberi G, et al: Cytokeratin expression and distribution in adamantinoma of the long bones and osteofibrous dysplasia of tibia and fibula. An immunohistochemical study correlated to histogenesis. Histopathology 25:71, 1994.
85. Cohen DM, Dahlin DC, Pugh DG: Fibrous dysplasia associated with adamantinoma of long bones. Cancer 15:515, 1962.
86. Unni KK, Dahlin DC, Beabout JW, et al: Adamantinomas of long bones. Cancer 34:1796, 1974.
87. Weiss SW, Dorfman HD: Adamantinoma of long bone. An analysis of nine new cases with emphasis on metastasizing lesions and fibrous dysplasia-like changes. Hum Pathol 8:141, 1977.
88. Levack B, Revell PA, Roper BA: Adamantinoma associated with fibrous dysplasia. Int Orthop 10:253, 1986.
89. Schajowicz F, Santini-Araujo E: Adamantinoma of the tibia masked by fibrous dysplasia. Report of three cases. Clin Orthop 238:294, 1989.
90. Adler CP: Case report 587: Adamantinoma of the tibia mimicking osteofibrous dysplasia. Skeletal Radiol 19:55, 1990.
91. Ueda Y, Roessner A, Bosse A, et al: Juvenile intracortical adamantinoma of the tibia with predominant osteofibrous dysplasia-like features. Pathol Res Pract 187:1039, 1991.
92. Ishida T, Iijima T, Kikuchi F, et al: A clinicopathological and immunohistochemical study of osteofibrous dysplasia, differentiated adamantinoma, and adamantinoma of long bones. Skeletal Radiol 21:493, 1992.
93. Springfield DS, Rosenberg AE, Mankin HJ, et al: Relationship between osteofibrous dysplasia and adamantinoma. Clin Orthop 309:234, 1994.
94. Moon NF: Adamantinoma of the appendicular skeleton in children. Int Orthop 18:379, 1994.
95. Czerniak B, Rojas-Corona RR, Dorfman HD: Morphologic diversity of long bone adamantinoma: The concept of differentiated (regressing) adamantinoma and its relationship to osteofibrous dysplasia. Cancer 64:2319, 1989.
96. Bridge JA, Dembinski A, DeBoer J, et al: Clonal chromosomal abnormalities in osteofibrous dysplasia. Implications for histopathogenesis and its relationship with adamantinoma. Cancer 73:1746, 1994.
97. Hardinge K: Congenital anterior bowing of the tibia. The significance of the different types in relation to pseudarthrosis. Ann Royal Coll Surg 51:17, 1972.
98. Brown GA, Osebold WR, Ponseti IV: Congenital pseudarthrosis of long bones: A clinical, radiographic, histologic and ultrastructural study. Clin Orthop 128:228, 1977.
99. Campanacci M, Nicoll EA, Pagella P: The differential diagnosis of congenital pseudarthrosis of the tibia. Int Orthop 4:283, 1981.
100. Riccardi VM: Neurofibromatosis and Albright's syndrome. Dermatol Clin 5:193, 1987.
101. Waldron A: Fibro-osseous lesions of the jaws. J Oral Surg 28:58, 1970.
102. Waldron CA, Giansanti JS: Benign fibro-osseous lesions of the jaws: A clinical-radiologic-histologic review of sixty-five cases: Part I. Fibrous dysplasia of the jaws. J Oral Surg Oral Med Oral Pathol 35:190, 1973.
103. Waldron CA, Giansanti JS: Benign fibro-osseous lesions of the jaws: A clinical-radiologic-histologic review of sixty-five cases. Part II. Benign fibro-osseous lesions of periodontal ligament origin. J Oral Surg Oral Med Oral Pathol 35:350, 1973.
104. Waldron CA, Giansanti JS: Sclerotic cemental masses of the jaws (so-called chronic sclerosing osteomyelitis, sclerosing osteitis, multiple enostosis and gigantiform cementoma). J Oral Surg 39:590, 1975.
105. Waldron CA: Fibro-osseous lesions of the jaws. J Oral Maxil Surg 43:249, 1985.
106. de Mello DE, Archer CR, Blair JD: Ethmoidal fibro-osseous lesion in a child: Diagnostic and therapeutic problems. Am J Surg Pathol 4:595, 1980.
107. Harrison DF: Osseous and fibro-osseous conditions affecting the craniofacial bones. Ann Otol Rhinol Laryngol 93:199, 1984.
108. Pecaro BC: Fibro-osseous lesions of the head and neck. Otolaryngol Clin North Am 19:489, 1986.
109. Fechner RE: Problematic lesions of the craniofacial bones. Am J Surg Pathol 13(Suppl 1):17, 1989.
110. Summerlin DJ, Tomich CE: Focal cemento-osseous dysplasia: A clinicopathologic study of 221 cases. J Oral Surg Oral Med Oral Pathol 78:611, 1994.
111. Zegarelli EV, Kutschner AH, Napoli N, et al: The cementoma: A study of 230 patients with 435 cementomas. J Oral Surg 17:219, 1964.
112. Krausen AS, Pullen PA, Gulmen S, et al: Cementomas: Aggressive or innocuous neoplasms. Arch Otolaryngol 103:349, 1977.
113. Margo CE, Ragsdale BD, Perman KI, et al: Psammomatoid (juvenile) ossifying fibroma of the orbit. Ophthalmology 92:150, 1985.
114. Margo CE, Weiss A, Habal MB: Psammomatoid ossifying fibroma. Arch Ophthalmol 104:1347, 1986.
115. Slootweg PJ, Panders AK, Nikkels PG: Psammomatoid ossifying fibroma of the paranasal sinuses. An

extragnathic variant of cemento-ossifying fibroma. Report of three cases. J Craniomaxil Surg 21:294, 1993.
116. Wenig BM, Vinh TN, Smirniotopoulos JG, et al: Aggressive psammomatoid ossifying fibromas of the sinonasal region: A clinicopathologic study of a distinct group of fibro-osseous lesions. Cancer 76:1155, 1995.
117. Nager GT, Kennedy DW, Kopstein E: Fibrous dysplasia: A review of the disease and its manifestations in the temporal bone. Ann Otol Rhinol Laryngol 92(Suppl): 1, 1982.
118. Slootweg PJ, Panders AK, Koopmans R, et al: Juvenile ossifying fibroma: An analysis of 33 cases with emphasis on histopathological aspects. J Oral Pathol Med 23:385, 1994.
119. Som PM, Lidov M: The benign fibroosseous lesion: Its association with paranasal sinus mucoceles and its MR appearance. J Comp Assist Tomogr 16:871, 1992.
120. Ferris NJ, Tien RD: Ethmoid mucocele in an infant with a benign fibroosseous lesion. Am J Neuroradiol 16:473, 1995.
121. Meister HP, Lufft W, Schlegel D: Differential diagnosis of fibro-osseous jaw lesions (fibrous dysplasia vs. ossifying fibroma). Beitr Pathol 148:221, 1973.
122. Kessel LJ, Milne AM: Fibro-osseous lesions of the mandible. Br J Oral Surg 6:84, 1968.
123. Boysen ME, Olving JH, Vatne K, et al: Fibro-osseous lesions of the cranio-facial bones. J Laryngol Otol 93:793, 1979.
124. Mohammadi-Araghi H, Haery C: Fibro-osseous lesions of craniofacial bones. The role of imaging. Radiol Clin North Am 31:121, 1993.
125. Higashi T, Iguchi M, Shimura A, et al: Computed tomography and bone scintigraphy in polyostotic fibrous dysplasia. J Oral Surg 50:580, 1980.
126. Dahlgren SE, Lind PO, Lindblom A, et al: Fibrous dysplasia of jaw bones. A clinical, roentgenographic and histopathologic study. Acta Otolaryngol 68:257, 1969.
127. Brown EW, Megerian CA, McKenna MJ, et al: Fibrous dysplasia of the temporal bone: Imaging findings. AJR Am J Roentgenol 164:679, 1995.
128. Cangiano R, Stratigos GT, Williams FA: Clinical and radiographic manifestations of fibro-osseous lesions of the jaws: Report of five cases. J Oral Surg 29:872, 1971.
129. Obwegeser HL, Freihofer HP, Horejs J: Variation of fibrous dysplasia in the jaws. J Maxil Surg 1:161, 1973.
130. Talbot IC, Keith DA, Lord IJ: Fibrous dysplasia of the cranio-facial bones. A clinico-pathological survey of seven cases. J Laryngol Otol 88:429, 1974.
131. Daly BD, Chow CC, Cockram CS: Unusual manifestations of craniofacial fibrous dysplasia: Clinical, endocrinological and computed tomographic features. Postgrad Med J 70:10, 1994.
132. Han MH, Chang KH, Lee CH, et al: Sinonasal psammomatoid ossifying fibromas: CT and MR manifestations. AJNR 12:25, 1991.
133. Cornelius EA, McClendon JL: Cherubism: Hereditary fibrous dysplasia of the jaws. Roentgenographic features. AJR Am J Roentgenol 106:136, 1969.
134. Johannsen A: Chronic sclerosing osteomyelitis of the mandible. Radiographic differential diagnosis from fibrous dysplasia. Acta Radiol (Diagn) 18:360, 1977.
135. Slootweg PJ, Muller H: Differential diagnosis of fibro-osseous jaw lesions. A histological investigation of 30 cases. J Craniomaxil Surg 18:210, 1990.
136. Wojno KJ, McCarthy EF: Fibro-osseous lesions of the face and skull with aneurysmal bone cyst formation. Skeletal Radiol 23:15, 1994.
137. Slow IN, Friedman EW: Osteogenic sarcoma arising in a pre-existing fibrous dysplasia. J Oral Surg 24:214, 1971.
138. Koury ME, Regezi JA, Perrott DH, et al: "Atypical" fibro-osseous lesions: Diagnostic challenges and treatment concepts. Int J Oral Maxil Surg 24:162, 1995.
139. Khosla V, Rosenfeld H, Berk L: Chronic osteomyelitis of the mandible. J Oral Surg 29:649, 1971.
140. Jacobsson S, Heyden G: Chronic sclerosing osteomyelitis of the mandible. J Oral Surg 43:357, 1977.
141. Jacobsson S, Hollender L, Lindberg S, et al: Chronic sclerosing osteomyelitis of the mandible. J Oral Surg 45:167, 1978.
142. Carillo R, Morales A, Rodriguez-Peralto JL, et al: Benign fibro-osseous lesions in Paget's disease of the jaws. J Oral Surg Oral Med Oral Pathol 71:588, 1991.
143. Davis GB, Sinn DP, Watson SW: Case 43, part II: Cherubism. J Oral Maxil Surg 41:119, 1983.
144. Jones WA, Gerrie J, Pritchard J: Cherubism: A familial fibrous dysplasia of the jaws. J Bone Joint Surg 32B:325, 1950.
145. Kaugars GE, Niamtu J, Svirsky JA, et al: Cherubism: Diagnosis, treatment, and comparison with central giant cell granulomas and giant cell tumors. J Oral Surg Oral Med Oral Pathol 73:369, 1992.
146. Patel JR: Cherubism: Report of three cases. ASDC J Dent Child 54:289, 1987.
147. Peters WJ: Cherubism: A study of twenty cases from one family. J Oral Surg Oral Med Oral Pathol 1979; 47:307.
148. Pina-Neto JM, Moreno AF, Silva LR, et al: Cherubism, gingival fibromatosis, epilepsy, and mental deficiency (Ramon syndrome) with juvenile rheumatoid arthritis. Am J Med Genet 25:433, 1986.

Chapter

14

EWING'S SARCOMA, LYMPHOMA, AND LANGERHANS' CELL PROLIFERATIONS

ELIZABETH J. PERLMAN

The last decade has been marked by considerable progress in the ability of pathologists to provide a specific diagnosis when faced with a primitive, cytoplasm-poor, and stroma-poor osseous neoplasm. These so-called "round cell" tumors of bone, which include tumors of unrelated histogenesis that are treated with divergent therapies, are considered together in this chapter because of their similar appearances and the resulting pathologic challenge. The prototypic round cell tumor of bone is Ewing's sarcoma. Other small round cell tumors of childhood may present with a single osseous lesion and therefore cause diagnostic difficulty; however, in reality they rarely do so. Neuroblastomas in bone are virtually all metastatic and the majority show overt neural differentiation by routine histology. Similarly, rhabdomyosarcomas arising in bone without a clinically evident soft tissue primary tumor are rare. Primary lymphoma of bone is also quite uncommon, particularly the histologic subtypes that resemble other round cell tumors of childhood. In addition, sensitive and specific immunohistochemical stains are readily available to aid in the diagnosis of neuroblastoma, rhabdomyosarcoma, and lymphoma. Therefore, the greatest diagnostic challenge when faced with a small round cell tumor of bone often lies in the recognition of unusual forms of osseous tumors, such as small cell osteogenic sarcoma, mesenchymal chondrosarcoma, and the poorly understood primitive sarcoma of bone. A precise histologic diagnosis is becoming more important as disease-specific therapeutic strategies continue to result in improvement in the prognosis of many neoplasms. The aim of this chapter is to examine the pathology of small round cell tumors primary to bone and related conditions, and the appropriate tests utilized in their diagnosis (Table 14–1). Not to be included in this discussion are tumors that show primarily a spindle cell morphology, even if highly undifferen-

Table 14–1. Synopsis of Chapter

- The Ewing's sarcoma/peripheral neuroectodermal tumor family
  - Clinical presentation
  - Pathology
  - Diagnostic methods
- Differential diagnosis of Ewing's sarcoma
  - Lymphoma of bone
  - Small cell osteosarcoma
  - Mesenchymal chondrosarcoma
  - Primary malignant mesenchymoma of bone
  - Rhabdomyosarcoma
  - Primitive round cell sarcoma of bone
  - Desmoplastic small round cell tumor
- Langerhans' cell histiocytosis

tiated and cellular. These spindle cell tumors present their own challenges and are considered in Chapter 12.

THE EWING'S SARCOMA / PERIPHERAL NEUROECTODERMAL TUMOR FAMILY

Ewing's sarcoma is an undifferentiated tumor of bone whose histogenesis has been avidly, and at times hotly, debated since its initial description by James Ewing in 1921.[1, 2] The concept most seriously questioned in the decades following its description was whether Ewing's sarcoma was truly an independent etiologic and histogenetic entity, or instead represented a collection of poorly differentiated tumors of diverse derivation. Simultaneously and independently, the concept of an extracranial primitive neuroectodermal tumor (PNET) was introduced by Stout,[3] and was fully accepted and developed in the following decades. PNETs were initially thought to be exclusively soft tissue lesions composed of small blue cells showing evidence of neural differentiation; these were variably called adult neuroblastoma, peripheral neuroepithelioma, and peripheral neuroblastoma. However, the histologic distinction between PNET and Ewing's sarcoma became blurred as it became apparent that some osseous lesions show overt evidence of neural differentiation and occasional soft tissue lesions show no differentiation.[4–7] The biologic distinction between Ewing's sarcoma and PNET became less clear when laboratory studies demonstrated the ability of undifferentiated Ewing's sarcoma cells to develop neural features following growth in tissue culture (see Chapter 3).[8–10] Soon thereafter, cytogenetic analyses of these apparently independent tumors demonstrated that both Ewing's sarcoma and PNET contain the same specific chromosomal translocation involving chromosomes 11 and 22.[11, 12] As a result, a consensus has developed that Ewing's sarcoma and PNET represent a family of tumors showing a range of neural differentiation. It has been proposed that Ewing's sarcoma/PNETs arise from postganglionic parasympathetic neurons dispersed throughout the body, in contrast to classic neuroblastoma, which originates from neurons populating the sympathetic nervous system. Despite this consensus, many questions remain concerning the prognostic significance of the degree of neural differentiation, and the possibility that the cell of origin of Ewing's sarcoma may be a primitive mesenchymal cell that is capable of differentiating along pathways other than neural. Lastly, other primitive tumors showing neuroectodermal differentiation exist that are clearly biologically and histologically distinct from the PNETs discussed previously, such as melanocytic progonoma. Such lesions are also often placed in the PNET category, but are not discussed in this chapter as they are quite rare and typically present in the soft tissue.

Clinical Presentation

Tumors in the Ewing's sarcoma family, including PNET, may arise in any part of the skeleton, although the long tubular bones and bones of the pelvic girdle are the most frequent sites.[13, 14] The age distribution shows these to be tumors predominately of adolescence and young adulthood, with two thirds of reported tumors occurring before the age of 20 years.[14–16] However, most large reports are derived from cooperative pediatric studies and may under-represent adult cases. Ewing's sarcoma/PNETs in infants and toddlers do rarely occur, although studies thus far show no significant differences in presentation, prognosis, or biology.[17] Over 10% of Ewing's sarcoma/PNETs arise in the chest wall.[16, 18, 19] These thoracopulmonary lesions were initially thought to represent a distinct clinicopathologic entity and were classified as Askin tumors and malignant small round cell tumors of the thoracopulmonary region.[20–22] Subsequent histologic, immunohistochemical, and cytogenetic studies have stressed the similarity between these chest wall tumors and Ewing's sarcoma/PNETs.[23–26] While the propensity for these tumors to arise in the chest wall is intriguing and unexplained, at this time there is no evidence to support a biologic, histologic, or therapeutic distinction from Ewing's sarcoma/PNET at other sites.

Patients with Ewing's sarcoma often present with constant pain of 6 to 12 months' duration, without a consistent pattern, accompanied by local tenderness, erythema, and swelling. This presentation overlaps significantly with that of osteomyelitis.[27, 28] Radiographically, Ewing's sarcoma/PNETs of bone do not show specific features and may be confused with osteosarcoma, lymphoma, or chondrosarcoma, as well as with benign lesions such as

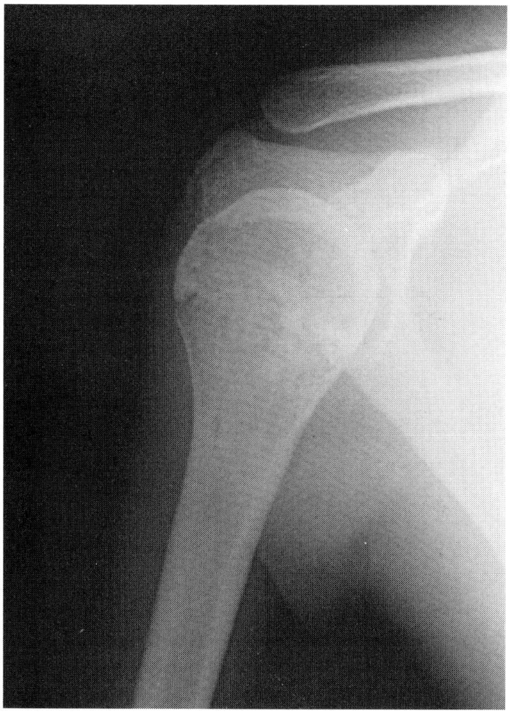

Figure 14–1. Typical Ewing's sarcoma. Radiograph showing the typical poorly marginated appearance, with subtle changes extending well into the diaphysis of the humerus.

osteomyelitis and eosinophilic granuloma. Common radiographic features of Ewing's sarcoma/PNET include poor margination, soft tissue involvement, and periosteal new bone formation in an onion-skin pattern (Fig. 14–1).[29] A minority of cases show a diffusely sclerotic pattern similar to that seen in osteomyelitis and osteogenic sarcoma.[30]

Pathology

The evidence suggests that the Ewing's sarcoma/PNET family of neoplasms demonstrates a continuum of neural differentiation. At one end of the spectrum is Ewing's sarcoma, an undifferentiated tumor; at the other extreme is the peripheral primitive neuroectodermal tumor, showing clear evidence of neural differentiation by histology, immunohistochemistry, and electron microscopy. The majority of tumors show a histologic appearance falling between these extremes, and the criteria utilized for nomenclature purposes are arbitrary and vary from report to report. Many observers have attempted to divide this continuum into three categories: (1) Ewing's sarcoma, representing those tumors with no evidence of differentiation; (2) PNET, representing those tumors with clear evidence of neural differentiation; and (3) atypical Ewing's sarcoma, representing an intermediate category. These will be discussed separately in the following sections; however, there is no agreement on what constitutes the boundaries of these categories or the level of diligence required in the search for neural differentiation.

Ewing's Sarcoma

Typical Ewing's sarcoma consists of sheets of tightly packed, spherical to ellipsoid cells with an indistinct cell wall, scant clear cytoplasm, a delicate nuclear membrane, faintly stippled, homogeneous chromatin, inconspicuous nucleoli, and no intercellular stroma. The mitotic rate is typically very low (fewer than two mitoses per 10 high-power fields). A feature that is highly characteristic of Ewing's sarcoma is the presence of a dimorphic population of cells, including the larger cells described earlier as well as smaller cells containing increasingly eosinophilic cytoplasm and densely hyperchromatic nuclei, probably representing effete cells (Fig. 14–2*A*). Although the presence of this dimorphic population is not specific for Ewing's sarcoma, its absence should prompt the consideration of other diagnoses. Geographic areas of coagulative necrosis, small or large, are another highly characteristic feature of Ewing's sarcoma (Fig. 14–2*B*). Unlike the areas of necrosis in neuroblastoma, those in Ewing's sarcoma are rarely accompanied by calcification. The Azzopardi phenomenon, a smearing out of chromatin that is an artifactual feature of nuclear fragility, is uncommon in Ewing's sarcoma.[6, 13, 14, 31–34]

Ewing's sarcomas show a number of architectural growth patterns. Many tumors show a diffuse pattern with broad fields of tumor lacking distinctive topographic features. Others have a lobular growth pattern characterized by multicellular aggregates separated by fibrovascular septa (Fig. 14–2*C*). A widely reported "filigree" pattern shows delicate anastomosing strands of tumor cells separated by fibrovascular stroma (Fig. 14–2*D*). The presence of the filigree pattern has been associated with a poor prognosis in some studies,[14, 35] although this has not been confirmed by others.[36] The possibility has been raised that the filigree pat-

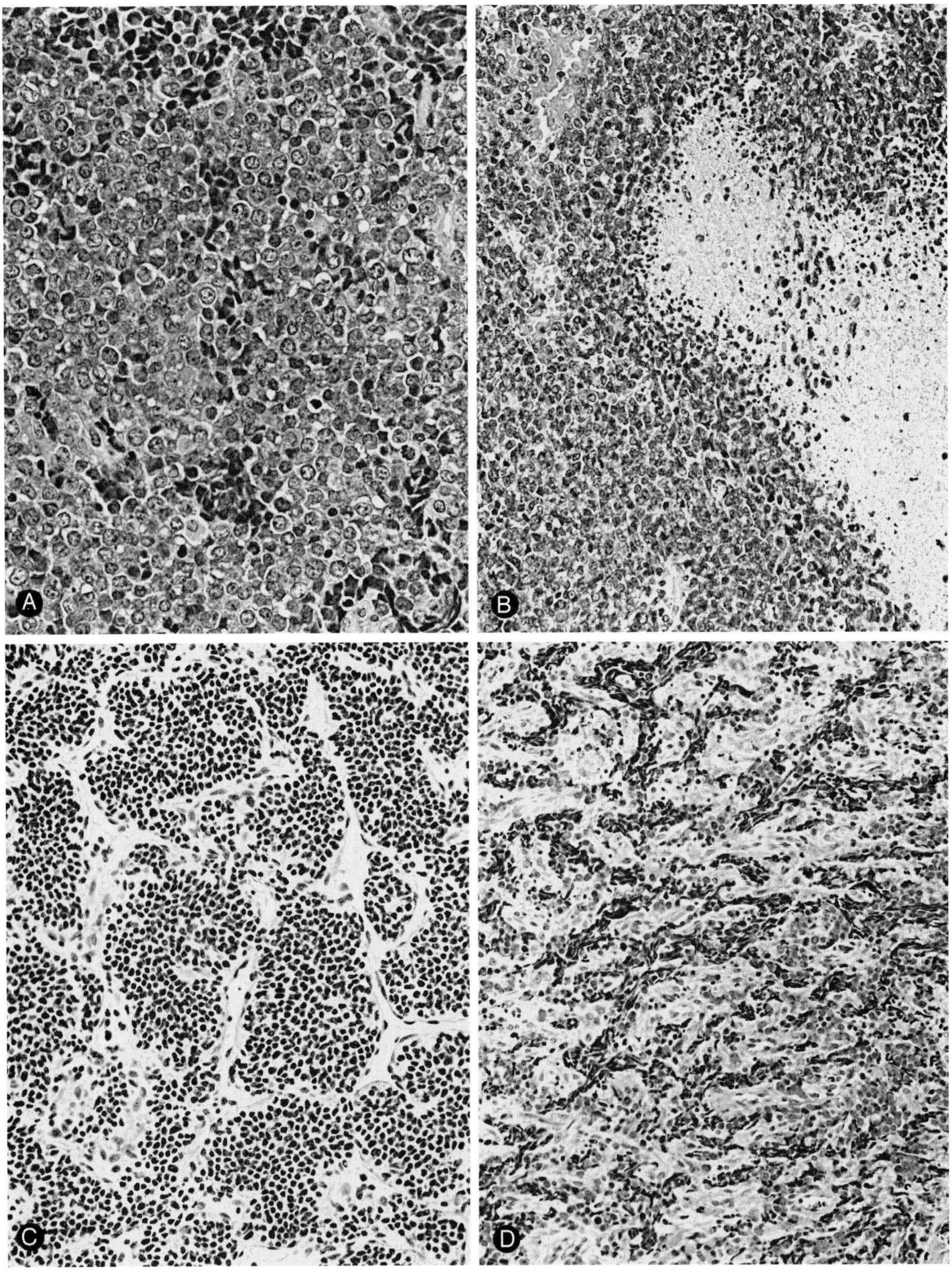

Figure 14–2. Features of Ewing's sarcoma. *A*, Rounded cells with scant cytoplasm, absence of significant stroma, low mitotic rate, and a dimorphic population of cells. *B*, Geographic areas of coagulative necrosis are highly characteristic of tumors in the Ewing's family. *C*, A minority of tumors in the Ewing's family show a prominent lobular architecture. *D*, The filigree pattern, with anastomosing strands of tumor cells separated by fibrovascular stroma, is a pattern present focally in many Ewing's sarcomas; the prognostic implications of this pattern have been debated.

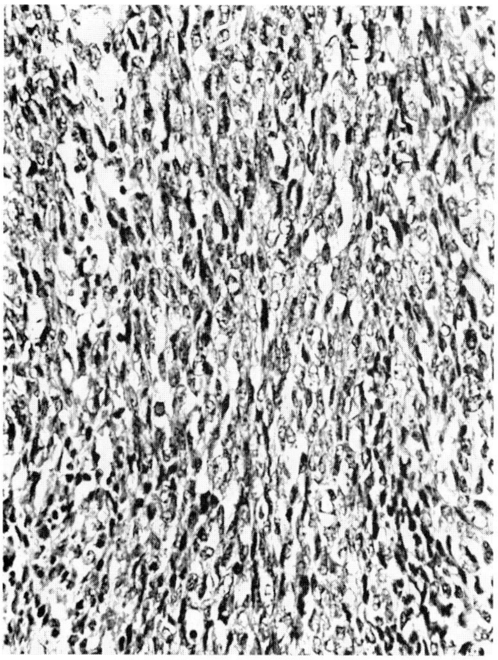

Figure 14–3. Rare Ewing's sarcoma showing significant, although focal, spindling. Although this alerts the pathologist to consider other diagnostic entities, it need not prevent the diagnosis of Ewing's sarcoma.

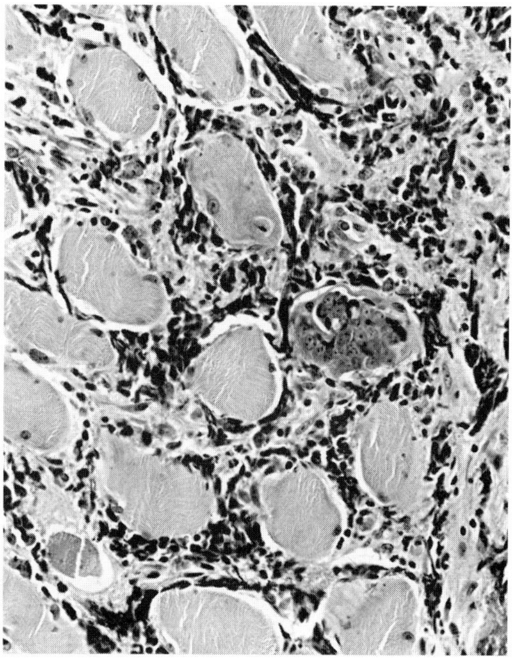

Figure 14–4. Intramyofibrillar colonization is a peculiar form of skeletal muscle invasion seen in Ewing's sarcoma that is a poor prognostic indicator.

tern is seen in areas of soft tissue invasion and that the poor associated prognosis is due to the higher stage rather than the histologic pattern itself. Rarely, tumors otherwise quite consistent with Ewing's sarcoma show areas with significant spindling (Fig. 14–3). While this should alert the pathologist to other diagnostic possibilities, the presence of spindling alone should not preclude the diagnosis of Ewing's sarcoma.

Ewing's sarcomas almost universally contain cytoplasmic glycogen, a feature that has historically been considered the light microscopic hallmark of Ewing's sarcoma. However, glycogen may be seen in almost all round cell tumors of childhood and is occasionally noted in both small cell osteosarcoma and mesenchymal chondrosarcoma.[13, 37] In addition, unless precautions are taken to preserve glycogen during processing, up to 40% of Ewing's sarcoma are glycogen negative. Therefore, the role of glycogen staining in the differential diagnosis of Ewing's sarcoma is limited. Reticulin stains may be diagnostically useful in that individual Ewing's sarcoma cells are not enmeshed by reticulin whereas lymphoma, small cell osteosarcoma, and mesenchymal chondrosarcomas often show significant reticulin deposition.[14] Rare cases of Ewing's sarcoma may show vague reticulin deposits encircling groups of cells, but reported cases have not shown well-defined lobular groupings.

Ewing's sarcoma commonly invades surrounding soft tissue and bone. Osseous invasion often extends further histologically than is indicated radiographically, and invasion of the tumor cells through the haversian canals is not infrequent. A peculiar pattern of skeletal muscle invasion has been reported in which the tumor cells are incorporated into the sarcoplasm (Fig. 14–4). This intramyofibrillar colonization is an uncommon finding and represents an ominous predictor of clinical outcome, with an increased rate of developing distant metastases and a decreased survival rate compared with cases not demonstrating this skeletal muscle parasitism.[38] Vascular involvement is frequently present, corresponding with the high rate of metastasis and requirement for systemic therapy.

Electron microscopic examination of typical Ewing's sarcoma reveals closely apposed, homogeneous round cells with smooth contours, and occasional small junctions bearing relatively thin cytoplasmic plaques, some of which show attached bundles of intermediate filaments. Fully developed desmosomes are not observed. The scant cytoplasm is devoid of cytoskeleton and contains only sparse organelles. The nuclei are typically small, round, and smooth with homogeneously distributed heterochromatin. Large pools of glycogen restricted to one or two areas of the cytoplasm are present in almost all Ewing's sarcomas. The presence of pools of glycogen and the paucity of cytoplasmic organelles constitute the most characteristic ultrastructural feature of Ewing's sarcoma.[31, 34, 39, 40]

Primitive Neuroectodermal Tumor

Extracranial PNETs are primitive small blue cell tumors that closely resemble Ewing's sarcoma. The predominant cell type of PNET is round, like that of Ewing's sarcoma, but may contain more cytoplasm, a round or elongated nucleus with fine or coarse chromatin, and inconspicuous or prominent nucleoli. Unlike typical Ewing's sarcoma, mitoses in PNETs may be moderate to numerous, and cellular pleomorphism may be present (Fig. 14–5*A*).[31] Like Ewing's sarcoma, PNETs may show a diffuse, lobular, organoid, or pseudoalveolar pattern. The diagnosis of PNET depends on the demonstration of neural differentiation; however, there is no agreement on the degree of neural differentiation required for this designation. Some observers consider true rosettes by histology to be mandatory for the diagnosis of a PNET. However, true rosettes containing a central lumen are extraordinarily uncommon in these lesions, even in those tumors that show abundant neural differentiation by electron microscopy. When present, the rosettes are more commonly of the Homer-Wright type or pseudorosettes, which lack a central lumen but instead show a center composed of amorphous material or the cytoplasmic portions of converging tumor cells (Fig. 14–5*B*).[16–19] Such pseudorosettes are often quite subtle and widely scattered. Many observers do not demand light microscopic evidence of neural differentiation and will classify tumors as PNET if they show evidence of neural differentiation by electron microscopy or if they show the expression of at least two neural markers by immunohistochemistry. PNETs do not commonly show mature neural elements such as ganglion cells and obvious neuropil, although ganglionic differentiation has been described in rare cases (Fig. 14–5*C*).[18, 19] When neuropil and ganglion cells are seen, the diagnosis of metastatic neuroblastoma should be considered. Alternatively, the presence of polyphenotypic differentiation should be searched for (utilizing muscle and epithelial markers in addition to neural markers), and, if positive, the most appropriate diagnosis may be malignant ectomesenchymoma.

The ultrastructural hallmark of PNET is the presence of cytoplasmic processes containing neurosecretory granules. The granules are much fewer in number and more variable in size than those seen in neuroblastomas, and the predominant cell population in most PNETs lacks processes and neurosecretory granules. Compared with Ewing's sarcoma, the cells of PNET show a more elaborate content of organelles with rough endoplasmic reticulum and mitochondria, as well as intermediate cytoplasmic filaments (Fig. 14–5*D*). Occasional cases show a basal lamina and extracellular matrix production.[15, 16, 19, 31]

Atypical Ewing's Sarcoma

Within the Ewing's family of tumors, some tumors exhibit greater pleomorphism, a higher mitotic rate, and more cytoplasm. By electron microscopy, these tumors often show an elaborate content of cytoplasmic organelles, a few intermediate filaments, well-developed attachments, irregular cell contours, and cytoplasmic processes with cell moulding, although, by definition, no dense core granules are present. Collagen bundles and a microgranular or amorphous extracellular matrix may be present.[36, 41] These tumors have been classified by many as *atypical* or *large cell* Ewing's sarcoma (Fig. 14–6). Metastases from these tumors may show clear neural differentiation,[33] supporting the hypothesis that atypical Ewing's sarcomas represent tumors with intermediate differentiation between Ewing's sarcoma and PNET. Atypical Ewing's sarcoma has been defined in several ways, using light microscopic features alone or in combination with electron microscopy or immunohistochemistry, or both. Depending on the definitions applied and the diligence used to search for neural differentiation, 6 to 30% of tumors in the Ewing's sarcoma family may fit into the atypical Ewing's category. No clinical differences have been seen in outcome between Ewing's sarcoma and atypical Ewing's sarcoma.[18, 41] The importance of recognizing atypical Ewing's sarcoma is the histologic similarity to large cell lymphoma and small cell osteosarcoma.

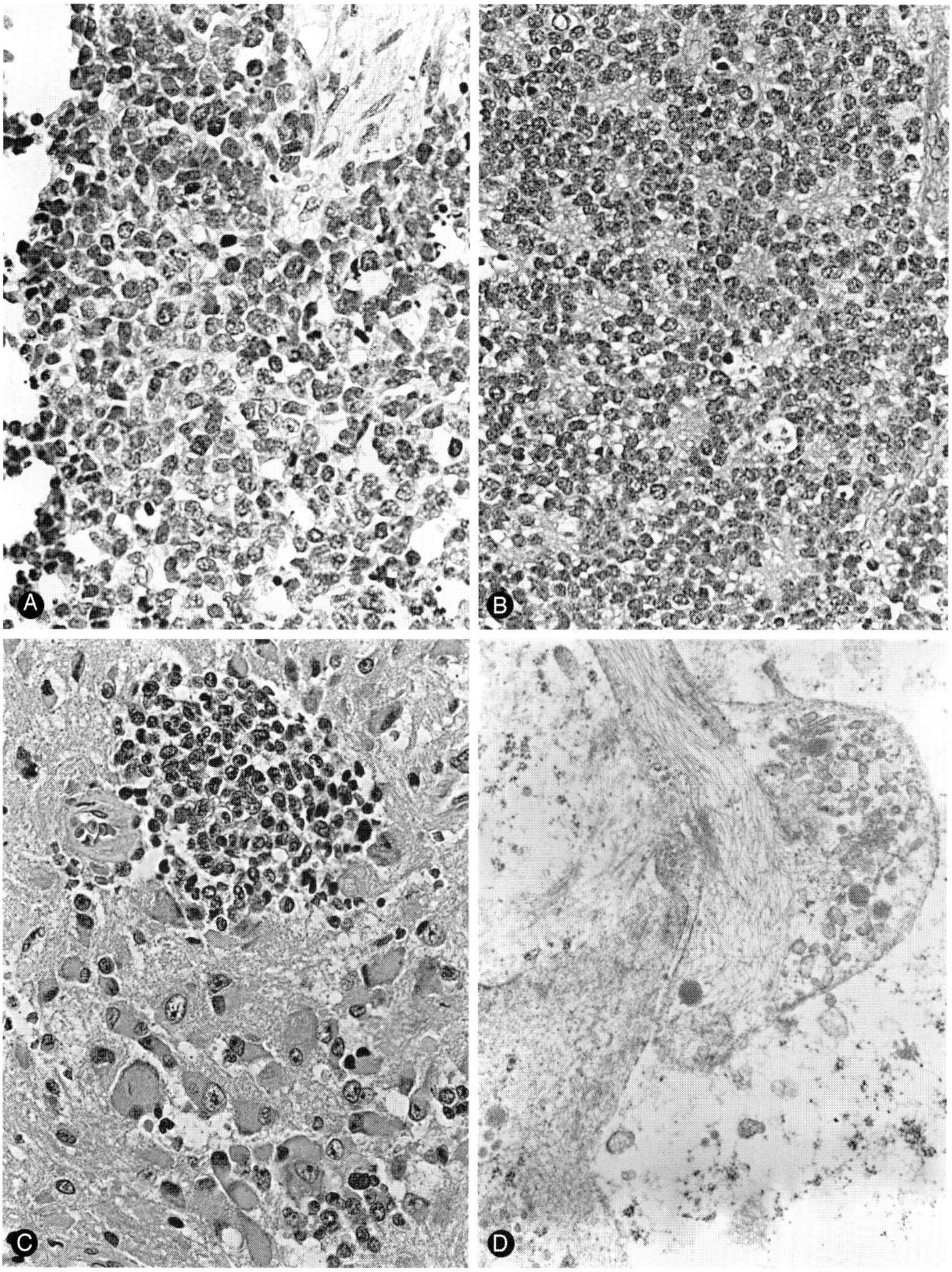

Figure 14–5. Peripheral neuroectodermal tumor. *A*, PNET showing many cytologic similarities to Ewing's sarcoma; however, more cellular pleomorphism and more mitotic activity is present when compared to the classic Ewing's sarcoma shown in Figure 14–2. *B*, Rare PNETs show numerous pseudorosettes, which lack a central lumen. *C*, An unusual PNET showing ganglionic differentiation in addition to the primitive cell component. Until proven otherwise, such tumors in young patients should be presumed to represent a neuroblastoma. This unusual histology presented in a PNET following therapy. *D*, Ultrastructurally, the vast majority of PNETs show scant and widely scattered evidence of neural differentiation. Rare tumors such as the one illustrated show defined processes with microtubules and neurosecretory granules.

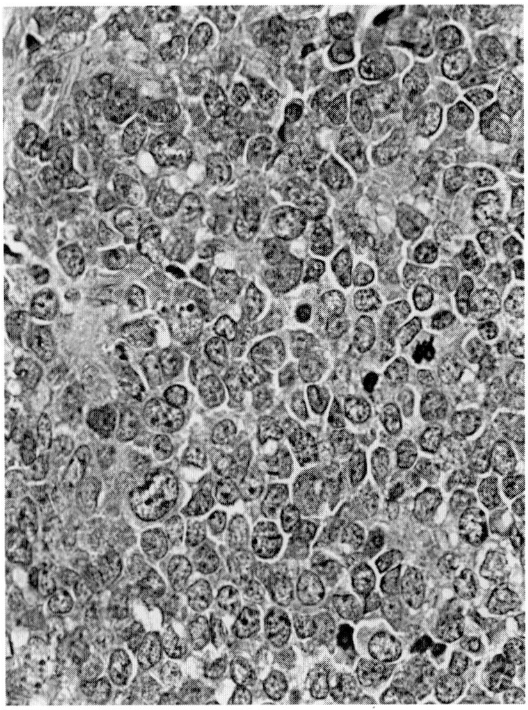

Figure 14–6. Atypical Ewing's sarcoma. The histologic appearance is similar to that of classic Ewing's sarcoma as well as PNET. The cells are often larger and more pleomorphic, with readily identifiable mitotic figures. Such lesions may be difficult to distinguish from large cell lymphomas.

Histology Following Therapy

The current management of Ewing's sarcoma/PNET, like that of osteosarcoma, includes chemotherapy followed by surgery. The prognostic predictive value of post-chemotherapy histologic grading of osteosarcoma has been reported and is currently utilized in cooperative clinical trials. Similar studies of Ewing's sarcoma/PNET have only recently been addressed. A preliminary examination of resection specimens from the Intergroup Ewing's Sarcoma protocols scored and graded 53 resection specimens for necrosis and fibrosis and compared this to 3-year survival rate. Those specimens showing 100% tumor destruction showed 100% survival, whereas those showing less than 10% tumor destruction showed a 30% 3-year survival.[42] A second study analyzed 31 patients with Ewing's sarcoma/PNET and found that the disease-specific survival rate at a median follow-up of 3.5 years was 87% for tumors showing greater than 70% necrosis and 35% for tumors showing less than 70% necrosis.[43] While these findings are preliminary, they suggest that histologic response to chemotherapy in osseous Ewing's sarcoma/PNET may be prognostically useful (see Chapter 8). Another uncommon post-chemotherapy observation is the presence of neural differentiation, most frequently characterized by rosettes. The development of alveolar features after chemotherapy has been reported on occasions and should not cause confusion with rhabdomyosarcoma or malignant mesenchymoma.

Histology and Prognosis in Ewing's Sarcoma/PNET

The impetus to characterize and clarify the histology of tumors in the Ewing's sarcoma/PNET family lies in the need to identify the optimal therapy for these aggressive neoplasms. Categorizing this family of tumors into Ewing's sarcoma, PNET, and atypical Ewing's sarcoma enables observers to determine the prognostic relevance of these categories and to correlate the degree of neural differentiation with prognosis. Several studies have associated neural differentiation with a poor outcome[15, 18, 36]; however, these findings are open to question due to the failure to correct for variables such as size of tumor, site, stage, and therapy received. More recent studies employing multiagent chemotherapy for both PNET and Ewing's sarcoma, and correcting for site and stage, have shown no difference in clinical behavior with neural differentiation.[44–46] The definitive answer to this dilemma resides in the forthcoming analysis of the recently closed Intergroup Ewing's Sarcoma study.

Other studies have related histologic features other than neural differentiation to prognosis. On multifactorial analysis, several large, retrospective studies of Ewing's sarcoma of bone found that the presence of necrosis or a filigree pattern were the only histologic characteristics to be of poor prognostic significance.[14, 32, 47] Other studies have failed to confirm that a filigree growth pattern implied a shorter survival,[36] but have suggested that tumors with a higher mitotic rate were associated with poor prognosis.[32] All studies of Ewing's sarcoma/PNET have demonstrated that the site of primary involvement is an important predictor of clinical behavior, with survival among patients with tumors of pelvic bones significantly less than those with lesions in distal bones.[14, 22, 48] The presence of metastases at the time of diagnosis is likewise a poor prognostic indicator, the most common site of metastases being lung and bone.[49]

Diagnostic Methods

Immunohistochemistry

Tumors in the Ewing's sarcoma/PNET family lack specific light microscopic features that enable a confident diagnosis. While the same is often true with other round cell tumors of childhood such as alveolar rhabdomyosarcoma and neuroblastoma, these diagnoses are aided by immunohistochemistry utilizing specific and sensitive antibodies. Unfortunately, until recent years, the role of immunohistochemistry in the diagnosis of Ewing's sarcoma/PNET has been to exclude other diagnoses. The available antibodies reacting with neural antigens either lack specificity or fail to stain the most primitive tumors in the group. Recently, antibodies to a protein encoded by the *MIC2* gene have provided a significant breakthrough in the diagnosis of Ewing's sarcoma/PNET.

Neural Markers. Neural markers can be characterized as neuronal or neuroendocrine. The most widely utilized neuronal marker is neuron-specific enolase (NSE), which consistently stains neural tumors regardless of the degree of differentiation. The utility of NSE, however, is diminished by its lack of specificity and wide interlaboratory variability. Decalcification often interferes with NSE immunoreactivity. As a general rule, NSE does not stain typical Ewing's sarcomas, whereas atypical Ewing's sarcomas are often positive and PNETs are usually positive.[16, 50, 51] Positivity for NSE has also been observed in primitive round cell sarcomas of bone,[52] mesenchymal chondrosarcomas,[53] and scattered cells of some rhabdomyosarcomas.[33] Fixation with B5 may result in diffuse, light staining of lymphomas with antibodies to many antigens, and NSE is among those. A second group of neuronal markers widely utilized are the neurofilaments, which form part of the neuronal cytoskeleton. Only 37% of PNETs are positive for neurofilaments.[16]

The most commonly utilized neuroendocrine markers are synaptophysin and chromogranin. Synaptophysin, a glycoprotein localized to the membrane of presynaptic vesicles of neurons, paraganglia, and several epithelial neuroendocrine cells, is present in neuroblastomas, paragangliomas, carcinoids, and neuroendocrine carcinomas. Many Ewing's sarcomas and most PNETs are positive for synaptophysin.[16, 50, 51] However, synaptophysin is very sensitive to formalin fixation for over 2 to 4 hours and the results are therefore quite variable. Synaptophysin positivity has also been described in rhabdomyosarcomas.[33] Antibodies to chromogranin react with cells containing dense core granules, so do not stain typical Ewing's sarcoma and stain only the most differentiated PNETs.[16, 50, 51]

Other commonly used neural markers are the S-100 protein (a marker of glial and Schwann cells) and *HNK*-1 (*Leu* 7). Antibodies to S-100 react in a patchy pattern with over 60% of PNETs.[19] Unfortunately, a similar pattern of S-100 staining may be seen in primitive round cell sarcomas of bone as well as in mesenchymal chondrosarcoma.[16, 33] Although the presence of S-100 positivity in PNET suggests differentiation to precursor Schwann cells, overt schwannian differentiation is absent. *HNK*-1, which recognizes glycoproteins belonging to the family of neural cell adhesion molecules, has been shown to react with 37 to 51% of both Ewing's sarcoma and PNETs.[16, 50] It also reacts with most mesenchymal chondrosarcomas and neuroblastomas.[33]

Intermediate Filaments. Vimentin positivity is widely reported in the vast majority of Ewing's sarcomas and PNETs, as well as in all tumors within the differential diagnosis. Therefore, the primary utility of vimentin staining in Ewing's sarcoma/PNET is as a positive control for general immunoreactivity of the individual specimen. Although vimentin positivity in a majority of Ewing's sarcomas and PNETs is well recognized, the expression of keratins is not widely appreciated. Studies of Ewing's sarcoma and PNET have shown a wide variability in keratin expression, with 9 of 11 tumors immunoreactive for broad-spectrum keratin antibodies,[51] 0 of 45 immunoreactive with CAM 5.2,[50] and 2 of 40 PNETs immunoreactive with AE1/AE3 cocktail.[16] Studies of Ewing's sarcoma cell lines treated with phorbol ester suggest that keratin expression may be gained with differentiation.[54] Those tumors with cytokeratin expression may show poorly formed cell junctions by electron microscopy. The significance of the ability of Ewing's sarcoma/PNET to express cytokeratin, as well as NSE, lies in the danger of automatically considering all keratin-positive primitive small cell tumors in the adult (soft tissue and osseous lesions) to be small cell carcinoma, either metastatic or of extrapulmonary origin. The therapy and prognosis of small cell carcinoma are quite different from those of Ewing's sarcoma/PNET.

***MIC2* Expression.** Monoclonal antibodies recognizing the product of the *MIC2* gene (now designated *CD99*) have transformed the diagnosis of Ewing's sarcoma/PNET. The *MIC2* gene, located on the pseudoautosomal region of the sex chromosomes, is not directly genetically related to the t(11;22) seen in most Ewing's sarcoma/PNET.[55, 56] The function of this cell membrane-bound glycoprotein is unknown, but it appears to be involved in cell adhesion processes.[57] The most commonly utilized antibodies that react with this protein are HBA71, 12E7, and the commercially available O13 (Signet).[58, 59] All these antibodies appear to bind to the same four peptide epitopes, and no differences in their staining pattern or quality have been reported.[60] Nearly all normal cells express the *MIC2* gene at very low levels; however, only a very few normal cell types show high enough levels to be detectable immunohistochemically. These include cortical thymocytes, pancreatic islet cells, Sertoli cells, and to a lesser extent granulosa cells. In addition, endothelial cells in some individuals stain positively. The utility of *MIC2* antibodies is their ability to strongly and reliably stain tumors in the Ewing's sarcoma/PNET family, regardless of fixation and decalcification variables.[61] Two large studies have reported the *MIC2* expression in Ewing's sarcoma and PNET as well as a wide variety of other tumors, only a few of which appear in Table 14–2.[62, 63] These studies and others show *MIC2* expression to be a very reliable marker for Ewing's sarcoma/PNET.[58, 61, 64] The *MIC2* staining pattern in Ewing's sarcoma/PNET is strong, homogeneous, and membranous (Fig. 14–7). All neuroblastomas, osteosarcomas, and mesenchymal chondrosarcomas analyzed have been negative. Of some concern is positive staining in a small subset of rhabdomyosarcomas and desmoplastic small round cell tumors; however, these show a staining pattern that is heterogeneous, quite different from the strong, homogeneous pattern seen in Ewing's sarcoma/PNET. Furthermore, in these cases, staining is characteristically confined to the most differentiated rhabdomyoblasts, and the primitive undifferentiated cells within a rhabdomyosarcoma are negative.[33] Of greater concern is the strong, homogeneous staining pattern seen exclusively in one type of lymphoma, lymphoblastic lymphoma.[65] This is of particular concern as lymphoblastic lymphomas show a histology that may overlap that of Ewing's sarcoma, may present in the bone, and may not show positivity for common leukocyte antigen. Importantly, small cell carcinomas,[66] esthesioneuroblastomas,[67] and Merkel cell carcinomas[68] do not react with these antibodies in the vast majority of cases.

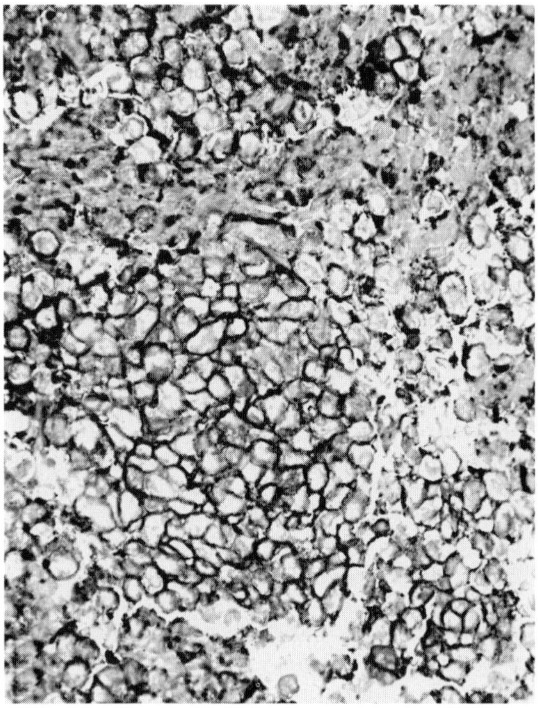

Figure 14–7. *MIC2* immunostaining of a Ewing's sarcoma showing the strong, membranous pattern required for the positive interpretation of this stain.

Table 14–2. *MIC2* Expression in Selected Human Tumors

	Fellinger et al., 1991[63]	Ambros et al., 1991[62]
Ewing's sarcoma	61/63	16/17
PNET	9/11	33/34
Neuroblastoma	0/24	0/12
Osteogenic sarcoma	0/2	0/8
Desmoplastic small round cell tumor	0/5	—
Rhabdomyosarcoma	3/15	1/9
Medulloblastoma	0/5	0/3
Mesenchymal chondrosarcoma	—	0/2
Synovial sarcoma	0/3	0/2

Despite the utility of *MIC*2 antibodies, care needs to be taken in the interpretation. Most reports in the literature predated the use of antigen retrieval systems, which are now used in many laboratories. *MIC*2 expression is present at low levels in all cells. Therefore, as the sensitivity of these procedures increases, the specificity will fall. However, only Ewing's sarcoma/PNET and lymphoblastic lymphoma show strong, homogeneous, membranous staining. Staining that is present in only scattered cells, or diffuse, low-level cytoplasmic staining, should not be relied on.

Cytogenetics and Molecular Genetics

Classic Cytogenetic Analysis. Ewing's sarcoma and PNET share a unique and specific chromosomal translocation involving chromosomes 11 and 22, t(11;22)(q24;q12) (Fig. 14–8), which is present in over 85% of all Ewing's sarcoma/PNET by classic cytogenetic analysis.[11, 12] An additional 5% of tumors show variant translocations involving 22q12 but with a chromosome other than chromosome 11.[11, 23, 69] Most tumors show other cytogenetic changes, the significance of which is unknown; over 50% of Ewing's sarcoma show trisomy for chromosome 8, and up to 20% show a translocation involving chromosomes 1 and 16, t(1;16)(q11;q11).[11, 70] The significance of these latter aberrations is unknown.

Shortly after the t(11;22) was first described, and before the characterization of the *MIC*2 immunoreactivity of Ewing's sarcoma/ PNET, cytogenetics represented the only positive diagnostic feature of these tumors. The diagnostic utility of cytogenetics in Ewing's sarcoma/ PNET, coupled with the description of the typical translocations for alveolar rhabdomyosarcomas and desmoplastic small round cell tumors (see Chapter 4), led many institutions to routinely submit all small blue cell tumors of childhood for cytogenetic analysis. However, the tissue, time, expense, and forethought necessary to perform cytogenetic analysis on all pertinent tumors is not available in many situations. In addition, the experience with *MIC*2 expression in rare entities is currently insufficient. Therefore, molecular techniques for the detection of the t(11;22) have been sought.

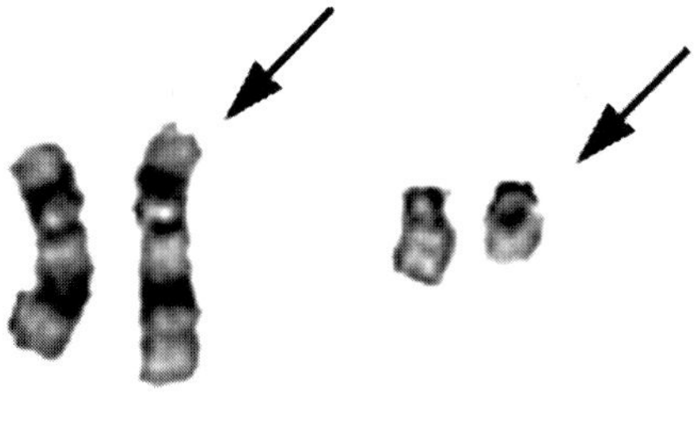

Figure 14–8. Partial karyotype of a Ewing's sarcoma showing the translocation involving chromosomes 11 and 22, t(11;22)(q24;12). The left chromosome of each pair represents the normal copy, and the right *(arrows)* the translocated chromosome.

Fluorescence In Situ Hybridization. Chromosomes and chromosomal abnormalities can be visualized in metaphase and interphase cells by utilizing DNA probes labeled with fluorescent dyes, a technique known as fluorescence in situ hybridization (FISH) (see Chapters 4 and 5). The t(11;22)(q24;q12) of Ewing's sarcoma/PNET can be detected using DNA probes recognizing sites on chromosomes 11 or 22, which can be applied to interphase cells of suspensions or touch preparations of Ewing's sarcoma/PNET.[71, 72] The specific probes include those that are closely linked to the translocation breakpoints and, more recently, probes that span the breakpoint site,[73] as illustrated in Figure 14–9. This technique is particularly useful when chromosome 22 breakpoint probes are utilized, as all the variant translocations are detected. However, the breakpoint at 22q12 is also found in the desmoplastic small round cell tumor (see discussion following) and will be detected by this method.[74] The advantage of FISH is that it requires only a small number of tumor cells and can be rapidly performed in an overnight test. Unlike other molecular techniques, it also enables the detection of a small population of tumor cells within a larger population of nonneoplastic cells.

Reverse Transcriptase Polymerase Chain Reaction (RT-PCR). In 1992, the translocation breakpoints on chromosomes 11 and 22 were cloned and the genes involved were identified.[75] The t(11;22) translocation results in the fusion of the *EWS* gene at 22q12 to the *FLI*-1 gene at 11q24 (see Fig. 14–8). In a small subgroup of tumors, a variant translocation has been detected, the t(21;22)(q22;q12), which fuses *EWS* to a different *ETS* family member, *ERG*, located on chromosome 21. The chimeric protein that results from the fusion of *EWS* to *ERG* is structurally similar to the *EWS/FLI*-1 protein.[77] These hybrid proteins may al-

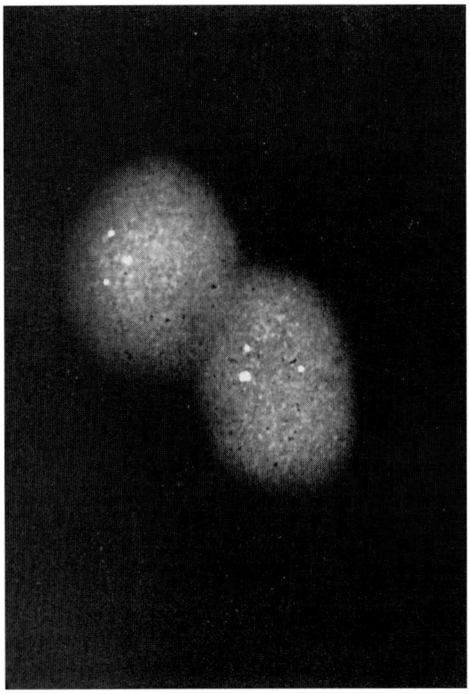

Figure 14–9. Interphase FISH with a cosmid probe spanning the breakpoint site. In cells having the 11;22 translocation, the large signal represents the residual normal chromosome 22, and the two smaller signals represent the separate portions of the translocated chromosome 22.

ter the transcriptional regulation of as yet unidentified target genes (for more details see Chapter 5).[75, 78]

These studies have increased our understanding of the possible pathogenesis of Ewing's sarcoma/PNET and have also defined sensitive and reliable diagnostic modalities for identifying the 11;22 translocation. Using RT-PCR with oligonucleotide primers derived from *EWS* and *FLI*-1, complimentary DNAs can be generated and amplified to detect this specific fusion transcript. These primers promote amplification only if their targeted regions are physically linked by the translocation (Fig. 14–10).[77–79] Thus far, the use of RT-PCR has resulted in a fusion transcript in nearly all Ewing's sarcoma/PNETs.[75, 77, 78] Recently, a malignant ectomesenchymoma has been shown to express *EWS-FLI*-1 fusion transcripts and chimeric proteins identical to those of Ewing's sarcoma/PNET.[80] In addition, two reported esthesioneuroblastoma cell lines and four of six primary esthesioneuroblastomas have shown the *EWS-FLI*-1 fusion transcript.[81]

The correlation between *MIC*2 expression and the presence of the *EWS-FLI*-1 fusion transcript has been assessed; 19 of 20 Ewing's family tumors showed *MIC*2 expression. The *MIC*2 negative tumor showed a variant 11;22 translocation, and three tumors with *MIC*2 expression did not show *EWS* alteration by Southern blot analysis.[82] Rare round cell tumors of bone have been described, but not classified, that are *MIC*2 positive and lack *EWS* fusion transcripts.[77] Whether or not rigorous membranous, homogeneous staining pattern was required for *MIC*2 positivity in these studies is not known. Clearly, more studies are needed that correlate these diagnostic modalities in difficult cases.

Summary

The availability of a wide range of molecular and cytogenetic investigations raises the important issue of the minimal or optimal criteria required to make a diagnosis of Ewing's sarcoma. The issue is difficult to address, because many of the tests are only available in a few institutions and often require a significant quantity of fresh or frozen tissue. Furthermore, the diagnostic criteria are highly dependent on a concordance of the diagnosis with the site and histopathology. The minimal diagnostic criteria for Ewing's sarcoma when analyzing an osseous lesion composed of small round blue cells with areas of geographic necrosis will differ considerably from the criteria required when analyzing a spindled, extra-osseous lesion. For all lesions, a full immunohistochemical panel should be performed including muscle markers (such as desmin and actin), neural markers (such as neurone specific enolase), CD45 (with CD3 and CD20 when necessary) and CD99 (*MIC*2). If the tumor is *MIC*2-positive, and is negative for muscle and hematopoietic markers, *and* if the histological and clinical settings are typical of Ewing's sarcoma/PNET, further tests are not necessary. Molecular tests are most useful when faced with histologically or immunohistochemically (*MIC*2 negative) atypical lesions in unusual clinical settings, particularly in extra-osseous sites.

DIFFERENTIAL DIAGNOSIS OF EWING'S SARCOMA

Lymphoma of Bone

Primary lymphoma of bone, first described as reticulum cell sarcoma, is a relatively rare disorder constituting only 3% of all primary

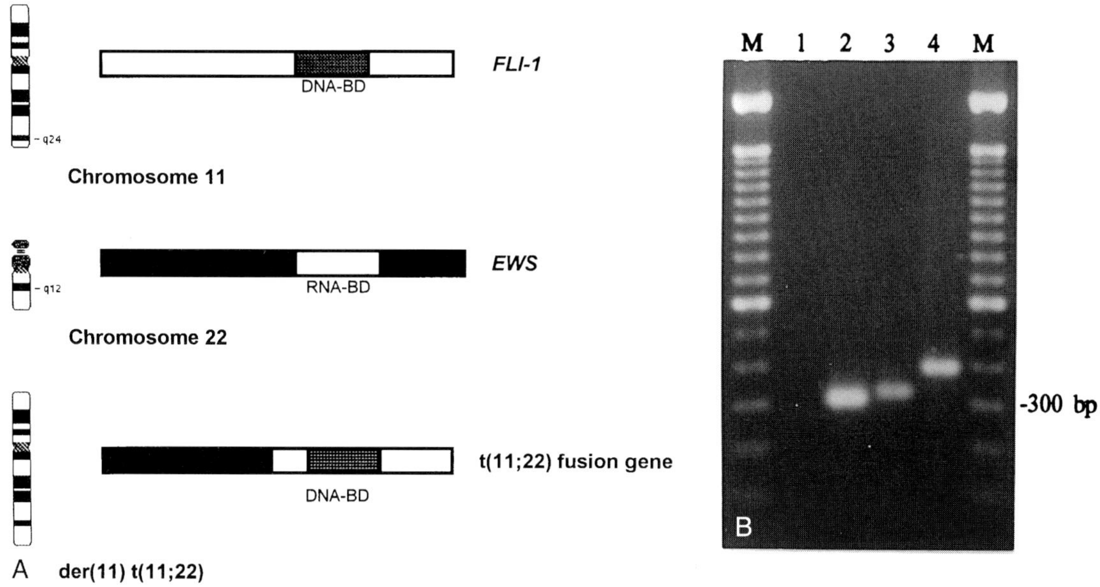

Figure 14–10. Pathogenesis of Ewing's sarcoma. *A*, Schematic diagram of the *EWS* and *FLI*-1 genes and the t(11;22) specific *EWS-FLI*-1 fusion product. The shaded region in *FLI*-1 corresponds to an *ets*-like DNA-binding domain, whereas the unshaded region of *EWS* corresponds to a domain homologous to RNA-binding proteins. *B*, RT-PCR analysis of *EWS/FLI*-1 chimeric transcript expression in a Ewing's sarcoma patient sample. PCR analysis was performed on oligo-dT reverse-transcribed total RNA samples with primers 22.3 and 11.3. Amplified PCR products were separated by electrophoresis on a 2% agarose gel and visualized with ethidium bromide staining. M = 100 bp marker. Lane 1: negative control (Ewing's sarcoma patient sample RNA without primers); Lane 2: Ewing's sarcoma patient sample RNA quality control with β-actin primers (314 bp); Lane 3: Ewing's sarcoma (patient sample) showing a type I fusion (328 bp); and Lane 4: positive control, Ewing's sarcoma cell line (SK-ES-1) with a type II fusion (394 bp). (From Bridge JA: Soft tissue sarcomas. *In* Wolman S, Sell S [eds]: Cytogenetic Markers of Human Disease. Clifton, NJ: Humana Press, Inc. 1997, p 425.)

malignant bone tumors.[83] The radiographic features of intraosseous lymphoma frequently mimic those of bone sarcoma; therefore, the diagnosis of lymphoma is often not considered before the initial biopsy. The pathologic interpretation at the time of initial biopsy is usually problematic due to the often small size of the biopsy, the frequent presence of necrosis, the heterogeneity of the cell composition, and the need to appropriately handle the specimen for lymphoid markers and molecular studies. These factors result in a high rate of re-biopsy. The management and prognosis of patients with osseous lymphoma are quite different from those with sarcomas; a correct diagnosis as well as subclassification is imperative.

Clinical and Radiologic Features

Large cell lymphomas of bone are usually tumors of middle-aged and elderly adults, with a median age of about 40 years.[84, 85] These lesions are more common in the appendicular skeleton. Patients commonly present with localized pain, often of more than a year's duration, and systemic symptoms such as fever, chills, and weight loss are rare. Radiographically, primary lymphoma of bone may be epiphyseal, diaphyseal, or metaphyseal and is most often lytic, but may be sclerotic in a minority of cases. These lesions differ from most osseous sarcomas in that they rarely show a periosteal response or extension into adjacent soft tissues.

Pathology and Prognosis

All studies of osseous lymphomas have shown that the overwhelming majority present in adult life (median age 53 years) are large cell lymphomas. A small group of undifferentiated (lymphoblastic) lymphomas presents in the pediatric population.[84–87] Large cell lymphomas in bone are usually polymorphic with varied proportions of a mixture of small and large lymphoid cells (Fig. 14–11*A*).[84, 86] The nucleus of the large cells characteristically exhibits grooves or foldings and prominent nucleoli, and there is often abundant intercellular reticulin; all features not commonly observed in Ewing's sarcoma cells.[37] Primary lymphomas of bone are of B cell immunophenotype.

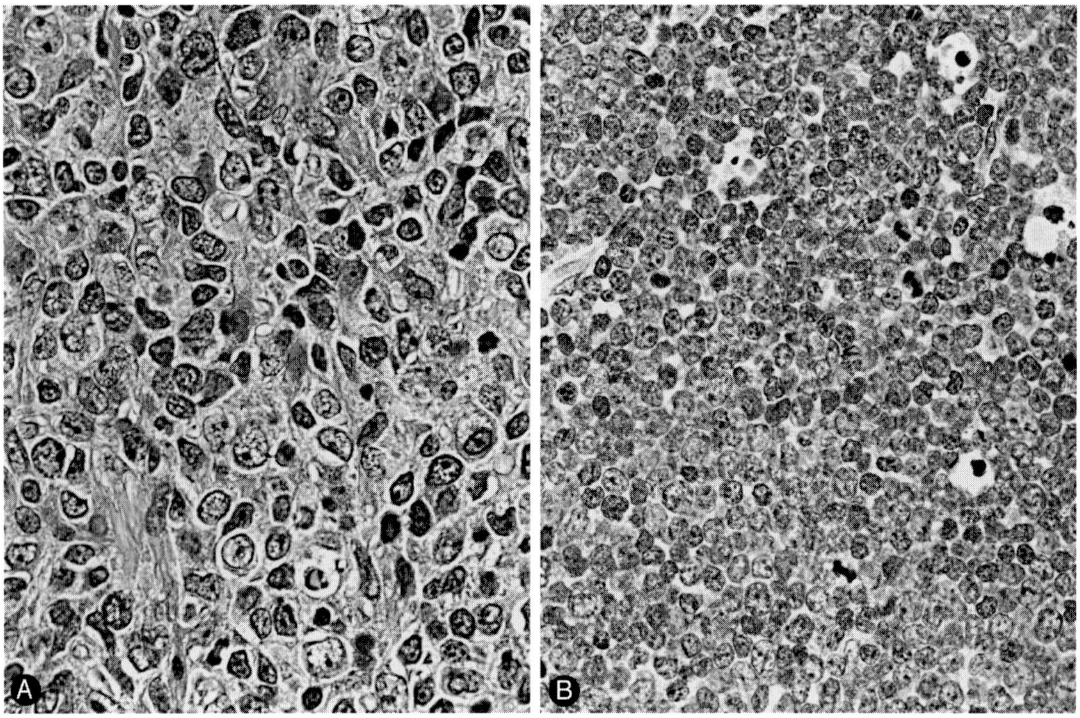

Figure 14–11. Lymphoma of bone. *A*, Large cell lymphomas of bone are commonly polymorphic, with large cells containing prominent nucleoli often apposed to the nuclear membrane. *B*, Lymphoblastic lymphomas may rarely present in the bone. While these share many features with Ewing's sarcoma, the cell borders are distinct, the cells are less cohesive, and more mitotic figures are present.

Studies of the prognosis of adult osseous lymphomas vary depending on whether the analysis includes all patients with lymphomas in bone, or is restricted to patients with lymphomas confined to bone or to patients with lymphomas presenting in bone.[84, 86] In the Mayo Clinic series, only about 40% of osseous lymphomas were confined to bone; the remainder were preceded by or associated with systemic involvement. By convention, a primary lymphoma of bone is defined as a tumor arising within the cavity of a single bone without the development of regional or visceral involvement within a 6-month period.[88] The current treatment regimes for adult lymphomas use radiation either alone or in combination with chemotherapy. The 5-year survival is significantly longer in patients treated with chemotherapy (including cyclophosphamide, vincristine, and prednisolone) and radiotherapy (88%) than for those receiving radiation alone (40%).[84] Risk factors for regional relapse include bulky disease and the use of limited radiation fields.

Pediatric osseous lymphomas usually present with disseminated disease, most commonly of the large cell type. However, many are lymphoblastic lymphomas, and these show a higher incidence of pre-B-cell phenotype than those arising in lymph nodes.[87, 89] This is of interest in that lymphoblastic lymphomas show histologic overlap with some Ewing's sarcomas, and both show strong membranous *MIC2* staining. While the nuclear features of Ewing's sarcomas and lymphoblastic lymphomas are similar, other histologic features differ; lymphoblastic lymphomas are less cohesive, show a distinct cell border, and have a higher mitotic rate (Fig. 14–11*B*). It is often helpful to perform B- and T-cell markers, such as CD20 and CD3, on histologically suspicious lesions, as CD45 staining performed on paraffinized tissue may be absent in some lymphoblastic lymphomas. A recently abstracted study of 33 Ewing's sarcoma/PNETs showed that all were negative for CD3 and CD20.[90]

Small Cell Osteosarcoma

Osteosarcomas can show a wide range of histologic patterns (see Chapter 9), but the small cell osteosarcoma (SCOS) is composed predominately of primitive, undifferentiated cells, similar to Ewing's sarcoma.

Clinical and Radiologic Features

Small cell osteosarcomas are rare tumors presenting in young adults (mean age, 15–19 years), and involving both sexes. The sites of involvement are similar to those of conventional osteosarcoma and include (in order of frequency) ilium, femur, humerus, and tibia.[37, 91] Radiographically, the majority show mixed lytic and sclerotic features.[91]

Pathology and Prognosis

The diagnosis of SCOS is dependent on the identification of osteoid production, which may be difficult in these lesions. SCOS is divided into two morphologic subcategories, Ewing's-like SCOS and lymphoma-like SCOS. Each is characterized by a lack of cohesion of the tumor cells and sharply defined cytoplasmic borders (Fig. 14–12). The Ewing's-like SCOS are generally relatively monomorphous, whereas the lymphoma-like are more pleomorphic. Mitotic rates in both groups vary from low to high, and foci of necrosis appear in all cases reported. Nucleoli range from indistinct to small to large, and the nuclear chromatin pattern is usually vesicular. Cartilaginous zones may be seen, and stainable glycogen has been reported in 3 of 16 cases. The reticulin pattern varies greatly in SCOS: in the majority, reticulin is virtually absent, whereas in others a well-defined reticulin network surrounds groups of two to 30 tumor cells, but does not surround individual cells, similar to the reticulin pattern seen in Ewing's sarcoma. Electron microscopic examination of SCOS may be indistinguishable from that of Ewing's sarcoma.[34, 92] Immunohistochemical studies of SCOS have shown S-100 protein staining in a minority of cases, *Leu*-7 staining in 4 of 16, and cytokeratin reactivity in 1 of 6 cases.[37] *HBA*71 (*MIC*2) has been reported to be negative in three cases of SCOS; however, the 11;22 translocation has been described following classic cytogenetic analysis of one case of putative small cell osteosarcoma.[93] Because the diagnosis of SCOS is based on the identification of osteoid, which may be problematic and varies from observer to observer, care should be taken before concluding that any relationship exists between Ewing's sarcoma and SCOS.

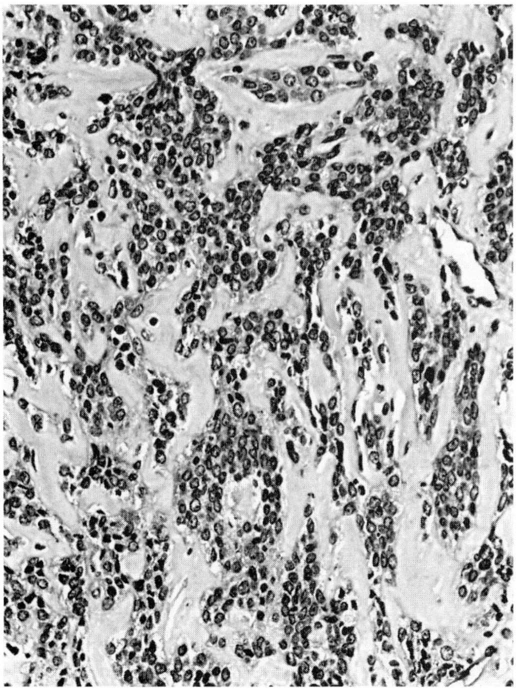

Figure 14–12. Small cell osteogenic sarcoma showing primitive cells adjacent to well-developed osteoid production. When the latter is small or absent, the distinction between this and Ewing's sarcoma may be difficult.

Mesenchymal Chondrosarcoma

Clinical and Radiologic Features

Mesenchymal chondrosarcoma is a rare, highly malignant tumor most frequently seen in the second to third decade of life (mean, 24 years; range, 6–70 years), and most commonly located in the ribs, jaw, or femur, although it can arise at extraskeletal sites.[94–98] Pain and swelling are the most common symptoms. The radiographic appearance varies and is nonspecific, although most mesenchymal chondrosarcomas are predominantly lytic and destructive lesions with irregular borders.[98]

Pathology and Prognosis

These are tumors composed of undifferentiated round to spindled mesenchymal cells with occasional small, discrete islands of well to moderately well differentiated cartilage (Fig. 14–13*A*). The undifferentiated component of mesenchymal chondrosarcoma is often arranged in an alveolar or hemangiopericytomatous pattern (Fig. 14–13*B*). The cartilagi-

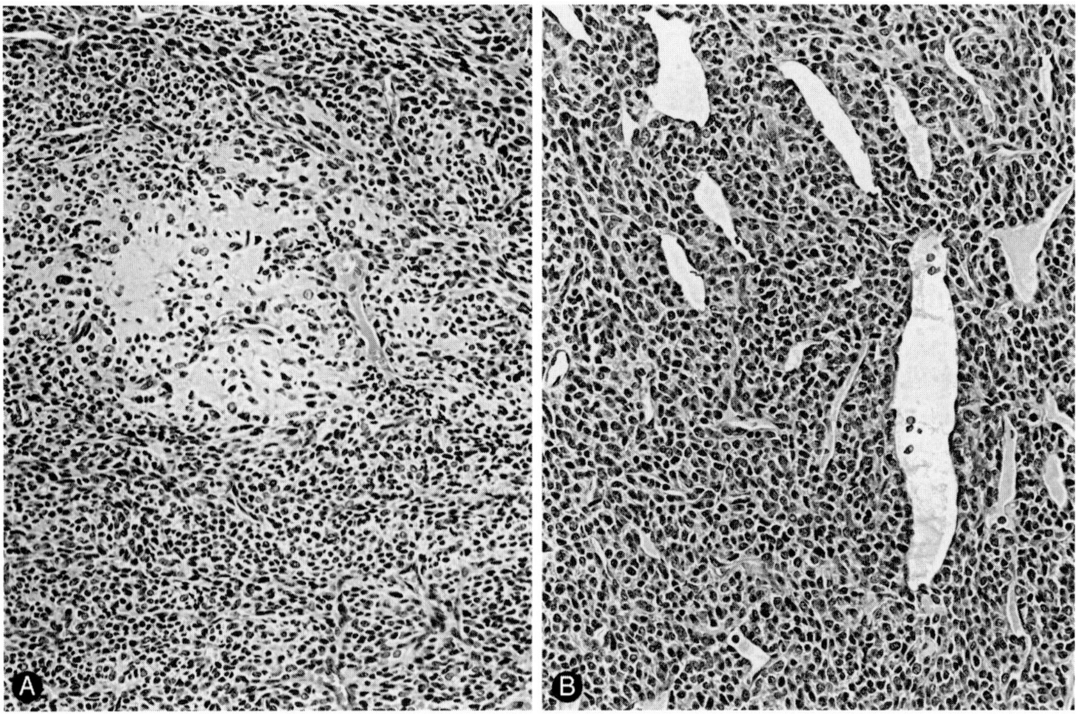

Figure 14–13. Mesenchymal chondrosarcoma. *A*, Composition is of undifferentiated primitive cells adjacent to small, discrete islands of well to moderately well differentiated cartilage. *B*, A prominent alveolar or hemangiopericytomatous pattern is often evident.

nous nodules are usually well defined, but they sometimes appear poorly circumscribed and blend in with the undifferentiated tumor cells. Biopsy specimens containing only the small cell regions of mesenchymal chondrosarcoma may easily be confused with Ewing's sarcoma or synovial sarcoma. However, unlike Ewing's sarcoma, a prominent reticulin network can be identified between the malignant cells of mesenchymal chondrosarcoma, encircling from one to 10 tumor cells.[37] Although S-100 protein staining in overtly differentiated cartilaginous tumors has been documented, the data concerning staining of the primitive round cells in mesenchymal chondrosarcomas are conflicting, varying from staining a few undifferentiated cells to positive staining of the majority of tumor cells.[37, 53, 95] Other immunohistochemical markers reported in mesenchymal chondrosarcoma include NSE positivity in 5 of 11, *Leu*-7 positivity in 8 of 11, and *HBA*71 negativity in both of two cases.[37]

A mesenchymal chondrosarcoma has been reported in the tibia of a 13-year-old boy that histologically showed a monotonous proliferation of small round cells with a hemangiopericytomatous pattern and areas of immature hyaline cartilage. Cytogenetic analysis of this tumor was characterized by t(11;22) (q24;q12).[99] This raises the possibility that at least some mesenchymal chondrosarcomas may be related to Ewing's sarcoma/PNET, and suggests that the cell of origin of Ewing's sarcoma may support differentiation other than neuroectodermal. However, the possibility that the translocation may not involve a fusion between *EWS* and *FLI*-1 needs to be considered.

Primary Malignant Mesenchymoma of Bone

Malignant mesenchymomas are sarcomas composed of two or more unrelated malignant cell types. Fewer than 10 cases of primary malignant mesenchymoma of bone have been described.[100] Histologically, the dominant pattern is that of pleomorphic storiform spindle cells resembling malignant fibrous histiocytoma. Regions showing only primitive round cells may also be present and therefore confused with Ewing's sarcoma when tumors are inadequately sampled. Regions of osteoid production and scattered cells with cross striations may be seen.

Rhabdomyosarcoma

Primary rhabdomyosarcoma of bone is rare. Those rhabdomyosarcomas of soft tissue that present with osseous metastases without a clinically evident primary tumor are also quite rare. Primary rhabdomyosarcomas are located most commonly in the metaphyses of the extremities and in the spine and display a destructive or diffusely permeative radiologic pattern without sclerotic margins. Histologically, metastatic rhabdomyosarcomas may present serious diagnostic difficulties, as the majority show an alveolar histologic pattern that is difficult to distinguish from Ewing's sarcoma.[101, 102] Immunohistochemical staining for muscle markers (such as desmin and actin) is quite sensitive and specific. Laboratories performing RT-PCR for the *EWS-FLI*-1 fusion transcript also commonly test for the fusion transcript resulting from the 2;13 translocation characteristic of alveolar rhabdomyosarcomas (see Chapter 4). Rarely, embryonal rhabdomyosarcomas may present in a leukemic fashion with diffuse marrow involvement.[102] Rhabdomyosarcomatous features may be present in non-rhabdomyosarcomas, including dedifferentiated chondrosarcoma and malignant mesenchymoma; these are more common than true rhabdomyosarcomas of bone.[103]

Primitive Round Cell Sarcoma of Bone

Rare primitive round cell tumors have been described that show areas of extracellular dense collagenous or myxoid matrix but lack the overt cartilaginous or osteoid differentiation necessary to make the diagnosis of mesenchymal chondrosarcoma or small cell osteosarcoma. These tumors have been grouped under the generic term *primitive round cell sarcoma of bone*.[32, 52] Whether these tumors constitute a nosologic entity separate from Ewing's sarcoma, malignant mesenchymoma, or small cell osteosarcoma has not yet been determined. Most primitive round cell sarcomas have a lobular architecture or filigree pattern, while others show a sinusoidal or pseudohemangiopericytomatous pattern. Cytologically, these tumors are reported to be composed of cells that are larger and more pleomorphic than those of Ewing's sarcoma. They also show abundant pink or clear cytoplasm, a coarse nuclear chromatin pattern, and often contain some spindle cells. The mitotic rate is variable, but is higher than that seen in typical Ewing's sarcoma. Electron microscopy demonstrates a spectrum of differentiation, with some showing only sparse organelles, and others showing a fair number of organelles, variable amounts of glycogen, and prominent nuclear pleomorphism. Prominent intracytoplasmic intermediate filaments and conspicuous intercellular attachments have been described, but neurosecretory granules have not been observed.

Desmoplastic Small Round Cell Tumor

Desmoplastic small round cell tumor is a rare soft tissue neoplasm that most commonly presents in the abdomen of adolescent males.[104, 105] The neoplasm is characterized histologically by small blue cells showing polyphenotypic expression of muscle, neural, and epithelial markers on immunohistochemistry. Genetic markers have confirmed this as a distinct entity by demonstrating a consistent (11;22)(p13;q12) translocation resulting in the fusion of *WT*1 and *EWS*, which is detectable by RT-PCR.[74, 106] This disease has been reported to arise in unusual sites, including bone.[107]

LANGERHANS' CELL HISTIOCYTOSIS

Langerhans' cell histiocytosis is a disorder of unknown etiology characterized by a proliferation of cells having the phenotype of normal epidermal Langerhans' cells. This proliferation may range from a spontaneously regressing, solitary lesion of bone to a multisystem, aggressive, and fatal disorder. The pathogenesis, pathology, and clinical features of Langerhans' cell histiocytosis have been extensively reviewed.[108–115] Historically, the inclusion of patients with various clinical syndromes into a single nosologic entity was first made by Lichtenstein in 1953, using the term *Histiocytosis X* to emphasize the unknown nature of the cell of origin and pathogenesis. Lichtenstein recognized the similarities between the entities previously known as Hand-Schüller-Christian disease (a triad of defects of membranous bones, exophthalmos, and polyuria), Letterer-Siwe disease (an acute disseminated disease characterized by hepatosplenomegaly, lymphadenopathy, and localized tumors in bones), and isolated eosinophilic granuloma of bone. Following the identification and description of the Langerhans' cell, Nezelof reported that the proliferating cells of all forms of Histiocytosis X were in fact histiocytic cells of the Langerhans' cell system.[116] As a result, the name of the disease was changed to Langerhans' cell histiocytosis (LCH). Research in the last decade has resulted in the standardization of nomenclature and establishment of clinical and pathologic criteria for diagnosis and treatment, allowing for the initiation of multi-institutional clinical protocols. In addition, hypotheses concerning the neoplastic or reactive nature of LCH have been investigated, including the role of cytokines, viruses, and genetic changes.

Pathogenesis

Langerhans' cells are mononuclear cells involved in immune and nonimmune inflammatory responses. These cells are derived from CD34+ bone marrow stem cells, which undergo maturation in the epidermis and can be distinguished from macrophages by phenotypic markers, the most noteworthy being CD1a.[111, 115] Langerhans' cells are poor phagocytes, but are efficient presenters of new antigens to CD4+ T-lymphocytes. Many features of LCH have led observers to regard the proliferation of Langerhans' cells as a reactive rather than neoplastic process. These include clinical observations (particularly the high rate of spontaneous remission), the histopathologic appearance (which usually lacks cytologic atypia and shows a low mitotic rate[117]), and biologic features (diploid DNA content and no cytogenetic abnormalities in most cases[118]). Such observations have resulted in divergent hypotheses concerning the pathogenesis of LCH, centering on cytokines, viruses, and genetic abnormalities.

Many local and systemic signs and symptoms of LCH may be caused by the elaboration of one or more cytokines. Levels of cytokines are increased in the affected tissues of patients with LCH, and cytokines are able to cause growth and differentiation of Langerhans' cells in vitro.[110, 119, 120] The pattern of cytokines detected in LCH lesions is consistent with the local activation of T-lymphocytes and suggests the possibility of LCH stimulation by super antigen stimulated Vβ-restricted T-lymphocytes.[110] Cytokines may account for the presence of multinucleated giant cells within LCH lesions, and hence the stimulation of bone resorption, producing the characteristic radiologic changes. Therefore, the hypothesis that cytokines may cause cell transformation or proliferation of Langerhans' cells may help to explain the pathogenesis of LCH at one particular point in time. However, there are features of LCH that have not yet been explained by this hypothesis, including the waxing and waning nature of the disease, its frequent chronicity, and the eventual burning out of the disease in many patients. Further in vivo and in situ studies are needed to clarify the role of cytokines and T-cells in the pathogenesis of the various clinical forms of LCH.

Mononuclear cells such as Langerhans' cells perform important roles in immune regulation. However, no consistent defect has been demonstrated in the immune system of patients with LCH. It has been postulated that LCH may be the result of a viral infection that causes the Langerhans' cells to proliferate, with or without cytokine involvement. This hypothetical virus may be capable of activating histiocytes and impairing the immune regulation of the subsequent histiocytic proliferation. Molecular studies have been applied to DNA extracted from LCH lesions in the search for specific viral DNA. No DNA specific to human T-cell viruses types I and II, human immunodeficiency virus, adenovirus, cytomegalovirus, Epstein-Barr virus, parvovirus, or herpes simplex virus have been found. However, DNA from human herpes virus type 6 has been identified in lesional tissue taken from 14 of 30 patients with LCH; 63% of patients with extraosseous disease and 29% of patients with disease limited to bone contained HHV-6 DNA.[121] This has not been confirmed in other studies using in situ hybridization, the polymerase chain reaction, and electron microscopy.[122] Because HHV-6 infection is common in children, further in situ hybridization studies of LCH are needed.

For decades it has been thought that LCH may be a reactive proliferation rather than a neoplastic process, but recent laboratory studies have demonstrated that the cells in some forms of LCH are clonal expansions. Willman et al.[123, 124] utilized X-linked polymorphic probes and detected clonal histiocytes in 9 of 10 females with LCH. Three had isolated eosinophilic granuloma of bone and six showed extensive disease with or without organ dysfunction. Subsequent studies confirmed clonality in LCH by analyzing CD1a+

cells isolated from the lesional tissues of three additional patients with extensive disease.[125] These studies support the hypothesis that LCH is a clonal neoplastic disorder arising from somatic mutations. However, the proliferation of rare progenitor cells may produce a non-neoplastic clonal proliferation of histiocytes. Clonality, therefore, does not necessarily indicate a neoplastic process. An important question remaining is whether clonality has prognostic implications.

Clinical Findings

Diffuse LCH is a rare condition, with an estimated prevalence of 1:50,000 and an annual incidence of 1.08 per 200,000 children under 15 years of age.[126] However, localized LCH of bone is a common disease that goes unreported and possibly undetected. While localized LCH can be present at birth and can occur in persons older than 75 years of age, over 50% of cases are found in children between 1 and 15 years of age, equally in males and females.[127] LCH can involve any bone in the body.[112] In an extensive review of 686 patients with eosinophilic granuloma of bone, 51% experienced pain as the single symptom.[128] Radiographically, osseous lesions have a characteristic punched-out lytic appearance with irregular margination (Fig. 14–14).

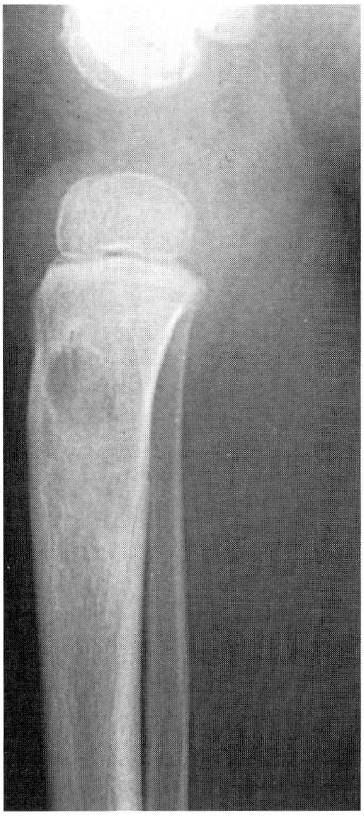

Figure 14–14. Langerhans' cell histiocytosis. Radiograph showing the typical punched-out appearance.

Pathology

The histopathology of LCH has been extensively reviewed.[112–114] Langerhans' cells have a moderate amount of homogeneous pink granular cytoplasm with distinct cell margins. Only rarely are cytoplasmic vacuoles or signs of phagocytic activity evident. The nucleus is often folded or indented, giving a characteristic "coffee-bean" shape (Fig. 14–15*A*). By electron microscopy, the Langerhans' cells show a very irregular border with common pseudopods. A variety of organelles are present in the cytoplasm, including rough endoplasmic reticulum, free polyribosomes, lysosomes, and mitochondria. Cytoplasmic organelles specific to Langerhans' cells were first described by Birbeck.[129] The Birbeck granule consists of lamellar plates of variable length (190–360 nm) and consistent width (33 nm), with a central striated line and an occasional terminal bulbous dilation, giving the so-called tennis racket appearance (Fig. 14–15*B*). Birbeck granules have been seen in continuity with the cytoplasmic membrane and are often clustered near the Golgi apparatus. Recent studies suggest that Birbeck granules arise from invaginations of the cytoplasmic membrane via receptor-mediated endocytosis.[130–132] Birbeck granules are resistant to formalin fixation and paraffin embedding, but cannot always be documented in otherwise typical LCH lesions, even after exhaustive searching. Mierau et al. found granules in 2 to 69% of lesional cells.[133]

Langerhans' cell histiocytosis lesions are very variable in their cellular composition, often causing diagnostic difficulty. The lesions often contain macrophages in addition to Langerhans' cells, and either may be the predominant cell type. The macrophages may show considerable hemophagocytic activity and may be granulomatous in appearance. Osteoclast-like giant cells are common and appear to arise from local macrophages, as they show macrophage enzymes and surface characteristics, lack CD1a and S-100 positivity, and do not contain Birbeck granules.[114] Eosinophils, though conspicuous in some lesions, may be

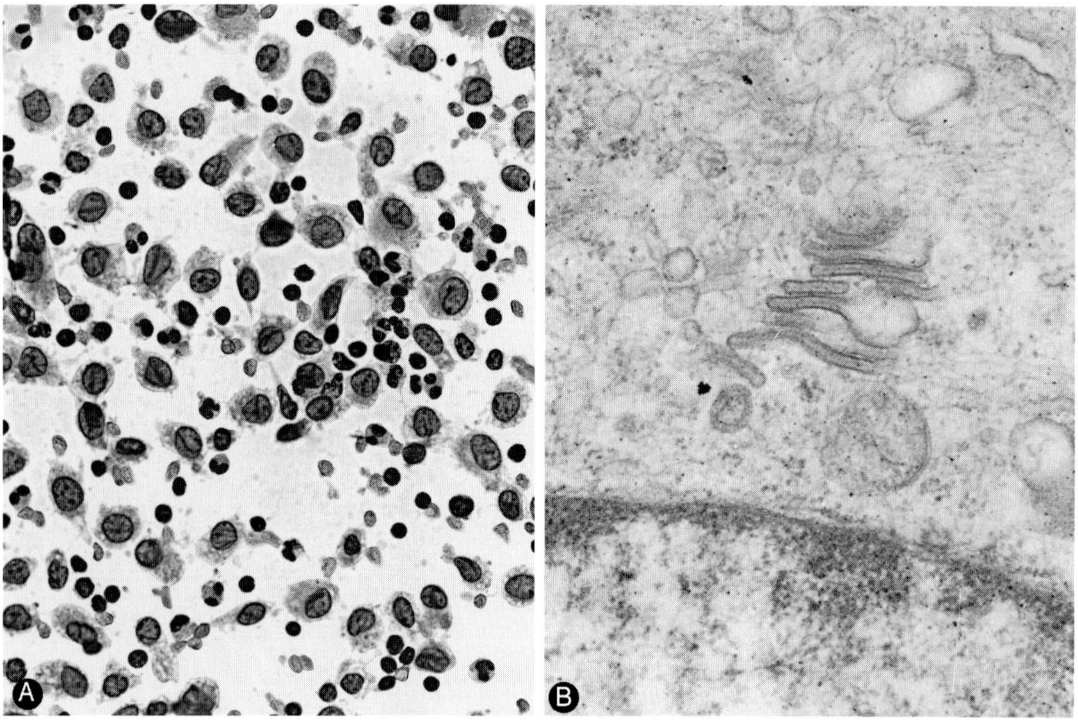

Figure 14–15. Langerhans' cell histiocytosis. *A,* A touch imprint of a fresh specimen shows numerous Langerhans' cells with the typical grooved, "coffee-bean" appearance. *B,* Electron microscopy showing a cluster of Birbeck granules, consisting of lamellar plates and a central striated line with occasional terminal bulbous dilatations.

absent and are not essential for a diagnosis of LCH.[114] Plasma cells are not usually obvious in LCH, and their presence should prompt the consideration of osteomyelitis.

Immunohistochemistry. Immunohistochemical features of LCH are of major importance in establishing the proper diagnosis. Important, albeit non-specific, markers found in Langerhans' cells and cells of LCH include peanut lectin and S-100 protein.[134] Studies have shown S-100 protein analysis to be useful and reliable in the diagnosis of LCH.[133, 135] However, S-100 staining is not positive in all tumors, and its utility is comparable to that of electron microscopy. The use of S-100 protein as a marker for LCH is also limited by its widespread tissue distribution and lack of specificity.[136] Peanut lectin has a characteristic staining pattern in LCH cells of a membranous halo with a paranuclear dot, unlike the diffuse cytoplasmic pattern seen with other histiocytes.[137]

Langerhans' cells and cells of LCH express the CD1a, or T6, antigen, which is a nonpolymorphic MHC class I–related cell surface glycoprotein that may be directly involved in immunologic reactions. CD1a is expressed in cortical thymocytes and Langerhans' cells of the skin, lymph nodes, and lung but in no other cell type tested.[111] Monoclonal antibodies recognizing CD1a are therefore useful in the diagnosis of LCH. While these antibodies have been used predominately on cytospins of fresh cells or cryostat sections,[135] more recently there have been reports of a monoclonal antibody to CD1a, O10, that can be used on paraffin-embedded tissues.[138–140] These studies show that O10 staining of archival tissue parallels that seen in frozen tissue, although there was no difference in the number of cells staining positive by O10 and for S-100 protein, both of which varied from 17 to 81% of cells.[114, 139] CD1a is a valuable marker not only for histologic identification of Langerhans' cells, but also to target radionuclides to LCH cells for imaging of disease.[141] Anti-CD1a antibodies potentially may also be useful for targeting therapy in patients with LCH.

Prognosis

The clinical course of LCH localized to bone is generally benign, and the lesions tend to resolve spontaneously over a period of months to years.[142] Those lesions involving bones that undergo cartilaginous ossification rather than direct ossification show more rapid healing.[143] Biopsy itself may be therapeutic, but curettage after biopsy is usually considered adequate therapy. Chemotherapy and radiation therapy do not appear to speed the healing process.[143] The approaches to the treatment of generalized LCH have been as varied as the clinical presentation of the disease. Although it is generally accepted that spontaneous healing and remission of multisystem LCH has been seen, systemic chemotherapy (steroids plus vinblastine or etoposide) is usually recommended.[112] Initially, the prognosis of generalized LCH was thought to directly correlate with the number of organ systems involved. More recently, it has become evident that dysfunction of certain crucial systems, such as hepatic, pulmonary, and hematopoietic systems, may be more important.[112] In a retrospective analysis of 83 patients, of the 33 patients who had evidence of dysfunction of one or more of the above three systems, only 10 responded to therapy and 22 (66%) died. In contrast, of the 50 patients without dysfunction, 33 (66%) responded to therapy and 2 (4%) died; neither death was directly attributable to the LCH.[144] In patients with disseminated LCH, the age at the time of onset is prognostically important: an age of less than 2 years at diagnosis significantly decreases the chances of prolonged survival. Patients with single system osseous disease have negligible mortality. Patents with bony involvement as part of multisystem disease had a significantly better outcome than those who did not, particularly in the youngest age group.[142] Studies of large numbers of localized and disseminated LCH have failed to identify histologic features that would correlate with outcome.[117]

REFERENCES

1. Ewing J: Diffuse endothelioma of bone. Proc NY Pathol Soc 21:17, 1921.
2. Stout AP: A discussion of the pathology and histogenesis of Ewing's tumor of bone marrow. AJR Am J Roentgenol 50:334, 1943.
3. Stout AP: A tumor of the ulnar nerve. Proc NY Pathol Soc 18:2, 1918.
4. Yunis EJ: Ewing's sarcoma and related small round cell neoplasms in children. Am J Surg Pathol 10:54, 1986.
5. Steiner GC, Graham S: Malignant round cell tumor of bone with neural differentiation (neuroectodermal tumor). Ultrastruct Pathol 12:505, 1988.
6. Marina NM, Etcubanas E, Parham DM, et al: Peripheral primitive neuroectodermal tumor (peripheral neuroepithelioma) in children. Cancer 64:1952, 1989.
7. Schmidt D, Mackay B, Ayala AG: Ewing's sarcoma with neuroblastoma-like features. Ultrastruct Pathol 3:143, 1982.
8. Llombart-Bosch A, Carda C, Peydro-Olaya A, et al: Soft tissue Ewing's sarcoma. Cancer 66:2589, 1990.
9. Noguera R, Navarro S, Peydro-Olaya A, et al: Patterns of differentiation in extraosseous Ewing's sarcoma cells. Cancer 73:616, 1994.
10. Noguera R, Triche TJ, Navarro S, et al: Dynamic model of differentiation in Ewing's sarcoma cells. Comparative analysis of morphologic, immunocytochemical, and oncogene expression parameters. Lab Invest 62:143, 1992.
11. Turc-Carel C, Aurias A, Mugneret F, et al: Chromosomes in Ewing's Sarcoma. I. An evaluation of 85 cases and remarkable consistency of t(11;22)(q24;q12). Cancer Genet Cytogenet 32:229, 1988.
12. Maletz N, McMorrow LE, Greco A, et al: Ewing's sarcoma: Pathology, tissue culture, and cytogenetics. Cancer 58:252, 1986.
13. Kissane JM, Askin FB, Nesbit ME, et al: Sarcomas of bone in childhood: Pathologic aspects. National Cancer Institute Monographs 56:29, 1981.
14. Kissane JM, Askin FB, Foulkes M, et al: Ewing's sarcoma of bone: Clinicopathologic aspects of 303 cases from the Intergroup Ewing's Sarcoma Study. Hum Pathol 14:773, 1983.
15. Kushner BH, Hajdu SI, Gulati SC, et al: Extracranial primitive neuroectodermal tumors. Cancer 67:1825, 1991.
16. Cavazzana AO, Ninto V, Roberts J, et al: Peripheral neuroepithelioma: A light microscopic, immunocytochemical, and ultrastructural study. Mod Pathol 5:71, 1992.
17. Maygarden SJ, Askin FB, Siegal GP, et al: Ewing sarcoma of bone in infants and toddlers. Cancer 71:2109, 1993.
18. Schmidt D, Herrmann C, Jurgens H, et al: Malignant peripheral neuroectodermal tumor and its necessary distinction from Ewing's sarcoma. Cancer 15:2251, 1991.
19. Schmidt D, Harms D, Burdach S: Malignant peripheral neuroectodermal tumours of childhood and adolescence. Virch Arch (A) 406:351, 1985.
20. Askin FB, Rosai J, Sibley RK, et al: Malignant small cell tumor of the thoracopulmonary region in childhood: A distinctive clinicopathologic entity of uncertain histogenesis. Cancer 43:2438, 1979.
21. Rao BN, Hayes FA, Thompson EL, et al: Chest wall resection for Ewing's sarcoma of the rib: An unnecessary procedure. Ann Thorac Surg 46:40, 1988.
22. Thomas PRM, Foulkes MA, Gilula LA, et al: Primary Ewing's sarcoma of the ribs. A report from the Intergroup Ewing's Sarcoma study. Cancer 51:1021, 1983.
23. Christiansen H, Altmannsberger M, Lampert F: Translocation (5;22) in an Askin's tumor. Cancer Genet Cytogenet 62:203, 1992.
24. Contesso G, Llombart-Bosch A, Terrier P, et al: Does malignant small round cell tumor of the thoracopulmonary region (Askin tumor) constitute a clinicopathologic entity? Cancer 69:1012, 1992.

25. Seemayer TA, Vekemans M, de Chadarevian J: Histological and cytogenetic findings in a malignant tumor of the chest wall and lung (Askin tumor). Virch Arch (A) 408:289, 1985.
26. Fuzesi L, Heller R, Schreiber H: Cytogenetics of Askin's tumour. Pathol Res Pract 189:235, 1993.
27. Wilson KS, Nyssen J, Alexander S: Ewing sarcoma: Phalangeal primary with fatal cardiac metastases. Med Ped Oncol 7:361, 1979.
28. Nance CL, Roberts WM, Miller GR: Ewing's sarcoma mimicking osteomyelitis. South Med J 60:1044, 1967.
29. Reinus WR, Gilula LA: Radiology of Ewing's sarcoma: Intergroup Ewing's Sarcoma Study (IESS). Radiographics 4:929, 1984.
30. Shirley SK, Gilula LA, Siegal GP, et al: Roentgenographic-pathologic correlation of diffuse sclerosis in Ewing sarcoma of bone. Skeletal Radiol 12:69, 1984.
31. Dehner LP: Primitive neuroectodermal tumor and Ewing's sarcoma. Am J Surg Pathol 17:1, 1993.
32. Daugaard S, Kamby C, Sunde LM, et al: Ewing's sarcoma. A retrospective study of histological and immunohistochemical factors and their relation to prognosis. Virch Arch (A) 414:243, 1989.
33. Tsokos M: Peripheral primitive neuroectodermal tumors: Diagnosis, classification and prognosis. Persp Pediat Pathol 16:27, 1992.
34. Navas-Palacios JJ, Aparicio-Duque R, Valdes MD: On the histogenesis of Ewing's sarcoma: An ultrastructural, immunohistochemical, and cytochemical study. Cancer 53:1882, 1984.
35. Siegal GP, Oliver WR, Reinus WR, et al: Primary Ewing's sarcoma involving the bones of the head and neck. Cancer 60:2829, 1987.
36. Hartman KR, Triche TJ, Kinsella TJ, et al: Prognostic value of histopathology in Ewing's sarcoma: Long-term follow-up of distal extremity primary tumors. Cancer 67:163, 1991.
37. Devaney K, Vinh TN, Sweet DE: Small cell osteosarcoma of bone: An immunohistochemical study with differential diagnostic considerations. Hum Pathol 24:1211, 1993.
38. Stratton B, Askin FB, Kissane JM: Intramyofiber skeletal muscle invasion in Ewing's sarcoma of bone: Clinicopathologic observations from the Intergroup Ewing's Sarcoma Study. Am J Pediatr Hematol 4:231, 1982.
39. Povysil C, Matejovsky Z: Ultrastructure of Ewing's tumour. Virch Arch (A) 374:303, 1977.
40. Hou-Jensen K, Priori E, Dmochowski L: Studies on ultrastructure of Ewing's sarcoma of bone. Cancer 29:280, 1972.
41. Nascimento AG, Unni KK, Pritchard DJ, et al: A clinicopathologic study of 20 cases of large-cell (atypical) Ewing's sarcoma of bone. Am J Surg Pathol 4:29, 1980.
42. Schoedel K, Dickman PS, Krailo M, et al: Histologic response to chemotherapy and prognosis in osseous Ewing's sarcoma/Primitive neuroectodermal tumor. XX International Congress of the International Academy of Pathology. Hong Kong, 1994.
43. Rosenberg AE, Amstalden EMI, Nielsen GP, et al: Ewing's sarcoma/PNET: Preoperative chemotherapy induced necrosis and outcome. Lab Invest 74:13A, 1996.
44. Llombart-Bosch A, Terrier-Lacombe MJ, Peydro-Olaya A, et al: Peripheral neuroectodermal sarcoma of soft tissue (peripheral neuroepithelioma): A pathologic study of ten cases with differential diagnosis regarding other small round-cell sarcomas. Hum Pathol 20:273, 1989.
45. Miser JS, Kinsella TJ, Triche TJ, et al: Treatment of peripheral neuroepithelioma in children and young adults. J Clin Oncol 5:1752, 1987.
46. Horowitz M, Meyer W, Wexler L, et al: Neuroectodermal differentiation does not play a role in the prognosis of Ewing's sarcoma versus primitive neuroectodermal tumor. Lab Invest 74:7A, 1996.
47. Llombart-Bosch A, Contesso G, Henry-Amar M, et al: Histopathological predictive factors in Ewing's sarcoma of bone and clinicopathological correlations. Virch Arch (A) 409:627, 1986.
48. Shirley SK, Askin FB, Gilula LA, et al: Ewing's sarcoma in bones of the hands and feet: A clinicopathologic study and review of the literature. J Clin Oncol 3:686, 1985.
49. Evans R, Nesbit M, Askin F, et al: Local recurrence, rate and sites of metastases, and time to relapse as a function of treatment regimen, size of primary and surgical history in 62 patients presenting with non-metastatic Ewing's sarcoma of the pelvic bones. Int J Radiat Oncol Biol Phys 11:129, 1985.
50. Dierick AM, Roels H, Langlois M: The immunophenotype of Ewing's sarcoma: An immunohistochemical analysis. Pathol Res Pract 189:26, 1993.
51. Moll R, Lee I, Gould VE, et al: Immunocytochemical analysis of Ewing's tumors. Patterns of expression of intermediate filaments and desmosomal proteins indicate cell type heterogeneity and pluripotential differentiation. Am J Pathol 127:288, 1987.
52. Tsokos M, Miser J, Horowitz M, et al: Primitive round cell sarcoma of bone: A group of tumors resembling Ewing's sarcoma by light microscopy, but with distinctive ultrastructural appearance. Lab Invest 58:96A, 1988.
53. Swanson PE, Lillemoe TJ, Manivel JC, et al: Mesenchymal chondrosarcoma. Arch Path Lab Med 114:943, 1990.
54. Dellagi K, Lipinski M, Paulin D, et al: Characterization of intermediate filaments expressed by Ewing tumor cell lines. Cancer Res 47:1170, 1987.
55. Goodfellow PJ, Darling SM, Thomas NS, et al: A pseudoautosomal gene in man. Science 234:740, 1986.
56. Darling SM, Banting GS, Pym B, et al: Cloning an expressed gene shared by the human sex chromosomes. Genetics 83:135, 1986.
57. Gelin C, Aubrit F, Phalipon A, et al: The E2 antigen, a 32kd glycoprotein involved in T-cell adhesion processes, is the MIC2 gene product. EMBO J 8:3253, 1989.
58. Fellinger EJ, Garlin-Chesa P, Su SL, et al: Biochemical and genetic characterization of the HBA71 Ewing's sarcoma cell surface antigen. Cancer Res 51:336, 1991.
59. Levy R, Dilley J, Fox RI, et al: A human thymus-leukemia antigen defined by hybridoma monoclonal antibodies. Immunology 76:6552, 1979.
60. Banting GS, Pym B, Darling SM, et al: The MIC2 gene product: Epitope mapping and structural prediction analysis define an integral membrane protein. Molec Immunol 26:181, 1989.
61. Perlman EJ, Dickman PS, Askin FB, et al: Ewing's sarcoma-routine diagnostic utilization of MIC2 analysis: A Pediatric Oncology Group/Children's Cancer Group Intergroup Study. Hum Pathol 25:304, 1994.
62. Ambros IM, Ambros PF, Strehl S, et al: MIC2 is a

specific marker for Ewing's sarcoma and peripheral primitive neuroectodermal tumors. Cancer 67:1886, 1991.
63. Fellinger EJ, Garin-Chesa P, Triche TJ, et al: Immunohistochemical analysis of Ewing's sarcoma cell surface antigen p30/32 mic2. Am J Pathol 139:317, 1991.
64. Kovar H, Dworzak M, Strehl S, et al: Overexpression of the pseudoautosomal gene MIC2 in Ewing's sarcoma and peripheral primitive neuroectodermal tumor. Oncogene 5:1067, 1990.
65. Riopel M, Dickman PS, Link MP, et al: MIC2 analysis in pediatric lymphomas and leukemias. Hum Pathol 25:396, 1994.
66. Lumadue JA, Askin FB, Perlman EJ: MIC2 analysis of small cell carcinoma. Am J Clin Pathol 102:692, 1994.
67. Nelson RS, Perlman EJ, Askin FB: Is esthesioneuroblastoma a peripheral neuroectodermal tumor? Hum Pathol 26:639, 1995.
68. Perlman EJ, Lumadue JA, Hawkins AL, et al: Primary cutaneous neuroendocrine tumors. Cancer Genet Cytogenet 82:30, 1995.
69. Davison EV, Pearson ADJ, Emslie J, et al: Chromosome 22 abnormalities in Ewing's sarcoma. J Clin Pathol 42:797, 1989.
70. Mugneret F, Lizard S, Aurias A, et al: Chromosomes in Ewing's sarcoma. II. Nonrandom additional changes, trisomy 8 and der(16)t(1;16). Cancer Genet Cytogenet 32:239, 1988.
71. Taylor C, Patel K, Kiely F, et al: Diagnosis of Ewing's sarcoma and peripheral neuroectodermal tumour based on the detection of t(11;22) using fluorescence in situ hybridisation. Br J Cancer 67:128, 1993.
72. Giovannini M, Selleri L, Biegel JA, et al: Interphase cytogenetics for the detection of the t(11;22) (q24;q12) in small round cell tumors. J Clin Invest 90:1911, 1992.
73. Monforte-Munoz H, Lopez-Terrada D, Rowland JM, et al: Documentation of EWS gene rearrangement by fluorescence in situ hybridization (FISH) in frozen sections of Ewing's sarcoma/pPNET biopsy material using a single EWS probe. Lab Invest 74:4P, 1996.
74. Biegel JA, Conard K, Brooks JJ: Translocation (11;22)(p13;q12): Primary change in intra-abdominal desmoplastic small round cell tumor. Genes Chrom Cancer 7:119, 1993.
75. Delattre O, Zucman J, Plougastel B, et al: Gene fusion with an ETS DNA-binding domain caused by chromosome translocation in human tumours. Nature 359:162, 1992.
76. Bridge JA: Soft tissue sarcomas. *In* Wolman S, Sell S (eds): Cytogenetic Markers of Human Disease. Clifton, N.J., Humana Press, Inc., 1997, p 425.
77. Delattre O, Zucman J, Melot T, et al: The Ewing family of tumors—a subgroup of small-round-cell tumors defined by specific chimeric transcripts. N Engl J Med 331:294, 1994.
78. Downing JR, Head DR, Parham DM, et al: Short communication. Detection of the (11;22)(q24;q12) translocation of Ewing's sarcoma and peripheral neuroectodermal tumor by reverse transcription polymerase chain reaction. Am J Pathol 143:1294, 1993.
79. Sorenson PHB, Liu XF, Biggs CH, et al: Reverse transcriptase PCR amplification of EWS/FLI1 fusion transcripts as a diagnostic test for peripheral primitive neuroectodermal tumors of childhood. Diagn Mol Pathol 2:147, 1993.
80. Sorenson PHB, Shimada H, Liu XF, et al: A subset of sarcomas with myogenic and neural differentiation express the Ewing's sarcoma EWS/FLI1 fusion gene. Cancer Res 55:1385, 1995.
81. Sorenson PHB, We JK, Berean KW, et al: Olfactory neuroblastoma is a peripheral primitive neuroectodermal tumor related to Ewing's sarcoma. Proc Natl Acad Sci 93:1038, 1996.
82. Ladanyi M, Lewis R, Garin-Chesa P, et al: EWS rearrangement in Ewing's sarcoma and peripheral neuroectodermal tumor. Molecular detection and correlation with cytogenetic analysis and MIC2 expression. Diagn Mol Pathol 2:141, 1993.
83. Reimer RR, Chabner BA, Young RC, et al: Lymphoma presenting in bone. Ann Int Med 87:50, 1977.
84. Rathmell AJ, Gospodarowicz MK, Sutcliffe SB, et al: The Princess Margaret Hospital Lymphoma Group: Localised lymphoma of bone: Prognostic factors and treatment recommendations. Br J Cancer 66:603, 1992.
85. Lewis SJ, Bell RS, Fernandes BJJ, et al: Malignant lymphoma of bone. Can J Surg 37:43, 1994.
86. Shannon JA, Bell DR, Levi JA, et al: Bone presentation of non-Hodgkin's lymphoma: Experience at the Royal North Shore Hospital, Sydney: highlighting primary bone lymphoma. Aust NZ J Med 24:701, 1994.
87. Wollner N, Lane JM, Marcove RC, et al: Primary skeletal non-Hodgkin's lymphoma in the pediatric age group. Med Ped Oncol 20:506, 1992.
88. Ostrowski M, Kuni K, Banks P, et al: Malignant lymphoma of bone. Cancer 58:2646, 1986.
89. Niemann TH, Thomas PA: Primary lymphoma of bone: Diagnosis by fine-needle aspiration biopsy in a pediatric patient. Diagn Cytopathol 12:165, 1995.
90. Ozdemirli M, Fanburg JC, Hartman D, et al: Differentiating lymphoblastic lymphoma and Ewing's sarcoma: lymphocyte markers and gene rearrangement. Mod Pathol 10:13A, 1997.
91. Edeiken J, Raymond AK, Ayala AG, et al: Small cell osteosarcoma. Skeletal Radiol 16:221, 1987.
92. Dickersin GR, Rosenberg AE: The ultrastructure of small-cell osteosarcoma, with a review of the light microscopy and differential diagnosis. Hum Pathol 22:267, 1991.
93. Noguera R, Navarro S, Triche TJ: Translocation (11;22) in small cell osteosarcoma. Cancer Genet Cytogenet 45:121, 1990.
94. Adler C: Case report 788. Skeletal Radiol 22:300, 1993.
95. Jacobs JL, Merriam JC, Chadburn A, et al: Mesenchymal chondrosarcoma of the orbit. Cancer 73:399, 1994.
96. Bottrill ID, Wood S, Barrett-Lee P, et al: Mesenchymal chondrosarcoma of the maxilla. J Laryngol Otol 108:785, 1994.
97. Crawford JG, Oda D, Egbert M, et al: Mesenchymal chondrosarcoma of the maxilla in a child. J Oral Maxil Surg 53:938, 1995.
98. Huvos AG, Rosen G, Pabska M, et al: Mesenchymal chondrosarcoma. A clinicopathologic analysis of 35 patients with emphasis on treatment. Cancer 51:1230, 1983.
99. Sainati L, Scapinello A, Montaldi A, et al: A mesenchymal chondrosarcoma of a child with the reciprocal translocation (11;22)(q24;q12). Cancer Genet Cytogenet 71:144, 1993.
100. Kessler S, Mirra JM, Ishii T, et al: Primary malignant

mesenchymoma of bone: Case report, literature review, and distinction of this entity from mesenchymal and dedifferentiated chondrosarcoma. Skeletal Radiol 24:291, 1995.
101. Beatty PT, Bjorkengern AG, Moore SG, et al: Case report 764. Skeletal Radiol 21:559, 1992.
102. Almanaseer IY, Trujillo YP, Taxy JB, et al: Systemic rhabdomyosarcoma with diffuse bone marrow involvement. Am J Clin Pathol 82:349, 1984.
103. Lamovec J, Zidar A, Bracko M, et al: Primary bone sarcoma with rhabdomyosarcomatous component. Pathol Res Pract 190:51, 1994.
104. Gerald WL, Miller HK, Battifora H, et al: Intra-abdominal desmoplastic small round cell tumor. Am J Surg Pathol 15:499, 1991.
105. Basade MM, Vege DS, Nair CN, et al: Intra-abdominal desmoplastic small round cell tumor in children: a clinicopathologic study. Pediat Hematol Oncol 13:95, 1996.
106. Argatoff LH, O'Connell JX, Mathers JA, et al: Detection of EWS/WT1 gene fusion by reverse transcriptase-polymerase chain reaction in the diagnosis of desmoplastic small round cell tumour. Am J Surg Pathol 20:406, 1996.
107. Mangham DC, Knight JC, Grimer RJ, et al: Desmoplastic small cell tumour of the tibia: the first report of this rare tumour in an intra-osseous location. J Pathol 181(Supplement):42A, 1997.
108. Egeler RM, D'Anglo GJ: Langerhans cell histiocytosis. J Pediatr 127:1, 1995.
109. Beverley PCL, Abbas AK: The scientific challenge of Langerhans cell histiocytosis. Br J Cancer 23(Suppl.):S61, 1994.
110. Kannourakis G, Abbas A: The role of cytokines in the pathogenesis of Langerhans cell histiocytosis. Br J Cancer 23(Suppl.):S37, 1994.
111. Chu T, Jaffe R: The normal Langerhans cell and the LCH cell. Br J Cancer 23(Suppl.):S4, 1994.
112. Egeler RM, Nesbit ME: Langerhans cell histiocytosis and other disorders of monocyte-histiocyte lineage. Crit Rev Oncol Hematol 18:9, 1995.
113. Favara BE, Jaffe R: Pathology of Langerhans cell histiocytosis. Hematol Oncol Clin N Am 1:75, 1987.
114. Favara BE, Jaffe R: The histopathology of Langerhans cell histiocytosis. Br J Cancer 23(Suppl.):S17, 1994.
115. Cline MJ: Histiocytes and Histiocytosis. Blood 84:2840, 1994.
116. Nezelof C, Basset F, Rousseau MF: Histiocytosis X. Histogenetic arguments for a Langerhans cell origin. Biomedicine 18:365, 1973.
117. Risdall RJ, Dehner LP, Duray P, et al: Histiocytosis X (Langerhans' cell histiocytosis). Arch Path Lab Med 107:59, 1983.
118. Ornvold K, Carstensen H, Larsen JK, et al: Flow cytometric DNA analysis of lesions from 18 children with Langerhans cell histiocytosis (Histiocytosis X). Am J Pathol 136:1301, 1990.
119. Reid CD, Stackpoole A, Meager A, et al: Interactions of tumor necrosis factor with granulocyte-macrophage colony-stimulating factor and other cytokines in the regulation of dendritic cell growth in vitro from early bipotent CD34 progenitors in human bone marrow. J Immunol 149:2681, 1992.
120. de Graaf JH, Tamminga RYJ, Dam-Meiring A, et al: The presence of cytokines in Langerhans' cell histiocytosis. J Pathol 180:400, 1996.
121. Leahy MA, Krejci SM, Friednash M, et al: Human herpesvirus 6 is present in lesions of Langerhans cell histiocytosis. J Invest Dermatol 101:642, 1993.
122. McClain K, Weiss RA: Viruses and Langerhans cell histiocytosis: Is there a link? Br J Cancer 23(Suppl.):S34, 1994.
123. Willman CL: Detection of clonal histiocytes in Langerhans cell histiocytosis: Biology and clinical significance. Br J Cancer 23(Suppl.):S29, 1994.
124. Willman CL, Busque L, Griffith BB, et al: Langerhans cell histiocytosis (Histiocytosis X)—A clonal proliferative disease. N Engl J Med 331:154, 1994.
125. Yu RC, Chu C, Buluwela L, et al: Clonal proliferation of Langerhans cells in Langerhans cell histiocytosis. Lancet 343:767, 1994.
126. Carstensen H, Ornvold K: The epidemiology of Langerhans cell histiocytosis in children in Denmark, 1975–1989. Med Ped Oncol 21:387, 1993.
127. Berry DH, Becton DL: Natural history of histiocytosis-X. Hematol Oncol Clin N Am 1:23, 1987.
128. Slater JM, Swarm OJ: Eosinophilic granuloma of bone. Med Ped Oncol 8:151, 1980.
129. Birbeck MS, Breathnach AS, Everall JD: An electron microscope study of basal melanocytes and high-level clear cells (Langerhans cells) in vitiligo. J Invest Dermatol 37:51, 1961.
130. Hanau D, Fabre M, Schmitt DA, et al: Appearance of Birbeck granule-like structures in anti-T6 antibody-treated human epidermal Langerhans cells. J Invest Dermatol 90:298, 1988.
131. Chu A, Eisinger M, Soo DVMJ, et al: Immunoelectron microscopic identification of Langerhans cells using a new antigenic marker. J Invest Dermatol 78:177, 1982.
132. Hanau D, Fabre M, Schmitt DA, et al: Human epidermal Langerhans cells internalize by receptor-mediated endocytosis T6 (CD1 "NA1/34") surface antigen, Birbeck granules are involved in the intracellular traffic of the T6 antigen. J Invest Dermatol 89:172, 1987.
133. Mierau GW, Favara BE: S-100 protein immunohistochemistry and electron microscopy in the diagnosis of Langerhans cell proliferative disorders: A comparative assessment. Ultrastruct Pathol 10:303, 1986.
134. Kahn HJ, Marks A, Thom H, et al: Role of antibody to S100 protein in diagnostic pathology. Am J Clin Pathol 79:341, 1983.
135. Beckstead JH, Wood GS, Turner RR: Histiocytosis X cells and Langerhans cells: Enzyme histochemical and immunologic similarities. Hum Pathol 15:826, 1984.
136. Cocchia D, Michetti F, Donato R: Immunochemical and immunocytochemical localization of S-100 antigen in normal human skin. Nature 294:85, 1981.
137. Ree HJ, Kadin ME: Peanut agglutinin. Cancer 57:282, 1986.
138. Cattoretti G, Pileri S, Parravicini C, et al: Antigen unmasking on formalin-fixed, paraffin-embedded tissue sections. J Pathol 171:83, 1993.
139. Krenacs L, Tiszalvicz L, Krenacs T, et al: Immunohistochemical detection of CD1A antigen in formalin-fixed and paraffin-embedded tissue sections with monoclonal antibody 010. J Pathol 171:99, 1993.
140. Emile J, Wechsler J, Brousse N, et al: Langerhans cell histiocytosis. Definitive diagnosis with the use of monoclonal antibody 010 on routinely paraffin-embedded samples. Am J Surg Pathol 19:636, 1995.
141. Kelly KM, Beverley PCL, Chu AC, et al: Successful in vivo immunolocalization of Langerhans cell histio-

cytosis with use of a monoclonal antibody NA1/34. J Pediatr 125:17, 1994.
142. Broadbent V: Favourable prognostic features in histiocytosis X: bone involvement and absence of skin disease. Arch Dis Child 61:1219, 1986.
143. Fiorillo A, Sadlie F, De Chiara C, et al: Bone lesions in Langerhans cell histiocytosis. Clin Pediatr 32:118, 1993.
144. Lahey ME: Histiocytosis X—comparison of three treatment regimens. J Pediatr 87:179, 1975.

Chapter

15

GIANT CELL TUMOR OF BONE AND GIANT CELL–CONTAINING LESIONS OF BONE

DAVID C. MANGHAM

If a careful search is made, virtually all bone lesions will be found to contain osteoclasts or osteoclast-like giant cells. This chapter discusses the nature of these cells and the spectrum of the lesions in which they are a prominent feature (Table 15–1). Giant cell tumor of bone (GCT), chondroblastoma, chondromyxoid fibroma, giant cell reparative granuloma, and the bone lesions of hyperparathyroidism are discussed in some detail and their important differential diagnoses considered.

WHAT ARE OSTEOCLAST-LIKE GIANT CELLS?

Osteoclasts are the specialized cells of the monocyte-macrophage system that are responsible for the resorption of bone. Osteoclasts may be mononucleate or multinucleate; multinucleate osteoclasts are formed by fusion of mononuclear osteoclasts rather than by nuclear division without cell division.[1] Osteoclasts differ from the macrophage polykaryons seen in foreign body and type 4 hypersensitivity reactions in their morphologic features, their immunophenotype,[2] and in their responsiveness to calcitonin (Table 15–2).[3]

Osteoclast-*like* giant cell (OLGC) is a term that describes a multinucleate cell that resembles an osteoclast morphologically and immunophenotypically but is not in the process of resorbing bone. These cells can be extracted from tumors and shown to resorb bone and respond to calcitonin in vitro (see Chapter 3).[4]

In tumors, it is important to distinguish between neoplastic multinucleate cells and OLGCs. OLGCs in tumors are always reactive, and no neoplastic proliferation of osteoclasts has been described (therefore, the term "osteoclastoma" is a complete misnomer). Many benign and malignant tumors, such as nevi, pleomorphic malignant fibrous histiocytoma, and clear cell sarcoma, contain multinucleate tumor cells (Fig. 15–1*A*). Reactive OLGCs can be readily distinguished from tumor giant cells by their nuclear features (Fig. 15–1*B*) and their strong immunoreactivity for CD68 (Fig. 15–1*C*), a pan-monocyte-macrophage system marker.

The number of nuclei in OLGCs is very often far greater than in osteoclasts involved in physiologic or pathologic bone resorption. Osteoclasts in the primary spongiosa (Fig. 15–1*D*), or involved in bone resorption adjacent to tumor rarely contain more than 10 nuclei, whereas OLGCs in GCT and chondroblastoma can contain 100 or more nuclei in a 4 μm thick section (see Fig. 15–1*C*). The appearance of multinucleate OLGCs can vary from cells

Table 15–1. Diseases in Which Osteoclast-like Giant Cells May Be a Prominent Feature

Benign lesions
Aneurysmal bone cyst
Brown tumor of hyperparathyroidism
Cherubism
Chondroblastoma
Chondromyxoid fibroma*
Eosinophilic granuloma*
Giant cell reparative granuloma
Nonossifying fibroma*
Osteoblastoma
Osteoid osteoma
Pigmented villonodular synovitis*
Simple bone cyst*
Intermediate malignancy
Clear cell chondrosarcoma*
Giant cell tumor
Giant cell tumor of Paget's disease
Malignant
Malignant giant cell tumor
Giant cell–rich osteosarcoma
Giant cell–rich telangiectatic osteosarcoma
Giant cell–rich fibrosarcoma
Giant cell–rich malignant fibrous histiocytoma
Dedifferentiated chondrosarcoma with osteoclast-like giant cell–dedifferentiated component
Metastatic carcinoma*

*These diseases usually lack significant numbers of osteoclast-like giant cells.

with pale pink cytoplasm and dispersed nuclear chromatin with small nucleoli, to cells with a more deeply staining eosinophilic and hyaline cytoplasm and dark staining, pyknotic nuclei (see Fig. 15–1*B*). It is assumed that the latter type is an older and degenerate cell. It is of interest that OLGCs have been reported in many varied types of extraosseous tumors including giant cell–rich carcinomas, sarcomas, and melanomas,[5–7] presumably recruited by an aberrantly expressed tumor cell product.

BONE LESIONS IN WHICH OSTEOCLAST-LIKE GIANT CELLS ARE OFTEN PROMINENT

Table 15–1 shows the primary bone tumors that characteristically contain numerous OLGCs. Some of these lesions may, and often do, lack significant numbers of OLGCs.

As is repeatedly stressed in this book, it is important for the histopathologist to work closely with clinicians and radiologists when presented with a bone lesion. Certain clinical features should always be reviewed when confronted with a bone lesion (Table 15–3). In particular, certain lesions characteristically affect certain age groups and anatomic sites (i.e., particular bones and regions within bones).

In general, a bone tumor can present with any or all of the following features: pain, swelling, deformity, limitation of movement, and fracture. The mode of presentation is not specific for any single entity or group of entities, although malignant tumors are likely to present with more severe and rapidly progressive symptoms. The presence of systemic symptoms should be noted, for example, night sweats in B-cell lymphoma and symptoms of hyperparathyroidism.

It is good practice to correlate all bone lesions with the radiologic features (see Chapter 6), ideally in discussion with a radiologist who has a special interest in bone tumors. Table 15–4 gives a brief overview of the key radiologic features of the OLGC-rich lesions.

As is evident from Table 15–1, the OLGC is promiscuous and keeps varied company. In a tumor, the recognition of OLGCs per se gives no clue as to the diagnosis or how a tumor is likely to behave and, having noted the presence and distribution of the OLGCs, a definitive diagnosis is reached by concentrating attention on the background features of the lesion.

GIANT CELL TUMOR OF BONE

Giant cell tumor of bone is a relatively common primary bone tumor of "borderline"

Table 15–2. Distinguishing Features of Osteoclasts and Macrophage Polykaryon

	Multinucleate Osteoclast	**Macrophage Polykaryon**
Nuclear distribution	Central cluster	Peripheral
Response to calcitonin	Present	Absent
Immunophenotype		
CD11a, b, c	−	+
CD13	+	+
CD14	−	+
CD15	+	+
CD16	−	±
CD25	−	±
CD31	−	+
CD35	−	+
CD36	−	+
CD37	−	+
CD43	−	+
CD44	+	+
CD45	+	+
CD54	+	+
CD68	+	+
CD71	+	+
HLA-DR	−	+

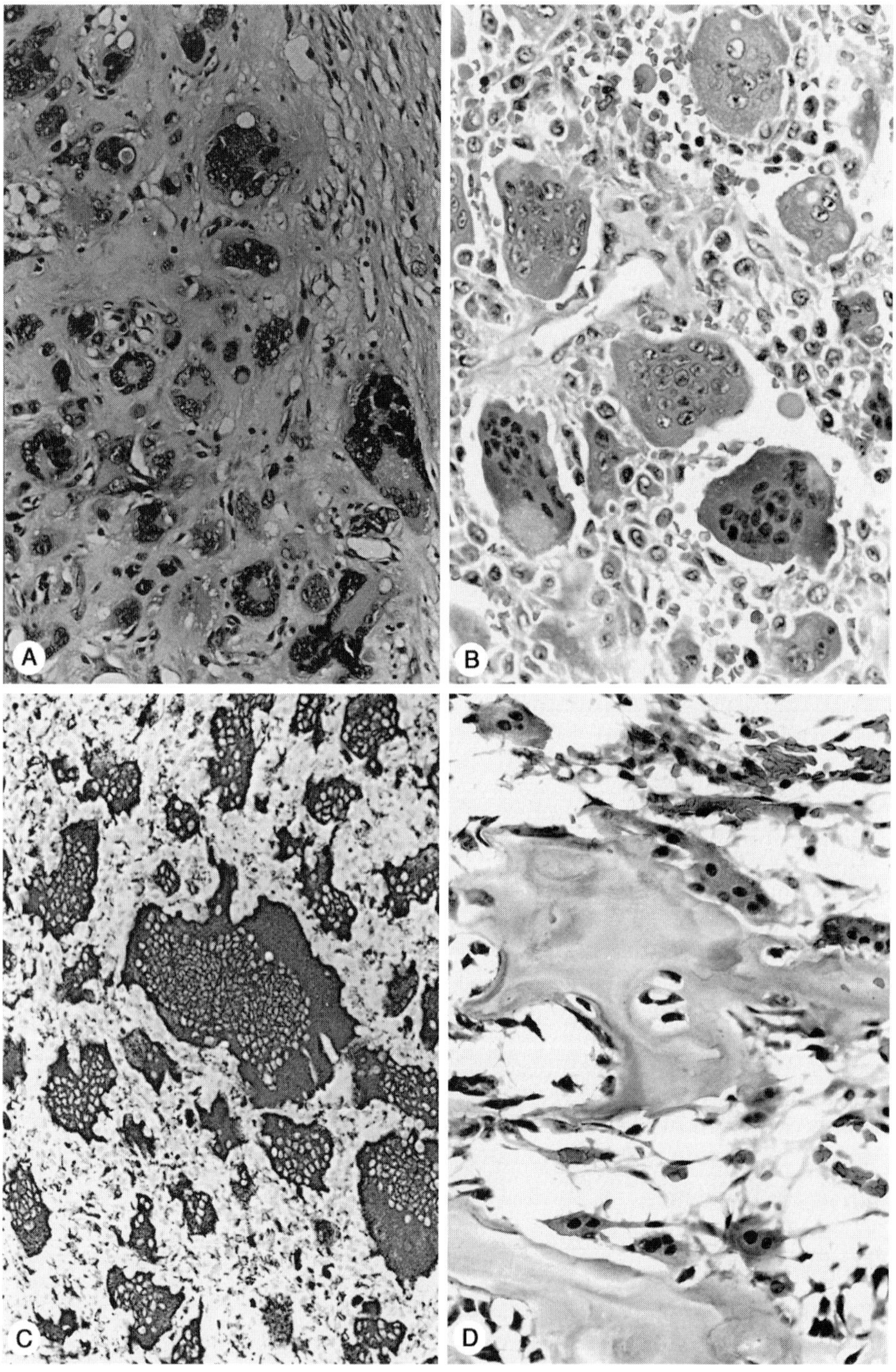

Figure 15–1. Multinucleate giant cells. *A*, Multinucleate tumor giant cells in a pleomorphic liposarcoma. Clear-cut nuclear atypia and pleomorphism distinguish these cells from osteoclast-like giant cells. *B*, Multinucleate osteoclast-like giant cells in a giant cell tumor of bone. There is mild variability in nuclear size, and nuclei tend to be centrally clustered. Nuclei often show small nucleoli. Some osteoclasts may show darkly stained, pyknotic nuclei undergoing apoptosis, and these cells tend to have darker staining cytoplasm. *C*, Multinucleate osteoclast-like giant cells in giant cell tumor of bone showing immunohistochemical labeling for CD68. Some osteoclast-like giant cells may contain hundreds of nuclei. *D*, Primary spongiosa showing bone formation and resorption. Multinucleate osteoclasts usually contain several nuclei. True osteoclasts rarely contain more than 10 nuclei in a routine histologic section (the important exception being the larger osteoclasts present in Paget's disease of bone).

Table 15–3. Clinical Features of Lesions that Can Contain Many Osteoclast-like Giant Cells

	Approximate % of Primary Bone Tumors	Peak Age of Incidence (y)	Principal Bones Involved	Area of Bone Involved
Benign				
Aneurysmal bone cyst	1–2	<20	Any, but mainly long bones and posterior spine	Metaphysis or diaphysis
Brown tumor of hyperparathyroidism	0.1–0.4	40–50	Often multiple	
Cherubism	Rare	Infancy	Mandible and maxilla	Symmetrical
Chondroblastoma	0.5–1.0	10–20	Long bones	Epiphysis ± metaphysis
Chondromyxoid fibroma	0.1–0.5	10–20	Long bones of leg and foot	Metaphysis
Eosinophilic granuloma	0.5–1.0	5–15	Flat bones (70%) Long bones (30%)	Veretebral body Long bones—metaphysis or diaphysis
Giant cell reparative granuloma	Rare	<30	Mandible and maxilla	
Nonossifying fibroma	2	5–20	Long bones	Metaphysis or diaphysis
Osteoblastoma	0.5–0.8	10–30	Long bones and spine	Metadiaphysis Posterior spine
Osteoid osteoma	2–3	10–20	Long bones or spine	Cortical
Pigmented villonodular synovitis		25–40	Joints	Juxta-articular
Simple bone cyst	3	5–15	Long bones—proximal humerus and femur	Metadiaphysis
Intermediate Malignancy				
Giant cell tumor	5	20–50	Long bones (90%)	Epiphysis ± metaphysis
Clear cell chondrosarcoma	0.1–0.2	30–50	Long bones (90%)	Epiphysis ± metaphysis
Giant cell tumor of bone in Paget's disease	<0.1	50–70	Skull (50%)	Any site
High-Grade Malignancy				
See text.				

Table 15–4. Radiologic Features of Lesions that Can Contain Significant Numbers of Osteoclast-like Giant Cells

	Typical Radiological Features
Benign	
Aneurysmal bone cyst	Eccentric, lucent, blown-out
Brown tumor of hyperparathyroidism	Purely lytic lesion lacking sclerotic border; any bone/area of bone may be affected
Cherubism	Bilateral, lucent, well defined
Chondroblastoma	Well defined, lucent, ± fluffy calcifications
Chondromyxoid fibroma	Eccentric, lucent, expanded cortex, ± trabeculations
Eosinophilic granuloma	Ill-defined, usually small lesion with mixed lysis/sclerosis
Giant cell reparative granuloma	Mandible or maxilla; radiolucent, well defined
Nonossifying fibroma	Metaphyseal; eccentric, oval, lucent, sclerotic margin
Osteoblastoma	Lucent or mineralized, well defined
Osteoid osteoma	Sclerotic rim, lucent with central nidus
Pigmented villonodular synovitis	Joint involvement with bone erosion either side of the joint
Simple bone cyst	Lucent with traversing bone trabeculae
Intermediate Malignancy	
Clear cell chondrosarcoma	Epiphyseal, usually well defined ± a sclerotic rim
Giant cell tumor	Epiphyseal ± metaphyseal extension; eccentric, expanded, lucent, ± soft tissue involvement
High-Grade Malignancy	
Malignant giant cell tumor	May be similar to typical giant cell tumor
Giant cell–rich osteosarcoma	Ill-defined mixed lucent and dense, soft tissue extension
Giant cell–rich telangiectatic osteosarcoma	Ill-defined mixed lucent and dense, soft tissue extension; possible fluid levels
Giant cell–rich fibrosarcoma	Ill-defined lucent, soft tissue extension
Giant cell–rich malignant fibrous histiocytoma	Ill-defined lucent, soft tissue extension
Dedifferentiated chondrosarcoma with giant cell tumor–like component	Area typical of chondrosarcoma + ill-defined lucent ± soft tissue extension

malignancy that typically affects the epiphysis, with or without metaphyseal extension, of long bones in the mature skeleton. It is characterized histologically by a fairly uniform scattering of often very large OLGCs set against a background of ovoid and spindled mononuclear cells.

Clinical Features

Several large series of GCTs have been reported.[8–13] Typically, the patient is a young to middle-aged adult. The median age is 30 years and the age range is 5 to 75 years. The tumor is rare in patients less than 15 years old, and the diagnosis should be carefully re-evaluated in any patient under 20 years of age. Females are affected slightly more commonly than males. Presentation is usually with increasing pain or swelling, or both, and, less commonly, with a pathologic fracture.

Most giant cell tumors affect the long bones. The approximate incidences of bones involved are as follows: distal femur (25%), proximal tibia (25%), distal radius (10%), pelvis and sacrum (10%), proximal humerus (5%), proximal femur (5%), distal tibia (4%), proximal fibula (4%), spine (3%), and other bones (9%). GCTs of the hands and feet are rare,[14, 15] and tumors of the skull are extremely rare.[16, 17]

There have been several reports of multicentric GCTs.[18–21] Such cases appear to be extreme rarities. Before accepting a case of apparent multifocal "GCT," it is essential to rule out brown tumors of hyperparathyroidism, multiple bony metastases from a giant cell–rich bone sarcoma or carcinoma, and, rarely, polyostotic Paget's disease complicated by multiple secondary giant cell tumors.[22] In all patients with a clinical or histologic diagnosis of GCT, a serum calcium and phosphate level should be measured to help exclude brown tumor of hyperparathyroidism. When GCT is a complication of Paget's disease of bone, the serum alkaline phosphatase level is raised.

Radiologic Features

Radiologically, GCT produces a lytic lesion that involves the epiphysis with or without metaphyseal extension (Fig. 15–2*A*). Most lesions are situated eccentrically, but they may be central. The lesion may be purely lytic or may show traversing coarse trabeculations due to persistent cortical bone. If the epiphysis is not involved, then the histology should be reappraised, considering the diagnoses of brown tumor of hyperparathyroidism or giant cell–rich osteosarcoma. The adjacent bone may show shallow permeation by tumor but usually appears normal. Only a minority (approximately 5%) of cases show peripheral reactive bone sclerosis. The lesion may erode the cortex completely but usually remains within the confines of the periosteum. The degree of cortical destruction and soft tissue extension is the basis for radiologic staging, the most important predictor of tumor aggressiveness.[23–25]

In the vertebral column, GCTs involve the cervical, thoracic, and lumbar regions equally. The vertebral body is the only area involved in 55% of cases; tumors involve the vertebral body and arch in 29% and the vertebral arch alone in only 16% of cases.[26, 27]

Gross Pathology

The diagnosis is usually made clinically with a high degree of confidence, and a diagnostic biopsy is not usually submitted for histopathologic interpretation. The pathologist is usually presented with curettage samples of the tumor. Curettages are often quite bulky and may measure up to 200 cm^3. The tissue is brown, soft, and friable, owing to rich vascularity, hemorrhage, and paucity of intralesional bone. Larger areas can contain cyst-like structures. Collagen-rich areas appear firmer and paler and are a more common feature of recurrent lesions.

Rarely, the size or location of a GCT necessitates an amputation. The intact specimen is usually confined by a periosteal capsule. The cut surface is heterogeneous, being mainly soft with hemorrhagic foci and occasional pale areas of collagenization (Fig. 15–2*B*). A fracture with or without reparative features may be present.

Microscopic Pathology

Invariable Features

1. Osteoclast-like giant cells. Most areas show an even distribution of OLGCs (Fig. 15–3*A*) that vary in size. Cells with 30 to 50 nuclei are typical, but huge OLGCs with literally hundreds of nuclei are not uncommon (see Fig. 15–1*C*).

2. Spindle-shaped and ovoid stromal cells with poorly defined cytoplasmic borders. The

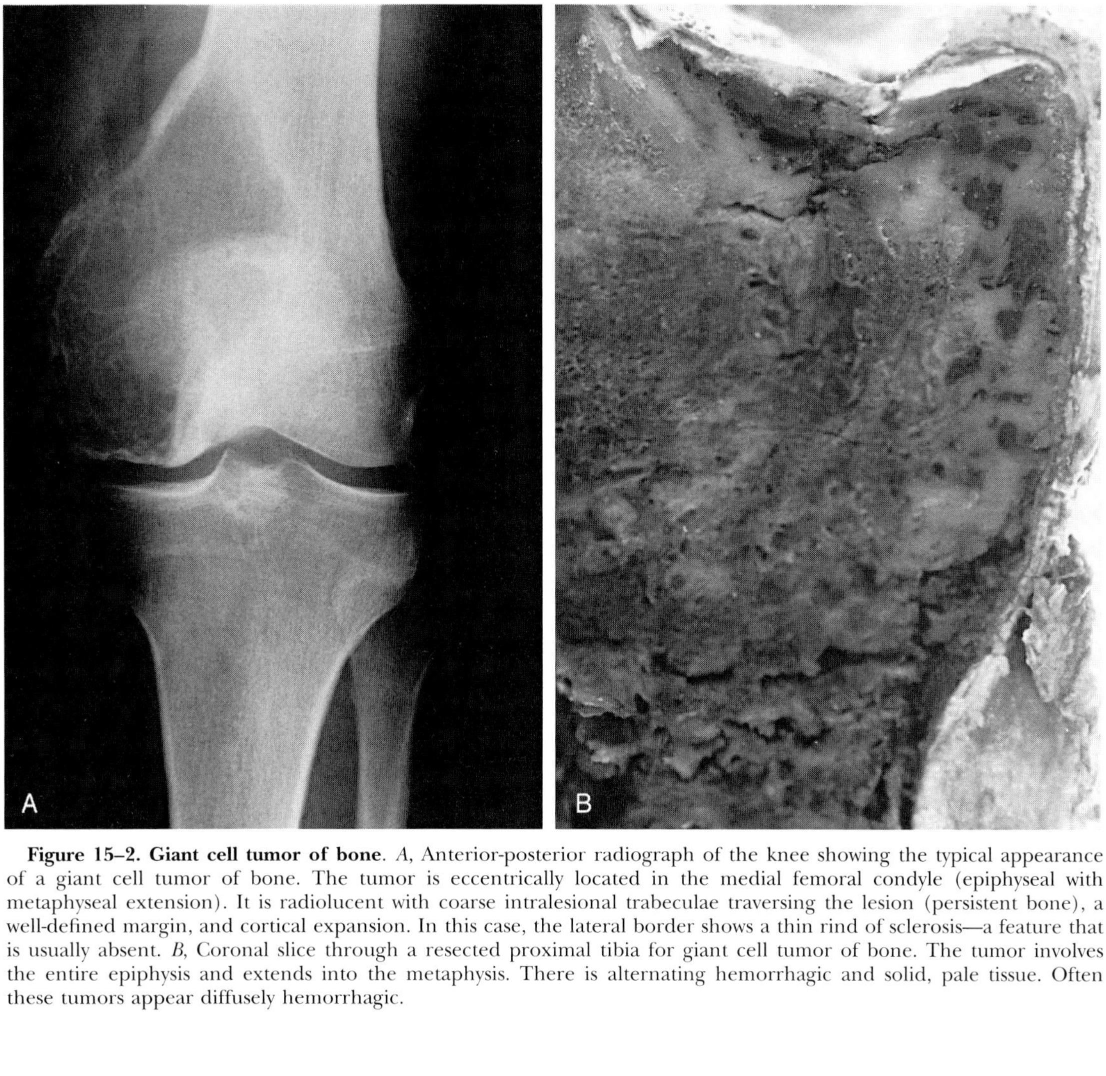

Figure 15–2. Giant cell tumor of bone. *A*, Anterior-posterior radiograph of the knee showing the typical appearance of a giant cell tumor of bone. The tumor is eccentrically located in the medial femoral condyle (epiphyseal with metaphyseal extension). It is radiolucent with coarse intralesional trabeculae traversing the lesion (persistent bone), a well-defined margin, and cortical expansion. In this case, the lateral border shows a thin rind of sclerosis—a feature that is usually absent. *B*, Coronal slice through a resected proximal tibia for giant cell tumor of bone. The tumor involves the entire epiphysis and extends into the metaphysis. There is alternating hemorrhagic and solid, pale tissue. Often these tumors appear diffusely hemorrhagic.

majority of nuclei resemble those of the reactive OLGCs; a useful internal comparison can thus be made when considering the degree of nuclear anaplasia of the stromal cells. The stromal cells are always mitotically active; the number of mitoses can range from two to three per 10 high-power fields (HPF) to 20 or rarely more per 10 HPF. In the absence of other worrying features, this high rate of mitotic activity is consistent with the diagnosis of GCT.

3. In a typical OLGC-rich field, there is little or no discernible extracellular matrix.

Variable Features

1. Areas relatively depleted of OLGC are often seen and occasionally may be very extensive, so a careful search may be required to identify foci of typical GCT. Such areas are often collagen rich and may be quite cellular with a storiform pattern that resembles benign fibrous histiocytoma or nonossifying fibroma (Fig. 15–3*B*). Areas of dense collagenization with no particular architectural pattern may be present.

2. Areas of hemorrhage are common and may be very extensive. OLGCs tend to accumulate and cluster around hemorrhage. Secondary aneurysmal bone cyst formation occurs in approximately 10% of GCTs (Fig. 15–3*C*). It is important to appreciate that the presence of such areas is completely consistent with the diagnosis of GCT.

3. Foam cells. Clusters of foamy histiocytes are often present, presumably indicating areas of previous hemorrhage (Fig. 15–3*D*). In such areas, a lymphocytic infiltrate may be prominent and OLGCs are relatively lacking.

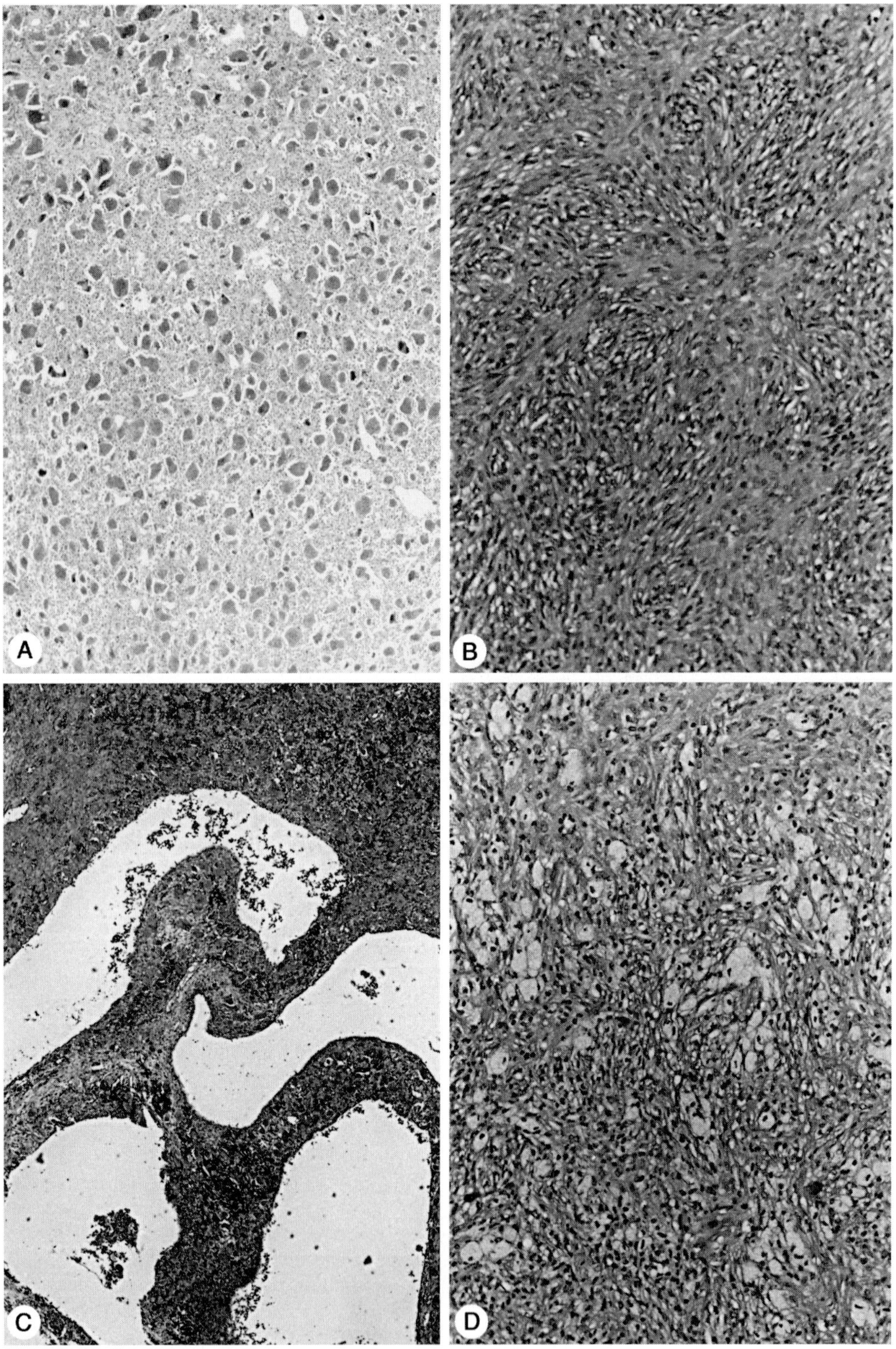

Figure 15–3. Giant cell tumor of bone. *A*, Typical low-power microscopic appearance showing evenly scattered, large osteoclast-like giant cells against a mononuclear cellular background. *B*, Fibrous histiocytoma-like cellular area composed of spindled cells arranged in a storiform pattern. *C*, Low-power view of secondary aneurysmal bone cyst arising in giant cell tumor of bone. *D*, Fibrous histiocytoma-like area with clusters of foamy histiocytes.

4. Reactive (woven) bone is usually present at the periphery of the lesion, but this may be difficult to appreciate on sections of curettage. Bone formation can occur intralesionally (Fig. 15–4*A*).[28] An important sign that the woven bone is reactive is the presence of a monolayer of osteoblasts rimming the bone/osteoid trabeculae (Fig. 15–4A and B). However, osteoblastic rimming of bone trabeculae may be difficult to appreciate in very immature reactive bone. Dense sheets of woven bone or a filigree pattern of woven bone deposition lacking osteoblastic rimming should alert one to the possible alternative diagnosis of osteosarcoma. If the amount of reactive bone/osteoid trabeculae is abundant, the diagnosis of osteoblastoma should be considered.

5. Necrosis is common and, on occasion, can be very extensive, especially if there has been a previous biopsy or pathologic fracture.

6. Intravascular OLGCs and intravascular tumor. This is a common feature and is not a sign of increased aggressiveness (Fig. 15–5).[29, 30]

7. Ancient change in conventional GCT. As is well recognized in many other mesenchymal tumors (e.g., schwannomas, nonossifying fibroma, chondromyxoid fibroma), so-called ancient changes can occur in GCTs. Although uncommon, it is important to be aware that GCTs can show these changes in order to avoid an overdiagnosis of high-grade malignancy (Fig. 15–6 [see also color Figure 15–6]). The changes take the form of large, bizarre nuclei. Such nuclei tend to be separated by clearly benign tumor nuclei, and they tend to show chromatin smudging, nuclear vacuolization, and a level of mitotic activity much lower than that seen in classic GCT.

Features that Are Inconsistent with the Diagnosis

1. Frankly malignant stromal cells. The presence of stromal cells in which nuclear atypia is marked excludes the diagnosis of

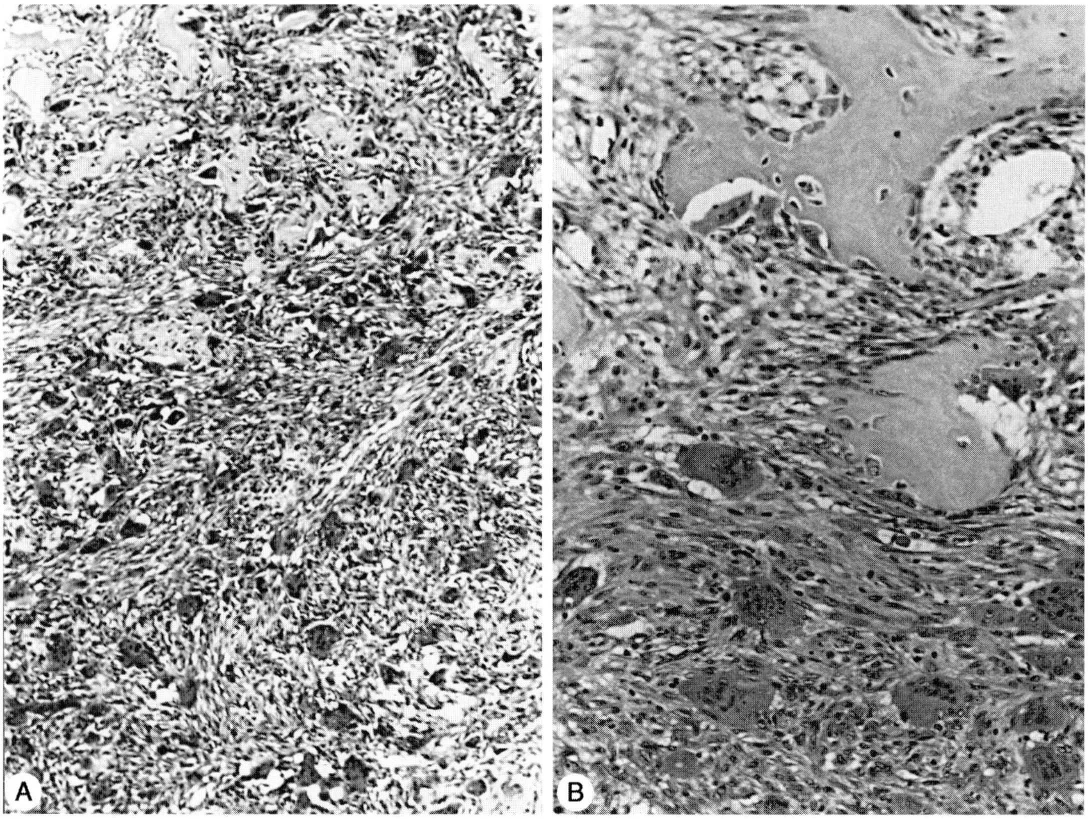

Figure 15–4. Giant cell tumor of bone. *A*, Intralesional reactive osteoid in the upper part of the field. *B*, Reactive woven bone trabeculae in a giant cell tumor of bone. The bone shows both osteoclastic resorption and a monolayer of active osteoblasts. Note the difference in the number of nuclei between true bone-phagocytosing osteoclasts and the much larger osteoclast-like giant cells.

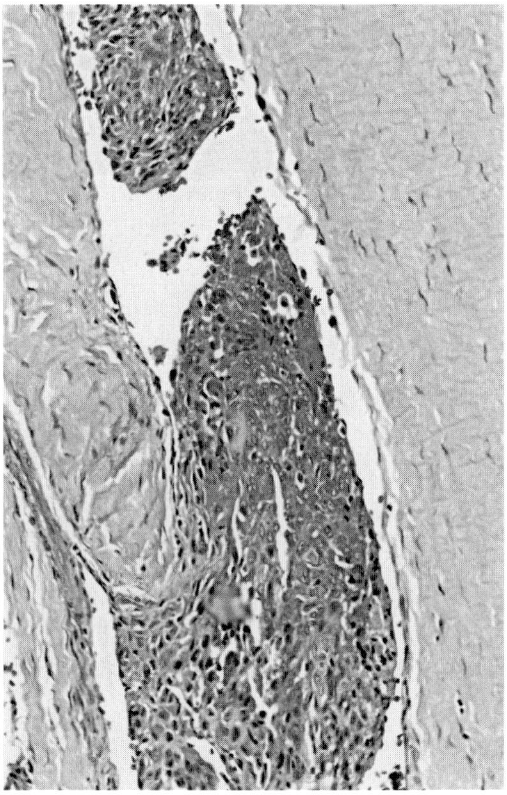

Figure 15–5. Giant cell tumor of bone within a dilated vascular channel. This is a common feature and does not indicate increased tumor aggressiveness.

GCT. When assessing the degree of stromal cell nuclear atypia, it is useful to compare their nuclei with those of the reactive OLGCs (Fig. 15–7).

2. Tumor cartilage and tumor chondroid. Cartilage can be present in GCTs when there is fracture callus. If noncallus, intralesional, neoplastic cartilage is present, the diagnosis of chondroblastoma, chondrosarcoma, or chondroblastic osteosarcoma should be considered.

Electron Microscopy

The ultrastructural characteristics of GCT[25, 26] are nonspecific and do not help in establishing the diagnosis.

Differential Diagnoses

Giant Cell Tumor of Hyperparathyroidism (Brown Tumor)

Histologically, the brown tumor of hyperparathyroidism can be identical to GCT. Any patient with a histologic diagnosis of GCT should be clinically investigated to exclude hyperparathyroidism.

Chondroblastoma

Histologic features present in chondroblastoma and absent from GCT are the presence of chondroid material, polygonal stromal cells with areas of chicken-wire calcification, and varying degrees of S-100 protein positivity by immunohistochemistry.

Giant Cell Reparative Granuloma

Giant cell reparative granuloma (GCRG) usually affects the jaw bones. Extragnathic GCRGs have been reported[31] but are probably best regarded as nonossifying fibromas[32] or a solid variant of aneurysmal bone cyst.[33, 34] Resemblence to GCT can be close, but generally the GCRG contains more spindled stromal

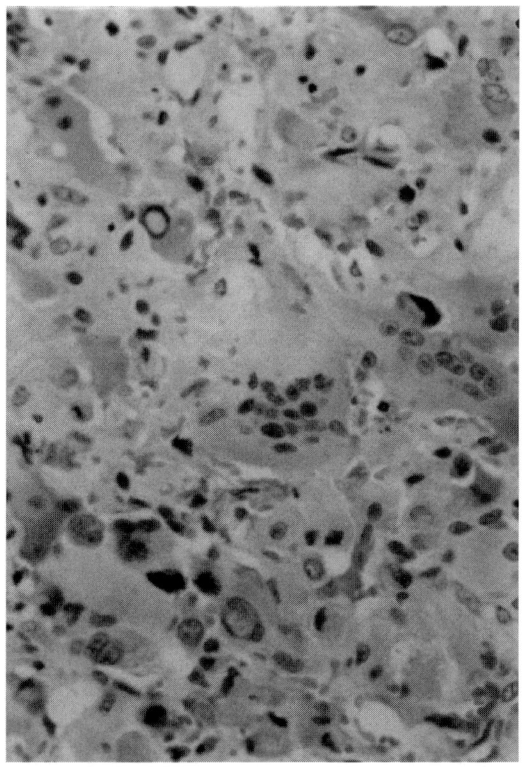

Figure 15–6. Area of giant cell tumor of bone showing degenerate nuclear features of the stromal cells. The nuclei show vacuolization, smudged chromatin, and hyperchromatism. No mitoses are present in this area of the tumor. The importance in recognizing this change is in the distinction from the nuclear pleomorphism of malignancy. (See also color figure.)

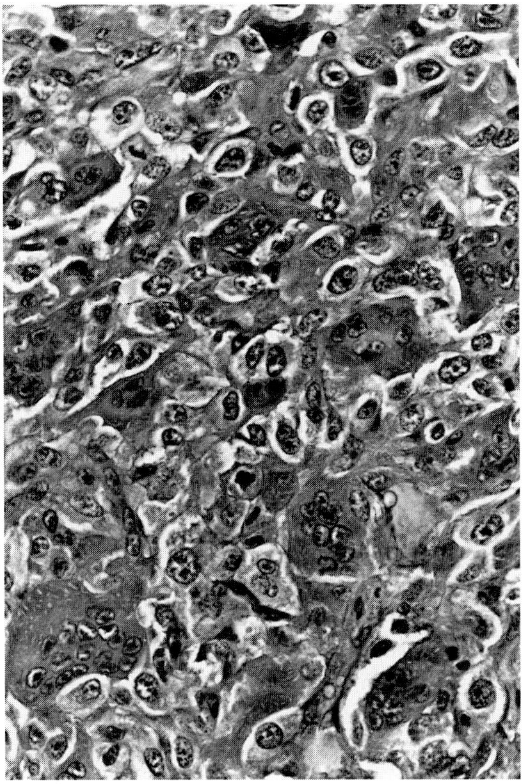

Figure 15–7. Osteoclast-like giant cells set against a frankly sarcomatous stromal background. A comparison of the nuclei in the osteoclast-like giant cells (reactive) and the stromal mononuclear cells (neoplastic) is a useful exercise in aiding the analysis of tumor cell nuclear atypia. In this case, the tumor showed no specific features of differentiation, and the osteoclast-like giant cells were evenly scattered throughout the tumor—a true malignant giant cell tumor of bone.

cells, unevenly scattered OLGCs, and a greater amount of collagen matrix. However, these are hardly reliable or distinctive discriminating features, and the diagnosis is made in the clinical setting. True GCT of the jaw is very rare, and reported cases should only be accepted as such when there are radiologic features of aggressive expansion with or without soft tissue extension and/or clinical recurrence.

Early-Phase Nonossifying Fibroma

Nonossifying fibroma (NOF) is an eccentrically located metaphyseal lesion that is often discovered incidentally when radiographs are taken for other reasons (see Chapter 12). They can, however, be symptomatic. Unlike GCT, the majority of NOFs are seen in patients under 20 years of age. If a confident diagnosis is made on radiologic examination, no further action is necessary other than clinical follow-up) as the lesion spontaneously regresses. Histologically, the lesion is composed of bland spindled cells with a usually uneven scattering of OLGCs and lymphocytes. With time, the lesion becomes more sclerotic and in late phase may resemble a fibrous histiocytoma. Resolution is achieved by the ingrowth of bone from the periphery.

Fibrous Histiocytoma

It is debatable whether fibrous histiocytoma of bone is a distinct entity (see Chapter 12). Areas of "fibrous histiocytoma" are often present within otherwise typical GCTs (see Fig. 15–3*B* and *D*) and are believed to be a reparative response to hemorrhage. Such an observation raises the possibility that a pure, epiphyseal fibrous histiocytoma is in fact an organized GCT. This is important, since an apparently recurrent fibrous histiocytoma may resemble a pure GCT. Before a diagnosis of fibrous histiocytoma is proffered on an epiphyseal lesion, all the tissue should be processed for examination to search for an area of GCT.

Solid Aneurysmal Bone Cyst

This variant of aneurysmal bone cyst (ABC) lacks the cavernous blood-filled spaces of the classic variety but otherwise contains all the elements seen in the walls of a classic aneurysmal bone cyst. These include an often florid proliferation of plump but benign fibroblasts and osteoblasts, scattered OLGCs and lymphocytes, and intralesional bone/osteoid formation. The bone is deposited in a trabecular fashion with osteoblastic rimming. Some areas are too immature to show clear osteoblastic rimming of trabeculae, and a gradual maturation of bone with rimming should then be sought emanating from the immature area. When present, the deposition of a peculiar material called lacy chondroid is a very useful diagnostic feature (see Chapter 16). Clinical features are often helpful in distinguishing GCT from solid ABC, as the latter are usually purely metaphyseal and affect patients less than 20 years old.

Giant Cell Tumor of Bone Associated with Paget's Disease

In GCT curettage, bone should be examined for the histologic features of Paget's disease. The coexistence of Paget's disease will explain an unusual location (e.g., nonepiphyseal) of the GCT. It is important to stress that a tumor arising in pagetic bone is most likely to be a high-grade sarcoma, and the diagnosis of GCT should be made with caution.

Osteoclast-like Giant Cell–Rich Sarcoma

True malignant GCT, OLGC-rich osteosarcoma, fibrosarcoma, and malignant fibrous histiocytoma can rarely enter the differential diagnoses of GCT. The clinical history and radiographic features will alert the pathologist to the possibility of these diagnoses in the majority of cases. True primary malignant GCT (see Fig. 15–7) is defined as a bone tumor in which there are areas of typical GCT as well as multiple foci showing clear-cut stromal nuclear atypia without features of specific differentiation.[35–37] The nuclear atypia may be subtle in some cases. Flow cytometry has been proposed as a useful adjunct to diagnosis.[38–42] Most GCTs are diploid, but the significance of aneuploidy in terms of biologic behavior is not entirely clear. The association of typical GCT and foci of malignant GCT underscores the importance of processing and examining all the curettage samples received.

A histologically bland GCT may rarely occur as the dedifferentiated component of dedifferentiated chondrosarcoma.[43] In spite of its appearance, it behaves as a highly malignant sarcoma. The correct diagnosis relies on a careful evaluation of the clinical and radiologic evidence. In particular, confusion may occur if the biopsy is sent for pathologic evaluation with little clinical information, especially the presence of an associated cartilaginous tumor radiologically.

Areas indistinguishable from GCT may also occur in dedifferentiated, low-grade chondrosarcomas in which the dedifferentiated component is an OLGC-rich osteosarcoma. If the frankly sarcomatous area is small, it may be undetected during tumor sampling. In any event, this appears to be an extremely rare entity.

Osteoclast-like Giant Cell–Rich Metastatic Carcinomas

Rarely, metastatic carcinoma can be rich in OLGCs (Fig. 15–8). In such cases, OLGCs are usually smaller than in GCT. A careful analysis will reveal the malignant cells, which can be highlighted by immunohistochemistry for cytokeratin expression. There are no reports of GCTs expressing cytokeratins.

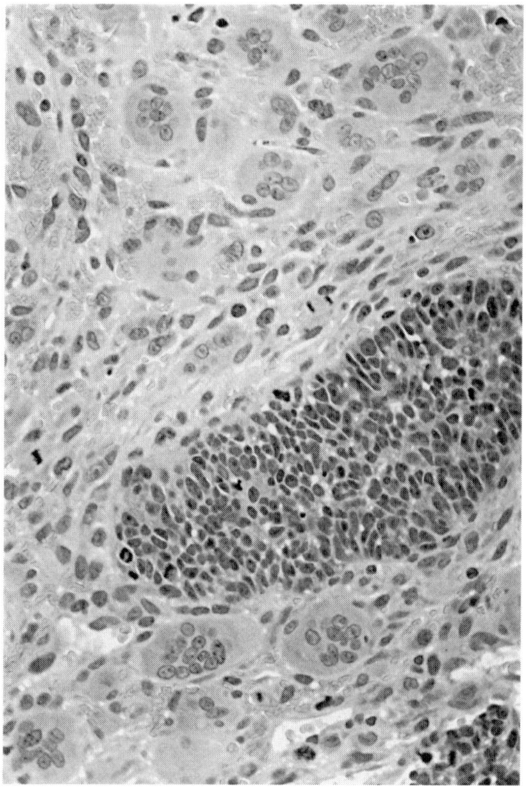

Figure 15–8. A humeral metastasis of a small cell carcinoma from the lung shows many osteoclast-like giant cells in the stroma.

Grading Systems for Giant Cell Tumor of Bone

The grading system introduced by Jaffe, Lichtenstein, and Portis[44] divided GCTs into grades 1, 2, and 3. Grades 1 and 2 separate tumors on subtle nuclear features, a difference in mitotic rate, and the ratio of the number of stromal cells relative to the number of OLGCs. Grade 3 tumors show nuclear atypia sufficient that they are regarded as frankly sarcomatous. It has become apparent that it is wise to distinguish frank sarcomas that are rich in OLGCs and classify them separately according to the specific features of the tumor (e.g., osteosarcoma, malignant fibrous histiocytoma, fibrosarcoma). It has been shown that classifying GCTs into grades 1 or 2 has no prognostic significance and this practice should therefore be abandoned.[11, 13] Neither proliferation rate nor vascularity appear to correlate with tumor aggressiveness.[35]

Treatment and Prognosis of Giant Cell Tumor of Bone

Vigorous curettage is the usual treatment for typical giant cell tumors. Some authors have advocated the use of adjuvant local chemical (e.g., phenol) or thermal (i.e., liquid nitrogen) treatment.[18, 45] The curettaged cavity may be packed with bone graft or methyl methacrylate. In large GCTs with extensive extracortical extension, it may be necessary to carry out an en bloc excision with either allograft or endoprosthetic replacement. If possible, curettage is favored over en bloc excision in terms of functional outcome.[46] Spinal GCTs may present special problems, and adjuvant radiotherapy is sometimes necessary. Radiation treatment of GCTs has become unpopular due to the risk of secondary, radiation-induced sarcoma.[47]

Widely varying data on the incidence of local recurrence have been reported[18]; the reported range in the larger series is between 20% and 40%. The risk of local recurrence is related to radiologic stage rather than any particular histologic characteristics and may be associated with soft tissue seeding.[23–25] Most recurrences occur within 2 years, and 5 years after curettage the risk of local recurrence is very low.[12] However, cases of GCT have recurred as late as 10 years after initial curettage.[13] Less than 5% of patients with GCT develop pulmonary metastases, and the risk increases with each recurrence. Resection of pulmonary metastases can be associated with long survival.[19, 20]

CHONDROBLASTOMA

Chondroblastoma is a rare, benign tumor that most often arises within the epiphysis of long bones. It is characterized histologically by polygonal tumor cells, which focally produce chondroid matrix, and by OLGCs. The very rare variant of malignant chondroblastoma is described at the end of this section. Although this tumor had been previously recognized, Jaffe and Lichtenstein coined the term *chondroblastoma* and clearly delineated the entity from GCT.[48]

Clinical Features

Several large series of chondroblastomas have been reported.[49–55] Typically the patient is young (75% of cases occur in the 10- to 20-year-old age group). The tumor is very rare in patients younger than 10 years or older than 60 years. The male-to-female ratio is approximately 3:2. Presenting symptoms are usually increasing pain or swelling, or both, and, rarely, pathologic fracture. A joint effusion may be present. The bones affected are the long bones (70%) and flat bones (30%). One tenth of chondroblastomas arise in the tarsal bones. The most common locations are the proximal tibia, the proximal humerus, and the distal femur. The entire axial skeleton accounts for about 15% of cases, and involvement of the tubular bones of the hands and feet is an extreme rarity. The epiphysis is involved in 98% of cases, and pure involvement of the metaphysis or metadiaphysis is an extreme rarity. The physis is open in the vast majority of cases and the lesion can, but usually does not, cross this structure into the metaphysis. When the physis is closed, metaphyseal involvement can occur.

Blood tests may show a slightly elevated ESR, but serum calcium, phosphate, and alkaline phosphatase levels are usually within normal limits.

Radiologic Features

Plain radiographs show a well-defined lesion in the epiphysis of the immature skeleton (Fig. 15–9). The lesion may be eccentrically placed and can involve the metaphysis. The lesion is either purely lucent or finely stippled due to fine calcifications within the tumor. The bone may or may not be expanded, and the cortex is, in most instances, intact. There is usually a thin sclerotic border, a feature that is usually absent in GCTs. Chondroblastomas are also usually smaller than GCTs. Uncommonly, chondroblastomas can reach a large size and show more coarse calcification, leading to the erroneous diagnosis of osteosarcoma. The magnetic resonance imaging features of chondroblastoma have been reported.[56, 57]

Gross Pathology

Because the surgical treatment of GCT and chondroblastoma is simple curettage, even if these two entities are considered as the clinical

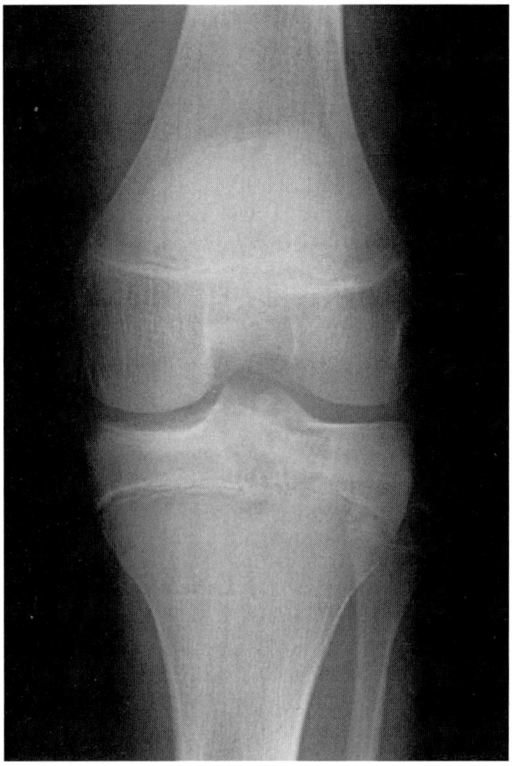

Figure 15–9. Anterior-posterior radiograph of the knee showing the typical appearance of a chondroblastoma. The growth plates are open. A predominantly lucent lesion involves the proximal tibial epiphysis. Fluffy calcifications are apparent within the tumor, which is well-defined and shows a rim of sclerosis.

differential diagnoses, curettage samples are the submitted specimen. The tissue is usually soft, granular, friable, and gray with areas of hemorrhage and possibly small, pale blue nodules (chondroid). There may be yellow foci of necrosis and gritty areas of calcification. Overall, the appearance is less hemorrhagic and more heterogeneous than that seen in GCT. Rarely, due to large size, chondroblastomas are excised en bloc, and there may then be a thin sclerotic margin of bone. Slight permeation of the surrounding trabecular bone may occasionally occur, but this should not be extensive. Cystic degeneration is sometimes apparent. In recurrent lesions excised en bloc, there may be several satellite nodules around the originally curettaged cavity.

Microscopic Pathology

Invariable Features

1. Chondroblasts. So-called "chondroblasts" are the neoplastic cells of the chondroblastoma (Fig. 15–10*A* [see also color Figure 15–10]). They are distinctive cells, being moderately sized, round or polygonal cells with a folded, clefted, or sometimes crenated nucleus. The cytoplasmic borders are conspicuous, and the cytoplasm is granular and eosinophilic. The nuclear chromatin is finely stippled and nucleoli are small and inconspicuous. The cells vary little in size or appearance throughout the tumor. A reticulin stain will demonstrate a fine network enveloping individual chondroblasts in the cellular areas. Mitoses are readily found but are not numerous (less than one per single HPF). Immunostaining for S-100 protein will show variably stained chondroblasts. Scattered chondroblasts stain for cytokeratin.[58]

2. Chondroid. Chondroid is a hyaline material, resembling cartilage mainly by the presence of distinct lacunae, which usually stains pink, but sometimes with a pale blue blush, with hematoxylin and eosin (see Fig. 15–10*A* [see color Figure 15–10]). The amount of chondroid is widely variable, ranging from less than 1% to as much as 30% of the tumor. Chondroid is present as small islands (<2 mm), which are surrounded by cellular areas. This arrangement of hypocellular chondroid and cellular intervening areas imparts a low-power lobularity to the tumor (Fig. 15–10*B* [see color Figure 15–10]). Even in areas where chondroid is lacking, at low power there is a vague lobularity to the tumor.

3. OLGCs are always present, but may vary greatly in size and in the number of nuclei, although they are generally smaller than those of GCT. They are admixed with the chondroblasts and often particularly numerous around islands of chondroid (Fig. 15–11*A*). Infrequently, there are cases in which osteoclasts are not numerous or are small and relatively inconspicuous. They can be highlighted by immunostaining for CD68.

Variable Features

1. "Chicken-wire" calcification. The pericellular reticulin network may become calcified to give the so-called pattern of chicken-wire calcification (see Fig. 15–10*A* and color Figure 15–10) that is virtually pathognomonic of chondroblastoma. Areas of calcification can fuse to give clumps of amorphous calcification.

2. Woven bone or osteoid trabeculae rimmed by osteoblasts may rarely be present in small amounts within a chondroblastoma (Fig. 15–

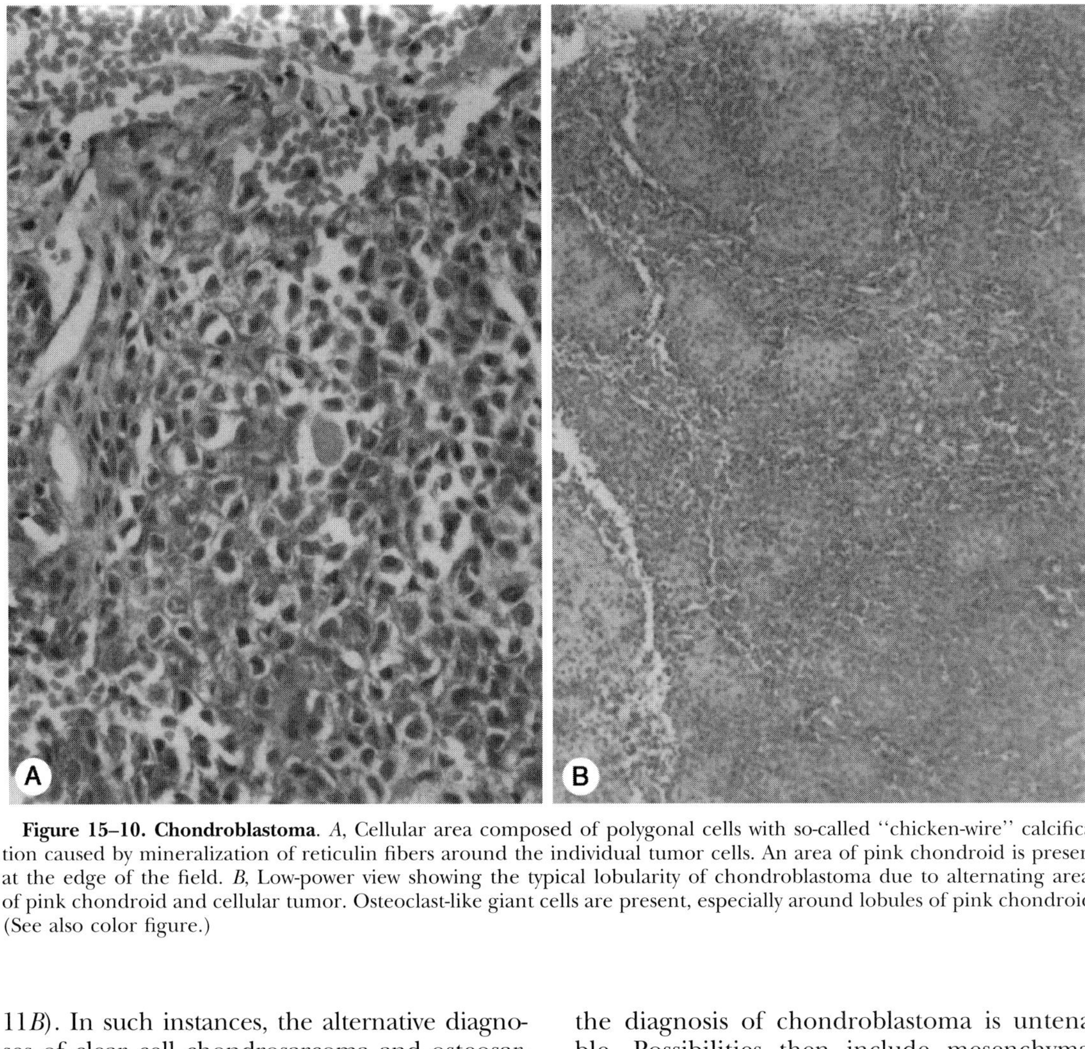

Figure 15–10. Chondroblastoma. *A*, Cellular area composed of polygonal cells with so-called "chicken-wire" calcification caused by mineralization of reticulin fibers around the individual tumor cells. An area of pink chondroid is present at the edge of the field. *B*, Low-power view showing the typical lobularity of chondroblastoma due to alternating areas of pink chondroid and cellular tumor. Osteoclast-like giant cells are present, especially around lobules of pink chondroid. (See also color figure.)

11*B*). In such instances, the alternative diagnoses of clear cell chondrosarcoma and osteosarcoma should be carefully considered.

3. Secondary aneurysmal bone cyst formation may occur, as in GCT.

4. Hemorrhage, small areas of necrosis, and collections of foamy cells can often be seen in chondroblastoma (Fig. 15–12). Around areas of hemorrhage, spindled fibroblasts and myofibroblasts are often present.

5. Ancient change, as seen in other benign bone tumors, has not been described in chondroblastomas.

Features Inconsistent with the Diagnosis of Chondroblastoma

1. Clear-cut nuclear atypia. The nuclei of chondroblastoma are plump and creased or folded and show only occasional mitoses. If the nuclei show features of malignancy, then the diagnosis of chondroblastoma is untenable. Possibilities then include mesenchymal chondrosarcoma, osteosarcoma, and possibly lymphoma (see Differential Diagnoses).

2. Extensive deposition of hyaline cartilage matrix never occurs in chondroblastomas. If present in a cellular lesion, the diagnosis is likely to be chondrosarcoma, mesenchymal chondrosarcoma, or clear cell chondrosarcoma.

3. Extensive permeation of lamellar bone trabeculae. Chondroblastomas may permeate host bone, but for a short distance only. Recurrent lesions may show satellite nodules around the original curettaged cavity. If there is extensive permeative growth, a malignant diagnosis is almost certainly correct.

Differential Diagnoses

Giant Cell Tumor

Areas of chondroblastoma can resemble GCT quite closely. A careful search should be

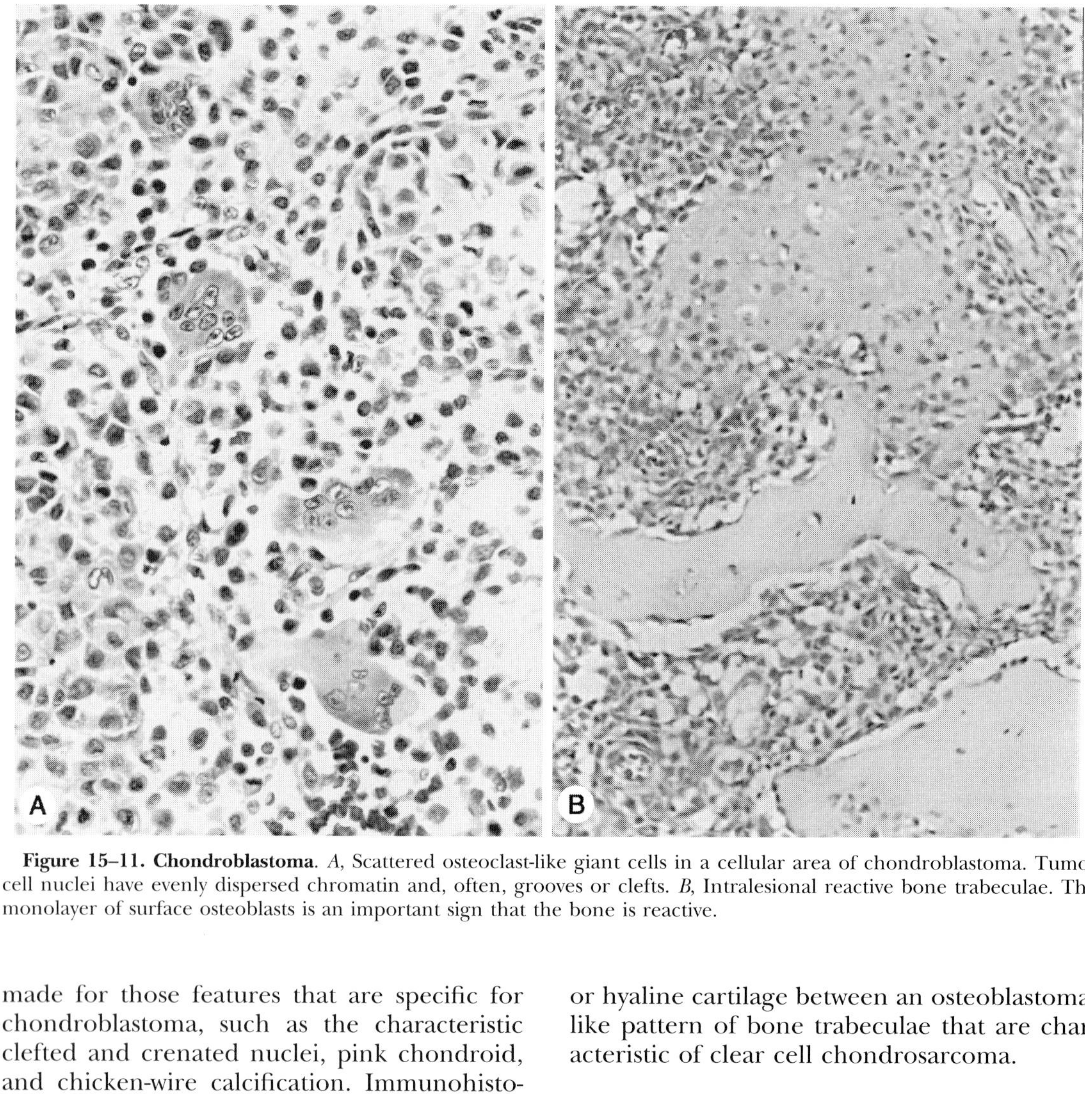

Figure 15–11. Chondroblastoma. *A,* Scattered osteoclast-like giant cells in a cellular area of chondroblastoma. Tumor cell nuclei have evenly dispersed chromatin and, often, grooves or clefts. *B,* Intralesional reactive bone trabeculae. The monolayer of surface osteoblasts is an important sign that the bone is reactive.

made for those features that are specific for chondroblastoma, such as the characteristic clefted and crenated nuclei, pink chondroid, and chicken-wire calcification. Immunohistochemistry for S-100 protein is useful in this situation, although it should be remembered that areas of chondroblastoma can stain very weakly.

Clear Cell Chondrosarcoma

Although discussed in detail in Chapter 10, clear cell chondrosarcoma deserves special mention. Like chondroblastoma, clear cell chondrosarcoma is epiphyseally located, radiologically can show a peripheral rind of sclerosis, but usually occurs in patients some 20 years older than those affected by chondroblastoma. However, it is important to be aware that clear cell chondrosarcoma can contain areas that, histologically, are virtually indistinguishable from chondroblastoma. Chondroblastomas do not show the clear cells producing chondroid or hyaline cartilage between an osteoblastoma-like pattern of bone trabeculae that are characteristic of clear cell chondrosarcoma.

Chondrosarcoma

A chondrosarcoma as cellular as a chondroblastoma would be at least a grade 2 tumor. Grade 2 chondrosarcomas display clear-cut lamellar trabecular bone entrapment caused by permeative growth and are often at least partly myxoid—features not seen in chondroblastoma. The tumor site and age of the patient are also useful distinguishing features.

Mesenchymal Chondrosarcoma

Mesenchymal chondrosarcoma is a malignant small spindle cell tumor characterized by scattered islands of hyaline cartilage (rarely seen in chondroblastoma). Mesenchymal chondrosarcomas usually lack significant numbers of OLGCs.

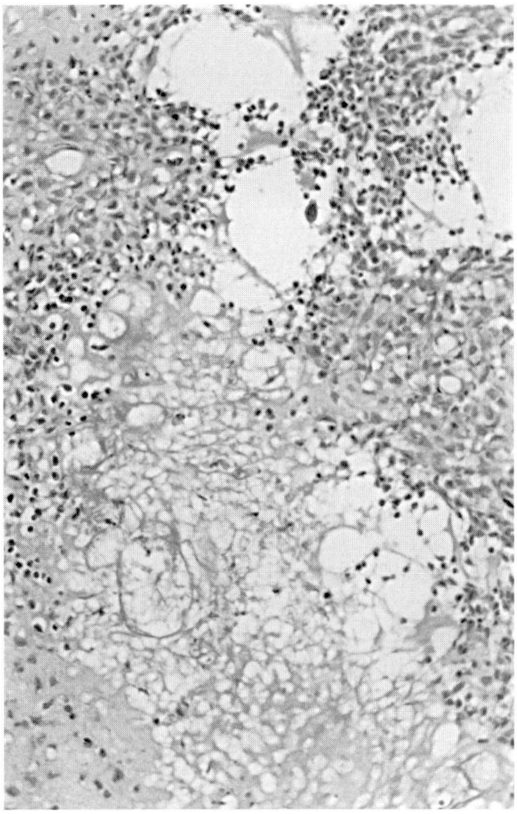

Figure 15–12. Chondroblastoma showing a small area of necrosis. Extensive necrosis, however, is uncommon and should alert one to the possibility of malignancy.

Osteosarcoma

Osteosarcomas can adopt a variety of appearances and mimic other primary bone tumors. The classic features of osteosarcoma should be sought. There are two reports of "chondroblastoma-like osteosarcoma,"[59, 60] one of which is in abstract form. If this entity exists, it appears to be an exceptionally rare disease.

Lymphoma

Lymphoma may mimic a chondroblastoma with sparse chondroid. Again, nuclear features should be carefully evaluated. Bone lymphomas are usually high-grade, B-cell non-Hodgkin's lymphomas. Lymphomas that are likely to be confused with chondroblastoma generally lack significant numbers of OLGCs and are more mitotically active. If the diagnosis of lymphoma is seriously being entertained, immunophenotyping should be carried out.

Malignant Chondroblastoma

Chondroblastomas can locally recur in about 5% of cases. However, for a lesion to be regarded as truly malignant, it should metastasize and the metastases should destroy local tissue aggressively.

There are a few reports of a malignant variant of chondroblastoma in which distant metastases have occurred. These rare cases have been reviewed,[61] and it was concluded that there were no morphologic differences between these malignant variants and their benign counterparts. Furthermore, the metastatic deposits appeared typical of benign chondroblastoma.

Treatment and Prognosis of Chondroblastoma

The first line of treatment should be simple curettage, with or without bone grafting or packing with methyl methacrylate. At times such treatment may be impossible, owing to the large size of the tumor, usually as a result of delayed presentation or diagnosis. Occasionally, aggressive growth with soft tissue extension necessitates an en bloc excision or amputation based on surgical feasibility. It is important to note that only rarely are chondroblastomas as locally aggressive as GCTs, and the diagnosis should be carefully re-evaluated if the lesion displays local aggressiveness. The worst prognosis appears to occur in patients with pelvic chondroblastomas (which also tend to be the largest). Matsuno et al.,[62] in a review of the literature of pelvic chondroblastomas, found that as many as 25% of patients died from their tumors or associated complications.

Local recurrence occurs in approximately 5% of cases. Recurettage is the preferred treatment. Radiotherapy is rarely necessary and carries the risk of post-irradiation sarcomatous transformation.

CHONDROMYXOID FIBROMA

Chondromyxoid fibroma (CMF) is a rare benign tumor (<1% of primary bone tumors) that usually affects the metaphysis of long bones in patients under 30 years old. Histologically it is a lobulated, noninvasive tumor composed of chondroid, myxoid, and fibrous tissue.

Clinical Features

Because of the rarity of this lesion, only a few substantial series of chondromyxoid fibroma have been reported.[63–66] In 1985, Kreicbergs et al.[67] reviewed the world literature of 400 cases. The reported age range is from 4 to 79 years, and approximately 65% of patients are less than 30 years old. There is a slight male predominance. Patients usually present with gradually increasing, localized pain and swelling. Half the cases affect the metaphyses around the knee, and the proximal tibial metaphysis is the single most common site. Three quarters of all cases affect the lower limbs, with approximately 20% affecting the bones of the feet. The hands and the axial skeleton are rarely involved, with the majority of axial cases affecting the pelvis and ribs.

Radiologic Features

Usually located in the metaphysis of long bones, CMF is a well demarcated, often eccentrically located, expansile, lytic lesion (Fig. 15–13*A*). Very rarely the lesion is diaphyseal. If large, there may be intralesional coarse trabeculations. There is usually a peripheral rind of sclerosis of variable thickness.

Gross Pathology

It is very rare to receive an intact, excised specimen. Most are curettaged with or without preceding biopsy. A very important feature is the complete separation of a CMF from the surrounding thickened bone. This separation aids curettage, and the surgeon may comment on the ease with which the lesion was curettaged out. The tissue is firm, slightly translucent, and has a rubbery quality. The color can vary from pale to blue-gray. Areas of cystic change and hemorrhage may be present.

Microscopic Features

Invariable Features

1. Lobularity, due to the alternating fibrous and chondromyxoid areas, is a feature of CMF seen at low magnification to a greater or lesser degree (Fig. 15–13*B*).

2. A sharp interface with the surrounding bone is present in cases subjected to vigorous curettage, although there is often no host bone present in a curettage specimen.

3. Chondromyxoid tissue is a myxoid tissue that falls short of achieving a cartilaginous appearance (see Fig. 15–13*B* and *C*). There is a variable amount of pink staining collagen present, sometimes so deficient that the matrix stains blue due to proteoglycan content. The cells do not occupy discrete lacunae, as is the case with true cartilaginous neoplasms. The nuclei can be quite large and angular, but the nucleoli are small and difficult to appreciate. The amount of chondromyxoid tissue present can vary markedly between cases.

4. Condensations of fibrous tissue are present in variable amounts, situated around, and merging with, the chondromyxoid areas (see Fig. 15–13*B* and *D*).

5. Low mitotic activity. Mitoses are always rare and should not exceed one per 50 HPF.

Variable Features

1. Microcystic degeneration of the chondromyxoid matrix often occurs (Fig. 15–14*A*). These areas may fuse to form quite large and distinctive macrocysts (often up to 1–2 mm diameter).

2. OLGCs are not a constant feature of CMF, despite the inclusion of this entity in this chapter. When present, OLGCs are situated in the peripheral condensations of fibrous tissue (Fig. 15–14*B*). They are more prominent if there is adjacent hemorrhage.

3. Matrix calcification may be seen focally in a minority of cases.

4. Ancient change in chondromyxoid fibroma may occur as degenerative nuclear features simulating malignancy, but mitotic figures will remain excessively rare.

Features Inconsistent with the Diagnosis

1. Significant mitotic activity. Mitotic rates as low as one per 5 HPF are inconsistent with the diagnosis of CMF. One should feel comfortable with the diagnosis of CMF only if the mitotic rate is around one per 50 HPF. If the mitotic rate is greater, the case should be carefully re-evaluated.

2. Cartilaginous matrix. When present, hya-

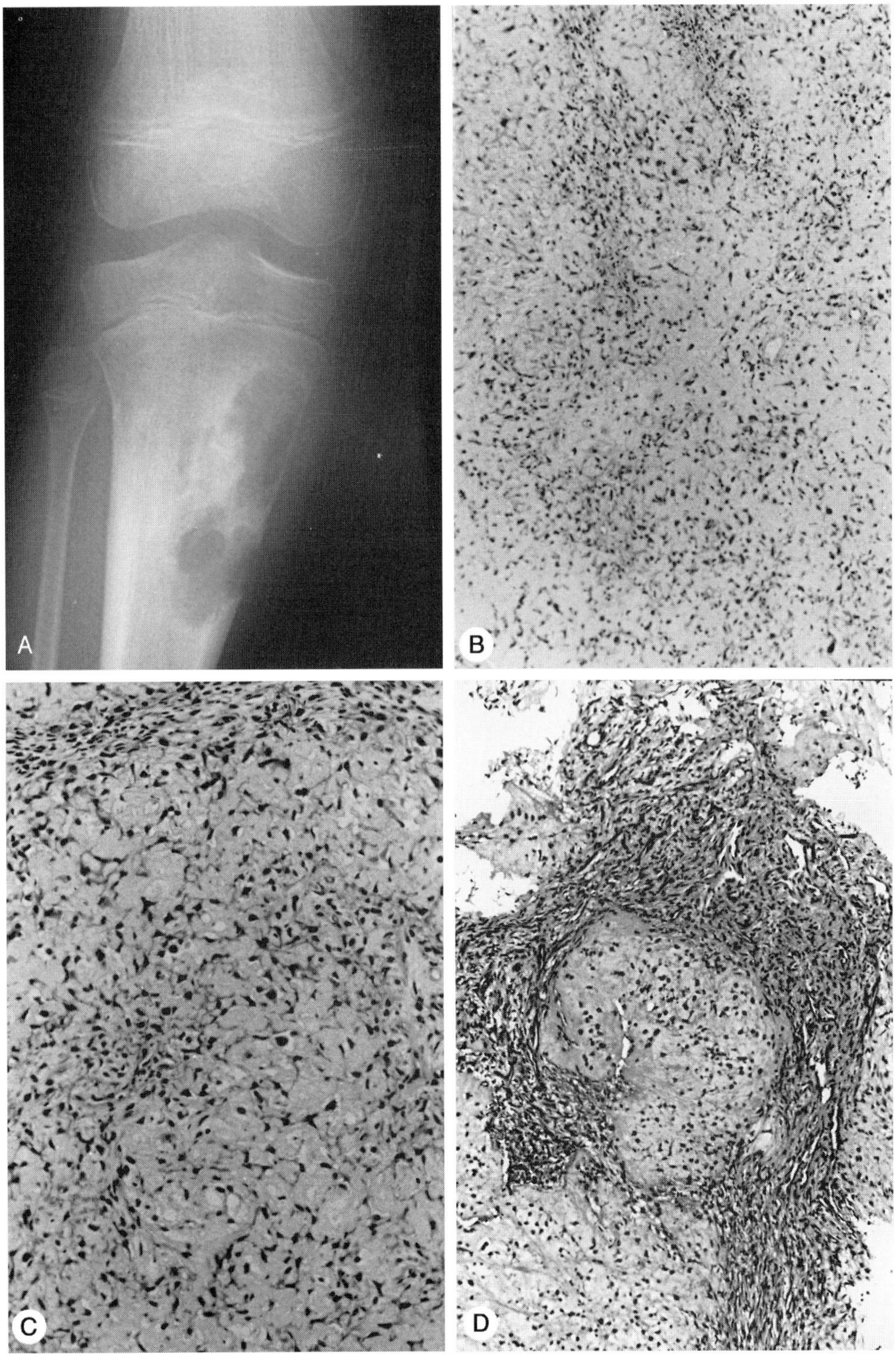

Figure 15–13. Chondromyxoid fibroma. *A*, Anterior-posterior radiograph showing an eccentrically located lesion in the proximal tibial metaphysis. The tumor is well defined and lobular, with a rim of sclerosis. The growth plates are open, but this lesion can affect patients in a wide age range. *B*, Low-power view showing vague lobularity caused by alternating cellular and hypocellular areas. *C*, Angular, often stellate cells set in a myxoid stroma that may appear chondroid. Cellularity can vary markedly, but mitoses are extremely rare. *D*, Cellular tissue merges with chondromyxoid lobules.

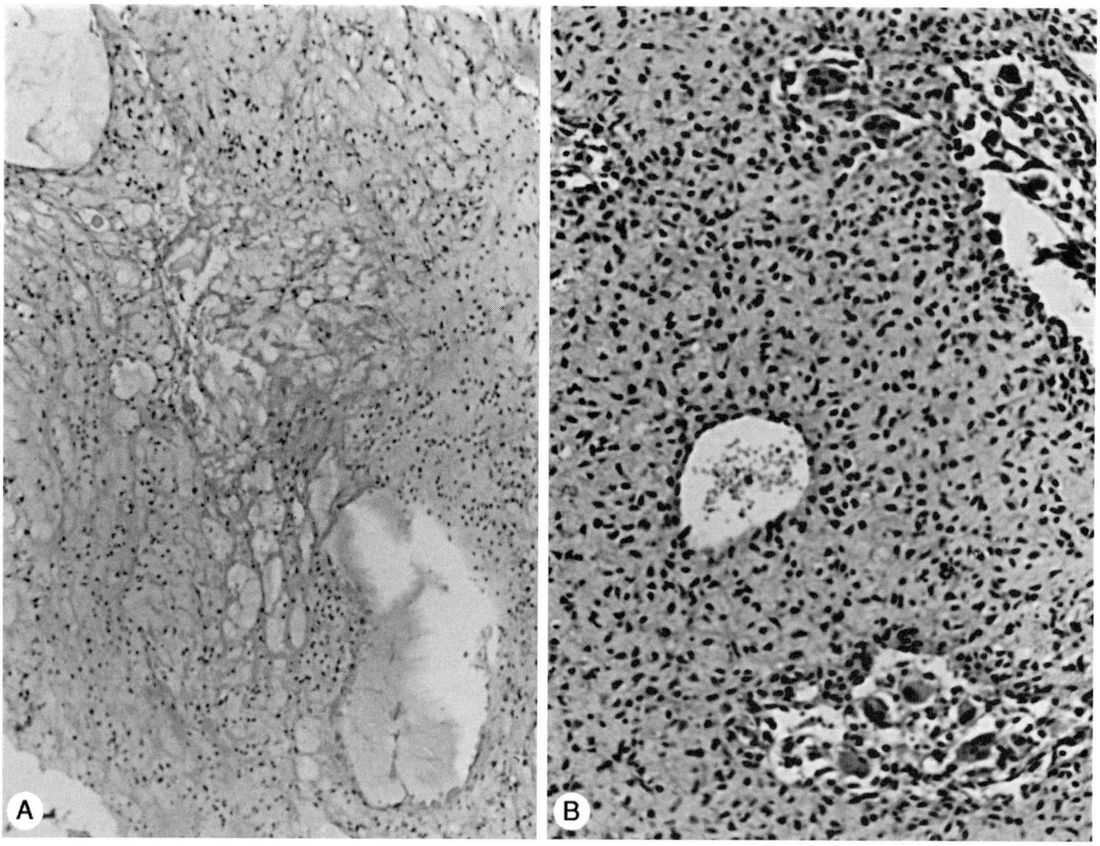

Figure 15–14. Chondromyxoid fibroma. *A*, Areas of microcystic degeneration. *B*, Clusters of osteoclast-like giant cells.

line cartilage is sparse and focal. If there is extensive, true hyaline cartilage matrix, then the lesion is likely to be either chondroma or chondrosarcoma.

3. Osteoid or bone production is reported as an extremely rare event in CMF. If present in a chondromyxoid lesion, the diagnosis is most likely an osteosarcoma (see Differential Diagnoses).

4. Permeative growth. If there is entrapped lamellar bone (i.e., a lamellar bone trabecula with lesional tissue on at least three sides) then the diagnosis is not CMF. Rarely, the presence of a pathologic fracture can cause difficulty in the interpretation of this feature.

Differential Diagnoses

Chondrosarcoma

The presence of pure hyaline cartilage should alert one to the diagnosis of a cartilaginous tumor, and additional features of chondrosarcoma should be sought. Lobules of chondrosarcoma can have a peripheral rim of fibrous tissue in some instances.

A dedifferentiated chondrosarcoma will show fields where there is a collision of a cartilage tumor (possibly myxoid) and a high-grade tumor that may be spindled. Such areas may mimic CMF. Distinction is possible by examining the spindle cell component for mitotic activity and nuclear features of malignancy.

Mesenchymal Chondrosarcoma

In contrast to CMF, the cellular phase of a mesenchymal chondrosarcoma is frankly malignant and the cartilaginous nodules are hyaline.

Low-Grade Osteosarcoma (Chondromyxoid Fibroma–Like)

This is a rare tumor and represents one of several variants of low-grade osteosarcoma. It is probably the most treacherous of the differential diagnoses of CMF. Areas may closely resemble CMF, but the important features that enable the diagnosis to be made are a radiologic pattern of permeative growth, intralesional radiopacities (i.e., bone), and cortical destruction with soft tissue involvement. A more resistant feel to the tumor on curettage and, histologically, the presence of intralesional bone should suggest the strong possibility of osteosarcoma. Both lesions may be hypercellular, but a CMF-like osteosarcoma will display nuclear atypia and usually a mitotic rate of greater than one mitosis per 5 HPF, a rate never seen in CMF.

Chondroblastoma

Chondromyxoid fibroma may contain pink chondroid matrix; however, CMF lacks the distinctive chondroblasts and the reticulin pattern surrounding individual cells in the cellular areas. Both lesions may express S-100 protein, but unlike in chondroblastoma, cytokeratin expression has not been demonstrated in CMF. A most useful distinguishing feature is the fact that CMFs are metaphyseal lesions, whereas chondroblastomas are centered on the epiphysis.

Malignant Transformation

Malignant transformation of CMF has been reported but appears to be an extremely rare occurrence, and some cases may be misdiagnosed myxoid chondrosarcomas or CMF-like osteosarcomas. The difficulty in reliably diagnosing the rare entity of CMF is highlighted by a report from the Karolinska Institute, Stockholm, where a review of nine patients with disease originally diagnosed as CMF resulted in only two fulfilling the diagnostic criteria.[67]

Treatment and Prognosis of Chondromyxoid Fibroma

The treatment of choice is simple curettage with or without bone grafting. Feldman et al.,[68] on reviewing the world literature, reported a recurrence rate of 12%. Several studies have shown that the recurrence rate is greater in young patients,[67] and tumors may recur many years after initial curettage. In a series of 27 cases, it was reported that recurrence rates were lower if bone grafting was performed.[66]

BROWN TUMOR OF HYPERPARATHYROIDISM

Hyperparathyroidism is a disease complex caused by excessive production of parathyroid hormone. One rare manifestation is the bone lesion known as brown tumor of hyperparathyroidism (BTH), a pseudotumor of bone.[69] BTH has become increasingly rare owing to the early diagnosis and treatment of hyperparathyroidism that now take place.[70, 71]

Clinical Features of Hyperparathyroidism

Patients are usually middle-aged, but people of any age can be affected. The male-to-female ratio is 1:3. Symptoms are varied and include general weakness, nausea, vomiting, weight loss, constipation, abdominal pain, polyuria, pruritus, loss of visual acuity, headaches, confusion, and, rarely, psychosis. BTH may present with bone pain, fracture, and swelling.

Radiologic Features of Hyperparathyroidism

Many of the general radiologic features of hyperparathyroid bone disease are best detected in high-resolution radiographs of the hands.

1. Subtle osteopenia may affect up to one third of patients.
2. Cortical resorption tunnels appear as linear tunnels due to osteoclasts excavating deeply through the bone. This is considered to be pathognomonic of hyperparathyroidism.
3. Multiple subperiosteal resorption concavities, and loss of the distal phalangeal cortical outline.
4. In secondary hyperparathyroidism, osteosclerotic densities are seen, especially in the spine.
5. The radiographic appearance of BTH is essentially similar to that of GCT. The lesion is lytic and sometimes expansile, often with coarse trabeculae (Fig. 15–15). There may or may not be a sclerotic rim. The important point radiologically is the location of the lesion, whether there are multiple lesions, and the presence of other radiologic features of hyperparathyroidism. If the lesion is solitary and epiphyseal, it is extremely unlikely that

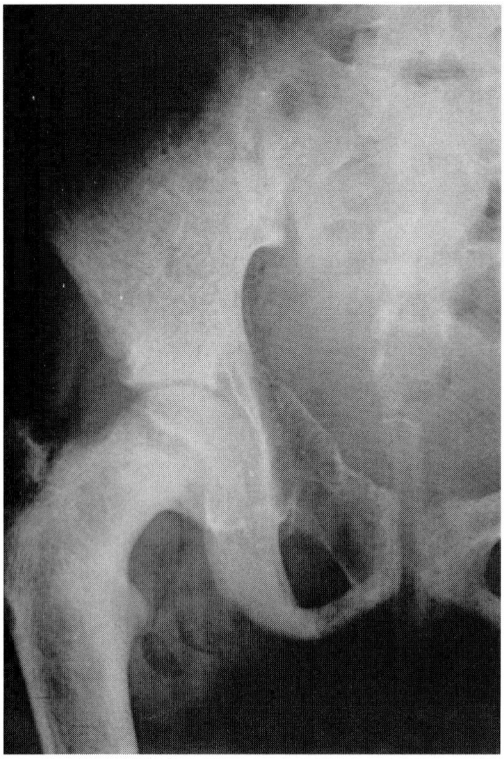

Figure 15–15. Radiograph of the right pelvis showing a brown tumor of hyperparathyroidism in a 17-year-old male patient. There is an expansile, lytic tumor in the superior pubic ramus with an intact cortex and a few intralesional bony trabeculae of persistent bone. The lesion has a similar appearance to that seen in giant cell tumor of bone. In addition, the proximal femur shows ill-defined lucencies typical of the bone changes in hyperparathyroidism.

BTH is the correct diagnosis. However, a serum calcium level should be measured whenever the histologic diagnosis of GCT is made.

Pathology

The gross appearance of brown tumors is identical to that of GCT. Histologically, the features of brown tumor overlap with those of GCT and GCRG (see relevant sections). If bone adjacent to the lesion is present, the features of hyperparathyroidism will be present. The differential diagnoses are as described in the section on GCT.

Prognosis and Treatment

The treatment is principally that of the underlying hyperparathyroidism. Small brown tumors will resolve once the underlying disorder is corrected. Large brown tumors may require local surgical treatment along similar lines as for GCT.

GIANT CELL REPARATIVE GRANULOMA

Giant cell reparative granuloma was initially described as a reactive lesion affecting the jaw bones,[72, 73] and subsequently has been described in extragnathic sites.[74–77] It is as a jaw lesion that the lesion represents a distinctive entity, composed of benign spindled and ovoid cells with scattered OLGCs and chronic inflammatory cells. A completely soft tissue (gingival) GCRG is termed a giant cell epulis (also known as peripheral GCRG).

Clinical Features

Only a few large series have been described in the jaw.[73, 78] The lesion affects the anterior portion of the mandible and maxilla, usually in young patients. Waldron and Shafer[73] found that 61% of patients were less than 20 years old, and 74% were younger than 30 years. Patients present with localized pain with or without a recognizable swelling. Females are affected twice as often as males.[73] The lesion may grow quite rapidly. An important feature is the low recurrence rate after curettage.[78]

Affected patients are usually in otherwise good health with normal biochemical indices (including calcium, phosphate, and parathyroid hormone levels).

Radiologic Features

Radiologically, GCRGs at any site are well demarcated, lytic lesions that may be divided into lobules by radiopaque septa of reactive bone (Fig. 15–16). There is usually endosteal scalloping of the cortex, and there may be expansion. Soft tissue involvement is distinctly uncommon. A rind of reactive peripheral sclerosis is often present and is best appreciated on CT imaging. The radiologic differential diagnoses of a lytic jaw lesion are apical cyst, dentigerous cyst, odontogenic tumors, giant cell tumor, and brown tumor of hyperparathyroidism.

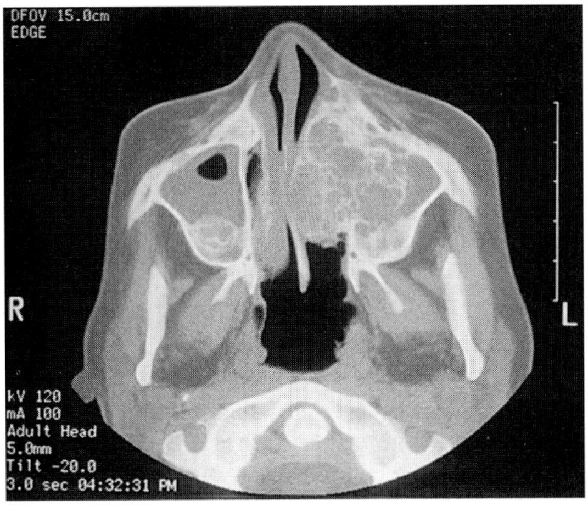

Figure 15–16. Giant cell reparative granuloma of the maxilla. Computed tomographic scan of the skull of a 14-year-old female patient, showing an expansile lesion of the maxilla with internal septation.

Gross Pathology

The lesion may be resected en bloc or may be curettaged. If a complete specimen is received, a sharp distinction from the surrounding bone is apparent. The tissue itself is soft, lobular, and tan to gray in color, with foci of hemorrhage. Yellow areas representing lipid-laden macrophages may be present.

Microscopic Pathology

Histologically, the lesion has a low-power vague lobularity (Fig. 15–17*A*) and is composed of OLGCs and ovoid and spindle-shaped cells (Fig. 15–17*B*).

Invariable Features

1. OLGCs are scattered throughout the lesion, but in a clustered distribution, and are particularly numerous around areas of hemorrhage. The OLGCs tend to be smaller than those seen in GCT, with individual cells containing up to 30 nuclei (Fig. 15–17*C*).
2. Predominantly spindle-celled with fewer ovoid fibroblast-like mononuclear cells (Fig. 15–17*D*). These cells are cytologically benign. The nuclear features can be usefully compared with those of the reactive OLGCs when examining for atypia. Mitotic rates are usually less than 4 per 10 HPF.
3. Hemorrhage and hemosiderin deposition.

Variable Features

1. Reactive bone formation may be present both peripherally and, in smaller amounts, within the lesion.
2. Especially in extragnathic sites, the deposition of a fibromyxoid stroma (also known as lacy chondroid), has been described.[33] The occurrence of this material, among other common features, has raised the possibility that this lesion is closely related to the solid variant of ABC (see Chapter 16). Unlike the typical ABC, the characteristic large blood-filled cavities are not seen in GCRG.
3. A variably intense lymphocytic infiltrate.
4. Variable amounts of collagenous matrix.

Features that Are Inconsistent with the Diagnosis

1. Nuclear atypia beyond the limits acceptable for a benign diagnosis.
2. Widespread entrapment of lamellar bone. If present, this feature is strongly suggestive of a malignant lesion.
3. Intralesional woven bone deposition may occur in GCRG, but the deposition of extensive amounts of woven bone, especially in a dense filigree pattern, should alert one to the possible diagnosis of osteosarcoma.
4. Hyaline cartilage matrix production by the tumor. However, fracture callus and lacy chondroid may be seen within these lesions.

Differential Diagnoses

Giant Cell Tumor

A few cases of true GCT of the jaw have been described.[79, 80] Radiologically, features that distinguish GCT from so-called GCRG are an aggressive growth pattern, especially marked cortical expansion, and soft tissue extension. Histologically, the OLGCs of GCT are on average larger (i.e., contain more nuclei) and are generally more evenly scattered.[81] The stromal cells of GCRG tend to be more spindled. There are cases in which the features overlap, and, in such areas, the distinction from GCT may not be possible. Fortunately, the treatment for the two conditions is the same.

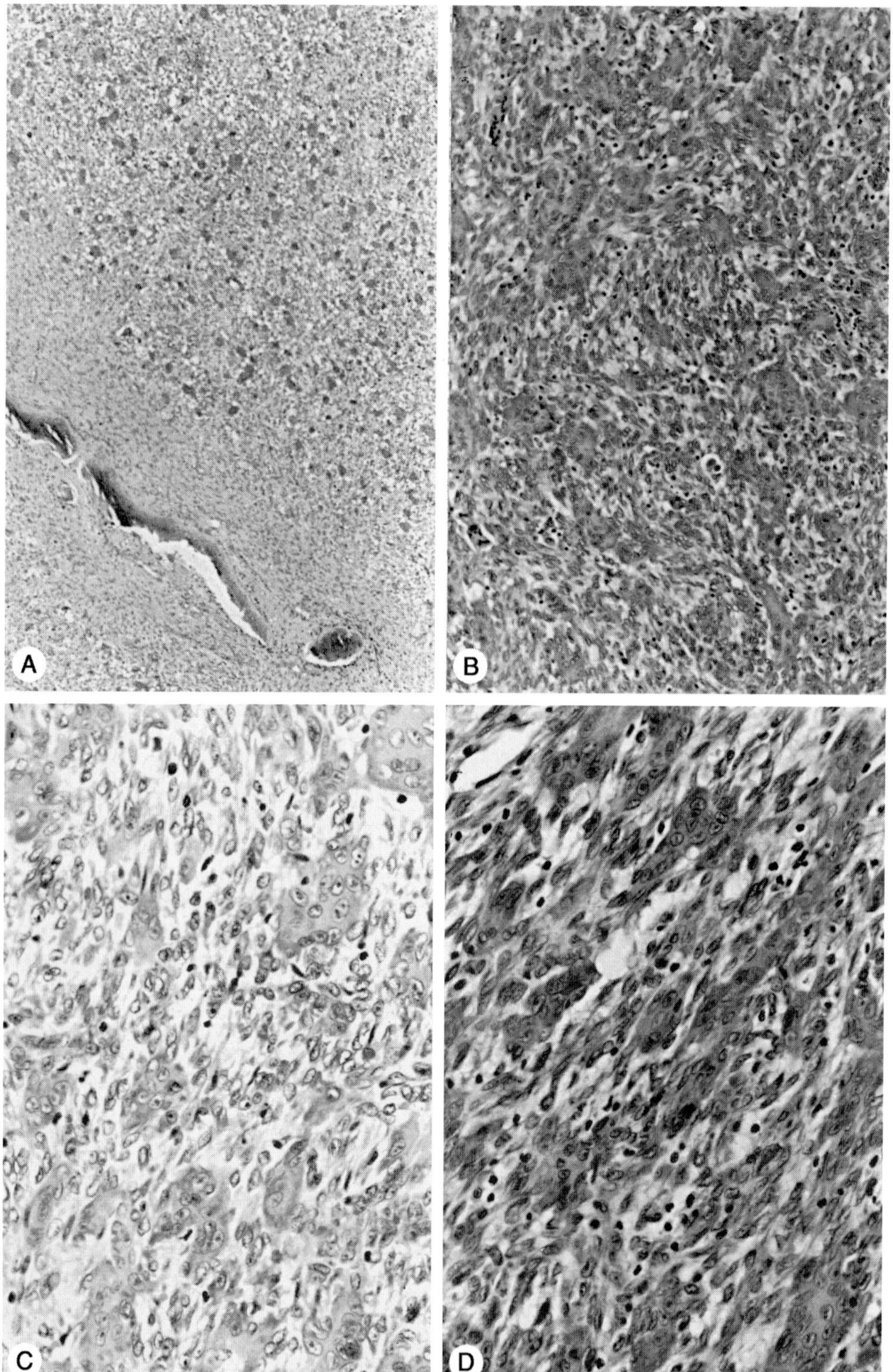

Figure 15–17. Giant cell reparative granuloma. *A,* Low-power view shows a fibro-osseous septum with many giant cells in the lesional tissue. *B,* Osteoclast-like giant cells are scattered against a background of spindled stromal cells. *C,* In this field, the features are very similar to giant cell tumor of bone. *D,* In typical areas, the stromal cells tend to be more spindle-shaped than those seen in giant cell tumor of bone.

Brown Tumor of Hyperparathyroidism

Brown tumor can affect any bone, including facial bones. The histologic appearances may be identical to those described for giant cell tumor.

Cherubism

Cherubism is a rare, hereditary condition (see Chapter 13), in which bilateral benign giant cell–rich lesions affect the molar and ramus areas of the mandible and, less commonly, the maxilla. The histopathologic appearance is indistinguishable from GCRG, but the lateral position and symmetry of the lesions should establish the diagnosis.

Nonossifying Fibroma and Benign Fibro-osseous Lesions of the Jaws

These lesions show many of the histologic features of GCRG (see Chapters 12 and 13).

Extragnathic Giant Cell Reparative Granuloma

The majority of cases of GCRG affecting non-jaw bones affect the hands and feet.[74–77] At these sites, the recurrence rate after simple curettage has been reported as between 23 and 70%. Reports of GCRG of the axial and long bones of the skeleton are less common.[33, 34] There appears to be some confusion in the literature about the nomenclature of these extragnathic benign giant cell rich lesions. Mirra[32] has argued that GCRG is identical to nonossifying fibroma (NOF), the histologic similarity being particularly convincing with the early phase of NOF. NOF has an active or formative phase, which is OLGC-rich against a background of fibroblastic spindle cells. Older NOFs show a gradual increase in fibrosis, a depletion of OLGCs, and peripheral reactive bone formation with eventual resolution. Most GCRG resemble the early phase of NOF (i.e., giant cell rich) and lesions from older patients show the same reparative features as are seen in NOF.

Oda et al.[33] reported a series of extragnathic, non-hand/foot GCRGs and argued that they should be considered as solid variants of ABC. Bertoni et al.[34] reached a similar conclusion. It is likely that all of these lesions represent morphologic variants of the same basic pathogenic process. It may be wise to retain the term GCRG for the distinctive jaw lesions, and, in an extragnathic location, to carefully consider the alternative diagnoses of solid ABC and NOF before labeling a lesion as extragnathic GCRG.

Prognosis and Treatment

Austin et al.[78] reported on 45 cases with an average follow-up of 10 years and found only two recurrences after local curettage. Waldron and Shafer,[73] however, in a series of 38 cases, found a higher recurrence rate of 16%. Recurettage of recurrent cases was curative. In some instances, it may be necessary to excise the lesion en bloc with reconstructive surgery.

REFERENCES

1. Chambers TJ: The cellular basis of bone resorption. Clin Orthop Rel Res 151:283, 1980.
2. Athanasou NA, Quinn J: Immunophenotypic differences between osteoclasts and macrophage polykaryons: Immunohistological distinction and implications for osteoclast ontogeny and function. J Clin Pathol 43:997, 1990.
3. Chambers TJ, Magnus CJ: Calcitonin alters the behaviour of isolated osteoclasts. J Pathol 136:27, 1982.
4. Grano M, Colucci S, De Bellis M, et al: New model for bone resorption study in vitro: Human osteoclast-like cells from giant cell tumors of bone. J Bone Min Res 9:1013, 1994.
5. Guccion JG, Enzinger FM: Malignant giant cell tumor of soft parts. An analysis of 32 cases. Cancer 29:1518, 1972.
6. Gaffey MJ, Lack EE, Christ ML, et al: Anaplastic thyroid carcinoma with osteoclast-like giant cells. Am J Surg Pathol 15:160, 1991.
7. Denton KJ, Stretch J, Athanasou N: Osteoclast-like giant cells in malignant melanoma. Histopathology 20:179, 1992.
8. Unni KK: Giant cell tumor (osteoclastoma). *In* Dahlin's Bone Tumors: General Aspects and Data on 11,087 Cases. 5th ed. Philadelphia, Lippincott-Raven, 1996, p 263.
9. Huvos AG: Giant cell tumor of bone. *In* Huvos AG (ed): Bone Tumors: Diagnosis, Treatment, and Prognosis. 2nd ed. Philadelphia, WB Saunders, 1991, p 429.
10. Mirra JM: Giant cell tumors. *In* Mirra JM (ed): Bone Tumors. Philadelphia, Lea & Febiger, 1989, p 941.
11. Goldenberg RR, Campbell CJ, Bonfiglio M: Giant cell tumor of bone: An analysis of two hundred and eighteen cases. J Bone Joint Surg 52A:619, 1970.
12. Campanacci M, Baldini N, Boriani S, et al: Giant cell tumor of bone. J Bone Joint Surg 69A:106, 1987.
13. McDonald DJ, Sim FH, McLeod RA, et al: Giant cell tumor of bone. J Bone Joint Surg 68A:235, 1986.
14. Mechlin MB, Kricun ME, Stead J, et al: Giant cell tumor of tarsal bones: Report of 3 cases and review of the literature. Skeletal Radiol 11:266, 1984.

15. Singhal RM, Mukhopadhyay S, Tanwar RK, et al: Case report. Giant cell tumor of metacarpals: Report of three cases. Br J Radiol 67:408, 1994.
16. Reed L, Willison CD, Schochet SS, et al: Giant cell tumor of the calvaria in a child. Case report. J Neurosurg 80:148, 1994.
17. Bertoni F, Unni KK, Beabout JW, et al: Giant cell tumor of the skull. Cancer 70:1124, 1992.
18. O'Donnell RJ, Springfield DS, Motwani HK, et al: Recurrence of giant cell tumors of the long bones after curettage and packing with cement. J Bone Joint Surg 76A:1827, 1994.
19. Kay RM, J EJ, Seeger LL, et al: Pulmonary metastases of benign giant cell tumor of bone. Six histologically confirmed cases, including one with spontaneous regression. Clin Orthop Rel Res 302:219, 1994.
20. Ladanyi M, Traganos F, Huvos AG: Benign metastasizing giant cell tumors of bone. A DNA flow cytometric study. Cancer 64:1521, 1989.
21. Peimer CA, Schiller AL, Mankin HJ, et al: Multicentric giant cell tumor of bone. J Bone Joint Surg 62A:652, 1980.
22. Potter HG, Schneider R, Ghelman B, et al: Multiple giant cell tumors and Paget disease of bone: Radiographic and clinical correlations. Radiology 180:261, 1991.
23. Merle D'Aubigne R, Tomeno B: The treatment of giant cell tumours. An analysis of 85 consecutive cases. Int Orthop 1:159, 1977.
24. Campanacci M, Giunti A, Olmi R: Giant cell tumours of bone. A study of 209 cases with long term follow up in 130. Ital J Orthop Traumatol 1:249, 1975.
25. Present D, Bertoni F, Hudson T, et al: The correlation between the radiologic staging studies and histopathologic findings in aggressive stage 3 giant cell tumor of bone. Cancer 57:237, 1986.
26. Sanjay BKS, Sim FH, Unni KK, et al: Giant-cell tumours of the spine. J Bone Joint Surg 75B:148, 1993.
27. Dahlin DC: Giant cell tumor of vertebrae above the sacrum: A review of 31 cases. Cancer 39:1350, 1977.
28. Shuffstall RM, Gregory JE: Osteoid formation in giant cell tumours of bone. Am J Pathol 29:1123, 1953.
29. Caballes RL: The mechanism of metastasis in the so-called 'benign giant cell tumor of bone.' Hum Pathol 12:762, 1981.
30. Sladden RA: Intravascular osteoclasts. J Bone Joint Surg 39B:346, 1967.
31. Panico L, Passeretti N, De Rosa N, et al: Giant cell reparative granuloma of the distal skeletal bones: A report of five cases with immunohistochemical findings. Virch Arch (A) 425:315, 1994.
32. Mirra JM: Non ossifying fibroma. *In* Mirra JM (ed): Bone Tumors. Philadelphia, Lea & Febiger, 1989, p 692.
33. Oda Y, Tsuneyoshi M, Shinohara N: 'Solid' variant of aneurysmal bone cyst (extra-gnathic giant cell reparative granuloma) in the axial skeleton and long bones. A study of its morphologic spectrum and distinction from allied giant cell lesions. Cancer 70:2642, 1992.
34. Bertoni F, Bacchini P, Capanna R, et al: Solid variant of aneurysmal bone cyst. Cancer 71:729, 1993.
35. Sulh MA, Greco MA, Jiang T, et al: Proliferation index and vascular density of giant cell tumors of bone: Are they prognostic markers? Cancer 77:2044, 1996.
36. Dahlin DC, Cupps RE, Johnson EW Jr: Giant cell tumor: A study of 195 cases. Cancer 25:1061, 1970.
37. Nascimento AG, Huvos AG, Marcove RC: Primary malignant giant cell tumor of bone: A study of eight cases and review of the literature. Cancer 44:1393, 1979.
38. Mankin HJ, Connor JF, Schiller AL, et al: Grading of bone tumors by analysis of nuclear DNA content using flow cytometry. J Bone Joint Surg 67A:404, 1985.
39. Fukunaga M, Nikaido T, Shimoda T, et al: A flow cytometric DNA analysis of giant cell tumors of bone including two cases with malignant transformation. Cancer 70:1886, 1992.
40. Ladanyi M, Traganos F, Huvos AG: Benign metastasizing giant cell tumors of bone: A DNA flow cytometric study. Cancer 64:1521, 1989.
41. Xiang J, Spanier SS, Benson NA, et al: Flow cytometric analysis of DNA in bone and soft tissue tumors using nuclear suspensions. Cancer 59:1951, 1987.
42. Bauer HCF, Kreicbergs A, Silfversward C, et al: DNA analysis in the differential diagnosis of osteosarcoma. Cancer 61:2532, 1988.
43. Mirra JM: False 'benign' giant cell tumor (GCT) ('Dedifferentiated' chondrosarcoma: false GCT variant). In Mirra JM (ed): Bone Tumors. Philadelphia, Lea & Febiger, 1989, p 565.
44. Jaffe HL, Lichtenstein L, Portis BR: Giant cell tumor of bone: Its pathologic appearance, grading, supposed variants and treatment. Arch Pathol 30:993, 1940.
45. Marcove RC, Weis LD, Vaghaiwalla MR, et al: Cryosurgery in the treatment of giant cell tumour of bone: A report of 52 consecutive cases. Cancer 41:957, 1978.
46. Gitelis S, Mallin BA, Piasecki P, et al: Intralesional excision compared with en bloc resection for giant cell tumors of bone. J Bone Joint Surg 75A:1648, 1993.
47. Boriani S, Sudanese N, Baldini N, et al: Sarcomatous degeneration of giant cell tumors. Ital J Orthop Traumatol 12:191, 1986.
48. Jaffe HL, Lichtenstein L: Benign chondroblastoma of bone: A reinterpretation of the so-called calcifying or chondromatous giant cell tumour. Am J Pathol 18:969, 1942.
49. Bloem JL, Mulder JD: Chondroblastoma: A clinical and radiological study of 104 cases. Skeletal Radiol 14:1, 1985.
50. Huvos AG, Marcove RC, Erlandson RA, et al: Chondroblastoma of bone: A clinicopathologic and electron microscopic study. Cancer 29:760, 1972.
51. Schajowicz F, Gallardo H: Epiphyseal chondroblastoma of bone: A clinico-pathological study of sixty-nine cases. J Bone Joint Surg 52B:205, 1970.
52. Springfield DS, Capanna R, Gherlinzoni F, et al: Chondroblastoma: A review of seventy cases. J Bone Joint Surg 67A:748, 1985.
53. Turcotte RE, Kurt AM, Sim FH, et al: Chondroblastoma. Hum Pathol 24:944, 1993.
54. Huvos AG: Chondroblastoma and clear cell chondrosarcoma. *In* Huvos AG (ed): Bone Tumors. Diagnosis, Treatment, and Prognosis. 2nd ed. Philadelphia, WB Saunders, 1991, p 295.
55. Mirra JM: Chondroblastoma. *In* Mirra JM (ed): Bone Tumors. Philadelphia, Lea & Febiger, 1989, p 589.
56. Weatherall PT, Maale GE, Mendelsohn DB, et al: Chondroblastoma: Classic and confusing appearance at MR imaging. Radiology 190:467, 1994.
57. Oxtoby JW, Davies AM: MRI characteristics of chondroblastoma. Clin Radiol 51:22, 1996.
58. Semmelink HJF, Pruszczynski M, Tilburg AWV, et al: Cytokeratin expression in chondroblastomas. Histopathology 16:257, 1990.
59. Mirra JM: Osseous tumors of intramedullary origin. *In* Mirra JM (ed): Bone Tumors. Philadelphia, Lea & Febiger, 1989, p 331.
60. Inwards C: Chondroblastoma-like osteosarcoma: A report of eight cases. Lab Invest 72:A7, 1995.

61. Kyriakos M, Land VJ, Penning HL, et al: Metastatic chondroblastoma: Report of a fatal case with a review of the literature on atypical, aggressive and malignant chondroblastoma. Cancer 55:1770, 1985.
62. Matsuno T, Hasegawa I, Masuda T: Chondroblastoma arising in the triradiate cartilage. Report of two cases with review of the literature. Skeletal Radiol 16:216, 1987.
63. Unni KK: Chondromyxoid fibroma. *In* Unni KK (ed): Dahlin's Bone Tumors. General Aspects and Data on 11,087 Cases, 5th ed. Philadelphia, Lippincott-Raven Publishers, 1996, p 59.
64. Huvos AG: Chondromyxoid fibroma. *In* Huvos AG (ed): Bone Tumors: Diagnosis, Treatment, and Prognosis. 2nd ed. Philadelphia, WB Saunders, 1991, p 319.
65. Mirra JM: Chondromyxoid fibroma. *In* Mirra JM (ed): Bone Tumors. Philadelphia, Lea & Febiger, 1989, p 623.
66. Gherlinzoni F, Rock M, Picci P: Chondromyxoid fibroma. The experience at the Instituto Ortopedica Rizzoli. J Bone Joint Surg 65A:198, 1983.
67. Kreicbergs A, Lonnquist PA, Willems J: Chondromyxoid fibroma. A review of the literature and a report of our own experience. Acta Pathol Mic Sc 93:189, 1985.
68. Feldman F, Hecht HL, Johnston AD: Chondromyxoid fibroma of bone. Radiology 94:249, 1970.
69. Lewis MM, Chew FSK, Scully RE, et al: A 74 year old woman with hyperparathyroidism and an osteolytic lesion in the humerus: Primary hyperparathyroidism with brown tumor of the right humerus. N Engl J Med 328:1031, 1993.
70. Heath H, Hodgson SF, Kennedy MA: Primary hyperparathyroidism: Incidence, morbidity and potential economic impact in a community. N Engl J Med 302:189, 1980.
71. Wilder RM: Hyperparathyroidism: Tumor of the parathyroid glands associated with osteitis fibrosa. Endocrinology 13:231, 1929.
72. Jaffe HL: Giant cell reparative granuloma, traumatic bone cyst, and fibrous (fibro-osseous) dysplasia of the jawbones. J Oral Surg Oral Med Oral Pathol 6:159, 1953.
73. Waldron CA, Shafer WG: The central giant cell reparative granuloma of the jaws: An analysis of 38 cases. Am J Clin Pathol 45:437, 1966.
74. Lorenzo JC, Dorfman HD: Giant-cell reparative granuloma of the short tubular bones of the hands and feet. Am J Surg Pathol 4:551, 1980.
75. Wold LE, Dobyns JH, Swee RG, et al: Giant-cell reparative granuloma of the small bones of the hands and feet. Am J Surg Pathol 10:491, 1986.
76. Glass TA, Mills SE, Fechner RE, et al: Giant cell reparative granuloma of the hands and feet. Radiology 149:65, 1983.
77. Picci P, Baldini S, Campanacci M: Giant cell reparative granuloma and other giant cell lesions of the hands and feet. Skeletal Radiol 15:415, 1986.
78. Austin LT, Dahlin DC, Royer RQ: Giant cell reparative granuloma and related conditions affecting the jawbones. Oral Surgery 12:1285, 1959.
79. Sentilles C, Michaud J: Giant cell lesions of the maxilla. The diagnostic difficulties. Rev Stomatol Chir Maxillofac 87:102, 1986.
80. Chuong R, Kaban LB, Kozakewich H, et al: Central giant cell lesions of the jaws: A clinico-pathologic study. J Oral Maxil Surg 44:708, 1986.
81. Abrams, Shear M: A histological comparison of the giant cells in the central giant cell reparative granuloma of the jaws and the giant cell tumour of long bone. J Oral Pathol Med 3:217, 1974.

Chapter

16

VASCULAR NEOPLASMS OF BONE

ALAN J. DARBY

The classification of vascular tumors of bone has failed to keep pace with that of tumors arising in soft tissues.[1, 2] In particular, the diagnostic term *hemangioendothelioma* has been applied to tumors ranging the whole gamut from benign to highly malignant endothelial neoplasms. As a result of this, much of the published work on the radiology and pathology of vascular lesions of bone is difficult to interpret. This has been the source of considerable confusion and has resulted in a lack of clear guidelines for the prognosis and treatment of these tumors.

In this chapter, as suggested by O'Connell et al.,[3] an attempt will be made to apply the World Health Organisation (WHO) soft tissue tumor classification where possible. There is an urgent need for this to be done by investigators with large series of bone tumors so that a better understanding of the clinical usefulness of such an approach can be assessed.

BENIGN TUMORS

Hemangioma

Clinical and Radiologic Features

Although reported as common at autopsy, hemangiomas are only occasionally symptomatic. Of the symptomatic cases, half are in the skull and nearly one quarter are in the vertebrae.[4] It is possible, however, that some of the vertebral lesions seen at autopsy are simply localized areas of vascular ectasia. Rarely, hemangiomas may be located on the cortical surface of the bone,[5] where they may mimic the radiologic appearance of an osteoid osteoma. Lysis of bone occurs, but the residual trabeculae are thickened, giving rise to the striations seen on radiographs (Fig. 16–1). It is said that this radiologic appearance may distinguish multiple hemangiomas from the more serious condition of hemangiomatosis, which lacks striations and is more diffuse on radiographs.[6]

Pathologic Features

Histologically, the majority of hemangiomas are cavernous in type, although areas of capillary hemangioma are often present (Fig. 16–2). Tumors containing thick-walled arteries and veins have also been described.[7] The vessels may be more widely spaced than in most soft tissue angiomas and, in a small biopsy specimen, can be difficult to distinguish from localized vascular ectasia. In such cases, the radiographic appearances are most helpful.

Epithelioid Hemangioma

Although Rosai's original account of histiocytoid (now better known as epithelioid) hemangiomas encompassed tumors in bone,[8] his concept has yet to gain wide acceptance in the world of bone tumors. It now seems likely that many of the tumors originally reported in the

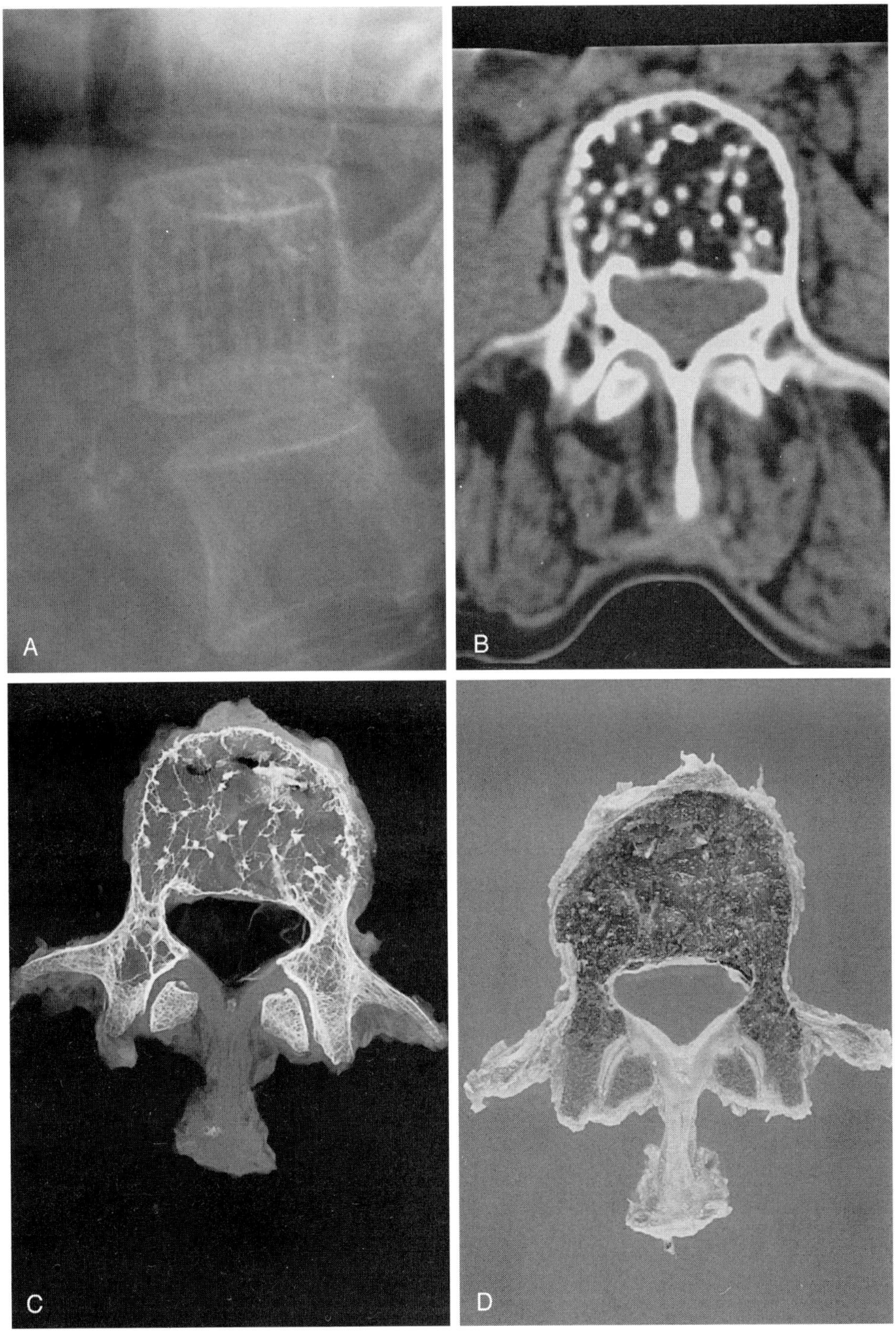

Figure 16–1. Hemangioma of vertebral body. *A*, The plain film shows a striated pattern due to thickening of vertically oriented residual bone trabeculae. *B*, The computed tomographic scan shows these sclerotic trabeculae in cross section. This is confirmed by the fine detail radiograph *(C)* of a 4 mm slice *(D)* of the same vertebral body removed at autopsy.

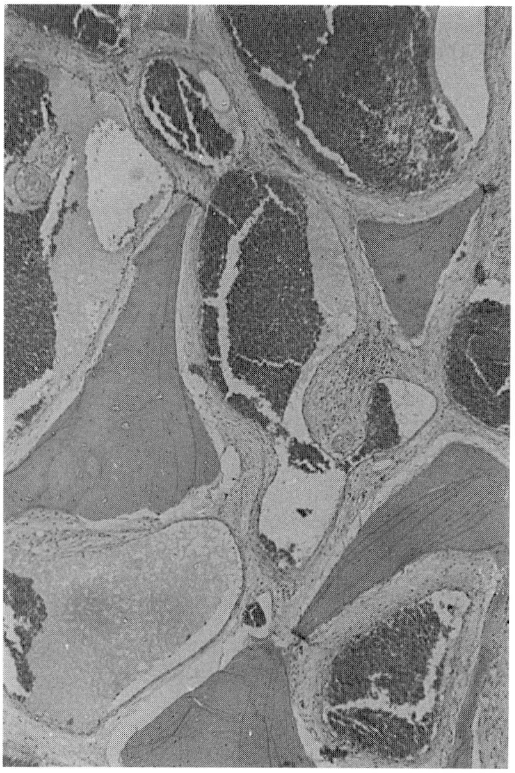

Figure 16–2. Hemangioma. Photomicrograph showing cavernous blood vessels infiltrating the marrow between sclerotic trabeculae.

literature as low-grade malignant hemangioendotheliomas or angiosarcomas, were in fact epithelioid hemangiomas, and this is borne out by their good prognosis.

Clinical and Radiologic Features

O'Connell et al.[3] reported a series of 12 patients with epithelioid hemangioma, ranging in age from 24 to 74 years. Three of the tumors had originally been classified as low-grade angiosarcomas. On plain radiographs, all the tumors were predominantly lytic with well-defined sclerotic margins (Fig. 16–3*A*). They varied in size from 2.5 to 15.0 cm and one case was multifocal. Although the follow-up period for these tumors was short, only one case recurred and none behaved aggressively.

Pathologic Features

Microscopically these tumors differ from ordinary hemangiomas by virtue of prominent epithelioid endothelial cells with abundant eosinophilic cytoplasm (Fig. 16–3*B*). The nuclei of the endothelial cells are often irregular and folded, a feature that led to Rosai's original use of the term "histiocytoid." Some tumors may be rich in eosinophils and plasma cells, and similar cases may have been reported previously as angiolymphoid hyperplasia of bone.[9] Immunohistochemistry reveals positive labeling for endothelial markers and, in most cases, for epithelial markers also.

Prognosis

The behavior of epithelioid hemangioma appears to be no different from that of classic cavernous or capillary hemangioma. However, it warrants separate recognition to distinguish it from epithelioid hemangioendothelioma and angiosarcoma. When Stout[10] described the histologic features of malignant vascular tumors, which he called hemangioendothelioma, the defining criterion was the presence of plump, atypical endothelial cells lining vascular channels. It is probable that many of his cases and those described by later authors as low-grade malignant tumors would be termed epithelioid hemangioma using current nomenclature. As a result of this, past papers on the prognosis of vascular tumors are difficult to assess, and the precise nature of the tumors under discussion must always be kept in mind.

Pyogenic Granuloma

Lesions similar in appearance to the pyogenic granuloma (lobular capillary hemangioma) of skin have rarely been described in bone.[5]

Lymphangioma

Purely intraosseous solitary lymphangioma of bone is extremely rare. Distinction on purely histologic grounds from hemangioma may be impossible, although ultrastructural differences have been described.[11] The surgeon's account of the type of fluid contained within the vessels may be the most helpful diagnostic feature. In practical terms, the distinction is of little clinical importance. Jumbelic et al.[12] reported an example involving most of the left humerus in a 2-year-old girl that responded well to curettage and bone grafting. Other cases have been described in the tibia,[13] spine,[14] and calvarium.[15]

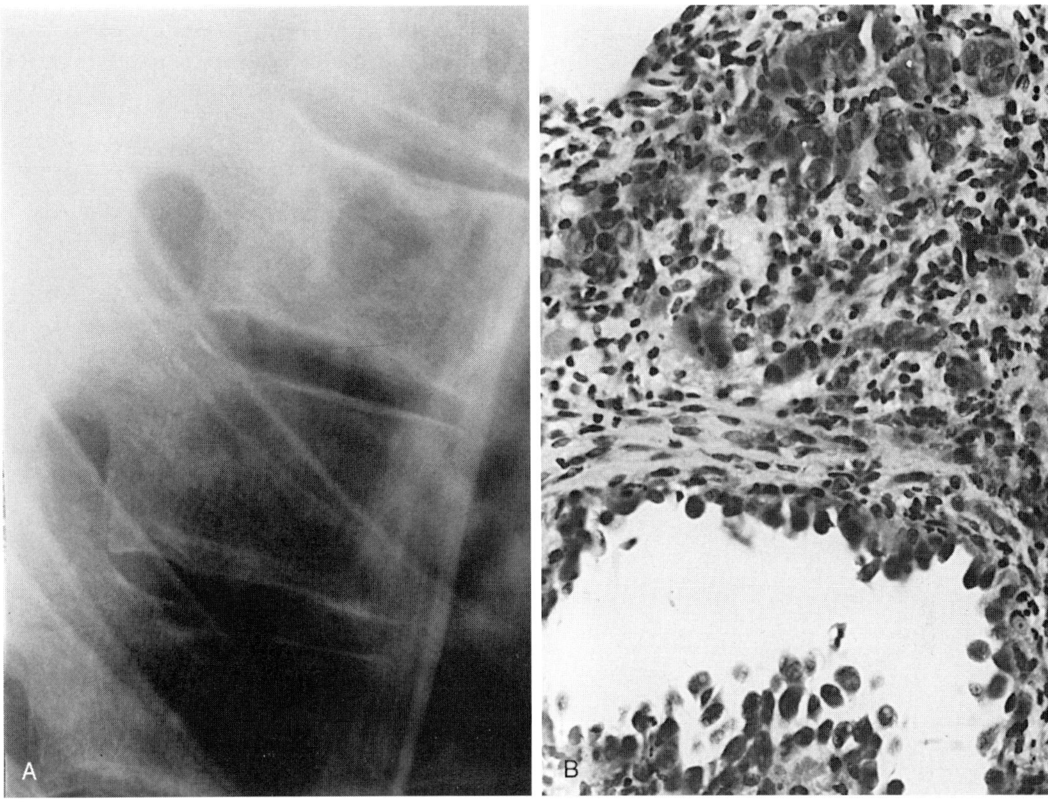

Figure 16–3. Epithelioid hemangioma. *A*, Plain radiograph showing an irregular lytic lesion with sclerotic margins. *B*, Photomicrograph showing a cavernous blood vessel lined by prominent epithelioid endothelial cells. Elsewhere, cords and clumps of endothelial cells lack vascular lumina. Inflammatory cells, including eosinophils, are prominent within the stroma. (The patient was alive and well with no evidence of recurrence 9 years following diagnosis.)

Angiomatosis of Bone

Clinical and Radiologic Features

Angiomatosis of bone is an abnormal proliferation of blood vessels, lymphatics, or both, which nearly always presents in childhood. Commonly, soft tissues are also involved and there may be generalized hypertrophy of the affected area. The skeletal lesions may be an asymptomatic incidental finding or may present with pain and or fracture.

The nomenclature of angiomatosis is confusing because a number of different clinicopathologic entities of variable prognosis have been included under this heading. Because of the difficulties in assessing prognosis and distinguishing angiomatosis from multiple hemangiomas of bone, or so-called cystic angiomatosis, Devaney et al.[16] have attempted to clarify the situation. They specify involvement of soft tissues as an essential component of the condition they call *skeletal-extraskeletal angiomatosis* (Fig. 16–4). This parallels angiomatosis of soft tissues, which is required to involve more than one tissue type or anatomic region. They use the term *cystic angiomatosis of bone* for multifocal lesions confined to the skeleton.

Cystic angiomatosis is essentially a radiologic term. In classic radiology, the hemangioma is a poorly defined lytic lesion lacking a sclerotic margin but with accentuation of the residual trabecular pattern. In hemangiomatosis involving the skeleton, the radiologic features are variable but may be purely lytic with clearly defined sclerotic margins. The reluctance of radiologists to accept such lesions as multicentric hemangiomas has led to the use of the term cystic angiomatosis to distinguish them from classic angiomas and, when evidence of soft tissue involvement is lacking, from skeletal-extraskeletal angiomatosis. From a pathologic viewpoint, however, it is clear that some such cases are indeed hemangiomas. It may be that cavernous hemangiomas account for the radiologically diagnosed hemangiomas and that cystic angiomatosis represents either skel-

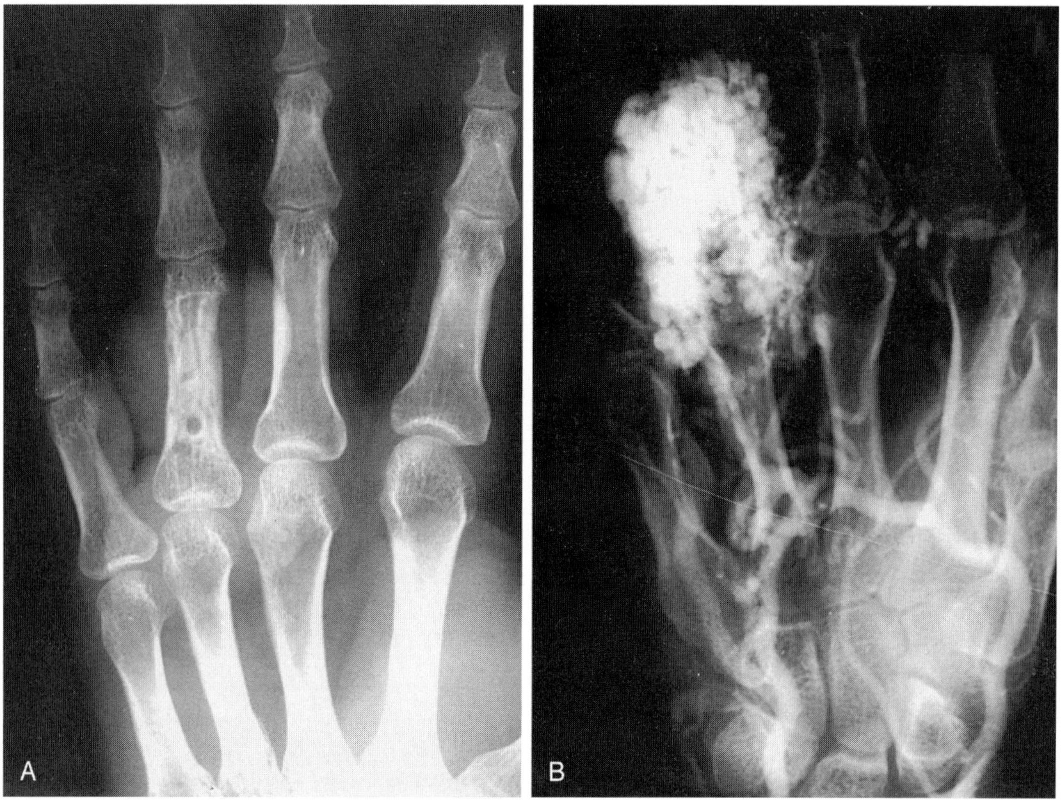

Figure 16–4. Skeletal-extraskeletal hemangiomatosis. *A*, The plain radiograph shows a mixed lytic and sclerotic lesion of the proximal phalanx with adjacent soft tissue swelling. *B*, Arteriography demonstrates involvement of bone and soft tissues.

etal-extraskeletal angiomatosis or multicentric epithelioid hemangiomas or hemangioendotheliomas. Further clarification of this point is needed.

Pathologic Features

The microscopic appearances are those of angiomas at any site. Cavernous or capillary spaces usually predominate. A few cases are composed mainly of thick-walled muscular vessels, and these may be true developmental abnormalities rather than neoplastic in nature. The identification of a lymphatic component is aided by the presence of small clusters of stromal lymphocytes.

Complications and Prognosis

The principal complication of skeletal involvement is fracture. Morbidity appears to increase in parallel with the extent of soft tissue involvement. Rare complications include malignant change and the Kasabach-Merritt syndrome.[17] The Kasabach-Merritt syndrome may also be seen in Klippel-Trenaunay syndrome, but here the skeletal changes are limited to hypertrophy and there is no true vascular involvement of bone.[18] Tumor-associated rickets has also been reported.[19]

Disappearing Bone Disease

The term *disappearing bone disease,* also known as massive osteolysis, vanishing bone disease, phantom bone disease, Gorham's disease, and Gorham-Stout disease, is a source of some confusion. These pathologically imprecise terms refer to what is probably a variant of angiomatosis and are based as much on clinical and radiologic findings as the underlying histology. Gorham et al.,[20] in 1954, described two cases in which the major pathologic change appears to have been hemangiomatosis of bone. One of the patients, a 16-year-old boy, also suffered a chylothorax presumably due to concomitant lymphatic involvement. The following year, Gorham and Stout[21] reviewed 24 cases in the literature and described the histology of eight cases, including Gorham's original two cases. They concluded that in all eight cases, the lysis of bone was accompanied by a hemangiomatous proliferation of blood vessels with varying degrees of fibrosis and that this could also have a lymphangiomatous component. Ensuing accounts in the literature appear to have included a somewhat broader range of conditions, but useful reviews of the clinical, radiologic, and pathologic aspects of the syndrome have been published recently.[22, 23]

Clinical and Radiologic Features

This disease usually presents in one bone, or part of a bone, and immediately adjacent soft tissue, but with the passage of time it spreads to adjacent areas of the skeleton. Significant extraskeletal involvement is rare, and eventually, sometimes after many years, the condition tends to stabilize. At the time of presentation, most patients are children or teenagers. The role of radiation therapy in halting the progression of the condition appears promising but has yet to be fully evaluated.

The radiologic presentation is usually that of an ill-defined lucency. This may be central in location, or resorption of bone may progress inward from the periosteal surface. Adjacent bones are eventually involved in the majority of cases.

Pathologic Features

Histologically, the syndrome cannot be distinguished from angiomatosis but is remarkable for its ability to absorb large areas of cortical and cancellous bone. In the early stages the lesion is highly vascular, but later the bone may be reduced to only a thin fibrous or fibrovascular remnant.

Lymphangiomatosis

As mentioned earlier, angiomatosis of bone commonly has a lymphatic component. In childhood, lymphatics may be the only or dominant type of vessel and in these cases the term *lymphangiomatosis* may be used.

Cohen and Craig[24] described the case of an 8-year-old girl who presented with multiple, progressive, destructive lesions of bone and died following spinal surgery. Macroscopically, there were multilocular cystic areas of bone destruction. Histology showed these to be lymphatic in origin. In addition there was involvement of the spleen and soft tissues. Since then, a number of case reports and small series have been reported.[25, 26] Like hemangiomatosis, prognosis appears to be related principally to the extent of visceral involvement.

A distinctive variant of lymphangiomatosis seems to be confined to boys and involves only the limbs.[27] It has a good prognosis.

Glomus Tumor

Although glomus bodies occur in the medullary cavity of bone, primary intraosseous glomus tumors are extremely rare. The most common site is within the phalanges, but it is not always clear from published reports whether the tumor was truly intraosseous or merely eroding bone from without. Kobayashi et al.[28] reported a case in the sacrum and reviewed 26 further cases in the literature. Histologically, these tumors are identical to their soft tissue counterparts.

INTERMEDIATE TUMORS

Epithelioid Hemangioendothelioma

Clinical and Radiologic Features

Following its description in the soft tissues,[29] epithelioid hemangioendothelioma was rapidly identified in other tissues, including bone. A series of 14 cases, drawn from a group of 29 malignant vascular tumors of bone, was described in 1986 by Tsuneyoshi et al.,[30] who also drew attention to previous cases described under the name of *myxoid angioblastoma*. Interestingly, although nine of his patients had multifocal tumors, only one of the 14 had extraosseous disease.

A larger series of 40 cases was recently reported from the Mayo Clinic.[31] The tumor was most common in the second decade but occurred throughout the age range. The great majority of tumors were in the lower limb and pelvis. It is noteworthy that 22 of the 40 patients had multiple tumors and 7 patients had additional extraskeletal tumors. In both series, there was a tendency for multicentric tumors

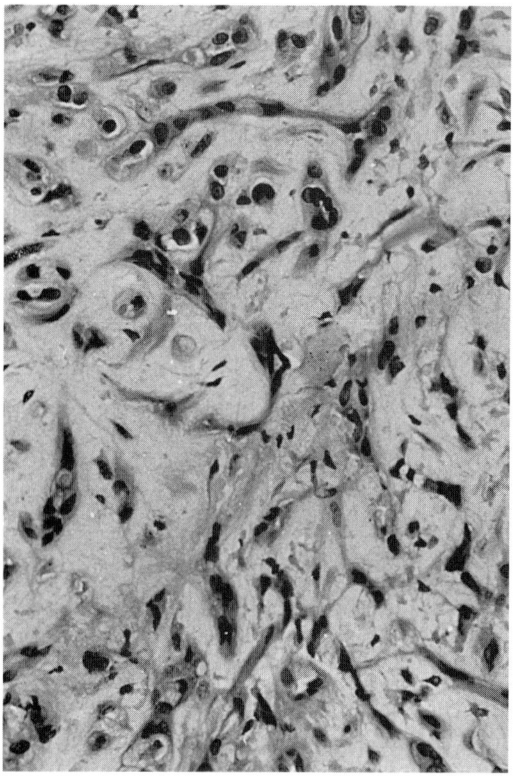

Figure 16–5. Epithelioid hemangioendothelioma. Photomicrograph showing a myxoid, sometimes hyaline, matrix containing attenuated cords and clusters of endothelial cells. Cytoplasmic vacuoles can be seen in some cells. (From a patient presenting with multiple lytic lesions of the pelvis. She later died with systemic involvement of lungs and liver.)

of bone to involve a particular anatomic area. The prognosis depended mainly on the presence or absence of visceral involvement and could not be predicted from histologic features.

Radiologically, these tumors present as lucent lesions with surrounding sclerosis, which can be surprisingly extensive. A periosteal reaction is absent or slight, but cortical expansion or destruction and soft tissue extension is not uncommon.

Pathologic Features

Histologically, the hallmark of the tumor is the presence of epithelioid endothelial cells in a myxoid matrix (Fig. 16–5). Recognizable vascular channels may be hard to find or absent, but all tumors contain cells with cytoplasmic vacuolation representing primitive lumen formation. The cells are commonly arranged in small nests or cords. The appearance may easily be confused with metastatic carcinoma or a myxoid cartilaginous tumor, but immunohistochemistry for endothelial markers is almost always positive.

A wide range of cellular pleomorphism and differentiation is possible in epithelioid hemangioendothelioma, and in some cases it may be difficult to distinguish from epithelioid hemangioma at one end of the spectrum and angiosarcoma at the other.

Spindle Cell Hemangioendothelioma

Spindle cell hemangioendothelioma of bone has not been reported. However, it has been claimed that this is the type of cutaneous hemangioma found in Maffucci's syndrome (Fig. 16–6).[32] This has been the author's experience with three hemangiomas from a single patient with Maffucci's syndrome.

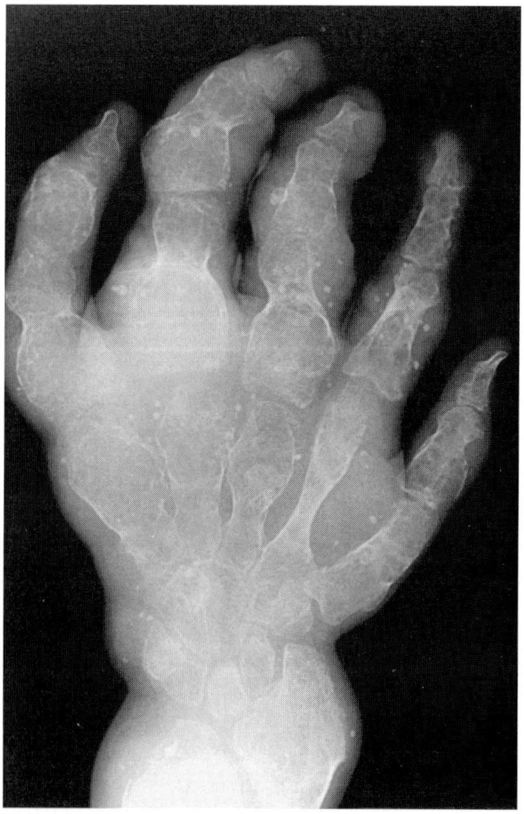

Figure 16–6. Radiograph of the hand of a 17-year-old boy with Maffucci's syndrome. Multiple chondromas are present. Calcified phleboliths mark the sites of spindle cell hemangioendotheliomas within the soft tissues.

MALIGNANT TUMORS

Angiosarcoma

In a series of 99 cases of angiosarcoma in Japan, only 4 were primary bone sarcomas but 44 tumors metastasized to bone.[33] In the literature, *hemangioendothelioma* is often used synonymously with *angiosarcoma of bone,* but many so-called low- or intermediate-grade hemangioendotheliomas probably include examples of epithelioid hemangiomas or epithelioid hemangioendotheliomas. This must be borne in mind when reading published series of vascular tumors of bone,[34–37] and only high-grade tumors should be regarded as full-fledged angiosarcomas. Such tumors have a poor prognosis.

Clinical and Radiologic Features

Angiosarcomas occur fairly uniformly across a wide age range but are rare in patients less than 30 years of age. Radiologic features are those of a lytic, poorly defined tumor proceeding to cortical destruction and invasion of soft tissues. Some tumors are multifocal.

Pathologic Features

The histologic appearance is that of a vasoformative tumor with vascular spaces lined by large pleomorphic endothelial cells (Fig. 16–7). Multilayering of cells and papillary structures may be present. Areas with minimal or no evidence of vascular differentiation are common. These undifferentiated areas may consist of spindle cells or sheets of epithelioid cells mimicking metastatic carcinoma.

Epithelioid Angiosarcoma

Epithelioid angiosarcoma[38] of bone has not been reported as such but is probably included with some of the high-grade tumors in the literature.

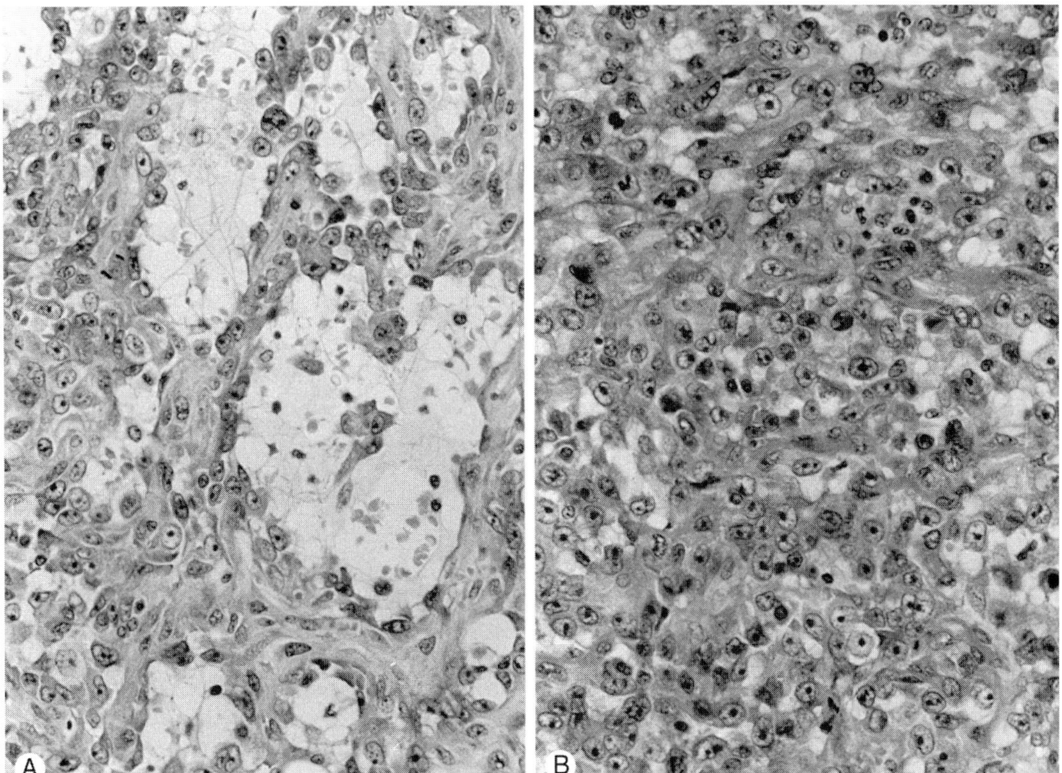

Figure 16–7. Angiosarcoma. *A,* Irregular vascular spaces are lined by pleomorphic endothelial cells with prominent nucleoli. Occasional papillary structures are present. *B,* In other areas from the same tumor, solid sheets of cells with an "epithelioid" appearance are seen.

Hemangiopericytoma

Clinical and Radiologic Features

Hemangiopericytoma of bone is rare. Patients of all ages are described, but the peak incidence is in the fourth and fifth decades. Its most common sites are the pelvis and lower limbs. Metastases to bone are seen more often than primary skeletal tumors. Of 94 patients with hemangiopericytoma of the central nervous system, bone was the most frequent site for metastasis.[39]

Radiographs show an irregular area of osteolysis, usually associated with cortical destruction and soft tissue extension.

Pathologic Features

The histologic features are identical to hemangiopericytoma of soft tissues. Monotonous spindle cells surround capillaries arranged in a branching "deer antler" pattern. Tumors may be graded according to nuclear pleomorphism and mitotic activity, but this is of limited value.

A major problem in diagnosis is the presence of hemangiopericytoma-like areas in other tumors, particularly mesenchymal chondrosarcoma of bone (Fig. 16–8). This possibility, or that of a metastasis, should always be considered as more likely than so rare a tumor as primary hemangiopericytoma of bone.

Prognosis

Tang et al.[40] reported four cases and reviewed a further 41 tumors in the world literature. They concluded that histologic grade correlated with prognosis and that late recurrence and distant metastases were common. Irrespective of grade, they are of the opinion that all osseous hemangiopericytomas should be regarded as malignant.

Kaposi's Sarcoma

Bone involvement has been reported in less than 10% of non-AIDS associated Kaposi's sarcoma in Africa.[41] Most, if not all, of these cases appear to have been by direct extension of cutaneous lesions. However, primary involvement of marrow has been reported in patients with and without AIDS.[42–44]

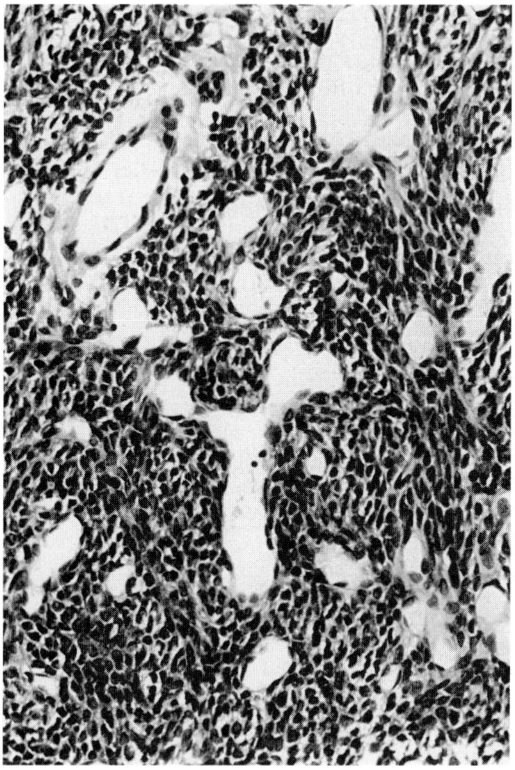

Figure 16–8. Hemangiopericytomatous area from a mesenchymal chondrosarcoma of bone.

PSEUDOVASCULAR LESIONS

Telangiectatic Osteosarcoma

Telangiectatic osteosarcoma has been well known as a variant of osteosarcoma since the paper from the Mayo Clinic in 1976.[45] In spite of this, these rare tumors may still be confused with aneurysmal bone cyst or even hemangioma. This is particularly the case if, as rarely happens, the tumor is accompanied by secondary aneurysmal bone cyst formation.

Clinical and Radiologic Features

The proportion of osteosarcomas reported as telangiectatic varies widely, but if the diagnosis is confined to tumors that radiologically are entirely lytic, it is undoubtedly rare. The clinical features are no different from those of conventional osteosarcoma. It is lytic on radiographs, usually with a permeative margin, cortical destruction, and a soft tissue extension. On occasion, it may resemble aneurysmal bone cyst and, like aneurysmal bone cyst, fluid-fluid levels are seen on computed tomography.

Pathologic Features

The macroscopic appearance is that of a hemorrhagic, often multicystic, tumor closely resembling aneurysmal bone cyst. Histologically, the typical appearance is that of irregular lakes of blood separated by cellular fibrous septa (Fig. 16–9). Cytologically malignant cells may not be readily apparent, further increasing the possibility of confusion with aneurysmal bone cyst.

Errors in histologic diagnosis are most likely to occur under low-power examination of biopsy material. It is essential to examine such tissue carefully for evidence of nuclear pleomorphism, abnormal mitoses, and the presence of small areas of lace-like osteoid formation. Unfortunately, osteoid may not be present in biopsy specimens[45] and can be hard to find even in a resection specimen. A further help to diagnosis is the presence of a permeative growth pattern in osteosarcoma, but again this may not be evident in biopsy material. Morphometric analysis has also been suggested as an aid to diagnosis.[46]

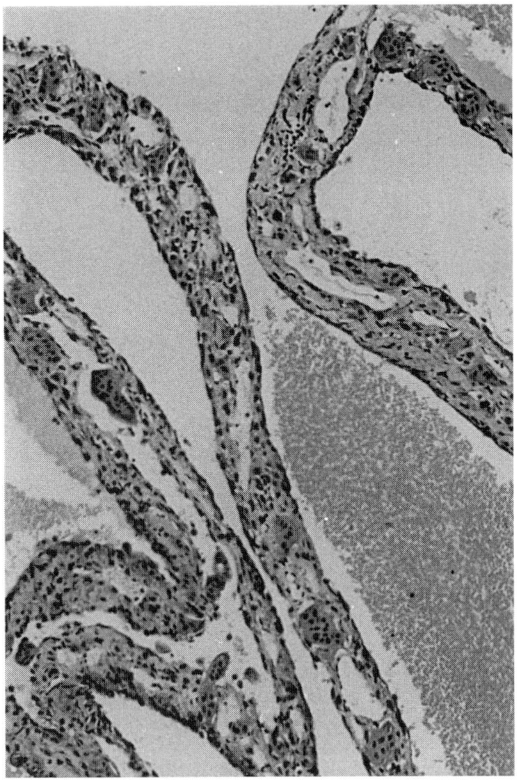

Figure 16–9. Telangiectatic osteosarcoma. Photomicrograph showing a pattern indistinguishable from that of an aneurysmal bone cyst, except for the degree of cellular pleomorphism. No osteoid is present in this field.

Aneurysmal Bone Cyst

Since its original description in 1942 by Jaffe and Lichtenstein[47] and subsequent fuller accounts by the same authors,[48, 49] the precise nature and pathogenesis of aneurysmal bone cyst has remained unknown. Nevertheless, its practical importance remains, firstly, as Lichtenstein made clear, in its distinction from hemangioma and osteosarcoma and secondly, because it is frequently associated with some underlying pathology. In one large series, 36 of 123 cases were secondary to some other bone pathology.[50] Fortunately, the great majority of associated lesions are benign, and in most cases a failure to recognize such lesions is of little clinical significance.

Clinical and Radiologic Features

Aneurysmal bone cyst may occur at any age but is usually seen in the first two decades. It is most common in the metaphyseal region of long bones or the vertebrae. Radiographically, it starts as an eccentric osteolytic lesion (Fig. 16–10*A* and *B*). Rapid expansion combined with extensive bone destruction may give an alarming but false impression of malignancy.

Pathologic Features

The low-power histologic picture is one of blood-filled spaces separated by fibrous septa without an endothelial lining (Fig. 16–10*C*). The septa contain variable numbers of osteoclast-like giant cells, which sometimes aggregate at the edge of the septa. Irregular trabeculae of osteoid tissue are usually seen, and, less commonly, a peculiar spiculated blue staining tissue sometimes referred to as fibromyxoid or chondroid tissue is seen (Fig. 16–10*D*). Mitoses may be frequent, but no abnormal forms are seen. Areas of more solid tissue, lacking the characteristic blood-filled spaces, may also be present.

Differential Diagnosis

Giant Cell Tumor. The presence of solid areas in aneurysmal bone cyst was alluded to earlier. If such areas contain many osteoclasts, a mistaken diagnosis of giant cell tumor can easily be made. Giant cell tumor is also one of the conditions in which secondary aneurysmal bone cyst formation is common. Consideration of the age of the patient and the radio-

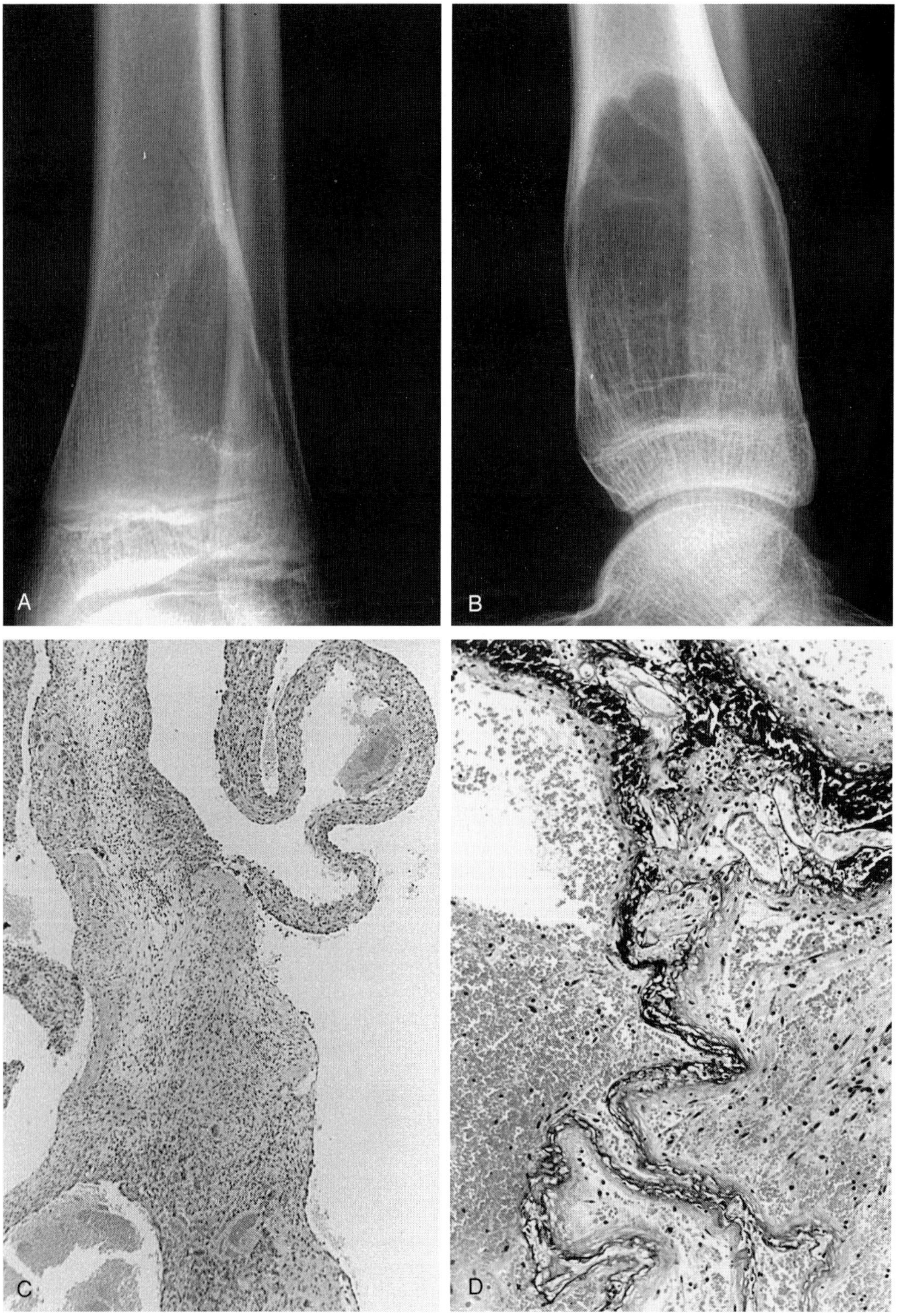

Figure 16–10. Aneurysmal bone cyst. *A*, Eccentric lytic lesion with a well-defined sclerotic margin. *B*, The same patient 8 months later following rapid growth of the lesion. *C*, Photomicrograph showing blood-filled spaces separated by fibrous septa containing occasional giant cells and trabeculae of woven bone. *D*, Spicules of hematoxyphilic, "chondroid" material are present in the septa.

graphic features, especially the precise location of the lesion, will usually enable the correct distinction to be drawn (see Chapter 15).

Telangiectatic Osteosarcoma. The difficulties in distinguishing between aneurysmal bone cyst and telangiectatic osteosarcoma have been discussed and errors can be made in both directions. It should be remembered that osteoid tissue is a normal component of the fibrous septa in aneurysmal bone cyst, and mitoses may be frequent. As always, the radiologic features may be of help, but one should be wary of the misleadingly aggressive appearances of some aneurysmal bone cysts and the rapidly expanding and destructive growth that can sometimes occur, particularly with recurrences.

Other Malignancies. A particularly difficult problem is the occurrence of aneurysmal bone cyst secondary to malignant tumors. In this instance, the biopsy histology can be entirely benign in appearance and the true nature of the condition will only be suspected if, as should always be done, the histology is considered in the full context of the clinical and radiologic findings.

Solid Aneurysmal Bone Cyst

This strangely named entity was described by Sanerkin et al. in 1983.[51] After some initial hesitation, due in no small part to its bizarre title, the term is now widely accepted. This lesion contains all the tissue components of aneurysmal bone cysts but lacks the prominent blood-filled lakes. Until the importance of Sanerkin's observations were recognized, such lesions were in danger of misdiagnosis as low-grade osteosarcomas.[52]

Clinical and Radiologic Features

The age range and anatomic sites of these lesions appear to mirror those of classic aneurysmal bone cysts. Radiologically, they are lytic but may contain faint foci of mineralization

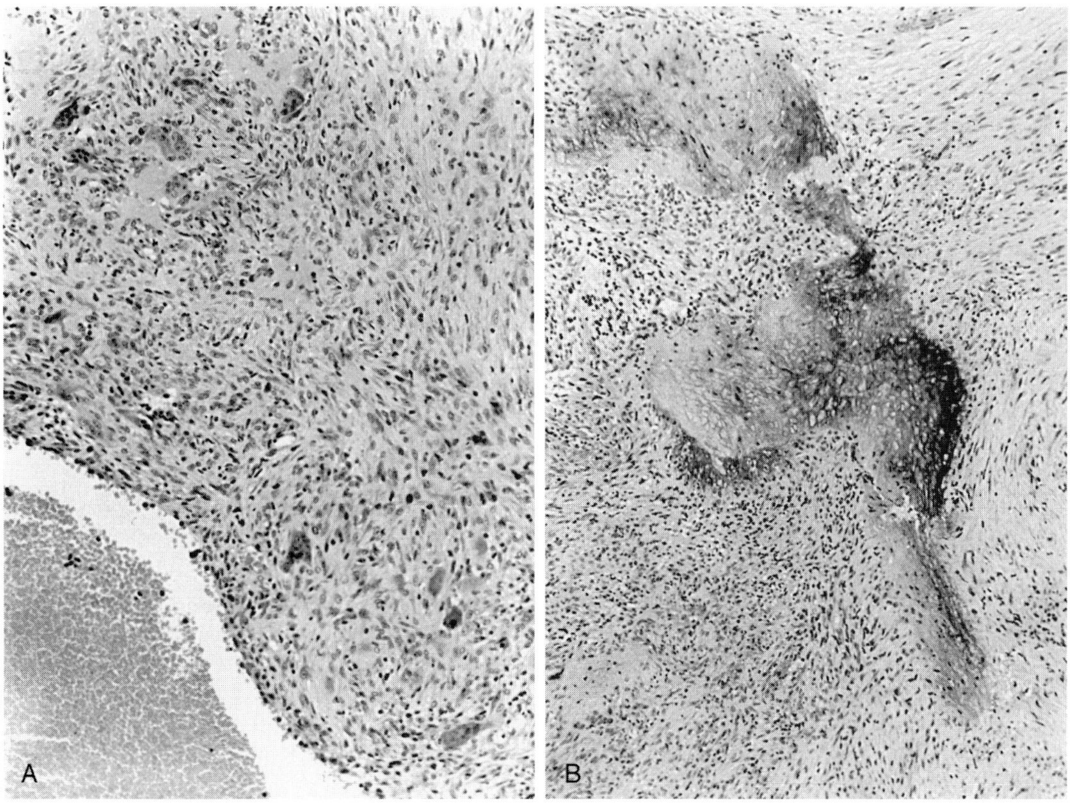

Figure 16–11. Solid aneurysmal bone cyst. *A*, Fibrous tissue containing scattered giant cells, a little osteoid, and the edge of a small sinusoidal space. *B*, Fibrous tissue containing a central focus of partially calcified "chondroid" tissue similar to that seen in the septa of some classic aneurysmal bone cysts.

that are best seen with computed tomography. Cortical destruction and soft tissue extension are seen in some cases and may give rise to a false impression of malignancy. Fluid-fluid levels are not seen.

Pathologic Features

The lesion consists of largely patternless fibrous tissue with irregularly distributed giant cells (Fig. 16–11*A*). Mitoses are present and may be numerous. There are irregular foci of immature osteoid and bone, which vary considerably in amount from case to case. Two features are of particular diagnostic help. One is the presence in most cases of small sinusoidal spaces, a sort of miniature version of the large blood-filled spaces of classic aneurysmal bone cysts (see Fig. 16–11*A*). The second, less common, finding is the presence of blue lace-like tissue, described by Sanerkin as "fibromyxoid" and by Mirra[52] as "chondroid" (Fig. 16–11*B*), which may also be seen in the fibrous septa of some ordinary aneurysmal bone cysts.

Differential Diagnosis

In cases with abundant mitoses and irregular foci of osteoid, it is tempting to make a diagnosis of low-grade osteosarcoma (see Chapter 9). However, once the particular conjunction of features described here is appreciated, the true diagnosis becomes apparent.

Solid aneurysmal bone cyst has many features in common with the giant cell–containing lesions of the sacrum reported by Dehner et al.,[53] lesions described as extragnathic giant cell reparative granuloma,[54] and giant cell reaction and giant cell reparative granuloma of the small bones of the hands and feet.[55, 56] It seems increasingly likely that all these are closely related, if not identical, conditions (see Chapter 15).

REFERENCES

1. Schajowicz F: Histological typing of bone tumours. 2nd ed. WHO International Histological Classification of Tumours Series. Berlin, Springer-Verlag, 1993.
2. Weiss SW: Histological typing of soft tissue tumours. 2nd ed. WHO International Histological Classification of Tumours Series. Berlin, Springer-Verlag, 1994.
3. O'Connell JX, Kattapuram SV, Mankin HJ, et al: Epithelioid hemangioma of bone. A tumor often mistaken for low-grade angiosarcoma or malignant hemangioendothelioma. Am J Surg Pathol 17:610, 1993.
4. Unni KK, Ivins JC, Beabout JW, et al: Hemangioma, hemangiopericytoma, and hemangioendothelioma (angiosarcoma) of bone. Cancer 27:1403, 1971.
5. Devaney K, Vinh TN, Sweet DE: Surface-based hemangiomas of bone. A review of 11 cases. Clin Orthop Rel Res 300:233, 1994.
6. Karlin CA, Brower AC: Multiple primary hemangiomas of bone. Am J Roentgenol 129:162, 1977.
7. Wold LE, Swee RG, Sim FH: Vascular lesions of bone. Pathol Annu 20(part 2):101, 1985.
8. Rosai J, Gold J, Landy R: The histiocytoid hemangiomas. A unifying concept embracing several previously described entities of skin, soft tissue, large vessels, bone, and heart. Hum Pathol 10:707, 1979.
9. Fornasier VL, Finkelstein S, Gardiner GW, et al: Angiolymphoid hyperplasia with eosinophilia: A bone lesion pathologically resembling Kimura's disease of skin. A report of two cases. Clin Orthop Rel Res 166:243, 1982.
10. Stout AP: Hemangioendothelioma: A tumor of blood vessels featuring vascular endothelial cells. Ann Surg 118:445, 1943.
11. Pearson JM, McWilliam LJ: A light microscopical, immunohistochemical, and ultrastructural comparison of hemangiomata and lymphangiomata. Ultrastruct Pathol 14:497, 1990.
12. Jumbelic M, Feuerstein IM, Dorfman HD: Solitary intraosseous lymphangioma: A case report. J Bone Joint Surg 66A:1479, 1984.
13. Bullough PG, Goodfellow JW: Solitary lymphangioma of bone: A case report. J Bone Joint Surg 58A:418, 1976.
14. Keenan TL, Buehler KC, Campbell JR: Solitary lymphangioma of the spine. Spine 20:102, 1995.
15. Kopperman M, Antoine JE: Primary lymphangioma of the calvarium. Am J Roentgenol 121:118, 1974.
16. Devaney K, Vinh TN, Sweet DE: Skeletal-extraskeletal angiomatosis: A clinicopathological study of fourteen patients and nosological considerations. J Bone Joint Surg 76A:878, 1994.
17. Anonymous: Case records of the Massachusetts General Hospital. A 76-year-old woman with multiple bone lesions and thrombocytopenia. N Engl J Med 320:854, 1989.
18. Samuel M, Spitz L: Klippel-Trenaunay syndrome: Clinical features, complications and management in children. Br J Surg 82:757, 1995.
19. Amir G, Boneh A, Tochner Z, et al: Widespread hemangiomatosis of bone associated with rickets: Recovery after irradiation. J Pediatr 123:269, 1993.
20. Gorham LW, Wright AW, Shultz HH, et al: Disappearing bones: A rare form of massive osteolysis. Am J Med 17:674, 1954.
21. Gorham LW, Stout AP: Massive osteolysis (acute spontaneous absorption of bone, phantom bone, disappearing bone), its relation to hemangiomatosis. J Bone Joint Surg 37A:985, 1955.
22. Kulenkampff H-A, Richter GM, Hasse WE, et al: Massive pelvic osteolysis in the Gorham-Stout syndrome. Int Orthop 14:361, 1990.
23. Shives TC, Beabout JW, Unni KK: Massive osteolysis. Clin Orthop Rel Res 294:267, 1993.
24. Cohen J, Craig JM: Multiple lymphangiectases of bone. J Bone Joint Surg 37A:585, 1955.
25. Ramani P, Shah A: Lymphangiomatosis. Histologic and immunohistochemical analysis of four cases. Am J Surg Pathol 17:329, 1993.
26. Canil K, Fitzgerald P, Lau G: Massive chylothorax

associated with lymphangiomatosis of the bone. J Paediatr Surg 29:1186, 1994.
27. Gomez CS, Calonje E, Ferrar DW, et al: Lymphangiomatosis of the limbs. Clinicopathologic analysis of a series with a good prognosis. Am J Surg Pathol 19:125, 1995.
28. Kobayashi Y, Kawaguchi T, Imoto K, et al: Intraosseous glomus tumor in the sacrum. A case report. Acta Pathol Jpn 40:856, 1990.
29. Weiss SW, Enzinger FM: Epithelioid hemangioendothelioma: A vascular tumor often mistaken for a carcinoma. Cancer 50:970, 1982.
30. Tsuneyoshi M, Dorfman HD, Bauer TW: Epithelioid hemangioendothelioma of bone: A clinicopathologic, ultrastructural, and immunohistochemical study. Am J Surg Pathol 10:754, 1986.
31. Kleer CG, Unni KK, McCleod RA: Epithelioid hemangioendothelioma of bone. Am J Surg Pathol 20:1301, 1996.
32. Fanburg JC, Meis-Kindblom JM, Rosenberg AE: Multiple enchondromas associated with spindle-cell hemangioendotheliomas: An overlooked variant of Maffucci's syndrome. Am J Surg Pathol 19:1029, 1995.
33. Naka N, Ohsawa M, Tomita Y, et al: Angiosarcoma in Japan. A review of 99 cases. Cancer 75:989, 1995.
34. Dorfman HD, Steiner GC, Jaffe HL: Vascular tumors of bone. Hum Pathol 2:349, 1971.
35. Wold LE, Unni KK, Beabout JW, et al: Hemangioendothelial sarcoma of bone. Am J Surg Pathol 6:59, 1982.
36. Campanacci M, Boriani S, Giunti A: Hemangioendothelioma of bone: A study of 29 cases. Cancer 46:804, 1980.
37. Volpe R, Mazabraud A: Hemangioendothelioma (angiosarcoma) of bone: A distinct pathologic entity with an unpredictable course? Cancer 49:727, 1982.
38. Fletcher CDM, Beham A, Bekir S, et al: Epithelioid angiosarcoma of the deep soft tissue. A distinctive tumor readily mistaken for an epithelial neoplasm. Am J Surg Pathol 15:915, 1991.
39. Mena H, Ribas JL, Pezeshkpour GH, et al: Hemangiopericytoma of the central nervous system: A review of 94 cases. Hum Pathol 22:84, 1991.
40. Tang JSH, Gold RH, Mirra JM, et al: Hemangiopericytoma of bone. Cancer 62:848, 1988.
41. Templeton AC: Kaposi's sarcoma. Pathol Annu 2:315, 1981.
42. Langford A, Pohle HD, Reichart P: Primary intraosseous AIDS-associated Kaposi's sarcoma. Int J Oral Maxil Surg 20:366, 1991.
43. Conran RM, Granger E, Reddy VB: Kaposi's sarcoma of the bone marrow. Arch Pathol 110:1083, 1986.
44. Ahluwalia C, Bernstein-Singer M, Beckstead J, et al: Kaposi's sarcoma in the bone marrow of a patient with AIDS. Am J Clin Pathol 95:561, 1991.
45. Matsuno T, Unni KK, McCleod RA, et al: Telangiectatic osteosarcoma. Cancer 38:2538, 1976.
46. Ruiter DJ, Cornelisse CJ, van Rijssel TG, et al: Aneurysmal bone cyst and telangiectatic osteosarcoma. A histopathological and morphometric study. Virch Arch (A) 373:311, 1977.
47. Jaffe HL, Lichtenstein L: Solitary unicameral bone cyst with emphasis on the Roentgen picture, the pathologic appearance and the pathogenesis. Arch Surg 44:1004, 1942.
48. Jaffe HL: Aneurysmal bone cyst. Bull Hosp Jt Dis 11:3, 1950.
49. Lichtenstein L: Aneurysmal bone cyst: A pathologic entity commonly mistaken for giant cell tumor, and occasionally for hemangioma and osteogenic sarcoma. Cancer 3:279, 1950.
50. Martinez V, Sissons HA: Aneurysmal bone cyst. A review of 123 cases including primary lesions and those secondary to other bone pathology. Cancer 61:2291, 1988.
51. Sanerkin NG, Mott MG, Roylance J: An unusual intraosseous lesion with fibroblastic, osteoclastic, osteoblastic, aneurysmal and fibromyxoid elements: "Solid" variant of aneurysmal bone cyst. Cancer 51:2278, 1983.
52. Mirra JM: Bone Tumors: clinical, radiologic and pathologic correlations, p 1307. Philadelphia, Lea & Febiger, 1989.
53. Dehner LP, Risdall RJ, L'Heureux P: Giant-cell containing "fibrous" lesion of the sacrum. A roentgenographic, pathologic, and ultrastructural study of three cases. Am J Surg Pathol 2:55, 1978.
54. Oda Y, Tsuneyoshi M, Shinohara N: "Solid" variant of aneurysmal bone cyst (extragnathic giant cell reparative granuloma) in the axial skeleton and long bones. A study of its morphologic spectrum and distinction from allied giant cell lesions. Cancer 70:2642, 1992.
55. Bertoni F, Bacchini MD, Capanna R, et al: Solid variant of aneurysmal bone cyst. Cancer 71:729, 1993.
56. Wold LE, Dobyns JH, Swee RG, et al: Giant cell reaction (giant cell reparative granuloma) of the small bones of the hands and feet. Am J Surg Pathol 10:491, 1986.

Chapter

17

BONE NEOPLASMS CONTAINING EPITHELIAL AND EPITHELIOID CELLS

JONATHAN R. SALISBURY

METASTATIC CARCINOMA

Metastatic carcinoma is the most frequently occurring malignant tumor in the adult skeleton.[1] Although the true incidence is unknown, up to 50% of patients coming to autopsy with disseminated carcinoma have skeletal metastases, although the likelihood of finding skeletal metastases at autopsy is proportional to the extent to which the bones are examined. Metastases are situated predominantly in the red marrow,[2] so that the usual practice in Britain of examining only the vertebral bodies by sawing or chiseling a "vertebral strip" will reveal some but not all metastases.

For the diagnostic surgical pathologist, the more important statistic is the probability that a solitary lesion found in an adult skeleton is a metastasis, rather than a primary bone tumor. Published frequency data are difficult to interpret because many benign bone tumors never present clinically, and significant numbers of solitary abnormalities found on isotope bone scans are due to benign disease processes, even in patients with proved extraosseous malignancies. Corcoran et al.[3] assessed the incidence and significance of solitary bone scan abnormalities in 1129 consecutive patients with extraskeletal primary malignancies. Solitary abnormalities were found in 15%. The cause of the abnormality was established in 90 of the 172 cases; 64% were due to metastatic disease, and 36% were secondary to a benign process.

Despite this, any surgical pathologist faced with a biopsy from a skeletal tumor should consider the possibility that the tumor may be a secondary deposit. Although skeletal deposits do occur in disseminated sarcomas,[4] melanomas, mesotheliomas,[5] and germ cell tumors,[6] these are comparatively rare and most secondary deposits in adults are metastatic carcinoma. Bone metastases from spindle-cell squamous carcinoma[7] can be particularly difficult to diagnose correctly.

More than 80% of all bone metastases originate in the lung, breast, prostate, kidney, and thyroid. Frisch et al.[8] examined 1810 bone marrow biopsy specimens from 1725 patients with known or suspected carcinomas. The frequency of positive biopsy results was 72% for unknown primaries, 42% for breast carcinoma, 32% for prostatic carcinoma, 14% for lung carcinoma, and 19% for other cancers; the overall rate of detection of metastases was 35%.

Clinical and Radiologic Features

If a patient with a skeletal tumor is already known to have a primary carcinoma, then the pathologist should be alerted to the possibility that the skeletal tumor represents a skeletal metastasis. In most cases, the deposits of metastatic carcinoma are multiple.

A more difficult problem arises when a solitary skeletal tumor is the first manifestation of a carcinoma. Again, there may be a clue from the clinical radiographs; for instance, a lesion in the metaphysis of a long bone in an adult is a good candidate for a metastasis. About 70% of bone metastases affect the axial skeleton alone (the cranium, spinal column including sacrum, and ribs). The remainder occur in the appendicular skeleton alone (the long bones) or in both the axial and the appendicular skeletons. Although bone tumors are often located in the knee area, patellar metastases are rare.[9] Metastases to long bones distal to the elbows and knees are unusual but are disproportionately well documented.[10–13] Metastases to the bones of the hands[14–16] and feet[17–19] are even rarer.

Hirshberg et al.[20] reviewed 390 cases of metastatic lesions to the jawbones. The primary site differed between the sexes: for women, it was the breast followed by the adrenal gland, colorectum, genital organs, and thyroid; for men, it was the lung, followed by the prostate, kidney, bone, and adrenal gland. The most common location of the metastatic tumors was the mandible, with the molar area the most frequent site involved. In 30% of cases, the oral lesion was the first sign of malignant disease.

Occasionally, pagetic bone can be the site of carcinomatous metastases, and such tumors should be distinguished from Paget's sarcoma.[21, 22]

Radiologically, most metastatic tumors are osteolytic, but some are osteoblastic (osteosclerotic) and some show a mixed osteolytic-osteoblastic pattern. Pure osteosclerotic metastases are usually prostatic adenocarcinoma, breast adenocarcinoma, or carcinoid tumor.[23]

Histopathology

The histologic features of carcinoma in a bone biopsy can show the same variation as carcinomas in their primary sites. Few problems are encountered with well or moderately differentiated adenocarcinoma or squamous cell carcinoma (Fig. 17–1*A, B*). Less differentiated and undifferentiated carcinoma can present more diagnostic difficulty (Fig. 17–1*C*). Immunohistochemistry for cytokeratins is invaluable here, ideally using a pancytokeratin antibody such as MNF116 (Dako Ltd) although, in practice, any of the commonly used low molecular weight anticytokeratin antibodies such as CAM 5.2 (Becton Dickinson) is usually adequate. Once the diagnosis of metastatic carcinoma has been established, the next step is to try to identify the likely site of the primary tumor. Further staining of the biopsy may be of help. Alcian blue and diastase-periodic acid-Schiff stains to detect acid and neutral mucins, respectively, are essential to establish the diagnosis of adenocarcinoma (Fig. 17–1*D*). In a man with a solitary skeletal deposit of adenocarcinoma, immunohistochemical staining of the biopsy with antibodies to prostate-specific antigen and prostatic acid phosphatase would be the next step (Fig. 17–2), although estimation of the serum prostatic acid phosphatase is also helpful. Immunohistochemical staining with an antibody to thyroglobulin may be useful for demonstrating that a solitary skeletal deposit of carcinoma is from a primary thyroid carcinoma, although in many cases this is clear from the appearance in the hematoxylin and eosin–stained section.

Sternal aspirates, iliac crest biopsy specimens, and biopsy imprints from 31 patients with verified metastatic cancer to bone marrow were reviewed by Bjorneklett et al.[23] All three methods were shown to be complementary in detecting metastases, as metastases were detected in some cases by one procedure and missed by the others (see Chapter 7).

The mechanisms of bone resorption around deposits of metastatic carcinoma are considered in Chapter 3.

Metastatic Patterns from Specific Primary Sites

Lung and Larynx

Auerbach et al.[24] reported on 662 autopsies of males with lung carcinoma. Metastases were found in 96.3% of the cases and the sites most frequently involved were regional lymph nodes, liver, brain, distant lymph nodes, adrenals, and bone. Metastases occurred most commonly from small cell carcinomas and least often from squamous cell carcinomas. Some cases of lung cancer metastatic to bone show a very unusual distribution of the skeletal metastases, such as solitary metastasis to the elbow[25] or polyostotic metastases to the phalanges.[26]

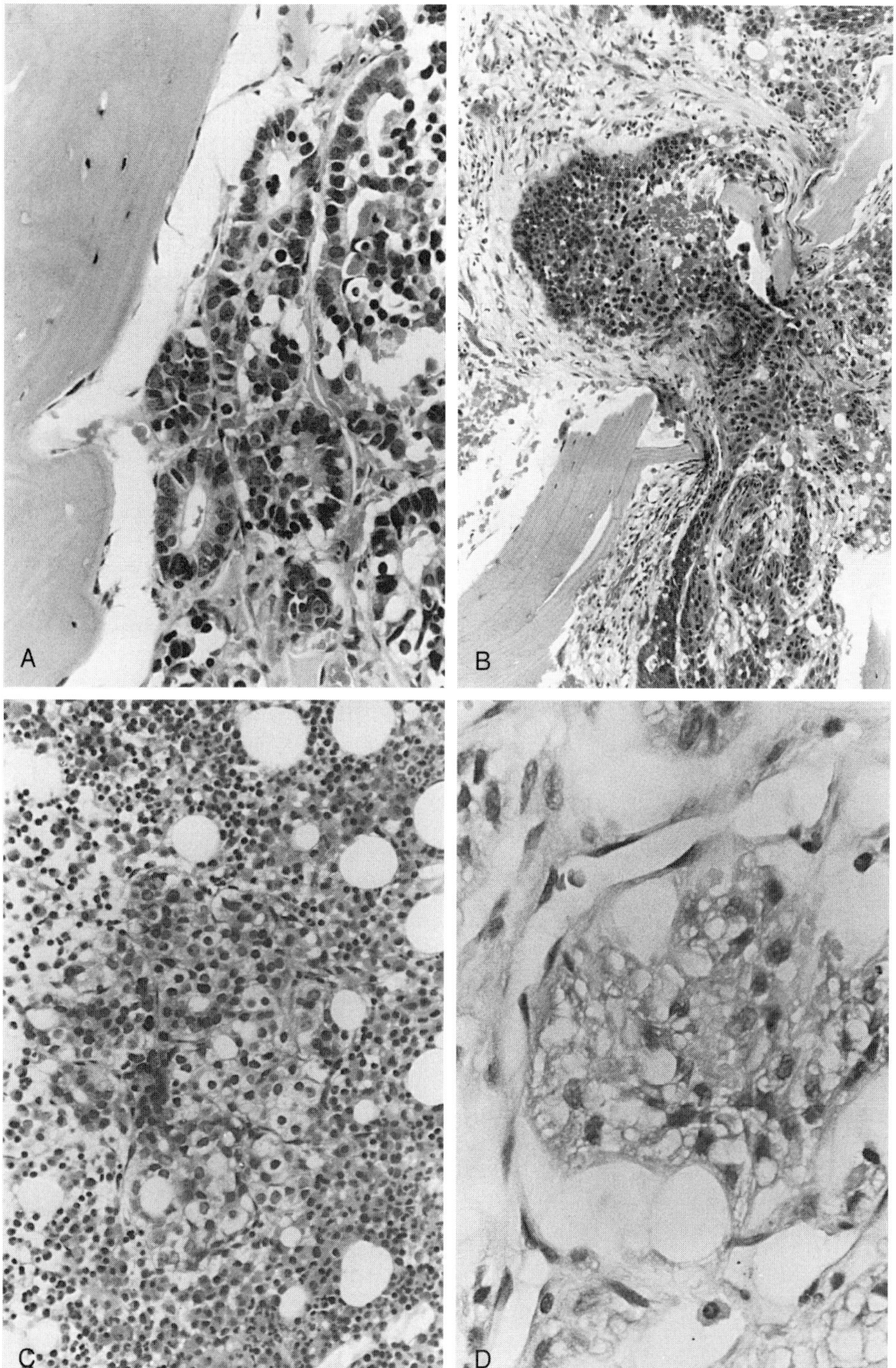

Figure 17–1. Metastatic carcinoma. *A*, Male, 64 years old. Vertebral bone is infiltrated by moderately differentiated metastatic adenocarcinoma forming glandular structures. The primary tumor was in the prostate. *B*, Male, 56 years old. Biopsy of radiologically destructive lesion in pelvis. Sheets of poorly differentiated squamous cell carcinoma are seen infiltrating the marrow and eroding a trabecula. The primary tumor was in the lung. *C*, Male, 48 years old. Multiple sclerotic bone lesions, raised serum acid phosphatase level, and clinically suspicious prostate on rectal examination. Biopsy of an iliac crest lesion shows clumps of moderately to poorly differentiated adenocarcinoma in the marrow. Subsequent biopsy of prostate confirmed prostatic adenocarcinoma. *D*, Male with lytic lesion in body of third thoracic vertebra. Biopsy shows a metastatic adenocarcinoma with moderate amounts of acid mucins. (Alcian blue.)

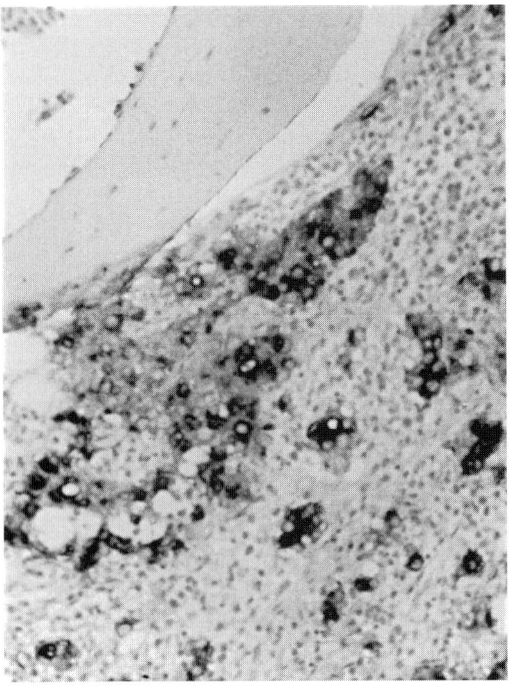

Figure 17–2. Male with previous history of colonic adenocarcinoma who presented with widespread sclerotic metastases in the pelvis and a subcapital fracture of the left femoral neck. The resected femoral head showed a moderately differentiated adenocarcinoma infiltrating the bone marrow. Immunohistochemical staining for prostate-specific antigen is strongly positive, demonstrating that the tumor is metastatic prostatic adenocarcinoma. (Immunoperoxidase with hematoxylin counterstain.)

Squamous cell carcinomas of the larynx metastasize to bone rarely.[27, 28] Merino et al.[29] reviewed 5019 patients with squamous cell carcinoma of the upper respiratory and digestive tracts who had no evidence of metastases at presentation. Of these, 10.9% developed clinical evidence of metastases, varying from 3.1% for vocal cord carcinomas to 28.1% for nasopharyngeal carcinoma. The lungs (52%) and bones (20.3%) were the most common metastatic sites.

Primary laryngeal small cell carcinomas behave similarly to their pulmonary counterparts. Most patients die of widespread metastases, including numerous skeletal metastases.[30]

Detection of Metastases

Hirsch et al.[31] studied bilateral bone marrow samples from the posterior iliac crests as a staging procedure in 89 patients with small cell anaplastic lung carcinoma. Marrow involvement was found in 22.5%, in 10.1% only on one side, and in 12.4% on both sides. Aspiration was found to be superior to biopsy. There is a lack of correlation between radionucleotide bone scan and bone marrow biopsy in identifying metastases of small cell anaplastic lung carcinoma,[32] probably because they identify independent patterns of osseous metastasis. Immunocytochemistry is superior to morphology in detecting bone marrow metastases from small cell anaplastic lung carcinoma.[33]

Breast

The frequency of bone metastases in patients with breast carcinoma has been examined in clinical and autopsy studies.[34] Between 35 and 40% of patients with operable breast carcinoma develop metastases after primary therapy.

Yablonski-Peretz et al.[35] described a patient with breast carcinoma, who developed a syndrome resembling agnogenic myeloid metaplasia. She had secondary myelofibrosis with bone marrow metastases, extramedullary hematopoiesis resulting in massive splenomegaly, and leukoerythroblastosis. Chronic monoarthritis of the elbow has been reported to be caused by a poorly differentiated metastatic breast adenocarcinoma in the radial head.[36]

Breast carcinomas produce more prostaglandin-like material than do benign tumors or normal breast tissue.[37] Greatest synthesis in vitro occurs with tumors associated with bone metastases, and the highest "basal" amounts occur in tumors showing histologic spread. It has been suggested that prostaglandins play a part in tumor spread and growth in bone.

Detection of Metastases

McNeil et al.[38] found that few patients with stage I or II carcinoma of the breast had a positive preoperative isotope bone scan, but that 16% of patients with stage III disease had evidence of bony metastasis at the time of operation. Bone marrow involvement by breast carcinoma in the absence of demonstrable bone lesions on isotope scans or radiographs is unusual. DiStefano et al.[39] reported six such patients, representing 2.8% of 213 patients with breast carcinoma in which marrow examination was performed and 6.2% of those in which marrow involvement was demonstrated. Deck and Lee[40] reported a woman with a mucinous lobular breast carcinoma with metastases to many bone sites whose terminal illness was the result of cerebral infarcts caused by emboli of mucin and emulsified fat.

Marrow micrometastases can be identified by immunocytochemistry using an antibody to anti–epithelial membrane antigen (EMA) in 26% of primary breast carcinoma patients at the time of initial surgery.[41] To determine the fate of these cells, Mansi et al.[42] repeated multiple marrow aspirates in 82 patients at a median time of 18 months after surgery. In surgically treated and untreated patients, micrometastases were only found in 2% and 3%, respectively. These results suggest that many micrometastases are the result of "shedding" of cells from the primary carcinoma and are not viable. Dearnaley et al.[43] showed that immunostaining of bone marrow aspirates with anti-EMA facilitated the detection of small numbers of carcinoma cells, and increased the yield of positive samples. Malignant cells were found in the marrow of breast carcinoma patients with no other evidence of metastasis. Gugliotta et al.[44] also demonstrated the value of antibodies to milk fat globule membrane antigen and carcinoembryonic antigen in the immunocytochemical identification of metastatic breast carcinoma cells in the bone marrow. Cote et al.[45] used monoclonal antibodies that recognized epithelial cell antigens (C26, T16, AE-1) in an immunohistochemical assay to find breast carcinoma cells in bone marrow aspirates. Their assay could detect one carcinoma cell among 50,000 to 100,000 hematopoietic cells. They found carcinoma cells in the bone marrow of 35% of breast carcinoma patients, even though none was identified by routine bone marrow cytology.

Prostate

Prostatic cancer commonly presents as obstructive uropathy, regional lymphatic metastases, or hematogenous metastases to the axial skeleton.[46] The pattern of dissemination of prostatic carcinoma varies, but skeletal metastasis is the single most common symptomatic mode of presentation. Viadana et al.[47] studied 58 autopsies of prostatic carcinoma to establish whether metastases spread at random from the primary tumor or whether the metastatic spread occurred in steps requiring intermediate disseminating sites. They showed that metastases appeared first in the skeleton and then in the lungs, before spread to other sites. Whether resection of the primary prostatic carcinoma is transurethral or radical has no effect on the subsequent incidence of osseous metastases.[48] Diethylstilbestrol causes extensive necrosis of metastatic prostatic carcinoma cells in the bone marrow.[49]

Neuroendocrine differentiation of prostatic adenocarcinoma has received considerable attention in recent years and can be demonstrated in both primary and metastatic carcinomas. Aprikian et al.[50] studied peptide hormone immunoreactivities of neuroendocrine differentiated tumor cells in prostatic carcinoma bone metastases and found chromogranin-A immunoreactive cells in 11 of the 21 metastases examined. Thyroid-stimulating hormone immunoreactive cells were found in all seven bone metastases examined.

Detection of Metastases

The biochemical examination of bone marrow aspirates may complement radiologic investigations in the detection of prostatic carcinoma metastases and will detect some extra cases (3 of 155 patients).[51] Boehme et al.[52] measured bone marrow acid and alkaline phosphatase, lactic dehydrogenase, and calcium levels in 18 patients with prostatic carcinoma and found that acid phosphatase was not significantly different between those with and those without bone metastases. Schaffer and Pendergrass[53] compared clinical, biochemical, and radiologic methods for detecting bone metastasis in 219 patients with prostatic adenocarcinoma classified as positive or negative by bone scans. Of those with proved metastases, 43% had no bone pain, 39% had normal acid phosphatase levels, 23% had normal alkaline phosphatase levels, 19% had normal levels of both enzymes, and 15% had normal enzyme levels without bone pain. Twenty-four per cent of patients with normal enzyme levels and clinically unsuspected bone metastases had bone scans that proved positive for metastasis; 62% of these had normal radiographs.

Oberneder et al.[54] used a monoclonal antibody against cytokeratin 18 for the detection of individual metastatic tumor cells in bone marrow aspirates from 84 patients with prostatic carcinoma. Tumor cells were detected in a sensitivity of 1 per 8×10^5 marrow cells using an alkaline phosphatase anti–alkaline phosphatase technique. They detected tumor cells in 33% of patients with stage N0M0 prostatic carcinoma. Simultaneous immunocytochemical labeling for cytokeratin 18 and prostate-specific antigen demonstrated double-labeling of cells in bone marrow aspirates from 5 of 14 patients.

Prediction of Metastasis in Prostatic Carcinoma

Wakui et al.[55] used a color image analysis system to assess tumor angiogenesis in prostatic carcinomas by determining the blood capillary density ratio (BCDR), defined as the ratio between the area of the blood capillaries and the area of the tumor. They showed that the BCDR may help in predicting tumor progression and bone marrow metastasis of carcinomas with low and intermediate Gleason's scores.

There is a statistically significant correlation between aneuploidy, as determined by flow cytometry, and bone marrow metastasis in prostatic carcinoma.[56]

Kidney

Forbes et al.[57] described bone metastases in 10% of 1668 patients with renal carcinoma. In 40% of patients with bone metastasis, this was the presenting lesion of an occult renal carcinoma and was associated with a poor prognosis. Most bone lesions were in the pelvis and lower lumbar spine, and some appeared 10 or more years after the initial tumor. The most common radiographic features were a lytic destructive lesion with indistinct margins, cortical erosion, and soft tissue expansion. Angiography often shows intense neovascularization in the metastatic deposits (Fig. 17–3). Pathologic long bone fractures were common, and calcifications were seen occasionally. The synovial joints were not affected.

Solitary metastasis is uncommon, occurring in 1.6% to 3.2% of patients with renal cell carcinoma.[58] However, resection of a metastatic deposit or amputation of an extremity with a metastasis is frequently advocated, particularly after successful nephrectomy, and the cure rate with amputation is at least 30%. Tobisu et al.[59] reviewed the clinical course and survival of 159 patients who underwent nephrectomy for renal cell carcinoma. Those with one to five lung or solitary bone metastases survived longer than those with more than six lung or multiple bone metastases. Spontaneous regression of a bone metastasis from renal cell carcinoma may rarely occur.[60]

Lawler and Marsden[61] found bone metastases in seven children in a survey of 132 children presenting with renal tumors using material from the Manchester Children's Tumour Registry. Bone metastases from nephroblastoma seem to be an exceptional finding, as only 1 of 117 Wilms' tumors developed bone metastases. The remainder included carcinoma (1 of 4), bone-metastasizing renal tumor of childhood (2 of 3), atypical tumors (2 of 2), and lymphosarcoma (1 of 1). Although bone-metastasizing renal tumor of childhood is primarily a mesenchymal neoplasm, occasional cases have a definite epithelial component, with epithelial cells present in groups, around either a central eosinophilic core or a small central lumen.[62]

Thyroid

Nemec et al.[63] analyzed a group of 840 patients with thyroid carcinomas (of all types) and found lung metastases in 14.6%. Lung metastases were the only metastases in 78 patients; in the remainder, other metastases were present, usually to bone (affecting 5.4% patients). The patients with both lung and bone metastases were older than those with lung metastases alone, and follicular carcinoma was the major histologic type. Evans[64] followed 44 patients with follicular thyroid neoplasms for at least 10 years. Of patients with follicular carcinoma, 67% died of tumor, and all had distant metastasis (affecting bone in 92% of cases).

Bone metastases from papillary carcinomas of the thyroid are very rare.[65] Lloyd and Beierwaltes[66] described a woman with a 6 mm occult sclerosing thyroid carcinoma that metastasized to the right humerus. Chetty et al.[67] described a patient who presented with a lesion of the iliac bone.

Gastrointestinal Tract and Liver

Symptomatic solitary bony metastasis as the first sign of asymptomatic gastric carcinoma or as the sole sign of recurrence after gastrectomy is very rare.[68] Koga et al.[69] analyzed the pathologic characteristics of 57 disseminated gastric adenocarcinomas and found that the carcinomas that developed bone metastases were mostly poorly differentiated. Schlimok et al.[70] detected tumor cells in the bone marrow of 34 of 97 patients at the time of primary surgery using an anti–cytokeratin 18 antibody. The in-

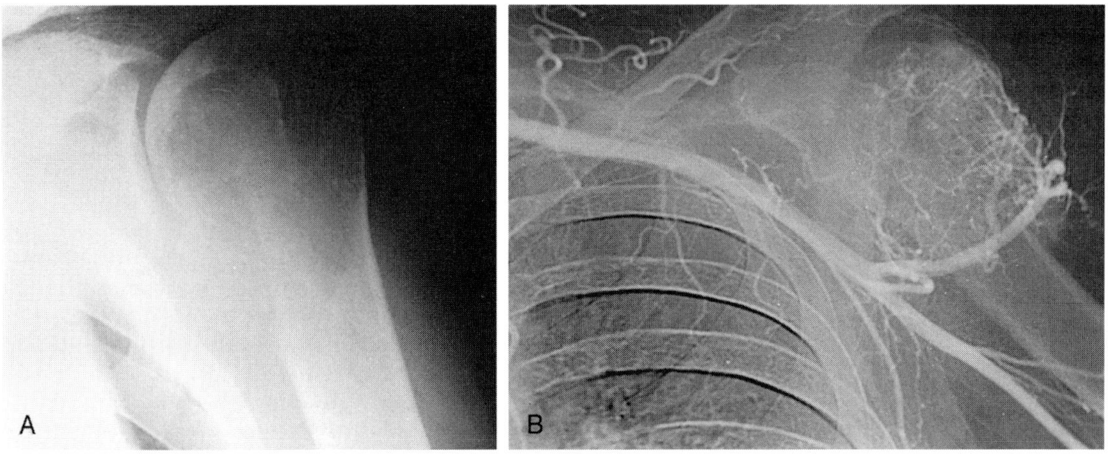

Figure 17–3. Metastatic renal carcinoma. *A*, Plain radiograph showing a poorly defined lytic lesion in the upper humerus. *B*, Digital subtraction angiogram showing the intense neovascularity of the metastatic carcinoma in the femur. (Courtesy of Dr D. Ritchie.)

cidence of positive findings was related to established risk factors. Rarely, gastric adenocarcinoma with widespread skeletal metastases can show high serum levels of human chorionic gonadotropin, carcinoembryonic antigen, and alkaline phosphatase.[71]

Primary hepatocellular carcinomas rarely give rise to skeletal metastases (Fig. 17–4).[72–76] An analysis of metastatic patterns of hepatocellular carcinoma has shown that bone metastases decrease in an age-dependent manner in men and are significantly more prevalent in men in their 40s and 50s. In an autopsy study of 350 cases of hepatocellular carcinoma, bone metastasis was more common in males with concomitant cirrhosis.[77]

Primary hepatic cholangiosarcomas may metastasize to bone.[78] Ali et al.[79] reported an unusual case of a fatal primary neuroendocrine carcinoma of the liver with metastases to porta hepatis lymph nodes and the pubic bone in which the patient suffered episodes of profound, intractable hypoglycemia. Imamura et al.[80] described a case of malignant insulinoma in a 53-year-old woman who presented with bony metastases 10 years after caudal pancreatectomy.

The distribution patterns of bone metastases from gut carcinomas can be most unusual.[81] Igarashi et al.[82] reported a rare case of bilateral sudden and profound hearing loss caused by bilateral temporal bone metastasis from a primary adenocarcinoma of the tail of the pancreas.

Studies of bone metastases in colorectal carcinoma by radionuclide scanning[83, 84] have shown a frequency of 33 to 75% compared with the frequency of 5 to 6% detectable by radiography or anatomic studies. Hoehn et al.[85] discuss colorectal carcinoma presenting clinically as a bone metastasis. These patients almost always have regional lymph node metas-

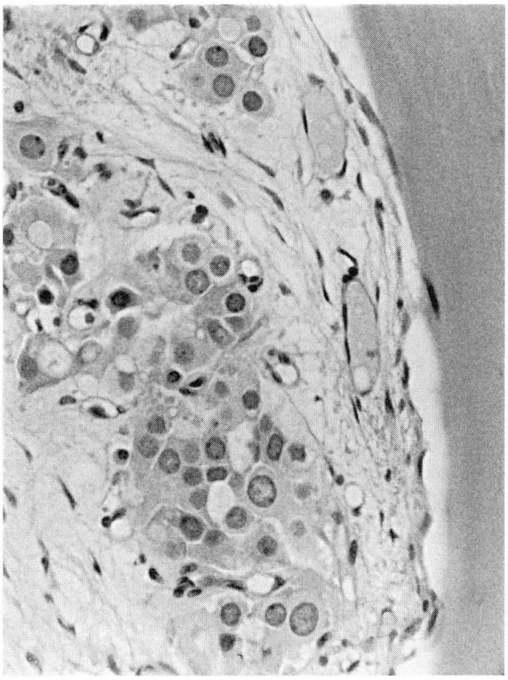

Figure 17–4. Hepatocellular carcinoma. Male, 60 years old. Pathologic fracture through left femoral neck in a patient known to have hepatocellular carcinoma. The bone marrow is infiltrated by hepatocellular carcinoma showing a pseudoglandular growth pattern.

tases but no liver or lung metastases, suggesting that the osseous metastases are occurring via the vertebral venous anastomotic networks (Batson's plexus). Yoshioka et al.[86] reported a patient with bone metastasis from a carcinoma in adenoma in the rectum.

Female Genital Tract

Brufman et al.[87] described four patients suffering from primary carcinoma of endometrium, cervix, ovary, and vulva in whom antemortem diagnoses of bone metastases were made. Among 713 patients followed after treatment for cancer of the uterine cervix, 6.6% had a metastasis to the bone, most frequently to the vertebral column, particularly the lumbar spine (48%) followed by the pelvic bones.[88] Onuba[89] described an unusual tibial metastasis from an endometrial adenocarcinoma.

Abdul Karim et al.[90] performed autopsies on 305 patients with primary carcinomas of the cervix, endometrium, ovaries, fallopian tubes, vulva, and vagina. Skeletal metastases were detected premortem and at autopsy in 16.1%: cervix 40.8%; endometrium 34.7%; ovary 14.3%; vulva 8.2%; fallopian tube 2%; and vagina 0%. This study demonstrated that osseous metastases are not uncommon, are more common than clinically appreciated, and correlate with advanced anatomic stage and histopathologic type and grade.

Skin

Cases of basal cell carcinoma metastasizing to bone occur rarely.[91–95] Christensen et al.[94] reviewed 95 previously recorded cases of metastasizing basal cell carcinomas with 20 of these metastatic to bone. Rare cases of basosquamous cell carcinoma of the skin with bone metastases are also reported. In the bone metastasis of one patient, there were rudimentary hair follicles and areas of matrical differentiation.[96]

Occasional sweat gland carcinomas metastasize to bones such as the tibia[97] or the foot.[98] Malignant eccrine poroma is a rare tumor that usually metastasizes to visceral organs. Exceptionally rare cases of bone metastasis occur, for example, in the femur and tibia.[99] Malignant pilomatrixoma may also metastasize to bone.[100, 101] Yeung and Stinson[102] reported an unusual case of an adenocystic carcinoma of the axillary sweat glands, in which after complete control of the primary tumor, metastases appeared in the skin and sacral and pelvic bones.

Salivary and Lacrimal Glands

Rare examples of salivary gland and lacrimal gland neoplasms metastasize to bones. Qureshi et al.[103] reported on a patient with a pathologic fracture through a lytic lesion in the left glenoid. Biopsy showed a pleomorphic adenoma. The patient had had a parotid pleomorphic adenoma removed 16 years previously. Pitman et al.[104] described two cases of salivary gland pleomorphic adenomas metastatic to bone diagnosed by fine-needle aspiration biopsy. The metastases contained benign epithelial, myoepithelial, and stromal components. Yamagiwa and Yatani[105] reported a case of lacrimal gland carcinoma with metastases to cervical vertebra and rib. Pierce et al.[106] reported on two patients with primary small cell carcinomas of the submandibular salivary gland and maxillary sinus. Both patients developed bone marrow metastases.

Thymus

Very rarely, malignant thymomas can metastasize to bones.[107]

CHORDOMA

Chordoma is a comparatively rare tumor that arises in the axial skeleton and is thought to be derived from persistent notochordal tissue. Data from the Mayo Clinic showed that it represented 4% of all malignant primary bone tumors,[108] but this included many referred patients. Schajowicz[109] quoted a figure of 1% of all malignant primary bone tumors. The mean annual (crude) incidence of chordoma in Finland has been shown to be $0.30/10^6$ in males, and $0.18/10^6$ in females.[110]

Notochord and Notochordal Remnants

The notochord is an embryonic, ectodermal structure that defines the midline of chordate embryos. In the human fetus, the notochord expands at the sites of the future intervertebral discs and contributes to the formation of the nuclei pulposi (Fig. 17–5).[111] The notochord regresses where it passes through the future

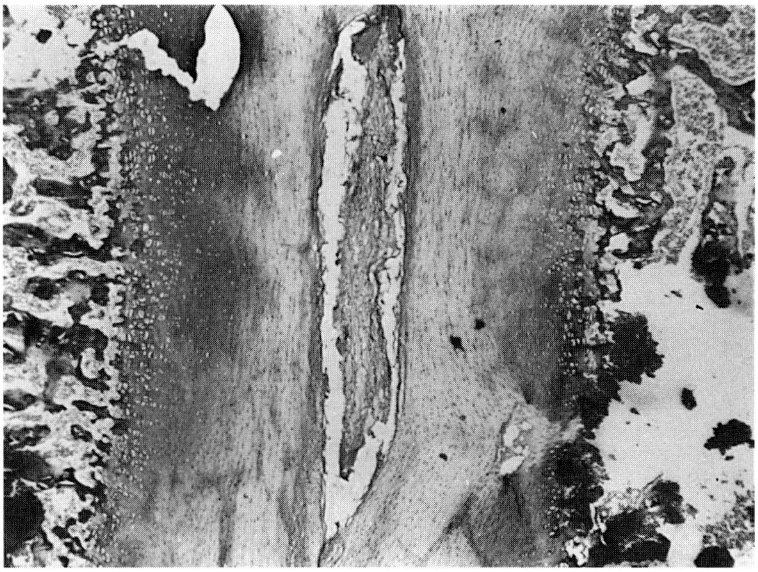

Figure 17–5. Human fetal notochord at 26 weeks gestational age. There is an expansion of notochordal tissue at the site of the future nucleus pulposus of the intervertebral disc. This is surrounded by fibrocartilage of the annulus pulposus. Ossification has occurred in the vertebral bodies on either side of the disc.

vertebral bodies, although an acellular notochordal sheath may persist. Three-dimensional reconstruction of serial sections of human embryos shows that the anatomy of the caudal and rostral ends of the notochord is complex.[112] Forking of the ends, with separate fragments of chordal tissue, can be demonstrated, and these fragments provide a way by which notochordal cell rests could be left behind in the basicranial and sacral regions when the notochord involutes elsewhere. Assuming the histogenesis of chordomas from notochordal cell rests would explain the observed skeletal distribution of chordomas, although not why the notochordal cell rests should transform into chordomas.

Notochordal cells resemble, both morphologically and immunophenotypically, those seen in chordomas (Fig. 17–6*A*). Notochordal cells are positive for S-100 protein (Fig. 17–6*B*),[113] cytokeratins (Fig. 17–6*C*)[114, 115] and epithelial membrane antigen.[116] Human notochord cells contain lysozyme (Fig. 17–6*D*), unlike chordoma cells.[117] Enzyme histochemical staining has shown that human notochord cells are positive for alpha-naphthyl acetate esterase.[117]

The spheno-occipital remnant is seen in 0.5 to 2.0% of autopsies on the anterior surface of the clivus when the dura is stripped from the base of the skull. These ecchordoses physaliphora were first described by Virchow,[118] who, believing them to be of a cartilaginous nature, named them ecchondroses physaliphora. Their true nature was recognized by Muller.[119] A rare case of ecchordosis physaliphora demonstrated by magnetic resonance imaging was described in a man who presented with hearing disturbance and reduction in facial sensation due to a schwannoma.[120] Magnetic resonance imaging revealed the schwannoma as well as a clival lesion, which histologically was an ecchordosis. The ecchordosis was not enhanced by gadolinium diethylenetriamine penta-acetic acid (Gd-DTPA) administration, which may be a characteristic finding, in contrast to chordoma that is generally enhanced.

Clinical Features

Most chordomas occur in adults, peak 55–65 years, although cases do occur both in children[121] and in old age. Males are affected about twice as frequently as females, the preponderance of males being greater in the sacral than in the cranial group.[108, 122] Chordoma is an uncommon neoplasm in the first two decades of life when it may be more variable histologically and may pursue a more aggressive clinical course than chordomas in adults. Oexle et al.[123] reported the first case of a congenital intracranial chordoma, which presented with hydrocephalus, sixth and seventh cranial nerve palsy, and torticollis shortly after birth. Coffin et al.[124] studied 12 chordomas presenting in six males and six females at age

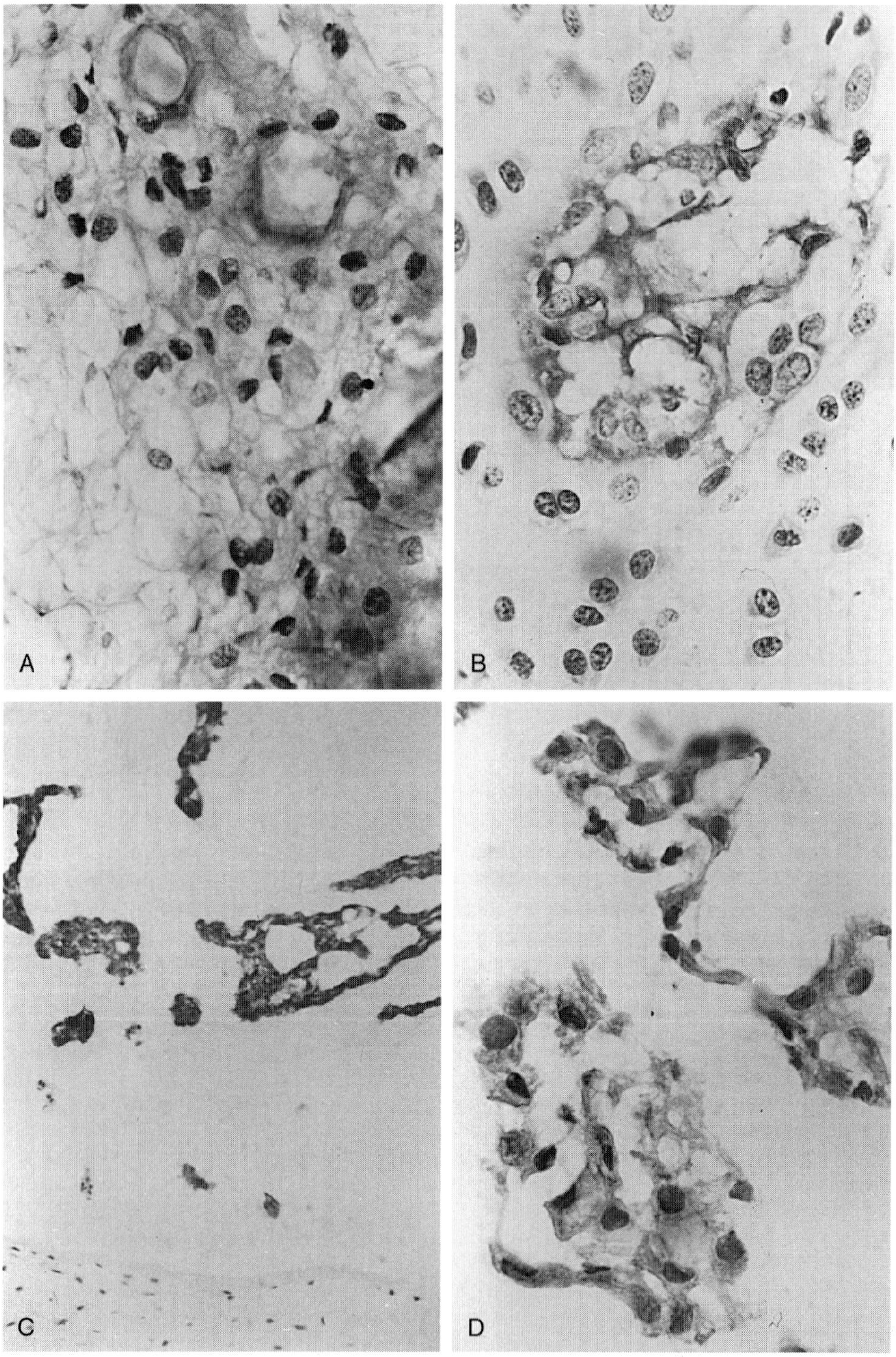

Figure 17–6. Human fetal notochord. *A*, 10 weeks gestational age. The morphologic similarity of the notochordal cells to those seen in chordoma is striking. *B*, 10 weeks gestational age. The notochordal cells stain positively for S-100 protein. There is weaker staining in some of the surrounding human fetal chondrocytes. (Immunoperoxidase with hematoxylin counterstain.) *C*, 26 weeks gestational age. The notochordal cells stain positively for cytokeratins. (Immunoperoxidase using CAM 5.2 as the primary antibody, hematoxylin counterstain.) *D*, 10 weeks gestational age. The notochordal cells stain positively for lysozyme. (Immunoperoxidase with hematoxylin counterstain.)

1 month to 20 years. Six tumors arose in the clivus, 4 in the cervical or thoracic vertebrae, and 2 in the lumbar and sacrococcygeal areas. Histologically, 6 cases were classic chordomas; the other 6 had nonclassic features of a round-cell or spindle-cell tumor. Ten children had died of tumor at intervals of 3 weeks to 4.5 years after treatment. Lung and lymph nodes were the most common metastatic sites.

Carson and Streib[125] described a patient with myasthenia gravis who had a chordoma of the clivus resected 16 years previously. Investigations suggested that the patient produced antibody to muscle-like antigens of the chordoma that subsequently cross-reacted with acetylcholine receptor and led to clinical myasthenia gravis.

The location of the tumor in the midline of the axial skeleton between the spheno-occipital region and the sacrum is an important diagnostic clue. In comparison, low-grade myxoid chondrosarcoma of the base of the skull usually originates off the midline.[126] Chordomas are more frequent at either end of the axial skeleton than in the intervening vertebrae, although tumors in that location do occur.[127, 128] Fewer than one sixth of chordomas arise in the mobile (cervical, thoracic, or lumbar) spine. Bjornsson et al.[129] studied 40 patients, 27 men and 13 women, with chordoma of the mobile spine. Of these, 19 tumors were located in the cervical spine, 7 in the thoracic spine, and 14 in the lumbar area. Variations in histologic appearance, including an occasional chondroid background, did not affect biologic behavior in this group.

Radiologic Features

Sacral chordomas show a midline, lobular, or geographic focus of osteolysis (Fig. 17–7). The tumors are occasionally associated with expansion, with or without osteosclerosis. An anterior or lateral soft tissue mass, best seen with a CT scan, is almost always present.[130, 131] The soft tissue mass, which usually shows patchy calcification or contains fragments of bone, protrudes anteriorly into the abdomen and may be of sufficient size to compress the intestines and bladder.[132] Chordomas appear hot on technetium 99m bone scans. Sacral chordomas are often difficult to visualize be-

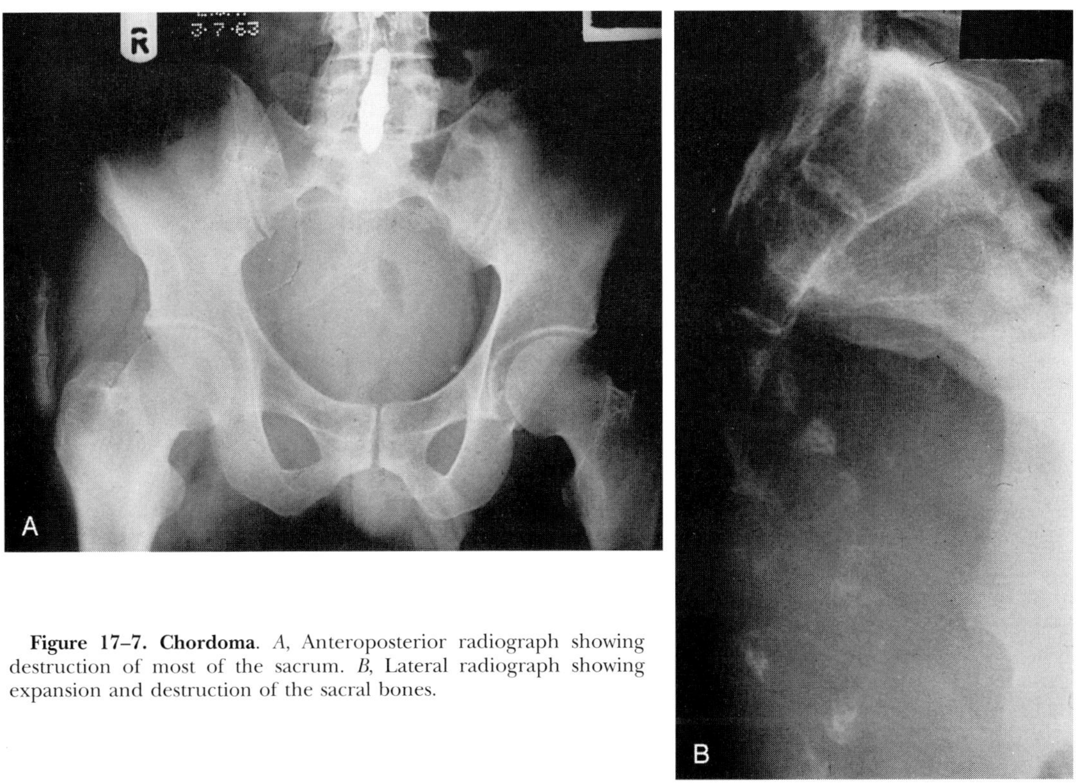

Figure 17–7. Chordoma. *A*, Anteroposterior radiograph showing destruction of most of the sacrum. *B*, Lateral radiograph showing expansion and destruction of the sacral bones.

cause of gas and fecal matter obscuring the bony destruction.

Intracranial chordomas characteristically destroy the clivus and parasellar parts of the middle fossa.[130] Occasionally, the clivus may remain intact despite extensive destructive lesions of the sellar region. Most intracranial chordomas are midline tumors but some are predominantly unilateral, and a nasopharyngeal mass is found in one third of cases at presentation. Calcification occurs in 50 to 70% of intracranial chordomas.[130]

Chordomas of the vertebral bodies lead to destruction and vertebral collapse. Vertebral chordomas often involve two or more vertebrae, producing destructive changes with a sclerotic rim. The intervertebral disc may be affected early in the course of the disease, unlike most primary or metastatic bone tumors. A paraspinal soft tissue mass containing calcification is often present.[130]

Pathologic Features

Macroscopic examination of chordomas shows them to be soft, gelatinous, lobulated tumors with areas of hemorrhage. The tumors often appear finely encapsulated, and the lobules of tumor are separated by thin bands of fibrous tissue. Foci of necrosis and cyst formation are common, but dystrophic calcification is rare. Size at presentation varies from 2 to 3 cm diameter for cranial chordomas to 7 to 15 cm for sacral chordomas. Intracranial chordomas are rarely large because of the involvement of vital structures—sella turcica, brain stem, and regional cranial nerves.[133] Recurrent sacral tumors can be as large as 80 cm in diameter and weigh 36 kg.

Histopathology

Chordomas are lobulated tumors formed of cells that grow in chords, nests, and trabeculae separated by variable amounts of extracellular mucins (Fig. 17–8*A* [see also color Figure 17–8]). Most chordomas have some areas where the cells show a syncytial arrangement. Recognition of this syncytial arrangement allows elimination of liposarcoma from the differential diagnosis as liposarcomas do not form cordlike or nesting patterns.[134]

Small spindle-shaped cells with little or no mucin are called stellate cells and are believed to be the precursor population. Larger cells containing abundant mucin with an open, basket-weave, or spider-web appearance with large vacuoles are called physaliphorous cells (from the Greek, meaning bubble) (Fig. 17–8*B*). Some of the vacuoles contain glycogen,[135] whereas others contain mucin. Occasional chordomas contain physaliphorous cells dominated by a single vacuole, which pushes the nucleus to one side and simulates signet ring adenocarcinoma. About 10% of chordomas do not contain physaliphorous cells despite extensive sampling. Cells intermediate between the stellate and physaliphorous cells are also found. Cultures of human sacral chordoma can be successfully maintained for up to 30 days.[136]

The differential diagnosis of chordoma includes metastatic carcinoma, chondrosarcoma (see later discussion) and meningioma. Meningioma is a relatively common intracranial tumor, occurring most frequently in adults, that is capable of a wide variety of growth patterns. Zuppan et al.[137] described a meningioma in a child that had a peculiar chordoma-like appearance.

Immunohistochemistry

Chordomas show positive immunohistochemical labeling for S-100 protein (Fig. 17–8*C*)[113] and for epithelial markers such as cytokeratins (Fig. 17–8*D* [see color Figure 17–8])[114, 115] and epithelial membrane antigen (Fig. 17–9*A* [see also color Figure 17–9]).[115, 116] This unusual combination is usually sufficient to establish the diagnosis in an appropriately sited tumor, although renal adenocarcinomas can show a similar immunophenotype. Touch preparations or cryostat sections of chordomas also stain positively for α-naphthyl acetate esterase (Fig. 17–9*B*).[117]

Heikinheimo et al.[138] described a detailed immunohistochemical characterization of different cytokeratin subclasses performed on three chordomas. Simple epithelial cytokeratins 8, 18, and 19 were detected in all tumors, while cytokeratin 7 was not found. Cytokeratins characteristic of squamous differentiation were generally lacking, with the exception of the variable expression of cytokeratin 4.

A study by Maiorano et al.[139] showed constant coexpression of cytokeratin, neurofilaments, and vimentin in chordomas, whereas desmin and glial fibrillary acidic protein are not demonstrable. Chordomas are positive

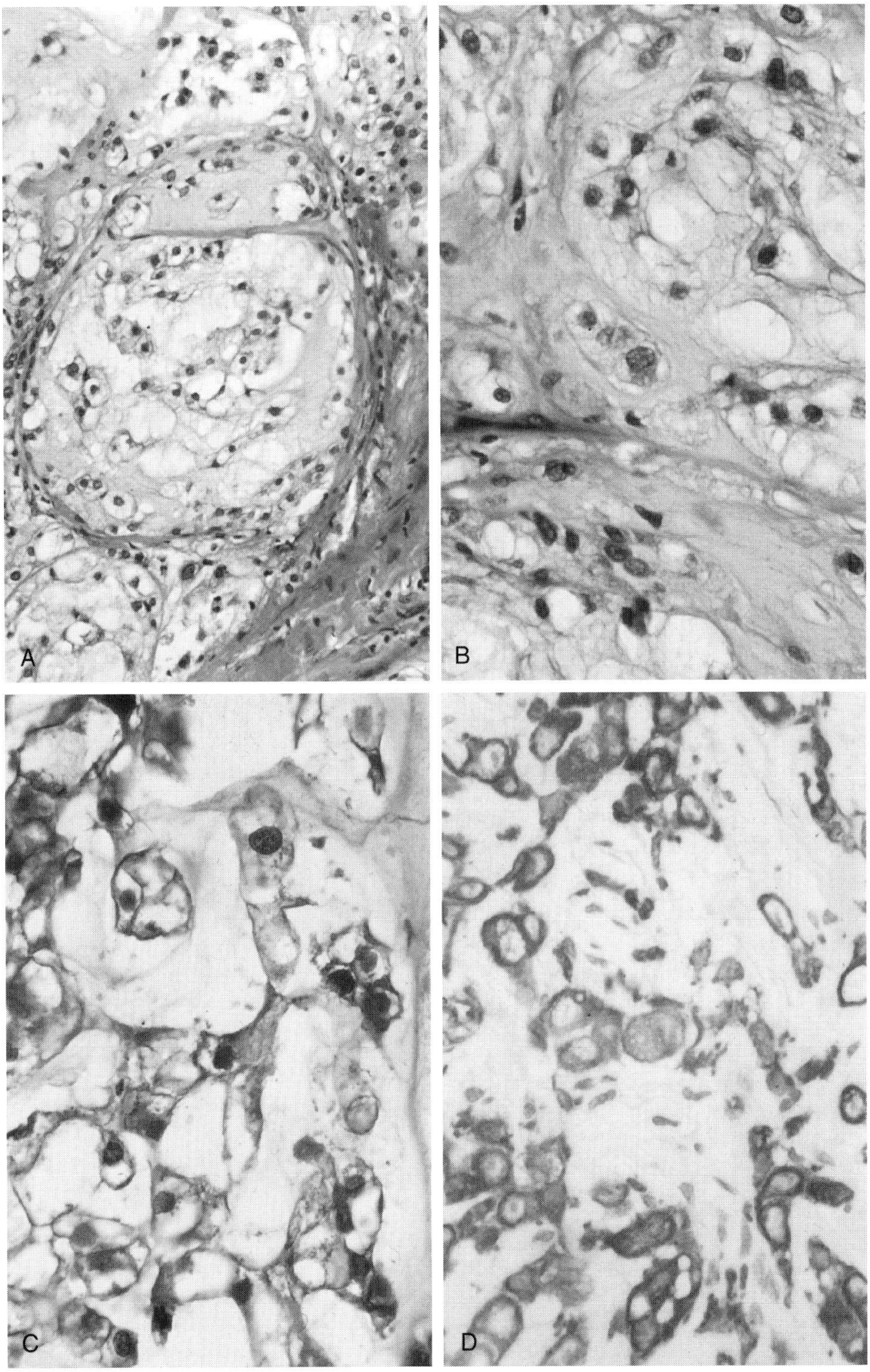

Figure 17–8. Chordoma. *A*, Low-power view of a typical chordoma showing the lobulated arrangement, with clusters of tumor cells surrounded by abundant extracellular mucin. *B*, High-power view of a typical chordoma. The clusters contain physaliphorous cells with numerous intracellular vacuoles. *C*, The nuclei and cytoplasm of the tumor cells stain strongly for S-100 protein. (Immunoperoxidase.) *D*, The cytoplasm of the tumor cells stains strongly for cytokeratins. (Immunoperoxidase using CAM 5.2 as the primary antibody, hematoxylin counterstain.) (See also color figure.)

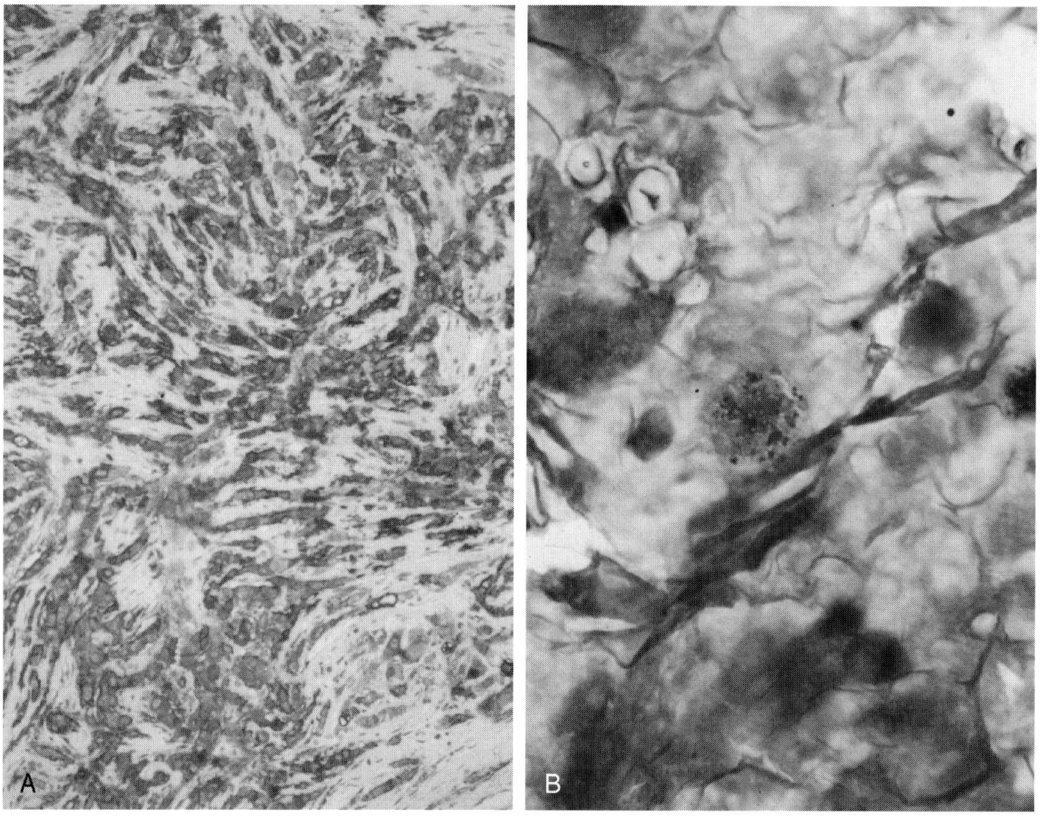

Figure 17–9. Chordoma. *A,* The cytoplasm, and especially the cell and vacuole membranes, stain for epithelial membrane antigen. (Immunoperoxidase using HMFG-2 as the primary antibody, hematoxylin counterstain.) *B,* Touch preparation stained for α-naphthyl acetate esterase showing positivity in the cell cytoplasm. (Simultaneous capture technique using hexazonium pararosaniline.) (See also color figure.)

with polyclonal, but not monoclonal, antibodies against glial fibrillary acidic protein.[140]

Human fetal notochords and chordomas both exhibit basement membrane proteins (such as type IV collagen and laminin) and type VI collagen. Type II collagen, a main structural protein of cartilage, is also present in both tissues. In chordomas, type II collagen is not so widespread as in notochords, and the main collagen is type I.[141]

Cytopathology

Cytologic examination shows syncytial clusters of hyperchromatic cells, often with abundant metachromatic extracellular matrix. Stellate and cuboidal cells often contain intracytoplasmic vacuoles (see Chapter 7). Intranuclear inclusions, mitotic figures, and anisonucleosis are prominent features.[142] That chordoma metastases may lack physaliphorous cells should also be recognized.[143] A number of chordomas have been diagnosed by fine-needle aspiration biopsy.[144, 145] Immunohistochemical studies are as useful in the cytologic diagnosis as in the histologic diagnosis of chordoma.[146]

Electron Microscopy

Peculiar granular endoplasmic reticulum-mitochondria complexes of unknown significance are present in many chordomas[147] but are not specific for this tumor, as they can be found in other neoplasms such as clear cell chondrosarcoma[148] and malignant fibrous histiocytoma.[149] The latter finding is consistent with the known transformation of chordoma into malignant fibrous histiocytoma. Jeffrey et al.[150] reported a clival chordoma that demonstrated many parallel bundles of 27 nm diameter microtubule aggregates within the rough endoplasmic reticulum. Such microtubule aggregates have been described in a number of different entities, and they are a nonspecific finding.

Cytogenetics

A specific or characteristic anomaly has not yet been identified in chordoma.[151–153] No recurrent structural rearrangement has been identified; the only chromosome bands involved more than once are 1q21, 3q11, 5p15, 20q13, and 21q22 (see Chapter 4).

Mertens et al.[151] described successful cytogenetic analysis in seven of eight sacral chordomas, with clonal chromosome aberrations detected in three cases. Gibas et al.[152] reported cytogenetic analyses of two sacral chordomas that showed clonal chromosome abnormalities, including numerical and structural aberrations. Both tumors showed translocations involving the same band of chromosome 21 (21q22) suggesting a specific association of this chromosome region with chordoma. Proto-oncogenes *ETS2* and *ERG* have been mapped to this chromosome band.

Chordomas with Malignant Spindle Cell Components

Sarcomatous transformation in chordoma *(dedifferentiated chordoma)* is a rare condition but has been emphasized as a distinct entity because of its more aggressive clinical course. Hruban et al.[154] described a recurrent lumbosacral chordoma with high-grade cartilaginous and spindle-cell components in additional to typical chordomatous tissue. This patient had undergone postoperative radiotherapy following resection of a histologically typical sacral chordoma. Tomlinson et al.[155] reported two anaplastic cranial chordomas in patients who had not received irradiation. The incidence of anaplastic transformation was 4% (2 of 52 cranial chordomas seen at the Mayo Clinic between 1966 and 1984). Immunohistochemistry showed the immunophenotype of chordoma in both tumors, but keratin and EMA reactivity was lost in the anaplastic areas.

Hruban et al.[156] studied four chordomas with malignant spindle cell components and 12 conventional chordomas by DNA flow cytometry and immunohistochemistry for a variety of epithelial and mesenchymal markers. Their results suggested that aneuploidy is more common in spindle-cell chordomas than in conventional chordomas, and that some spindle-cell chordomas are multipotential neoplasms in which the cells are capable of differentiation along both epithelial and mesenchymal pathways.

Choi and Kim[157] described a case of dedifferentiated chordoma (chordoma associated with malignant fibrous histiocytoma) arising from the sacrococcygeal region. Immunohistochemistry in the chordomatous area showed cytokeratin, EMA, and S-100 protein positivity. The spindle and giant cells in the transitional areas of chordoma and malignant fibrous histiocytoma were cytokeratin, EMA, vimentin, and α_1-antichymotrypsin positive. The spindle and giant cells in the central area of malignant fibrous histiocytoma were cytokeratin and EMA negative, but vimentin and α_1-antichymotrypsin positive. These results support the pathogenesis of sarcomatous transformation from chordoma.

Chondroid Chordomas

A seemingly distinct group of predominantly spheno-occipital neoplasms, which are histologically composed of both typical chordomatous and abundant cartilaginous tissue, is known as chondroid chordomas.[158] In the chondromatous areas, chordoma cells within lacunae are surrounded by stroma resembling cartilage. The tumors share ultrastructural features with both typical chordoma and chondrosarcoma[159] but have the immunophenotype of chordomas.[160] Rare cases of chondroid chordoma have been reported in the sacrococcygeal region. The mean age of patients with chondroid chordomas is 40 years and the male-to-female ratio is 1.8:1.[161]

It is important to distinguish between chondroid chordomas and other similar tumors in the skull base (chordoma, chondrosarcoma) because of the better prognosis and survival associated with chondroid chordomas. The mean survival time for 19 patients at the Mayo Clinic with chondroid chordomas was 15.8 years, compared with 4.1 years for 36 patients with typical chordomas.[158]

Rosenberg et al.[162] used light microscopy and immunohistochemistry to study 12 chondroid chordomas, 38 classic chordomas, and 28 chondrosarcomas that arose in the skull base or spine. All chondroid and nonchondroid chordomas were positive for cytokeratin, and the majority were also positive for EMA and carcinoembryonic antigen. In contrast, none of the chondrosarcomas stained for cytokeratin, EMA, or carcinoembryonic antigen. Vimentin and S-100 were positive in more than 95% of both classic and chondroid chordomas and chondrosarcomas. The authors concluded that chondroid chordoma is a variant of chordoma and should not be confused with chondrosarcoma.

Ishida and Dorfman[163] have discussed the classification of cartilaginous tumors of the skull base, including chondroid chordoma and chondrosarcoma. They concluded that chondrosarcoma of the skull base is a distinct clinicopathologic entity that can be distinguished from chordoma by the immunohistochemical staining pattern. They also suggested that the chondroid chordomas originally described by Heffelfinger et al.[158] may have included some true chondrosarcomas with focal areas of myxoid chordoma-like appearance. Focal chondroid differentiation in chordoma is not a rare phenomenon. Further study is needed to define whether chordoma with chondroid foci should be separated out from conventional chordoma as a distinct entity with a better prognosis. Jeffery et al.[164] proposed that chondroid chordomas should be classified as *hyalinized chordomas* to clarify their histogenesis and avoid confusion with chondrosarcomas of the skull base.

Treatment and Prognosis

The treatment of choice for chordoma usually consists of radical surgery, sometimes followed by radiotherapy. Extensive surgical resection is difficult because of local invasion, and the local recurrence rate remains high. Kaiser et al.[165] described the results of en bloc excision by the posterior approach for sacral chordomas. For 25 patients who had complete excision of the tumor without contamination of the surgical wound, the recurrence rate was 28%. For 25 patients whose tumor was entered at surgery, the recurrence rate was 64%.

Base of skull chordomas usually are not amenable to complete surgical resection, and most require postoperative radiotherapy. The natural history of skull base chordoma is typified by slow locally invasive tumor progression and eventual death, although few parameters are known that allow stratification of patients into prognostic groups. O'Connell et al.[166] described 62 patients with skull base chordomas treated by proton beam irradiation therapy with at least 2 years follow-up. Female sex, tumor necrosis in preradiation biopsy, and tumor volume in excess of 70 mL were each independent predictors of shortened overall survival. The striking difference in survival between the sexes suggests that further investigations of these tumors should include hormonal receptors status determination and consideration of hormonal manipulation in their management.

Metastases from chordomas are a late event. Chambers and Schwinn[167] reviewed the incidence of distant metastases in 30 cases of chordoma. The incidence of metastases was approximately 30%, mainly to skin and bone, with fewer in the lungs and lymph nodes. Mitchell et al.[161] have published Kaplan-Meier survival curves for both classic and chondroid chordomas. Classic chordomas have a 5-year survival rate of about 50% and a 10-year survival rate of 25 to 30%. Chondroid chordomas have 5- and 10-year survival rates of 80%. Forsyth et al.[168] showed that patients undergoing resection live longer, that patients who undergo postoperative radiotherapy tended to have longer disease-free survival times, and that overall and disease-free survival data were the same for classic and chondroid chordomas. Multivariate analysis showed that young age was the factor most strongly associated with longer survival, diplopia was associated with longer survival, and a high mitotic rate was associated with shorter disease-free survival.

There are several reports of chordomas with cutaneous metastases.[169–171] Zukerberg and Young[172] reported a case of sacral chordoma in which an ovarian metastasis was the first sign of recurrence 3.5 years after initial excision. The ovarian metastasis had to be differentiated from histologically similar primary ovarian neoplasms, particularly a juvenile granulosa cell tumor and an epithelioid smooth muscle tumor.

Accurate prediction of which chordomas will eventually metastasize is difficult. Clinically, local aggressiveness and the use of radiotherapy are related to metastasis, while histologically, more anaplastic chordomas are more likely to metastasize.

Schoedel et al.[173] evaluated predictors of survival in 36 chordomas and found that silver-staining nucleolar organizing region counts, fibrosis, and inflammatory response were not related to prognosis, but that aneuploid chordomas had a worse prognosis.

ADAMANTINOMA

Clinical Features

Adamantinoma of long bones is a rare, primary bone tumor of controversial histogenesis (see Chapters 4 and 13), usually arising in the anterior midshaft of the tibia. Most patients are teenagers or young adults, with 74% of patients in the second and third decades of life.[174] The literature suggests a very slight male predominance in the male-to-female ratio.[175, 176] Pain is the most common symptom, occasionally local swelling is seen, but pathologic fracture is uncommon. The duration of symptoms before diagnosis is very variable, from a few months to 50 years.[174]

This slowly growing, expansile tumor eventually causes thinning or destruction of overlying cortical bone. Occasional tumors arise in bones other than the tibia, such as the ischium,[177] rib,[178] and humerus.[179] The features of adamantinoma have been reviewed by Campanacci et al.,[180] Mori et al.,[175] and most recently by Moon[176] who has reviewed the 260 cases described in the world literature with emphasis on the case histories of 60 patients up to the age of 16 years. The case histories in children seemed to mirror those of adults, and the mortality rate was 20% in both groups.

Tibial adamantinoma may show the two apparently balanced translocations t(1;13;22)(q22;q12;p13) and t(15;17)(q12;p13) by cytogenetic analysis.[181]

Radiologic Features

Radiographs usually show an oval, well-circumscribed, multilocular cystic lesion (see Fig. 6–6).

Pathologic Features

The tumor consists of epithelial islands with palisading at the periphery and a loose reticular pattern in the center of the tumor cell nests, bearing a close resemblance to ameloblastoma of the jaw. Four histologic patterns have been described: spindle, basaloid, squamoid, and tubular.[182] Most tumors have a "basaloid" or "spindled" pattern (Fig. 17–10*A*). A squamoid pattern with keratinization or an

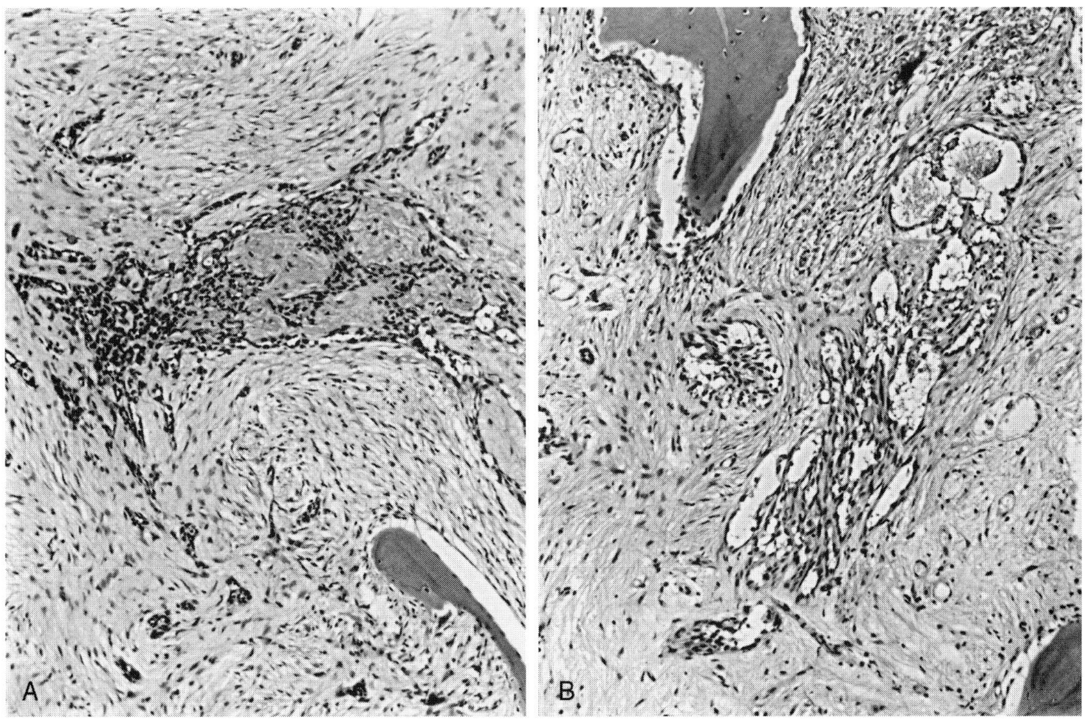

Figure 17–10. Adamantinoma of the tibia. *A*, Darkly stained clusters and strands of basaloid cells are present within a fibrous stroma. *B*, In this area, the epithelial cells show spaces within the clusters producing the so-called "angioblastic" appearance. (Courtesty of Dr T. Helliwell.)

"angioblastic" pattern[183, 184] is less common (Fig. 17–10*B*). In most cases with adequate material there is an associated fibrous dysplasia-like lesion,[185] which is interpreted as being a part of the spectrum of mesenchymal differentiation of which the tumor is capable (see Chapter 13).

Hales and Ferrell,[186] Tabei et al.,[187] and Galera-Davidson et al.[188] have described the cytologic features of primary, metastatic, and recurrent tibial adamantinomas, respectively. The smears contain single cells and cells arranged in small clusters and narrow strands, with some nuclear molding (see Chapter 7). Three cell types are described: large polygonal cells with abundant euchromatin, smaller cells with poorly defined cytoplasm and dense chromatin, and fusiform cells. The first two cell types are interpreted as epithelial and the third one as being derived from the stroma.

Immunohistochemistry

Adamantinomas show immunohistochemical labeling for cytokeratins and carcinoembryonic antigen.[189] They are negative for coagulation factor VIII–related antigen and blood group antigens.[189–193] The enzyme staining of the tumor cells for alkaline phosphatase and leucine aminopeptidase shows some correlation with normal eccrine glands, suggesting that adamantinoma may show eccrine differentiation.[189]

Electron Microscopy

Ultrastructural examination confirms the epithelial nature of the tumor with tonofilament bundles, moderate numbers of mitochondria, scattered rough endoplasmic reticulum, occasional Golgi bodies and lysosomes, dispersed glycogen granules, and microvillous processes.[189, 194] Well-formed basement laminae surround palisading tumor cell nests but not individual cells. The peripheral cells of the nests are bound to each other by desmosomes, and incomplete hemidesmosomes are seen in the outermost cells of the nests.[192] Features of endothelial differentiation (Weibel-Palade bodies, micropinocytotic vesicles, and tight junctions) are absent.[190]

Treatment and Prognosis

The clinically and histologically benign appearance of adamantinoma is deceptive, for the recurrence rate is high unless surgical extirpation is complete. Wide excision with bone grafting is the ideal treatment. The prognosis depends on the adequacy of therapy. Metastases to the lungs are not uncommon[195] and may present as pneumothorax.[196, 197] Van Schoor et al.[198] described the case of a woman who died of pulmonary metastases of an adamantinoma of the tibia in association with hypercalcemia. Terminal paraneoplastic severe hypercalcemia leading to coma and pancreatitis has also been reported.[197] Adamantinoma can also metastasize to other bones.[199]

OTHER BONE NEOPLASMS THAT MAY CONTAIN EPITHELIAL OR EPITHELIOID CELLS

Epithelioid Osteosarcoma

Uncommonly, osteosarcomas may contain epithelioid cells and should be considered in the appropriate age group (see Chapter 9).

Epithelioid Hemangioendothelioma

These rare tumors are discussed with the other vascular neoplasms in Chapter 16. In brief, histologic examination of these tumors shows epithelioid tumor cells with frequent intracytoplasmic vacuoles arranged in small nests or cords in hyalinized stroma. Immunohistochemical and lectin-histochemical studies for factor VIII–related antigen and *Ulex europaeus* I lectin confirm the endothelial nature of the tumor cells.

Sarcomas of Soft Tissues Involving Bone

Synovial sarcoma is the most common soft tissue sarcoma to directly invade bone from the adjacent soft tissues. The pathology of this sarcoma is discussed briefly in Chapter 18.

Epithelioid sarcoma of soft tissues[200] rarely can extend into the medullary cavity of adjacent bones, a finding that carries a worse prognosis.[201] Rosenberg et al.[202] reported on a patient with a recurrent epithelioid sarcoma of the hand who was observed for 5 years with a diagnosis of "nodular fasciitis." Eventually, the patient had a pulmonary metastasis and diffuse bone marrow spread, which was associated with a leukemoid reaction.

Epithelioid Leiomyosarcoma Metastatic to Bone

Wei et al.[203] reported a woman who presented with an epithelioid leiomyosarcoma in the breast that was treated by radical mastectomy. Brain and multiple bony metastases occurred 10 months later. The tumor was composed of nodules of small spindle and large round cells showing abundant eosinophilic, vacuolated cytoplasm, and prominent nucleoli. Glandular or ductular differentiation was absent. Tumor cells were vimentin and desmin positive, but cytokeratin, S-100 protein, EMA, actin, myoglobin, and α_1-antichymotrypsin negative. Electron microscopy showed focally cohesive large cells, with poorly defined intercellular junctions, surrounded by thin basal laminae.

Pituitary Adenomas and Carcinomas in Bone

Walker et al.[204] reported a malignant prolactinoma of the pituitary treated with external beam radiotherapy, bromocriptine, trans-sphenoidal hypophysectomy, and chemotherapy. Fifteen years after the original diagnosis, the patient developed bone metastases.

Very rarely, pituitary adenomas (developing from ectopic pituitary tissue) are found within the bones of the base of the skull. Borit and Blanshard[205] described a woman with the multiple endocrine neoplasia syndrome who died of a chromophobe pituitary adenoma of the sphenoid bone. A normal pituitary gland was present within the sella turcica.

Epidermoid Cysts Within Bones

These uncommon lesions are usually found in the terminal phalanges, although cases do occur at other sites. In a recent series of intraosseous epidermoid cysts, six cases were in the distal phalanges of the hand, one was in the distal phalanx of the foot with invasion of the adjacent joint, and one was in the skull.[206] The stratified squamous epithelium lining the cysts shows hyperkeratosis, occasionally with parakeratosis or dyskeratosis, and the cyst cavity is filled with keratin scales. In five of these eight cases, there was a history of previous local trauma.

REFERENCES

1. Simon MA, Bartucci EJ: The search for the primary tumor in patients with skeletal metastases of unknown origin. Cancer 58:1088, 1986.
2. Berrettoni BA, Carter JR: Mechanisms of cancer metastasis to bone. J Bone Joint Surg 68A:308, 1986.
3. Corcoran RJ, Thrall JH, Kyle RW, et al: Solitary abnormalities in bone scans of patients with extraosseous malignancies. Radiology 121:663, 1976.
4. Caffey J, Andersen DH: Metastatic embryonal rhabdomyosarcoma in the growing skeleton. Clinical radiographic and microscopic features. Am J Dis Child 95:581, 1958.
5. Machin T, Mashiyama ET, Henderson JA, et al: Bony metastases in desmoplastic pleural mesothelioma. Thorax 43:155, 1988.
6. Kulkarni JN, Kamat MR: Solitary metastasis to pubic bone from germ cell tumor of the testis: A case report. Tumori 77:271, 1991.
7. Schantz HD, Ramzy I, Tio FO, et al: Metastatic spindle-cell carcinoma: Cytologic features and differential diagnosis. Acta Cytol 29:435, 1985.
8. Frisch B, Bartl R, Mahl G, et al: Scope and value of bone marrow biopsies in metastatic cancer. Invasion Metastasis 1:12, 1984.
9. Urvoy P, Mestdagh H, Butin E, et al: Patellar metastasis from a large bowel adenocarcinoma. Acta Orthop Belg 59:409, 1993.
10. Seltzer VL, Beckman EM: Pathologic fracture of the ulna secondary to metastatic vulvar carcinoma: Report of a case. Gynaecol Oncol 4:232, 1976.
11. Gottlieb PD, Parikh SJ, Singh JK: Case report 295. Metastatic disease of the carpus (primary site: bronchogenic carcinoma). Skeletal Radiol 13:154, 1985.
12. Huber DF, Weis LD: Metastatic carcinoma of the distal ulna from an occult pancreatic carcinoma. J Hand Surg Am 10:725, 1985.
13. Morris DM, House HC: The significance of metastasis to the bones and soft tissues of the hand. J Surg Oncol 28:146, 1985.
14. Guttmann G, Stein I: Metastatic tumor of the thumb from adenocarcinoma of the colon. Internal Surgery 49:217, 1968.
15. Hayes MM, Jones EC, Verma AK, et al: Transitional cell carcinoma of the renal pelvis metastatic to the metacarpal: A case report correlating cytologic and histologic findings. Acta Cytol 36:946, 1992.
16. Knapp D, Abdul-Karim FW: Fine needle aspiration cytology of acrometastasis. A report of two cases. Acta Cytol 38:589, 1994.
17. Anderson EE, Leitner WA, Boyarsky S, et al: Renal-cell carcinoma metastatic to great toe. J Bone Joint Surg 50A:997, 1968.
18. Paul GR, Leach RE, Beetham WP: Pulmonary carcinoma metastasis to great toe. JAMA 208:2163, 1969.
19. Freedman DM, Henderson RC: Metastatic breast carcinoma to the os calcis presenting as heel pain. South Med J 88:232, 1995.
20. Hirshberg A, Leibovich P, Buchner A: Metastatic tumors to the jawbones: Analysis of 390 cases. J Oral Pathol Med 23:337, 1994.

21. Nicholas JJ, Srodes CH, Herbert D, et al: Metastatic cancer in Paget's disease of bone. A case report. Orthopedics 10:725, 1987.
22. Schajowicz F, Velan O, Santini-Araujo E, et al: Metastases of carcinoma in the pagetic bone. A report of two cases. Clin Orthop 228:290, 1988.
23. Bjorneklett A, Stavem P, Elgjo K: Relative value of sternal aspiration iliac crest biopsy and biopsy imprint in the diagnosis of secondary cancer involvement of the bone marrow. Acta Med Scand 203:279, 1978.
24. Auerbach O, Garfinkel L, Parks VR: Histologic type of lung cancer in relation to smoking habits, year of diagnosis and sites of metastases. Chest 67:382, 1975.
25. Philipson JD, Birkhead R, Phillip PE: Arthritis of the elbow caused by metastatic bronchogenic carcinoma. Clin Exp Rheumatol 1:165, 1983.
26. Nagendran T, Patel MN, Gaillard WE, et al: Metastatic bronchogenic carcinoma to the bones of the hand. Cancer 45:824, 1980.
27. Garciga CE, Bischoff ME: Uncommon metastases from cancer of the endolarynx. Rocky Mtn Med J 65:60, 1968.
28. Routh A, Lockey MW, Hickman BT: Metastases to bone as primary sign of laryngeal cancer. J Mississippi State Med Assoc 25:291, 1984.
29. Merino OR, Lindberg RD, Fletcher GH: An analysis of distant metastases from squamous cell carcinoma of the upper respiratory and digestive tracts. Cancer 40:145, 1977.
30. Kyriakos M, Berlin BP, DeSchryver-Kecskemeti K: Oat-cell carcinoma of the larynx. Arch Otolaryngol 104:168, 1978.
31. Hirsch FR, Hansen HH, Hainau B: Bilateral bone-marrow examinations in small-cell anaplastic carcinoma of the lung. Acta Pathol Microbiol Scand A 87:59, 1979.
32. Levitan N, Byrne RE, Bromer RH, et al: The value of the bone scan and bone marrow biopsy staging small cell lung cancer. Cancer 56:652, 1985.
33. Beiske K, Myklebust AT, Aamdal S, et al: Detection of bone marrow metastases in small cell lung cancer patients. Comparison of immunologic and morphologic methods. Am J Pathol 141:531, 1992.
34. Cifuentes N, Pickren JW: Metastases from carcinoma of mammary gland: An autopsy study. J Surg Oncol 11:193, 1979.
35. Yablonski-Peretz T, Sulkes A, Polliack A, et al: Secondary myelofibrosis with metastatic breast cancer simulating agnogenic myeloid metaplasia: Report of a case and review of the literature. Med Ped Oncol 13:92, 1985.
36. Garcia-Morteo D, Lema B, Maldonado-Cocco JA, et al: Carcinomatous arthritis of the elbow caused by metastatic breast carcinoma. Clin Rheumatol 6:273, 1987.
37. Bennett A, Charlier EM, McDonald AM, et al: Prostaglandins and breast cancer. Lancet 2:624, 1977.
38. McNeil BJ, Pace PD, Gray EB, et al: Preoperative and follow-up bone scans in patients with primary carcinoma of the breast. Surg Gynaecol Obstet 147:745, 1978.
39. DiStefano A, Tashima CK, Yap HY, et al: Bone marrow metastases without cortical bone involvement in breast cancer patients. Cancer 44:196, 1979.
40. Deck JH, Lee MA: Mucin embolism to cerebral arteries: A fatal complication of carcinoma of the breast. Can J Neurol Sci 5:327, 1978.
41. Mansi JL, Berger U, Easton D, et al: Micrometastases in bone marrow in patients with primary breast cancer: Evaluation as an early predictor of bone metastases. BMJ 295:1093, 1987.
42. Mansi JL, Berger U, McDonnell T, et al: The fate of bone marrow micrometastases in patients with primary breast cancer. J Clin Oncol 7:445, 1989.
43. Dearnaley DP, Sloane JP, Ormerod MG, et al: Increased detection of mammary carcinoma cells in marrow smears using antisera to epithelial membrane antigen. Br J Cancer 44:85, 1981.
44. Gugliotta P, Botta G, Bussolati G: Immunocytochemical detection of tumor markers in bone metastases from carcinoma of the breast. Histochem J 13:953, 1981.
45. Cote RJ, Rosen PP, Hakes TB, et al: Monoclonal antibodies detect occult breast carcinoma metastases in the bone marrow of patients with early stage disease. Am J Surg Pathol 12:333, 1988.
46. Matsumoto I, Furusato M, Inomata I, et al: Prostatic cancer presenting as metastatic adenocarcinoma of sphenoid sinus. Acta Pathol Jpn 36:1753, 1986.
47. Viadana E, Bross ID, Pickren JW: The metastatic spread of kidney and prostate cancers in man. Neoplasma 23:323, 1976.
48. Kuban DA, el Mahdi AM, Schellhammer PF, et al: The effect of transurethral prostatic resection on the incidence of osseous prostatic metastasis. Cancer 56:961, 1985.
49. Bjoorneklett A, Stavem P, Ly B, et al: Bone marrow metastases from prostatic cancer: Marked cytolytic effect after only a few days of treatment with diethylstilbestrol. Scand J Haematol 17:227, 1976.
50. Aprikian AG, Cordon-Cardo C, Fair WR, et al: Neuroendocrine differentiation in metastatic prostatic adenocarcinoma. J Urol 151:914, 1994.
51. Duchek M, Lingardh G, Saterborg NE, et al: Bone marrow examination as a diagnostic tool in carcinoma of the prostate. Int Urol Nephrol 7:59, 1975.
52. Boehme WM, Augspurger RR, Wallner SF, et al: Lack of usefulness of bone marrow enzymes and calcium in staging patients with prostatic cancer. Cancer 41:1433, 1978.
53. Schaffer DL, Pendergrass HP: Comparison of enzyme clinical radiographic and radionuclide methods of detecting bone metastases from carcinoma of the prostate. Radiology 121:431, 1976.
54. Oberneder R, Riesenberg R, Kriegmair M, et al: Immunocytochemical detection and phenotypic characterization of micrometastatic tumor cells in bone marrow of patients with prostate cancer. Urology Research 22:3, 1994.
55. Wakui S, Furusato M, Itoh T, et al: Tumour angiogenesis in prostatic carcinoma with and without bone marrow metastasis: A morphometric study. J Pathol 168:257, 1992.
56. Furusato M, Allsbrook W Jr, Kato H, et al: Flow cytometric analysis of prostatic carcinoma with and without bone marrow metastasis. Adv Exp Med Biol 324:189, 1992.
57. Forbes GS, McLeod RA, Hattery RR: Radiographic manifestations of bone metastases from renal carcinoma. Am J Roentgenol 129:61, 1977.
58. Marcove RC, Searfoss RC, Whitmore WF, et al: Cryosurgery in the treatment of bone metastases from renal cell carcinoma. Clin Orthop 127:220, 1977.
59. Tobisu K, Kakizoe T, Takai K, et al: Prognosis in renal cell carcinoma: Analysis of clinical course following nephrectomy. Jpn J Clin Oncol 19:142, 1989.

60. Kerbl K, Pauer W: Spontaneous regression of osseous metastasis in renal cell carcinoma. Aust N Z J Surg 63:901, 1993.
61. Lawler W, Marsden HB: Bone metastases in children presenting with renal tumors. J Clin Pathol 32:608, 1979.
62. Schmidt D, Harms D, Evers KG, et al: Bone metastasizing renal tumor (clear cell sarcoma) of childhood with epithelioid elements. Cancer 56:609, 1985.
63. Nemec J, Pohunkova D, Zamrazil V, et al: Pulmonary metastases of thyroid carcinoma. Czech Med 2:78, 1979.
64. Evans HL: Follicular neoplasms of the thyroid. A study of 44 cases followed for a minimum of 10 years with emphasis on differential diagnosis. Cancer 54:535, 1984.
65. Girelli ME, Casara D, Rubello D, et al: Severe hyperthyroidism due to metastatic papillary thyroid carcinoma with favorable outcome. J Endocrinol Invest 13:333, 1990.
66. Lloyd RV, Beierwaltes WH: Occult sclerosing carcinoma of the thyroid: Potential for aggressive biologic behavior. South Med J 76:437, 1983.
67. Chetty R, Learmonth GM, Kalan MR: The significance of nuclear grooves and phagocytosis in the diagnosis of metastatic papillary carcinoma of the thyroid. Cytopathology 2:43, 1991.
68. Birla RK, Bowden L: Solitary bony metastasis as the first sign of malignant gastric tumour or of its recurrence. Ann Surg 182:45, 1975.
69. Koga S, Takebayashi M, Kaibara N, et al: Pathological characteristics of gastric cancer that develop hematogenous recurrence with special reference to the site of recurrence. J Surg Oncol 36:239, 1987.
70. Schlimok G, Funke I, Pantel K, et al: Micrometastatic tumour cells in bone marrow of patients with gastric cancer: Methodological aspects of detection and prognostic significance. Eur J Cancer 27:1461, 1991.
71. Uchida T, Shikata T, Shimizu SI, et al: Gonadotropin and alkaline phosphatase producing occult gastric carcinoma with widespread metastasis of generalized bone. Cancer 48:140, 1981.
72. Schweitzer G, Villet W: Skeletal metastasis in primary carcinoma of the liver. S Afr Med J 45:476, 1971.
73. Shuffett WL, Richardson JD, McGee EM, et al: Hepatoma metastatic to rib. JAMA 215:120, 1971.
74. Sidhu GS: Hepatoma metastasis to bone. JAMA 218:1305, 1971.
75. Chakravorty RC, Makoui C: Symptomatic bony metastases from occult primary liver cancer. Am J Dig Dis 22:471, 1977.
76. Alavi AH: The clinic presentation of hepatocellular carcinoma by bone secondaries: A report of 25 cases. Ethiop Med J 24:71, 1986.
77. Fukusato T, Aoyama H, Mori W: Age and sex differences in bone metastasis of hepatocellular carcinoma in Japanese autopsy cases. Gastroenterol Jpn 24:127, 1989.
78. Perianes J, Pelaez JL, Lopez-Varela J, et al: Osseous metastasis as the only clinical manifestation of primary cancer of the liver. Bull Inst Med Res Univ Madrid 18:185, 1965.
79. Ali M, Fayemi AO, Braun EV: Malignant apudoma of the liver with symptomatic intractable hypoglycemia. Cancer 42:686, 1978.
80. Imamura M, Miyashita E, Miyagawa K, et al: Malignant insulinoma with metastasis to gallbladder and bone accompanied by past history of peptic ulcer and hyperthyroidism. Dig Dis Sci 32:1319, 1987.
81. Sworn MJ, Reasbeck P, Buchanan R: Rectal carcinoma presenting as massive metastatic involvement of foot bones. BMJ 2:98, 1978.
82. Igarashi M, Card GG, Johnson PE, et al: Bilateral sudden hearing loss and metastatic pancreatic adenocarcinoma. Arch Otolaryngol 105:196, 1979.
83. Antoniades J, Croll MN, Walner RJ, et al: Bone scanning in carcinomas of the colon and rectum. Dis Colon Rectum 19:139, 1976.
84. Vider M, Maruyama Y, Narvaez R: Significance of the vertebral venous (Batson's) plexus in metastatic spread in colorectal carcinoma. Cancer 40:67, 1977.
85. Hoehn JL, Ousley JL, Avecilla CS: Occult carcinoma of the colon and rectum manifesting as osseous metastasis. Dis Colon Rectum 22:129, 1979.
86. Yoshioka K, Shimizu H, Yokoo S, et al: Disseminated carcinomatosis of bone marrow from submucosal carcinoma in adenoma of the rectum. Intern Med 31:1056, 1992.
87. Brufman G, Krasnokuki D, Biran S: Metastatic bone involvement in gynecological malignancies. Radiol Clin Basel 47:456, 1978.
88. Matsuyama T, Tsukamoto N, Imachi M, et al: Bone metastasis from cervix cancer. Gynaecol Oncol 32:72, 1989.
89. Onuba O: Pathological fracture of right tibia, an unusual presentation of endometrial carcinoma: A case report. Injury 14:541, 1983.
90. Abdul Karim FW, Kida M, Wentz WB, et al: Bone metastasis from gynecologic carcinomas: A clinicopathologic study. Gynaecol Oncol 39:108, 1990.
91. Assor D: Basal cell carcinoma with metastasis to bone. Report of two cases. Cancer 20:2125, 1967.
92. Cornelius CE: Bone. A site of metastatic basal cell carcinoma. Arch Surg 104:848, 1972.
93. Lildholdt T, Sogaard H: Metastasizing basal cell carcinoma. Case report. Scand J Plast Reconstr Surg 9:170, 1975.
94. Christensen M, Briggs RM, Coblentz MG, et al: Metastatic basal cell carcinoma: A review of the literature and report of two cases. Am Surg 44:382, 1978.
95. McCrea ES, Coker DD, Hafiz MA: Metastatic basal cell carcinoma. South Med J 76:686, 1983.
96. Lopes de Faria J, Nunes PH: Basosquamous cell carcinoma of the skin with metastases. Histopathology 12:85, 1988.
97. Leslie BM, Kazes J, Ferrone JD: Sweat gland carcinoma metastatic to the tibia: A case report. Orthopedics 11:1189, 1988.
98. Morrissey K, Ward MD, Stadecker MJ, et al: Metastatic sweat gland carcinoma in an adolescent: A case report. Foot Ankle 9:96, 1988.
99. Grober A, Goldberg I, Rotem A: Malignant eccrine poroma with metastatic involvement of the long bones. Clin Orthop 223:303, 1987.
100. O'Donovan DG, Freemont AJ, Adams JE, et al: Malignant pilomatrixoma with bone metastasis. Histopathology 23:385, 1993.
101. Cross P, Richmond I, Wells S, et al: Malignant pilomatrixoma with bone metastasis [letter]. Histopathology 24:499, 1994.
102. Yeung KY, Stinson JC: Mucinous (adenocystic) carcinoma of sweat glands with widespread metastasis. Case report with ultrastructural study. Cancer 39:2556, 1977.
103. Qureshi AA, Gitelis S, Templeton AA, et al: "Benign" metastasizing pleomorphic adenoma. A case report and review of literature. Clin Orthop 308:192, 1994.

104. Pitman MB, Thor AD, Goodman ML, et al: Benign metastasizing pleomorphic adenoma of salivary gland: Diagnosis of bone lesions by fine-needle aspiration biopsy. Diagn Cytopathol 8:384, 1992.
105. Yamagiwa H, Yatani R: Adenocarcinoma of the lacrimal gland with metastases to the liver, bones and skin. Mie Med J 17:21, 1967.
106. Pierce ST, Cibull ML, Metcalfe MS, et al: Bone marrow metastases from small cell cancer of the head and neck. Head Neck 16:266, 1994.
107. Minkowitz S, Solomon L, Nicastri AD: Cytologically malignant thymoma with distant metastasis. Cancer 21:426, 1968.
108. Dahlin DC, Unni KK: Chordoma. *In* Bone Tumors: General Aspects and Data on 8542 Cases. Springfield, IL, Charles C Thomas, 1986, p 379.
109. Schajowicz F: Other tumors. 1. Chordoma. *In* Tumors and Tumorlike Lesions of Bones and Joints. New York, Springer Verlag, 1981, p 377.
110. Paavolainen P, Teppo L: Chordoma in Finland. Acta Orthop Scand 47:46, 1976.
111. Pazzaglia UE, Salisbury JR, Byers PD: Development and involution of the notochord in the human spine. J Roy Soc Med 82:413, 1989.
112. Salisbury JR, Deverell MH, Cookson MJ, et al: Three-dimensional reconstruction of human embryonic notochords: Clue to the pathogenesis of chordoma. J Pathol 171:59, 1993.
113. Nakamura Y, Becker LE, Marks A: S-100 protein in human chordoma and rabbit notochord. Arch Path Lab Med 107:118, 1983.
114. Miettinen M, Lehto V-P, Dahl D, et al: Differential diagnosis of chordoma chondroid and ependymal tumours as aided by anti-intermediate filament antibodies. Am J Pathol 112:160, 1983.
115. Salisbury JR, Isaacson PG: Demonstration of cytokeratins and an epithelial membrane antigen in chordomas and in human fetal notochord. Am J Surg Pathol 9:791, 1985.
116. Imrie SF, Sloane JP, Ormerod MG, et al: Detailed investigation of the diagnostic value in tumour histopathology of ICR2, a new monoclonal antibody to epithelial membrane antigen. Histopathology 16: 573, 1990.
117. Salisbury JR, Isaacson PG: Application of immunohistochemistry to the differential diagnosis of chordomas. J Pathol 143:330A, 1984.
118. Virchow R: Untersuchungen über die Entwicklungen des Schadelgrundes im gesunden und krankhaften Zustände und über den Einfluss derselben auf Schadelform Gesichtsbildung und Gehirnban. Berlin, G. Reimer, 1857.
119. Muller H: Ueber das Vorkommen von Resten der Chorda dorsalis bei Menschen nach der Geburt und über ihr Verhältniss zu den Gallertgeschwulsten am Clivus. Zeitschr Ration Med 2:202, 1858.
120. Watanabe A, Yanagita M, Ishii R, et al: Magnetic resonance imaging of ecchordosis physaliphora—case report. Neurol Med Chir Tokyo 34:448, 1994.
121. Sibley RK, Day DL, Dehner LP, et al: Metastasizing chordoma in early childhood: A pathological and immunohistochemical study with review of the literature. Pediat Pathol 7:287, 1987.
122. Willis RA: The Borderland of Embryology and Pathology. London, Butterworths, 1962.
123. Oexle K, Dammann O, Bechmann B, et al: Intracranial chordoma in a neonate. Eur J Pediat 151:336, 1992.
124. Coffin CM, Swanson PE, Wick MR, et al: Chordoma in childhood and adolescence. A clinicopathologic analysis of 12 cases. Arch Path Lab Med 117:927, 1993.
125. Carson HJ, Streib EW: Myasthenia gravis in a man with a history of chordoma: Observations of muscle-like antigens in carcinoma. Hum Pathol 24:339, 1993.
126. Bourgouin PM, Tampieri D, Robitaille Y, et al: Low-grade myxoid chondrosarcoma of the base of the skull: CT, MR and histopathology. J Comp Assist Tomogr 16:268, 1992.
127. Stoker DJ, Pringle J: Case report 205: Chordoma of mid-cervical spine. Skeletal Radiol 8:306, 1982.
128. Coraddu M, Floris F, Nurchi GC, et al: Chordoma of the cervical spine. Case report. J Neurol Sci 38:51, 1994.
129. Bjornsson J, Wold LE, Ebersold MJ, et al: Chordoma of the mobile spine. A clinicopathologic analysis of 40 patients. Cancer 71:735, 1993.
130. Firooznia H, Pinto RS, Lin JP, et al: Chordoma: Radiologic evaluation of 20 cases. Am J Roentgenol 27:797, 1976.
131. Utne JR, Pugh DG: The roentgenologic aspects of chordoma. Am J Roentgenol 74:593, 1955.
132. Smith J, Ludwig RL, Marcove RC: Sacrococcygeal chordoma. A clinicoradiological study of 60 patients. Skeletal Radiol 16:37, 1987.
133. Jaffe HL: Chordoma. Tumours and Tumourous Conditions of Bones and Joints. London, Kimpton, 1958, p 451.
134. Mirra JM: Intramedullary cartilage- and chondroid-producing tumours. *In* Mirra JM, Picci P, Gold RH (eds): Bone Tumors: Clinical Radiologic and Pathologic Correlations. Philadelphia, Lea & Febiger, 1989, p 648.
135. Crawford T: The staining reactions of chordoma. J Clin Pathol 11:110, 1958.
136. Horten BC, Montague SR: In vitro characteristics of a sacrococcygeal chordoma maintained in tissue and organ culture systems. Acta Neuropathol 35:13, 1976.
137. Zuppan CW, Liwnicz BH, Weeks DA: Meningioma with chordoid features. Ultrastruct Pathol 18:29, 1994.
138. Heikinheimo K, Persson S, Kindblom LG, et al: Expression of different cytokeratin subclasses in human chordoma. J Pathol 164:145, 1991.
139. Maiorano E, Renzulli G, Favia G, et al: Expression of intermediate filaments in chordomas. An immunocytochemical study of five cases. Pathol Res Pract 188:901, 1992.
140. Wittchow R, Landas SK: Glial fibrillary acidic protein expression in pleomorphic adenoma chordoma and astrocytoma. A comparison of three antibodies. Arch Path Lab Med 115:1030, 1991.
141. Ueda Y, Oda Y, Kawashima A, et al: Collagenous and basement membrane proteins of chordoma: Immunohistochemical analysis. Histopathology 21:345, 1992.
142. Finley JL, Silverman JF, Dabbs DJ, et al: Chordoma: diagnosis by fine-needle aspiration biopsy with histologic immunocytochemical and ultrastructural confirmation. Diagn Cytopathol 2:330, 1986.
143. Elliott EC, McKinney S, Banks H, et al: Aspiration cytology of metastatic chordoma. A case report. Acta Cytol 27:658, 1983.
144. Walaas L, Kindblom LG: Fine-needle aspiration biopsy in the preoperative diagnosis of chordoma: A

study of 17 cases with application of electron microscopic histochemical and immunocytochemical examination. Hum Pathol 22:22, 1991.
145. Hughes DE, Lamb J, Salter DM, et al: Fine-needle aspiration cytology in a case of chordoma. Cytopathology 3:129, 1992.
146. Plate KH, Bittinger A: Value of immunocytochemistry in aspiration cytology of sacrococcygeal chordoma. A report of two cases. Acta Cytol 36:87, 1992.
147. Erlandson RA, Tandler B, Lieberman PH, et al: Ultrastructure of human chordoma. Cancer Res 28:2115, 1968.
148. Povysil C, Matejovsky Z: A comparative ultrastructural study of chondrosarcoma, chordoid sarcoma, chordoma and chordoma periphericum. Pathol Res Pract 179:546, 1985.
149. Oliveira P, Clode AL, Simoe-Raposo J, et al: Mitochondria-rough endoplasmic reticulum complexes in a malignant fibrous histiocytoma. Ultrastruct Pathol 18:433, 1994.
150. Jeffrey PB, Davis RL, Biava C, et al: Microtubule aggregates in a clival chordoma. Arch Path Lab Med 117:1055, 1993.
151. Mertens F, Kreicbergs A, Rydholm A, et al: Clonal chromosome aberrations in three sacral chordomas. Cancer Genet Cytogenet 73:147, 1994.
152. Gibas Z, Miettinen M, Sandberg AA: Chromosomal abnormalities in two chordomas. Cancer Genet Cytogenet 58:169, 1992.
153. Bridge JA, Pickering D, Neff JR: Cytogenetic and molecular cytogenetic analysis of sacral chordoma. Cancer Genet Cytogenet 75:23, 1994.
154. Hruban RH, Traganos F, Reuter VE, et al: Chordomas with malignant spindle cell components. A DNA flow cytometric and immunohistochemical study with histogenetic implications. Am J Pathol 137:435, 1990.
155. Tomlinson FH, Scheithauer BW, Forsythe PA, et al: Sarcomatous transformation in cranial chordoma. Neurosurgery 31:13, 1992.
156. Hruban RH, May M, Marcove RC, et al: Lumbosacral chordoma with high-grade malignant cartilaginous and spindle cell components. Am J Surg Pathol 14:384, 1990.
157. Choi YJ, Kim TS: Malignant fibrous histiocytoma in chordoma—immunohistochemical evidence of transformation from chordoma to malignant fibrous histiocytoma. Yonsei Med J 35:239, 1994.
158. Heffelfinger MJ, Dahlin DC, MacCarty CS, et al: Chordomas and cartilaginous tumours at the skull base. Cancer 32:410, 1973.
159. Valderrama E, Kahn LB, Lipper S, et al: Chondroid chordoma: Electron-microscopic study of two cases. Am J Surg Pathol 7:161, 1983.
160. Salisbury JR: Demonstration of cytokeratins and an epithelial membrane antigen in chordoid chordomas. J Pathol 153:37, 1987.
161. Mitchell A, Scheithauer BW, Unni KK, et al: Chordoma and chondroid neoplasms of the sphenoocciput. An immunohistochemical study of 41 cases with prognostic and nosologic implications. Cancer 72:2943, 1993.
162. Rosenberg AE, Brown GA, Bhan AK, et al: Chondroid chordoma—a variant of chordoma. A morphologic and immunohistochemical study. Am J Clin Pathol 101:36, 1994.
163. Ishida T, Dorfman HD: Chondroid chordoma versus low-grade chondrosarcoma of the base of the skull: Can immunohistochemistry resolve the controversy? J Neurooncol 18:199, 1994.
164. Jeffrey PB, Biava CG, Davis RL: Chondroid chordoma. A hyalinized chordoma without cartilaginous differentiation. Am J Clin Pathol 103:271, 1995.
165. Kaiser TE, Pritchard DJ, Unni KK: Clinicopathologic study of sacrococcygeal chordoma. Cancer 53:2574, 1984.
166. O'Connell JX, Renard LG, Liebsch NJ, et al: Base of skull chordoma. A correlative study of histologic and clinical features of 62 cases. Cancer 74:2261, 1994.
167. Chambers PW, Schwinn CP: Chordoma. A clinicopathologic study of metastasis. Am J Clin Pathol 72:765, 1979.
168. Forsyth PA, Cascino TL, Shaw EG, et al: Intracranial chordomas: A clinicopathological and prognostic study of 51 cases. J Neurosurg 78:741, 1993.
169. Gagne EJ, Su WP: Chordoma involving the skin: An immunohistochemical study of 11 cases. J Cutan Pathol 19:469, 1992.
170. Peramezza C, Cellini A, Berardi P, et al: Chordoma with multiple skin metastases. Dermatology 186:266, 1993.
171. Jones B, Ghosh BC, Skelton HG: Chordoma with cutaneous metastasis. Cutis 54:250, 1994.
172. Zukerberg LR, Young RH: Chordoma metastatic to the ovary. Arch Path Lab Med 114:208, 1990.
173. Schoedel KE, Martinez AJ, Mahoney TM, et al: Chordomas: Pathological features, ploidy and silver nucleolar organizing region analysis. A study of 36 cases. Acta Neuropathol 89:139, 1995.
174. Unni KK: Adamantinoma of long bones. *In* Dahlin's Bone Tumors: General Aspects and Data on 11,087 Cases. 5th ed. Philadelphia, Lippincott-Raven, 1996, p 333.
175. Mori H, Shima R, Nakanishi H, et al: Adamantinoma of the tibia—a case report and a statistical review of reported cases. Acta Pathol Jpn 31:701, 1981.
176. Moon NF: Adamantinoma of the appendicular skeleton in children. Int Orthop 18:379, 1994.
177. Lasda NA, Hughes EC Jr: Adamantinoma of the ischium. Case report. J Bone Joint Surg 61A:599, 1979.
178. Plump D, Haponik EF, Katz RS, et al: Primary adamantinoma of rib: Thoracic manifestations of a rare bone tumour. South Med J 79:352, 1986.
179. Clarke RP, Leonard JR, von Kuster L, et al: Adamantinoma of the humerus with early metastases and death. A case report with autopsy findings. Orthopedics 12:1121, 1989.
180. Campanacci M, Giunti A, Bertoni F, et al: Adamantinoma of the long bones. The experience at the Istituto Ortopedico Rizzoli. Am J Surg Pathol 5:533, 1981.
181. Mandahl N, Heim S, Rydholm A, et al: Structural chromosome aberrations in an adamantinoma. Cancer Genet Cytogenet 42:187, 1989.
182. Weiss SW, Dorfman HD: Adamantinoma of long bone. An analysis of nine new cases with emphasis on metastasizing lesions and fibrous dysplasia-like changes. Hum Pathol 8:141, 1977.
183. Huvos AG, Marcove RC: Adamantinoma of long bones. A clinicopathological study of fourteen cases with vascular origin suggested. J Bone Joint Surg 57A:148, 1975.
184. Muretto P, Raspugli P: "Angioblastic" adamantinoma of the tibia. An immunohistochemical study. Tumori 71:387, 1985.
185. Levack B, Revell PA, Roper BA: Adamantinoma asso-

ciated with fibrous dysplasia. Int Orthop 10:253, 1986.
186. Hales MS, Ferrell LD: Fine-needle aspiration biopsy of tibial adamantinoma: A case report. Diagn Cytopathol 4:67, 1988.
187. Tabei SZ, Abdollahi B, Nili F: Diagnosis of metastatic adamantinoma of the tibia by pulmonary brushing cytology. Acta Cytol 32:579, 1988.
188. Galera-Davidson H, Fernandez-Rodriguez A, Torres-Olivera FJ, et al: Cytologic diagnosis of a case of recurrent adamantinoma. Acta Cytol 33:635, 1989.
189. Eisenstein W, Pitcock JA: Adamantinoma of the tibia. An eccrine carcinoma. Arch Path Lab Med 108:246, 1984.
190. Knapp RH, Wick MR, Scheithauer BW, et al: Adamantinoma of bone. An electron microscopic and immunohistochemical study. Virch Arch (A) 398:75, 1982.
191. Rosai J, Pinkus GS: Immunohistochemical demonstration of epithelial differentiation in adamantinoma of the tibia. Am J Surg Pathol 6:427, 1982.
192. Mori H, Yamamoto S, Hiramatsu K, et al: Adamantinoma of the tibia. Ultrastructural and immunohistochemic study with reference to histogenesis. Clin Orthop 190:299, 1984.
193. Perez-Atayde AR, Kozakewich HP, Vawter GF: Adamantinoma of the tibia. An ultrastructural and immunohistochemical study. Cancer 55:1015, 1985.
194. Rosai J: Adamantinoma of the tibia. Electron microscopic evidence of its epithelial origin. Am J Clin Pathol 51:786, 1969.
195. Lokich J: Metastatic adamantinoma of bone to lung. A case report of the natural history and the use of chemotherapy and radiation therapy. Am J Clin Oncol 17:157, 1994.
196. Winter WG, Jr: Spontaneous pneumothorax heralding metastasis of adamantinoma of the tibia. Report of two cases. J Bone Joint Surg 58A:416, 1976.
197. Altmannsberger M, Poppe H, Schauer A: An unusual case of adamantinoma of long bones. J Cancer Res Clin Oncol 104:315, 1982.
198. Van Schoor JX, Vallaeys JH, Joos GF, et al: Adamantinoma of the tibia with pulmonary metastases and hypercalcemia. Chest 100:279, 1991.
199. Law WB: Secondary adamantinoma of the ischium. Aust N Z J Surg 38:265, 1969.
200. Enzinger FM, Weiss SW: Soft tissue tumors. 2nd ed. St Louis, CV Mosby, 1988, p 936.
201. DeLuca FN, Neviaser RJ: Epithelioid sarcoma involving bone. Clin Orthop 107:168, 1975.
202. Rosenberg AE, Garber JE, Bennett W, et al: Epithelioid sarcoma with diffuse bone marrow metastases and associated leukemoid reaction. A case report and brief literature review. Am J Clin Pathol 90:723, 1988.
203. Wei CH, Wan CY, Chen A, et al: Epithelioid leiomyosarcoma of the breast: Report of a case. J Formosa Med Assoc 92:379, 1993.
204. Walker JD, Grossman A, Anderson JV, et al: Malignant prolactinoma with extracranial metastases: A report of three cases. Clin Endocrinol Oxford 38:411, 1993.
205. Borit A, Blanshard TP: Sphenoidal pituitary adenoma. Hum Pathol 10:93, 1979.
206. Hoessly M, Lagier R: Anatomico-radiological study of intraosseous epidermoid cysts. ROFO Fortschr Geb Rontgenstr Nuklearmed 137:48, 1982.

Chapter

18

TUMORS AND TUMOR-LIKE LESIONS OF JOINTS AND JUXTA-ARTICULAR BONE

Timothy R. Helliwell and David A. Ritchie

When a patient presents with a soft tissue swelling near to a joint, it is necessary to consider not only the uncommon primary neoplasms and tumor-like processes that may affect synovium but also the changes associated with inflammatory and degenerative arthropathies that may mimic some aspects of neoplasia and the possibility of disease spreading from the adjacent soft tissue or bone. Clinical and imaging investigations should narrow the differential diagnosis before a biopsy sample is taken, but, on occasion, the pathologist is presented with tissue from a clinically unsuspected disease process. Most primary neoplasms that may affect the juxta-articular bone (e.g., clear cell chondrosarcoma, giant cell tumor of bone, chondroblastoma, osteoid osteoma) are discussed in other chapters, although it should be noted that juxta-articular tumors such as osteoid osteoma may be associated with a proliferative synovitis.[1]

The general principles of imaging techniques are described in Chapter 6, and only pertinent details are included here. Plain radiography should be the initial imaging investigation. Although the lesion may be difficult to define radiographically, the presence of mineralization and adjacent bone changes may be important in the differential diagnosis. In addition, because many juxta-articular lesions may be related to an arthropathy, vital clues as to the type of arthropathy may be obtained from the radiograph (e.g., chondrocalcinosis and calcium pyrophosphate dihydrate disease). Although other imaging techniques, including ultrasonography, computed tomography (CT), and magnetic resonance imaging (MRI) may be helpful in the diagnosis of some juxta-articular lesions, many lesions have a wide range of appearances; and, therefore, tumor differentiation is not usually possible on imaging appearances alone, and histologic examination of the tissue is required.

STRUCTURE OF NORMAL SYNOVIUM

The structure of normal synovial tissue depends on the type of joint and the underlying tissue. The surface of a joint cavity or tendon sheath is lined by a layer of intimal cells that may be flattened in joints subjected to high intra-articular pressure (e.g., the hip) or may be cuboidal or columnar in joints that are under less mechanical stress. The intimal cells are supported by fibroadipose and vascular tissue, but there is no basement membrane and fluid, and solutes are readily exchanged between the synovial and intra-articular compartments.[2] Electron microscopic studies demonstrate two intimal cell types: type A cells with a phagocytic phenotype and type B cells, which show a fibroblastic phenotype with abundant endoplasmic reticulum.[2–4] These types probably represent the ends of a spectrum of cytologic differentiation, and transitional forms are also present.[4] Immunocytochemical studies support these concepts and suggest that fibroblast-like cells may have proliferative capacity.[5]

SYNOVIAL CHONDROMATOSIS

Synovial chondromatosis (synovial osteochondromatosis, synovial chondrometaplasia) is characterized by the formation of multiple cartilaginous nodules within the synovium, which may become detached to form intra-articular loose bodies. The disease was first described in 1813 by Leanac, with detailed descriptions provided by Jones in 1924, Freund in 1937, and Lichtenstein in 1955.[6, 7] "Primary" synovial chondromatosis should be distinguished from secondary synovial chondrometaplasia and from other causes of intra-articular loose bodies.

Clinical Features

Synovial chondromatosis presents as pain, stiffness, swelling, and limitation of movement between the ages of 14 and 67 years, with a peak incidence in the fifth decade, and with males affected twice as often as females.[8] Only rarely is the disease familial.[9] Fifty to 60% of cases involve the knee, with other common sites including the hip, shoulder, and elbow; 10% of cases are bilateral. Less common sites are the wrist, ankle, tarsal, and mandibular joints.[10] Extra-articular chondromatosis in a bursa may coexist with intra-articular disease.[11, 12]

Etiology and Pathogenesis

The etiology is unknown, although it is generally accepted that a metaplastic transformation of synovial myofibroblasts into a cartilaginous phenotype is the earliest abnormality.[6, 13] Milgram[14] described the disease as progressing through phases of metaplasia within the synovium without loose bodies, synovial metaplasia with loose bodies, and inactive synovial disease with intra-articular loose bodies.

Synovial chondromatosis tends to have a progressive course, although it may be self-limiting and may occasionally resolve spontaneously. Removal of loose bodies and the involved synovial membrane is the preferred treatment. Recurrence is uncommon.

The condition described as "snowstorm knee," in which hundreds of cartilaginous bodies up to 5 mm diameter occur in the knee joints of patients with normal synovial tissue, probably represents a different disease entity arising from the growth of aggregates of chondrocytes in the culture medium of the synovial fluid.[15]

Radiologic Features

The radiographic appearances vary with the stage of the disease. In early disease, nodule mineralization may be absent and radiographs may show only a nonspecific soft tissue density mass. However, most cases present as mineralized nodules that vary from small calcific foci to larger, rounded, ossified bodies (Fig. 18–1*A*). The loose bodies are usually multiple and of similar size, although a large dominant nodule may be present. Well-defined bony erosions and scalloping are occasionally evident, particularly in joints with a relatively tight capsule such as the hip and wrist.[16] In long-standing disease, secondary degenerative changes are usually present in the joint.

Arthrography may be useful in demonstrating unmineralized intra-articular lesions and can be combined with CT in the evaluation of the more complex joints.[10] The MR images reflect the components of the metaplastic nodules.[17, 18] Unmineralized nodules give a uniform intermediate signal intensity on T1-weighted images and a high signal intensity on T2-weighted images similar to that of hyaline cartilage. Because synovial fluid may have similar signal characteristics, a joint effusion may hide unmineralized nodules. If the nodules are attached to the synovium then, unlike synovial fluid, they may enhance with gadolinium. When calcification is present, foci of low signal intensity will be noted on all sequences. If the loose bodies ossify, the signal characteristics may show fatty marrow or trabecular bone internally and dense cortical bone peripherally.

Pathologic Features

Macroscopically, the synovium has an irregular surface with bluish white, rounded pedunculated nodules 0.1 to 3 cm in diameter (Fig. 18–2*A* [see also color Figure 18–2]). Usually the

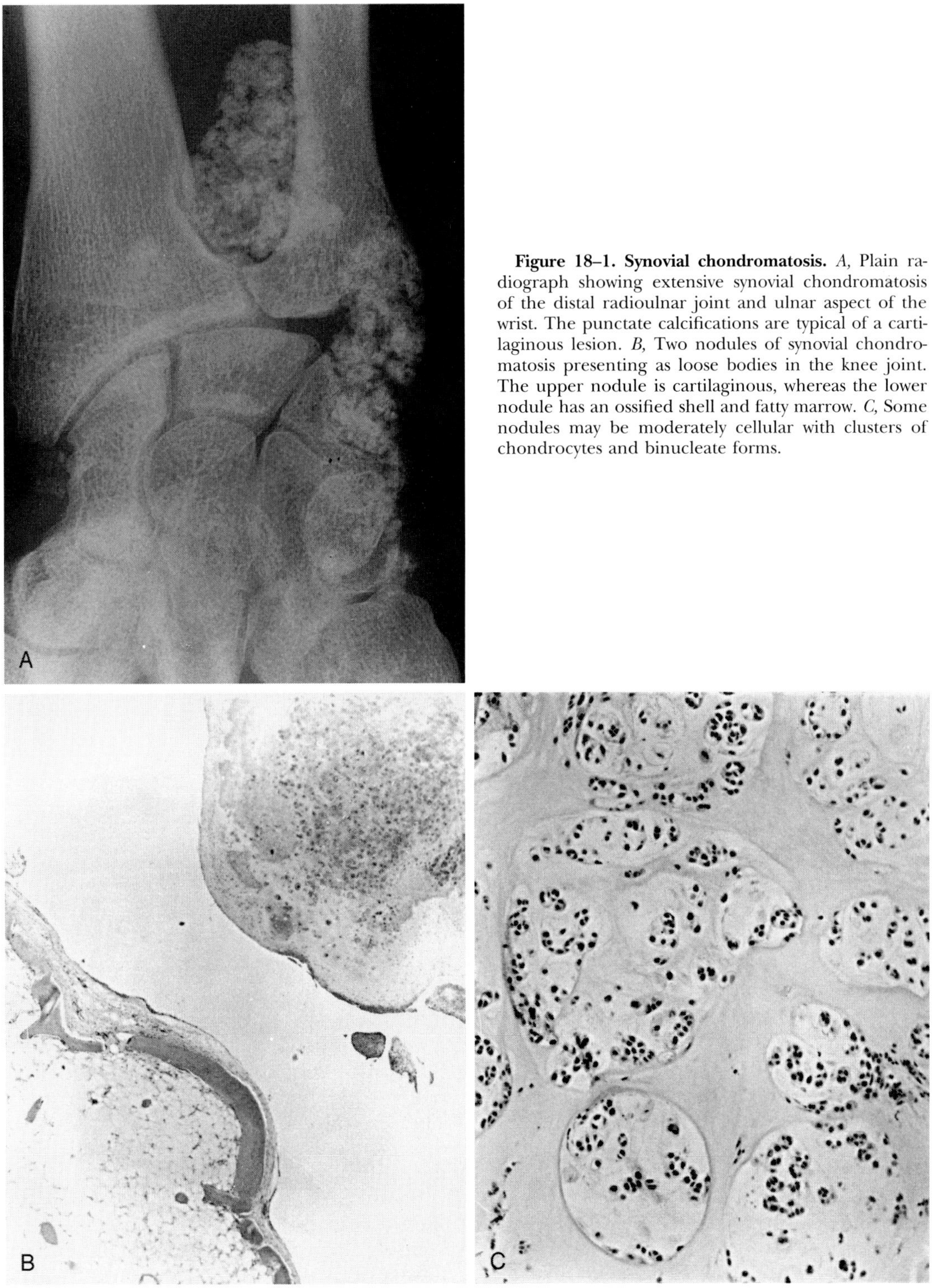

Figure 18–1. Synovial chondromatosis. *A,* Plain radiograph showing extensive synovial chondromatosis of the distal radioulnar joint and ulnar aspect of the wrist. The punctate calcifications are typical of a cartilaginous lesion. *B,* Two nodules of synovial chondromatosis presenting as loose bodies in the knee joint. The upper nodule is cartilaginous, whereas the lower nodule has an ossified shell and fatty marrow. *C,* Some nodules may be moderately cellular with clusters of chondrocytes and binucleate forms.

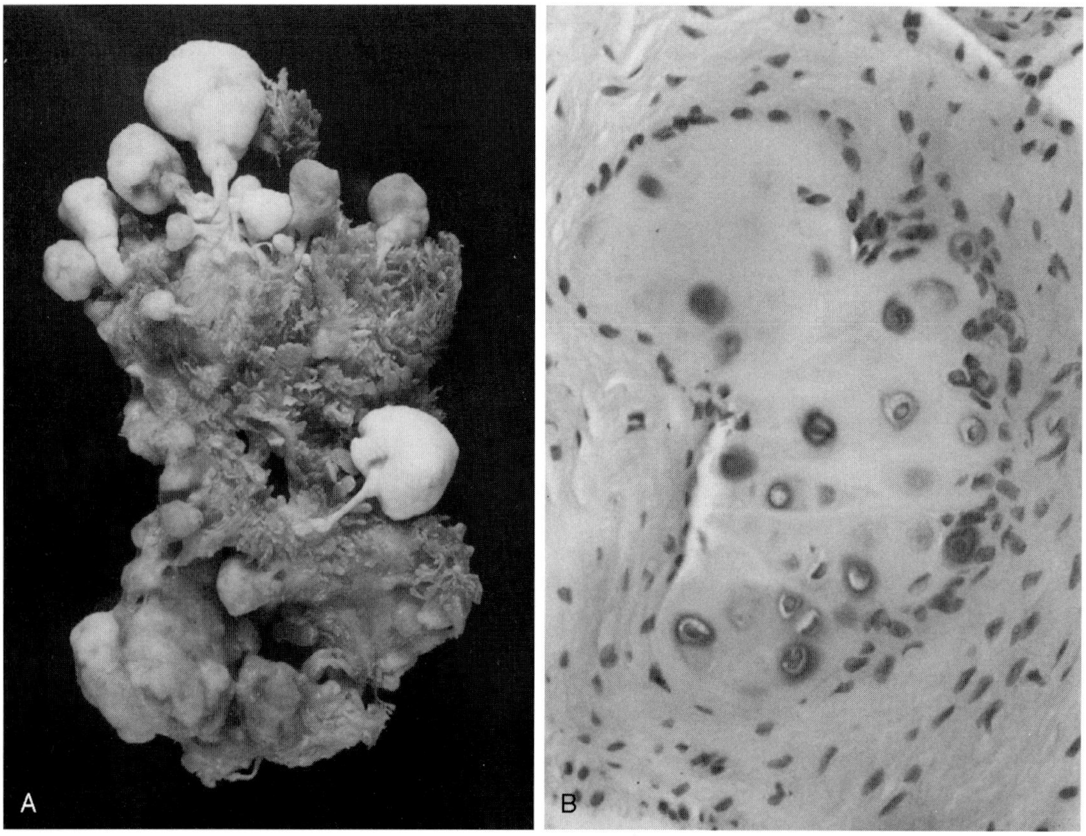

Figure 18–2. Synovial chondromatosis. *A,* Macroscopic appearance of typical synovial chondromatosis with pale cartilaginous nodules projecting from the synovial surface. *B,* A small chondroid nodule in synovial tissue is one of the earliest manifestations of synovial chondromatosis. (See also color figure.)

whole synovium is involved, but occasionally the changes may be restricted to a small area.

The earliest histologic changes are the formation of nodular aggregates of spindle cells in the synovium. These cells produce a chondroid matrix, which may be recognized by metachromatic staining with toluidine blue. As the nodules enlarge their cartilaginous nature becomes more evident (Fig. 18–2*B* [see color Figure 18–2]), and they tend to coalesce into multinodular aggregates. Calcification and ossification ultimately result in nodules of mature, lamellar bone with fatty marrow (Fig. 18–1*B*). Loose bodies, floating free within the synovial fluid, may show a covering of viable cartilage, even if the bone and marrow have undergone necrosis.

The cartilaginous nodules often show moderate cellularity with binucleate cells (Fig. 18–1*C*), features that in the appropriate intraosseous context would suggest chondrosarcoma. Provided the overall architecture is consistent, cytologic atypia is not a worrying feature in synovial chondromatosis.

Massive Synovial Chondromatosis

Uncommonly, the continued growth or fusion of smaller nodules results in a solitary intra-articular or extra-articular soft tissue mass.[19, 20] These patients tend to be slightly older (age range, 33 to 87 years) than the patients with typical synovial chondromatosis.[20] The knee is the most common site, but the disease may also affect the wrist, hand, shoulder, ankle, or elbow joints.

Radiologic and macroscopic examination show a large, lobulated soft tissue mass, 1.5 to 9 cm in diameter, adjacent to a joint and with focal calcification (Figs. 18–3 and 18–4 [see also color Figure 18–4]). Bone destruction does not occur, but "pressure" erosion of bone is described.

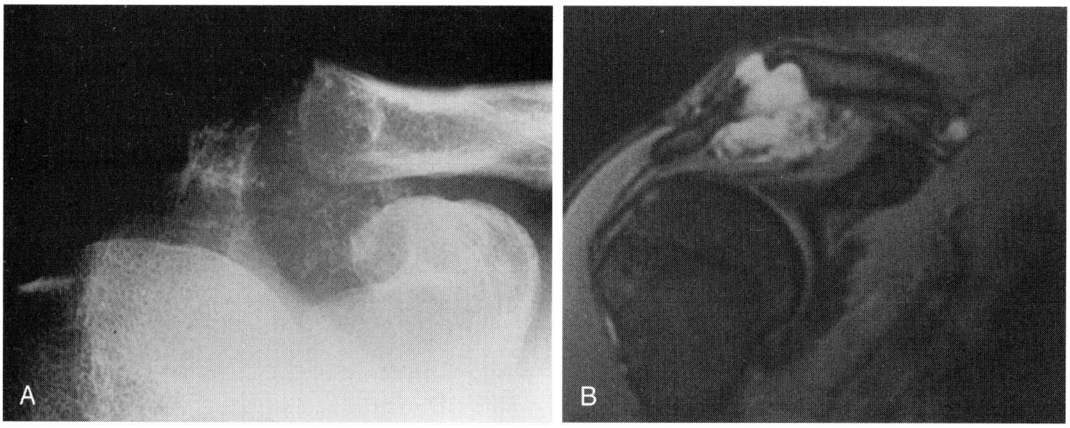

Figure 18–3. Massive synovial chondromatosis of the acromioclavicular joint. *A*, Plain radiograph showing a partly mineralized mass in the region of the acromioclavicular joint. *B*, T2-weighted MR image of the shoulder showing the mass has an inhomogeneous, mainly high signal intensity on T2-weighted sequences. The mass erodes the articular margins of the acromioclavicular joint and impinges on the supraspinatus muscle.

Microscopically, lobulated masses of hyaline cartilage are present and separated by birefringent collagenous strands (Fig. 18–5). The cartilage has a predominantly benign appearance, but foci of plump chondrocytes and binucleate cells are usually present. Focal clustering of chondrocytes into so-called brood capsules (reactive clustering) (see Fig. 18–1*C*) and the demonstration of metaplasia from fibrous tissue to cartilage should suggest the correct diagnosis.

The prognosis is good, with only 3 of 19 published cases recurring after local resection.

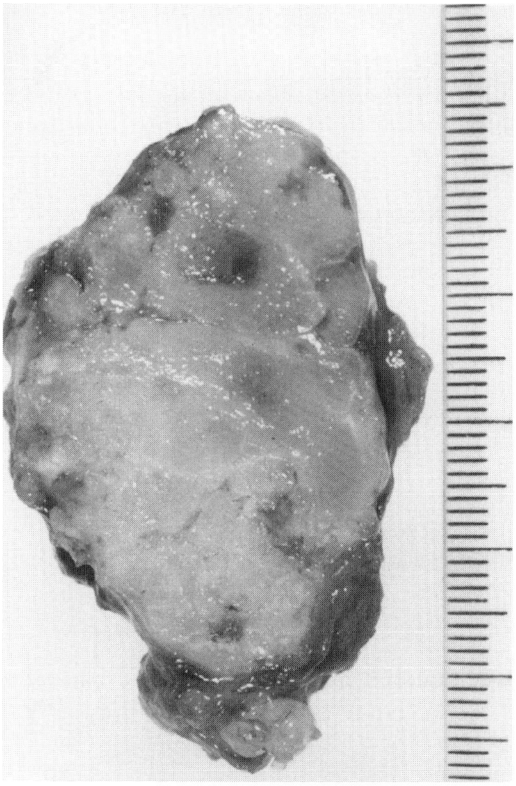

Figure 18–4. Massive synovial chondromatosis. Macroscopic appearance of a lesion of the shoulder that is up to 50 mm in diameter in this aspect (see also color figure).

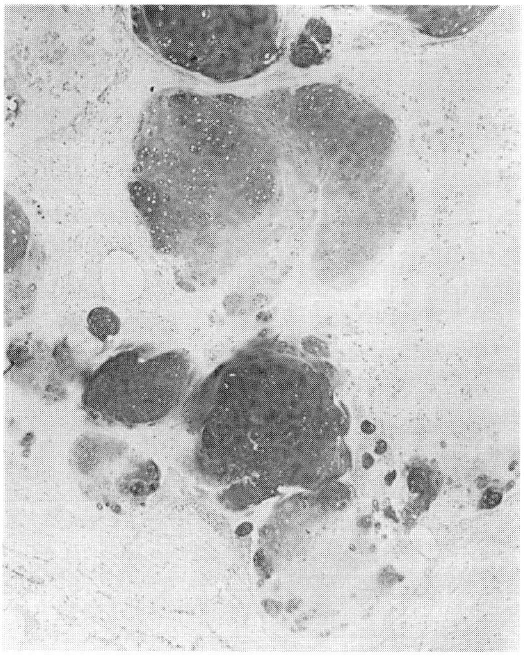

Figure 18–5. Massive synovial chondromatosis. Conglomerate nodules of chondroid tissue are the typical feature of this condition.

Differential Diagnosis

Synovial chondrosarcoma is the most important consideration. Malignancy is suggested by the presence of sheets of chondrocytes without the multinodularity seen in chondromatosis; crowding of cells, especially with spindle or undifferentiated cells at the edges of the sheets; myxoid change; necrosis; and mitotic figures.[21] Extension beyond the joint capsule or invasion of adjacent bone should also raise the suspicion of malignancy, although this has been reported in some cases of chondromatosis.[14]

Secondary synovial chondrometaplasia refers to the implantation of bony and cartilaginous debris as a result of degenerative joint disease that stimulates secondary cartilaginous metaplasia of the synovial tissues. The implanted fragments show a concentric layering of cartilage with endochondral ossification and lack of nuclear atypia.[22] In this situation, the radiologic appearance of gross joint destruction will be helpful, because this is only seen in the late stages of true synovial chondromatosis.[23] Secondary synovial chondrometaplasia may also occur in calcium pyrophosphate deposition disease[24] and after trauma or bone necrosis.

Intra-articular osteochondroma is the term used to describe a solitary, large (up to 5 cm) osteocartilaginous mass that is attached to the synovium by a pedicle. The surface is covered with cartilage, showing central endochondral ossification.[25] This appears to be a different process to that of multifocal synovial chondromatosis.

SYNOVIAL CHONDROSARCOMA

A malignant cartilaginous neoplasm arising in synovial tissues is a rare phenomenon and is much less common than synovial chondromatosis.

Clinical and Radiologic Features

By 1993, 19 cases of synovial chondrosarcoma arising in chondromatosis had been reported.[26] There is a wide age range (28–70 years) at presentation with a slight male predominance. Symptoms are usually present for at least 1 year (1 month to 25 years). Most cases occur at the knee, and rarely at the hip, elbow, or ankle joints. About half the cases show evidence of concurrent and presumably pre-existing synovial chondromatosis.[27]

Imaging studies are similar to those of synovial chondromatosis, the main distinguishing feature being the extension of the calcific deposits into the juxta-articular soft tissues or bone, although this is not always apparent.[28, 29]

Pathologic Features

In addition to the macroscopic features of chondromatosis (if present), resected cartilaginous tissue invades soft tissues and/or bone. The cartilage is often more mucinous than seen in chondromatosis, and necrosis may be present.

The microscopic architectural pattern is similar to that of chondrosarcomas at other sites (see Chapter 10) with a lobular growth pattern and chondrocytes dispersed in sheets with hypercellularity and spindling of the cells at the periphery of lobules.[21] Synovial chondrosarcomas may be Grade 1 through 3, although Grade 1 sarcomas are difficult to distinguish from synovial chondromatosis and unequivocal invasion beyond the joint capsule is required for diagnosis.

The differential diagnosis includes synovial chondromatosis and periosteal chondrosarcoma (see Chapter 11). Synovial chondromatosis is a more common disease with histologic differences (see earlier). In lesions with mild atypia, the diagnosis is more likely to be chondromatosis. It is important not to overdiagnose chondrosarcoma and therefore avoid unnecessarily radical surgery.

Treatment is usually radical surgery or amputation. Approximately one third of patients have developed pulmonary metastases, usually within 30 months of diagnosis.

FIBROHISTIOCYTIC PROLIFERATIONS OF SYNOVIAL TISSUES

A group of locally destructive fibrohistiocytic proliferations may affect the synovial tissues of joints, bursae, and tendon sheaths. These disorders are uncommon (two cases per million population), show similar histologic appearances, and are separated into three clinicopathologic entities with prognostic differences. These entities include diffuse villous and nodular synovial thickening of large joints (pigmented villonodular synovitis [PVNS]), a single lesion or cluster of nodular masses affecting a large joint or tendon sheath (localized nodular synovitis or localized tenosynovial giant cell tumor [L-TGCT]), and a soft tissue mass arising from a large joint or bursa that appears to be a more aggressive form of the disease (diffuse variant of tenosynovial giant cell tumor [D-TGCT]).[30, 31] Terms such as *benign synovioma* (suggesting a benign form of synovial sarcoma), *fibroxanthoma,* or *xanthogranuloma* have been superseded.[31]

Pigmented Villonodular Synovitis and Localized Tenosynovial Giant Cell Tumor

Although descriptions of L-TGCT and of PVNS are present in the literature of the late 19th and early 20th centuries,[32, 33] Jaffe et al.[32] were the first to recognize that the lesions affecting large and small joints and tendon sheaths were manifestations of the same cellular process and provided a detailed histologic description of the changes, recognizing the nonmalignant nature of the proliferation.

Clinical Features

Pigmented villonodular synovitis is most common between the ages of 20 and 40 years and affects females as frequently as males. The presentation is usually with progressive discomfort that may be associated with a nontraumatic hemorrhagic effusion. If untreated, secondary degenerative changes occur in the joint.

The L-TGCT more commonly affects females and is most common at age 30 to 50 years. The hand is the most common site, but lesions also occur around the feet, ankles, and knees. These nodular swellings grow slowly over several years and may present as mechanical derangement of large joints.

Etiology and Pathogenesis

The earliest descriptions considered these lesions to be a form of sarcoma, although most authors regarded the changes as those of a disturbance of lipid metabolism, a response to synovial hemorrhage, a benign neoplasm, or a reactive/inflammatory process.[34] Although lipid-laden macrophages are a prominent component of this group of lesions and may represent a localized disorder of lipid metabolism, there is no consistent systemic abnormality of triglyceride or cholesterol metabolism. The presence of intracellular and extracellular hemosiderin deposition has inevitably led to speculation on the possible role of repeated hemorrhage in the genesis of PVNS. However, the cellular changes are unlike those seen in hemophilia (see later) and are not identical to those evident after the injection of blood into the joints of experimental animals.[34]

Jaffe et al.[32] considered that the mixture of cells in these lesions and some similarity to the changes after traumatic or experimental hemarthrosis suggested that the lesions were of a reactive or inflammatory nature. The balance of evidence is now more in favor of a benign neoplastic process.[31] The nodular and centrifugal growth pattern of PVNS together with a difference between lesional tissue and adjacent synovium and a tendency to local invasion and recurrence are more suggestive of a benign intra-articular neoplasm.[30, 35, 36] Flow cytometric studies have shown that PVNS and L-TGCT have a diploid DNA profile, whereas three of seven cases of D-TGCT showed DNA aneuploidy, supporting a neoplastic hypothesis for the latter lesion.[37] Cytogenetic studies of a few cases of PVNS and L-TGCT have shown clonal chromosomal abnormalities, including trisomies 5 and 7[38–40]; and one case of D-TGCT showed trisomies 5 and 7 and clonal rearrangements involving chromosomes 1, 3, and 15.[41]

Radiologic Features

Plain radiographs of PVNS typically show periarticular soft tissue swelling without calcification, a normal bone density, preservation of cartilage until late in the disease, and well-corticated erosions, especially where the capsule is tight (e.g., in the hip or elbow joints). Arthrography may demonstrate a solitary mass (localized form) or multiple filling defects (diffuse form).[42] L-TGCT typically presents with a soft tissue mass commonly on the volar aspect of the finger, and associated osseous erosions are present in 10 to 25% of patients.[43]

Hemosiderin within the synovium can be detected by CT owing to its increased density.[44, 45] Although CT may be useful in demonstrating bone erosion and cyst formation, MRI is now the imaging method of choice for assessing both the localized and diffuse forms of PVNS (Fig. 18–6). Synovial hemosiderin is characterized by regions of low signal intensity on all MRI sequences[46, 47]; and although this is consistent with the diagnosis of PVNS, it also occurs in patients with a chronic hemarthrosis. MRI reveals the extent of bone involvement and allows assessment of any extra-articular or bursal extension of the disease.

Pathologic Features

The pathologic features of these conditions have been well described.[32–34] Macroscopically, PVNS of a large joint presents as a mixed, nodular, and villous thickening of the synovial tissues that have a yellow or red-brown color according to the amount of lipid and hemosiderin present (Fig. 18–7*A* [see also color Figure 18–7]). Villi may be fine or coarse and are often matted together to form a meshwork of tissue. Individual nodules may be several centimeters in diameter and may erode bone. Fibrinous masses ("rice seed bodies") may adhere to the surface or form loose bodies within the joint.

Localized tenosynovial giant cell tumor presents with rounded nodules or lobulated masses 0.4 to 4 cm diameter within tendon sheaths or in large joints. These nodules have a mottled yellow or red brown coloration on their cut surface, which is often crossed by bands of fibrous tissue.

Microscopic Features

The predominant cellular population is that of round or ovoid, histiocytic cells with a variable amount of cytoplasm that may be distended with lipid or hemosiderin (Fig. 18–7*B* [see color Figure 18–7]). There is often an uneven, zonal arrangement of lipid and hemosiderin-laden cells (Fig. 18–8*A*). The lipid and hemosiderin are always intracellular, and hemosiderin also accumulates in synovial intimal cells.

Osteoclast-like multinucleate giant cells are scattered through the lesions, although with variation in their number from one part to another. Fibroblasts, lymphocytes, and plasma cells are present in variable numbers and are

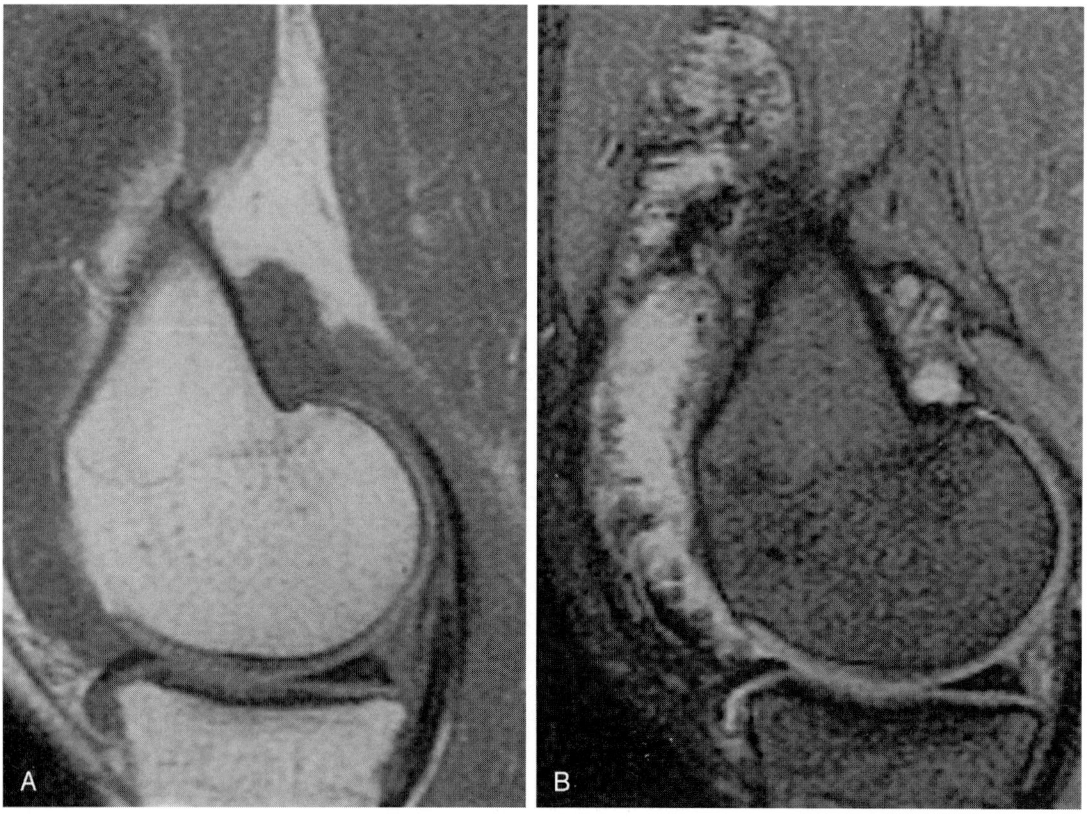

Figure 18–6. Pigmented villonodular synovitis of the knee joint. Sagittal T1-weighted *(A)* and T2-weighted *(B)* MR images demonstrate extensive synovial proliferation and a large joint effusion. On the T2-weighted image, some of the synovial proliferation has a very low signal intensity, owing to the paramagnetic effect of hemosiderin.

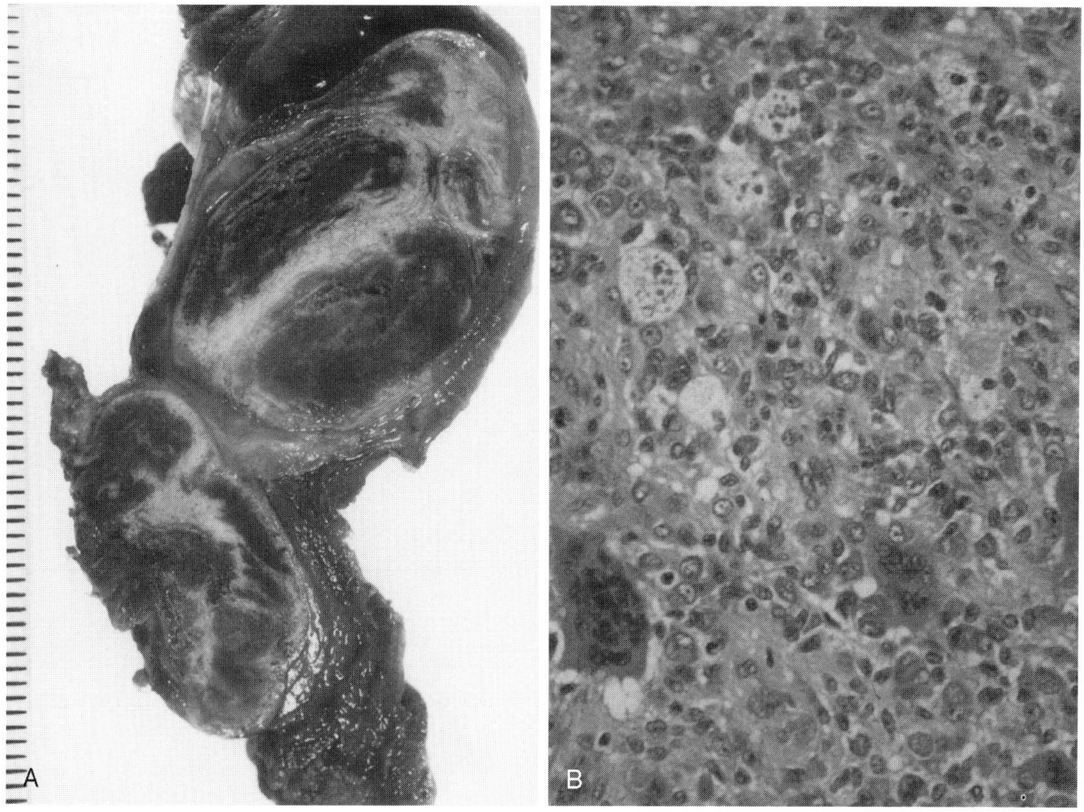

Figure 18–7. Pigmented villonodular synovitis of the elbow. *A,* Macroscopic appearance of predominantly nodular PVNS of the elbow showing the characteristic golden-brown and yellow coloration. *B,* Fibrohistiocytic mononuclear cells contain hemosiderin granules. Two osteoclast-like multinucleate cells are present. (See also color figure.)

often more prevalent toward the edge of the lesions. The more highly cellular and recurrent lesions tend to have fewer giant cells. Villous areas contain little reticulin or collagen, but nodular lesions have a more collagenous stroma including collagenous bands that may superficially resemble osteoid. Some lesions, particularly near their periphery, are highly vascular.

Many lesions are highly cellular, and it is usual to find mitotic figures of normal type in PVNS, with up to 3 or more mitoses in 10 high-power fields described in 10% of cases.[30] Nuclear pleomorphism and atypical mitoses are not features of these lesions. Immunocytochemical labeling for proliferating cell nuclear antigen (PCNA) is present mainly in fibroblastic cells, with little in fibrohistiocytic cells.[48] Tumor thrombi are identified in small veins in 1 to 5% cases.[31] Neither the presence of many mitoses nor vascular permeation predicts recurrence or metastasis. In older lesions, the vascularity and cellularity decrease and fibrosis increases.

At the edge and base of the lesions, the cellular infiltrate is usually clearly demarcated from the surrounding synovial tissues, although in some cases, particularly L-TGCT type, small nests of lesional tissue can be found in the adjacent synovium. Pedunculated lesions may undergo infarction. Bone erosion and the formation of subchondral cysts may be due to a variety of mechanisms, including direct erosion of the osteocartilaginous junction, extension into vascular foramina, and increased intra-articular pressure leading to focal osteoporosis.[34] The production of metalloproteinases, collagenase, and stromelysin by the stromal cells may contribute to the erosion of bone.[49]

In PVNS, partial fusion of the synovial villi results in spaces lined by synovial intima (Fig. 18–8*B*).[50] These spaces may contain mucopolysaccharide ground substances but are morphologically and immunophenotypically distinct from the epithelial-lined spaces seen in synovial sarcoma (see later).

Ultrastructural studies show that the cells in

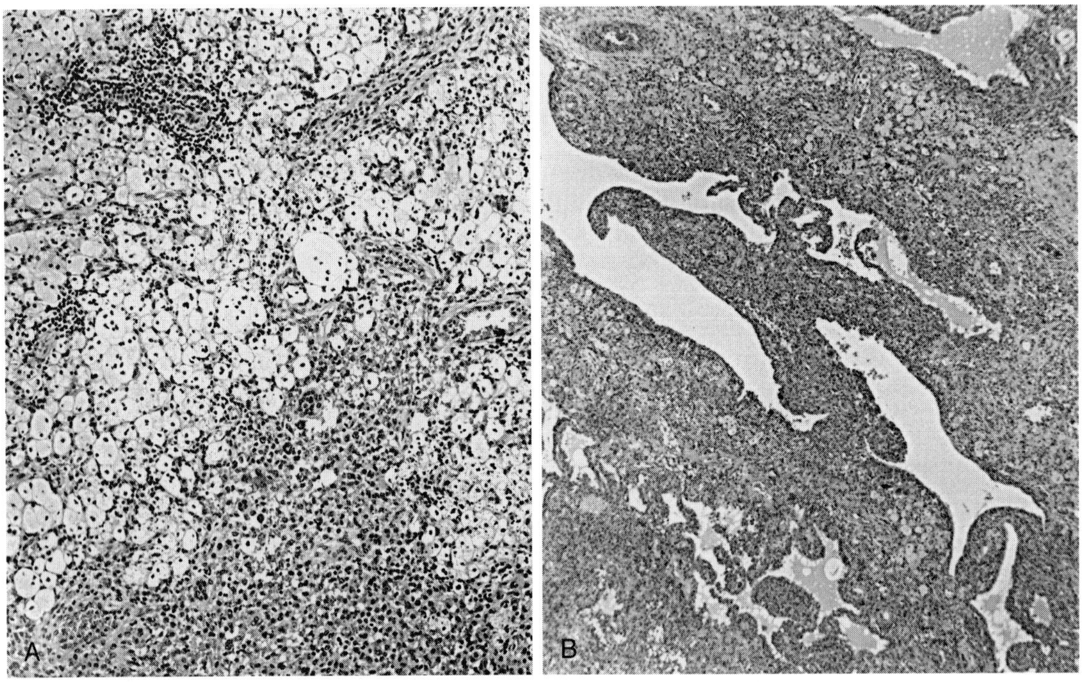

Figure 18–8. Pigmented villonodular synovitis. *A,* Zonal distribution of pale, lipid-laden histiocytes. *B,* Fusion of villous processes leads to cleft-like spaces within the synovial tissue.

PVNS are similar to normal synovial intimal cells and are a mixture of fibroblasts producing collagen and macrophages that contain lipid and/or hemosiderin.[51, 52]

Immunocytochemical labeling for CD68 and vimentin is present in both mononuclear cells and intimal surface cells, with fibroblastic cells labeling for fibronectin and the multinucleate cells labeling for leukocyte common antigen.[48, 53] It is thought that the osteoclast-like cells are formed by fusion of some of the mononuclear stromal cells, because most forms of each cell type express the receptor for parathormone-related peptide.[48] The giant cells in one case of PVNS have been shown to possess all the antigenic and functional characteristics of osteoclasts.[54]

Treatment and Prognosis

Surgical excision of the affected tissue is the treatment of choice for PVNS and L-TGCT, and the risk of recurrence reflects the technical ease of excision. L-TGCT may recur in 10 to 20% of patients,[30, 55] although lesions of high cellularity removed by enucleation may recur in up to 44% of cases.[56] PVNS recurs after synovectomy in up to one third of patients.[33, 35] Complete arthroscopic synovectomy may be an alternative to open surgery, with a lower risk of recurrence.[57, 58] In patients with PVNS for whom surgery is not appropriate for technical reasons, moderate-dose radiotherapy has been used to reduce disease bulk, preserve function, and avoid amputation, although concern about long-term joint damage and the risk of a radiation-induced sarcoma limit its use to problematic cases.[59]

Malignant transformation of a TGCT is an exceedingly rare phenomenon,[60] and the term *malignant giant cell tumor of tendon sheath* should be reserved for lesions in which there are areas of frankly malignant tissue in association with, or preceded by, a typical benign TGCT.[31] Malignant neoplasms affecting synovial tissue without other features are usually examples of clear cell sarcoma, epithelioid sarcoma, or malignant fibrous histiocytoma.

Diffuse Tenosynovial Giant Cell Tumor

The D-TGCT is an uncommon lesion that presents as a large soft tissue mass in association with a joint or bursa and affects the knee, ankle, or foot most commonly.[31] The presence of aneuploidy and of cytogenetic abnormalities in some cases (see earlier) suggests that these are true neoplasms. Macroscopically, these lesions often have a white, yellow, or brown cut surface, and histologically they grow as sheets of polygonal and spindle-shaped cells with scattered giant cells, lymphocytes, and plasma cells. The polygonal cells tend to contain rather less lipid and hemosiderin than their articular counterparts, and giant cells are also less prominent. Although mitoses and areas of necrosis may be present, there is no frank cytologic atypia and the overall pattern is that of a polymorphic cellular population with a tendency to maturation and lower cellularity at the edges of the lesion. Some cases show pseudoglandular spaces, which may be artifactual or may represent residual synovium. These are locally aggressive lesions that require treatment by wide local excision to avoid recurrence.

Differential Diagnosis

Chronic Hemarthrosis

Bleeding into the joint cavity most commonly occurs in the arthropathy that accompanies deficiency of factor VIII and less frequently with von Willebrand's disease.[61] Other causes of chronic intra-articular hemorrhage are trauma,[62] gout,[63] psoriatic arthritis, pseudogout, multiple myeloma, sickle cell disease,[64] and synovial hemangioma (see later). In hemophiliac arthropathy, the main hinge joints (elbows, knees, and ankles) are affected.

In all situations, the pathologic processes are similar to those described in experimental hemarthrosis[65] and in hemochromatosis.[61] The breakdown of erythrocytes in the joint space and synovial tissues leads to hemosiderin accumulation in macrophages in the synovial intimal and subintimal tissues (Fig. 18–9). The presence of blood in the joint initially results in thickened, hypervascular synovial tissue. In some patients, repeated damage leads to the formation of vascular pannus that destroys cartilage, leading to secondary osteoarthrosis.[64]

The concentration of the changes in the subintimal zone and the absence of obliteration of the synovial tissue by macrophages, including foam cells, giant cells, and inflammatory cells, are the main features distinguishing this condition from PVNS.

Hemophiliacs may also develop a hemorrhagic pseudotumor due to bleeding within bone, leading to its expansion and destruction; histologic examination shows organizing hematoma.[8]

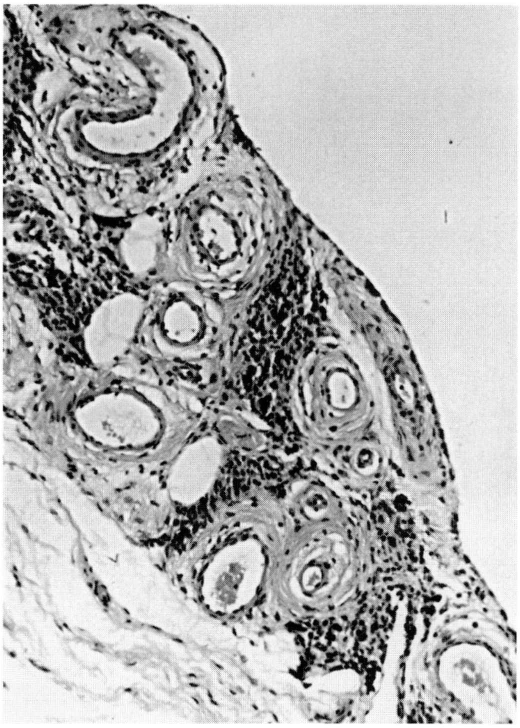

Figure 18–9. Hemophiliac synovium. The dark material in the synovial intima is hemosiderin granules within macrophages. Note the lack of a significant cellular infiltrate.

Rheumatoid Disease

The synovial tissues in rheumatoid disease are often bulky and have a villous appearance but are not usually pigmented. Histologically, the main cellular population is lymphocytes and plasma cells, with few macrophages and little hemosiderin accumulation (Fig. 18–10*A*). Small multinucleate cells are often seen (Fig. 18–10*B*), but they do not have the morphology of osteoclasts.

Degenerative Joint Disease

Patients with severe degenerative joint disease may have bulky synovial tissue, owing to the fibrotic and inflammatory changes associated with the accumulation of osteocartilaginous debris. Although this tissue may appear to be lightly pigmented macroscopically, the histologic features are unlike those of PVNS in the great majority of cases.[35] Vigorita described five cases of end-stage joint disease

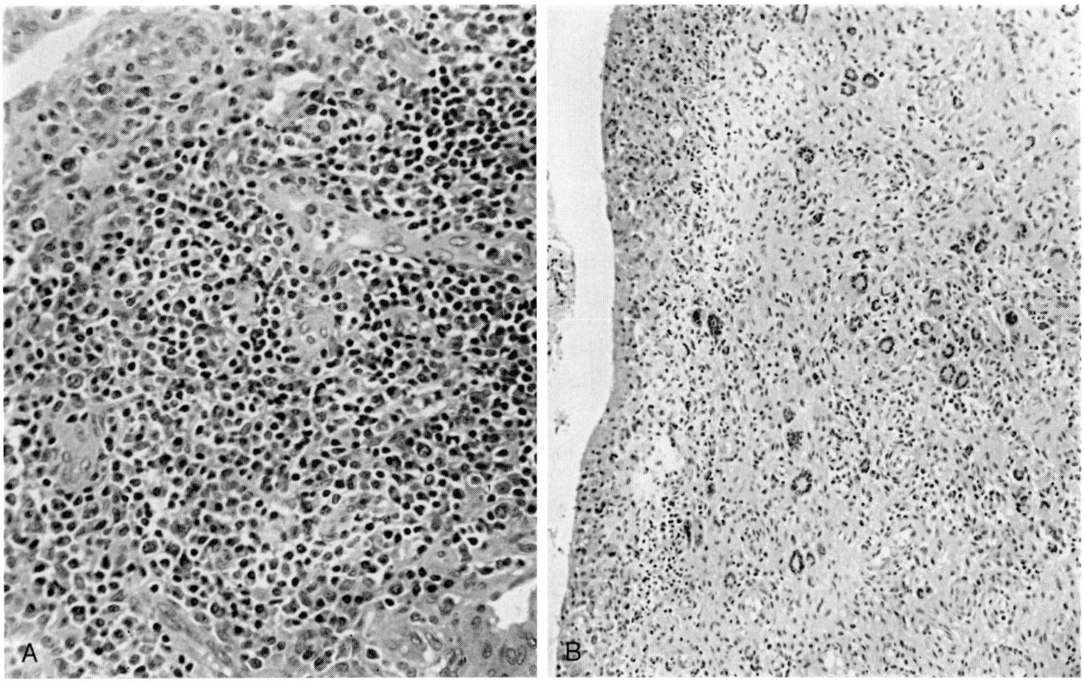

Figure 18–10. Rheumatoid disease. *A*, The cellular infiltrate is mainly by plasma cells and lymphocytes with few histiocytes and little hemosiderin. *B*, Scattered multinucleate cells with rosettes of nuclei are present.

due to rheumatoid arthritis or osteoarthritis in which the synovial tissue showed small subintimal nodules resembling PVNS[66]; it is unclear whether these represented true PVNS or an unusual reaction to joint degeneration.

Tendinous Xanthoma

The L-TGCT with a predominant component of foamy macrophages may closely resemble a tendinous xanthoma. In addition to the strong association of tendinous xanthoma with hyperlipidemia, these lesions are often multiple, occur within the tendon rather than arising from the tendon sheath, and are composed almost entirely of xanthomatous cells with very few multinucleate or inflammatory cells.[31]

Fibroma of Tendon Sheath

These lesions are composed of lobulated tissue with a hyalinized fibrous stroma. Because some fibromas may arise by sclerosis occurring in a L-TGCT, one can occasionally see lesions with features of both diseases.[31]

Synovial Sarcoma and Other Sarcomas

If careful attention is paid to the cytologic features of the cells in PVNS and tenosynovial giant cell tumors, there should be little risk of making an erroneous diagnosis of malignancy. Nevertheless, the possibility of a synovial sarcoma is often mentioned in referred material and so warrants further discussion.

Synovial sarcoma is a malignant soft tissue neoplasm that usually shows a biphasic, epithelial, and spindle cell morphology, although the proliferation may be monophasic for either component. The name is a misnomer because these neoplasms do not show synovial differentiation and are best regarded as carcinosarcomas of soft tissues.[67] They show a characteristic t(X;18) translocation that can be detected on routinely processed materials by fluorescent in situ hybridization.[68, 69]

Synovial sarcomas account for approximately 10% of soft tissue sarcomas and present most commonly between the ages of 15 and 40 years as a slow-growing painful mass around the knee, foot, or ankle joints that may secondarily involve the joint itself. Synovial sarcomas arising within a joint are extremely rare.[8, 70]

Imaging studies show an inhomogeneous, irregular soft tissue mass that may displace or infiltrate adjacent structures, including bone. Calcifications are found in up to 30% of cases and vary from fine stippling to dense opacities.

Histologically, both the epithelial and spindle cell populations show cytologic atypia (Fig. 18–11*A*) and mitoses, including atypical forms. The epithelial component shows strong immunocytochemical labeling for cytokeratin (Fig. 18–11*B*) and epithelial membrane antigen, with vimentin in the spindle cells. This contrasts to PVNS and the tenosynovial giant cell tumors in which immunocytochemical labeling for epithelial markers is not present.

Localized lesions may be cured by local resection, but usually diffusely infiltrating sarcomas require radical surgery. Despite improvements in staging and treatment, the 5-year survival rate is 36 to 51%, with death due mainly to pulmonary metastases. Favorable factors include young age, size less than 5 cm, a distal location, prominent mineralization, and a low mitotic rate.

SYNOVIAL HEMANGIOMA

Clinical Features

A hemangioma is a benign process characterized by an increase in the number of blood vessels, which may be histologically normal or abnormal. Synovial hemangiomas may affect joints, bursal spaces, or tendon sheaths. True synovial hemangiomas are uncommon, being first described by Bouchut in 1856,[71] and the first definitive series was published by Bennett and Cobey in 1939.[72] Approximately 150 cases have been described.

Hemangiomas of large joints affect children and young adults, with an age range of 9 to 49 years and a male predominance (65%), and may be associated with cutaneous hemangiomas.[72] The most common site is the knee (60%), followed by the elbow and finger joints, causing pain or swelling with an average duration of 2 years. Generalized lesions often present as a painful atraumatic hemarthrosis, whereas localized lesions may cause locking of the joints. Local resection is curative in almost all cases.

Hemangiomas of tendon sheaths mainly affect the distal upper extremity and are less likely to be confined within the synovial tissue or to produce a clinically discrete nodule.

Large lesions, which may involve bone, skeletal muscle, and subcutis in addition to the synovium, should be regarded as cases of angiomatosis,[73] with the implication that they have a high likelihood of recurrence after surgical resection.

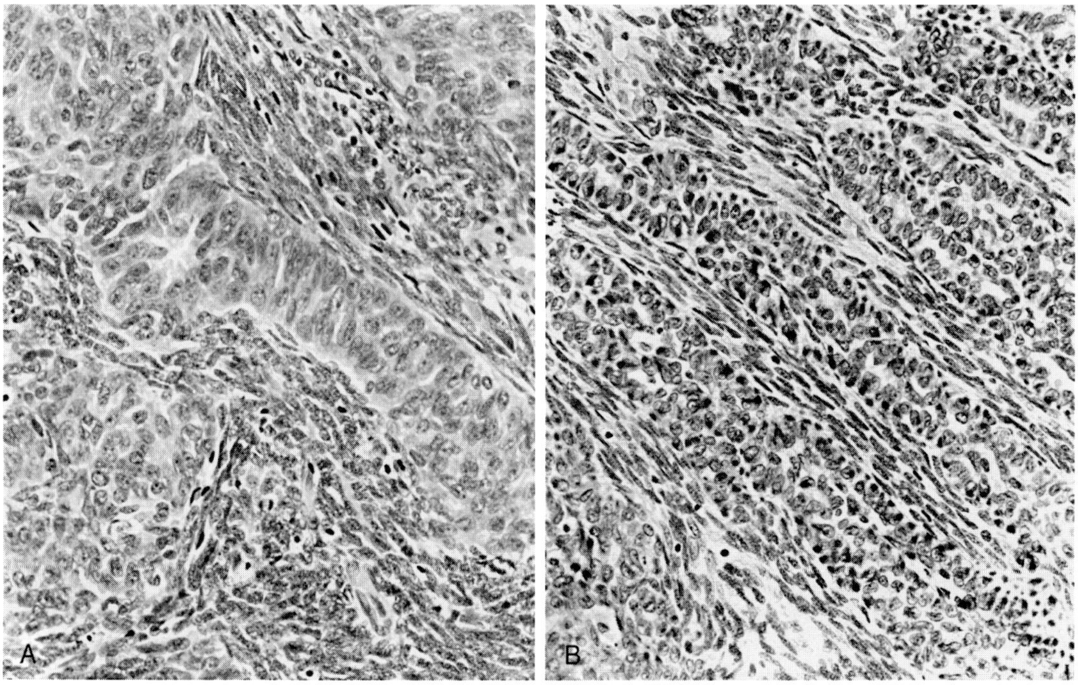

Figure 18–11. Synovial sarcoma. *A*, Biphasic pattern of larger, paler epithelioid cells and smaller, darker spindle cells. *B*, Epithelioid cells show immunohistochemical labeling for cytokeratins in the perinuclear cytoplasm.

Radiologic Features

Radiography usually shows a soft tissue mass, occasionally with phleboliths, periosteal new bone, and articular destruction. In the immature skeleton there may be advanced maturity and overgrowth of the epiphysis and limb-length discrepancy. Arthrography shows multiple intra-articular filling defects with a villous configuration that are hypervascular on angiography.[74] MRI may be nonspecific, although characteristic fibrous septa have been noted in some cases.[75]

Pathologic Features

Seventy per cent of hemangiomas are discrete nodular or sessile lesions, 0.8 to 6 cm in diameter, whereas the others are diffuse. Pigmentation may be visible.

Three histologic patterns occur[71]: 50% of hemangiomas are composed of dilated, thin-walled vascular spaces typical of a cavernous hemangioma; 25% are composed of groups of capillaries associated with larger vessels and are described as lobular capillary ("pyogenic granuloma-like") hemangiomas; whereas 20% are composed of thick-walled muscular vessels typical of arteriovenous hemangiomas. Cytologic atypia is not a feature, except for areas of papillary endothelial hyperplasia in which mild hyperchromasia and normal mitotic figures can be found. This is often associated with thrombosis and phlebolith formation.[76] Nodular lesions may show focal infarction. Hemosiderin deposition is commonly seen and very variable in its prominence, affecting either superficial or deep synovial tissue. Lymphoid follicles and a chronic inflammatory infiltrate are not features, nor are sheets of macrophages or multinucleate cells.

Differential Diagnosis

Reactive vascular proliferation in granulation tissue is usually associated with a myxoid stroma and inflammatory cells. Immunocytochemistry will identify the vascular nature of the spaces in the tissues but will not discriminate between reactive and neoplastic vessels. This will only be achieved by recognizing that the vessels tend to be orientated toward the synovial surface and do not show the lobular arrangement of vessels in a capillary hemangioma.

PVNS and similar conditions are characterized by sheets of macrophages and giant cells that do not occur in hemangiomas.

Post-traumatic and hemophilic hemarthrosis show hemosiderin deposition in the synovial tissues and are therefore indistinguishable on this basis. The presence of an abnormal vascular component is required to diagnose a hemangioma.

SYNOVIAL LIPOMA AND LIPOMA ARBORESCENS

Clinical Features

Localized, rounded nodules of mature adipose tissue occurring within synovial tissues may be regarded as *lipomas.* Only 16 cases of intra-articular lipoma have been reported, 13 of which affected the knee, causing pain, swelling, and/or locking of the joint.[77] Lipoma of tendon sheaths is also rare, usually affecting the wrist or hand of young adults aged 15 to 35 years.[78, 79] About half the cases are bilateral and often symmetrical and lead to pain, which may be severe and present for several years at diagnosis.

Lipoma arborescens (villous lipomatous proliferation of the synovium) is also a rare condition but is more common than other lipomatous proliferations. The disease affects males more than females, usually occurs in the knee joint, including the suprapatellar pouch, but may affect the wrist and hip[80] or the subdeltoid bursa.[81] This is a diffuse process, and although it may occur spontaneously, it is usually found as a reactive condition in older patients with joint trauma, degenerative joint disease, chronic synovitis, or diabetes mellitus. Lipoma arborescens should be distinguished from the localized synovial proliferation and inflammation replacing juxtapatellar fat after trauma or meniscal injury,[82] which is believed to be an unrelated condition.[80, 83, 84]

Hoffa[85] described lipomatous hyperplasia of the infrapatellar synovial tissues associated with secondary calcification in osseous and chondroid tissue, probably occurring after local trauma. The relationship between Hoffa's disease and other forms of lipoma arborescens is uncertain.

Complete synovectomy is almost always curative. There is no risk of malignant change.

Radiologic Features

Synovial lipoma and lipoma arborescens may both show low density intra-articular masses on plain radiographs.[86] The fatty nature of the lesions can be established by both CT and MRI.[87] The typical frond-like appearance of lipoma arborescens outlined by an accompanying joint effusion (Fig. 18–12*A*) differentiates it from a true synovial lipoma, in which the mass is smooth and lobular.[83, 84, 88, 89]

Pathologic Features

Synovial lipomas are rounded masses, usually less than 5 cm in diameter, formed by mature adipose tissue that occasionally shows osseous metaplasia.[77, 90] Pedunculated lesions may undergo necrosis.

Lipoma arborescens is a villous proliferation of the synovial membrane in which there is diffuse infiltration of the subintimal tissues by mature adipose tissue cells (Fig. 18–12*B*). The surface layer is often formed by fibrinous debris with scattered inflammatory cells (see Fig. 18–12*B*).[81, 83, 84, 91, 92] We have encountered one case in which multivacuolated adipocytes that resembled lipoblasts were found in the subintimal tissue of an otherwise typical lipoma arborescens.

JUXTA-ARTICULAR CYSTS, GANGLIA, AND MYXOMAS

Cystic structures may occur in the soft tissues in and around joints as well as in the juxta-articular bone. Most "cysts" near joints are the result of myxoid degeneration to form a ganglion or are synovial fluid spaces representing bursal sacs or herniations of the articular synovium into adjacent tissue; the variety of anatomic presentations of soft tissue juxta-articular cysts has been reviewed.[93] Many diseases may present radiologically with "cystic" radiolucencies in the subchondral or juxta-articular bone (Table 18–1). Soft tissue cystic lesions tend to be well defined and homogeneous on imaging, appearing transonic on ultrasonography and of water density on CT. On MRI they usually have a low signal intensity on T1 weighting, a very high signal intensity on T2 weighting, and, apart from the capsule, do

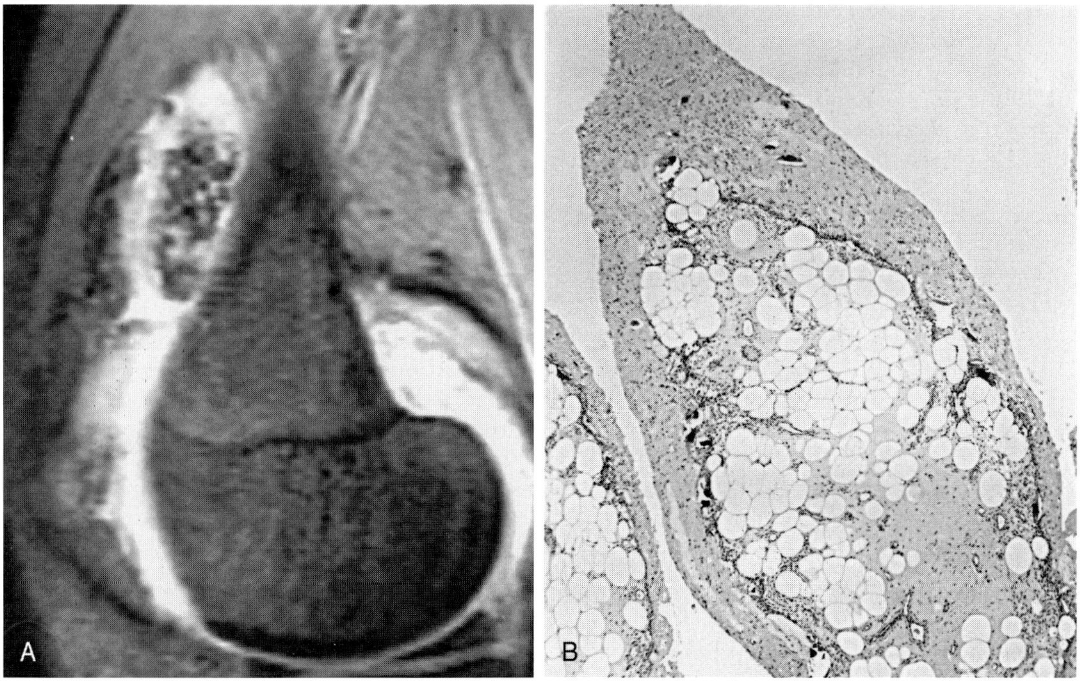

Figure 18–12. Lipoma arborescens. *A,* Axial T1-weighted MR image. Inhomogeneous irregular masses in the suprapatellar bursa are surrounded by synovial fluid. Note the masses contain foci of tissue isointense with subcutaneous and marrow fat (Courtesy of Dr. A. M. Davies, Birmingham). *B,* A villous process is formed by adipose tissue and has a surface covering of fibrinous material with bony debris.

Table 18–1. Juxta-articular Cystic Lesions of Soft Tissue and Bone

Ganglia and meniscal cysts
Myxomas of bone and soft tissue
Synovial cysts and bursae
Inflammatory and infectious arthropathies
Rheumatoid disease and osteoarthrosis
Mycobacterial infection
Crystal arthropathies
Gout
Calcium pyrophosphate deposition disease
Hydroxyapatite deposition disease
Amyloidosis
Silicone synovitis

not enhance with intravenous contrast agent instillation. Juxta-articular bony lesions can be detected by plain radiographs, but CT or MRI may be required to confirm their cystic nature. Some cysts may become inhomogeneous in the presence of internal septation or complications including hematoma, inflammation, gas, and loose bodies.

Ganglia and Meniscal Cysts

Ganglia are cystic masses that are usually attached to the tendon sheaths of the hands and feet and are formed by myxoid degeneration of connective tissues, rarely communicating with the synovium of the tendon sheath or joint in the unoperated patient. Histologically, the central cystic space has a fibrous wall within which are foci of myxoid degeneration, rich in acid mucopolysaccharides. The absence of a synovial lining distinguishes a ganglion from a bursa.

Cysts of the meniscal cartilages of the knees are associated with a horizontal tear of the meniscus, through which synovial fluid extends through to form a cyst at the capsulomeniscal junction.[94, 95]

Periosteal ganglia are rare lesions found beneath the periosteum. They are well-defined cystic lesions that may cause scalloping of the adjacent cortex and have typical fluid characteristics on CT and MRI.[96]

Ganglia occurring within bone may represent an extension from an adjacent soft tissue ganglion but may rarely occur as a primary, intramedullary lesion, presumably as a result of excessive production of acid mucopolysaccharides by fibroblast-like cells.[97, 98] Intraosseous ganglia tend to affect adults aged 30 to 60 years and occur most frequently in the distal or proximal tibia, the proximal femur, and ulna. These lesions affect the juxta-articular bone, forming eccentric, well-defined, lytic areas adjacent to a normal joint. Histologically, a central area of myxoid tissue containing spindle cells is surrounded by a fibrous capsule. The differential diagnosis includes subchondral cysts due to joint disease, chondromyxoid fibroma (which has a lobulated architecture, and cellular and chondroid areas [see Chapter 15]) and with extragnathic fibromyxoma (see later). Curettage is almost always curative.

Juxta-articular Myxoma of Soft Tissue

This term has been applied to a group of lesions that range between cysts of the lateral meniscus of the knee to large soft tissue masses up to 12 cm in diameter.[99] Although smaller lesions, especially those associated with traumatic or degenerative joint disease, are considered to be reactive in nature, other larger but histologically similar lesions may be neoplastic and show a tendency for local recurrence in up to one third of cases. The histologic features are those of spindle or stellate cells floating in a matrix rich in mucopolysaccharides. Cysts may form centrally, whereas fibrosis is often seen at the periphery. Some lesions may show more cellular spindle cell areas, but there is no cytologic atypia.

Myxoma of Bone

Myxoma of bone is an uncommon lesion, most commonly occurring in the jaw, where it is thought to be of odontogenic origin, and rarely in extragnathic sites. The diagnostic criteria for myxoma of bone are a benign, unicentric tumor composed of stellate cells set in a loose mucoid stroma, with only occasional areas of fibrosis; there should be no chondroblasts, lipoblasts, or rhabdomyoblasts present, and the tumor should be poorly vascularized.[100, 101] In all myxomas or fibromyxomas, a careful search should be made for other tissue elements, suggesting that myxoid change has occurred in another lesion such as chondrosarcoma, osteosarcoma, fibrosarcoma, fibrous dysplasia, or chondromyxoid fibroma.

Myxomas of the Mandible and Maxilla

Myxomas at these sites usually present as a painless swelling in a young adult, although children and middle-aged adults can be affected.[101–103] A case report of a mandibular myxoma in a monkey provides an excellent morphologic description of this lesion.[104] Radiologic features are of a well-defined unilocu-lated or multiloculated lucency with residual bony trabeculations giving a "soap bubble" appearance. The margin is usually well defined with some reactive sclerosis, and the cortex is expanded, is thinned, and may be completely eroded.

Histologically, stellate cells and fibroblasts are set in a large amount of mucinous, slightly basophilic, matrix. Occasional fibrous areas are often seen and may lead to the diagnosis of "fibromyxoma." Some myxomas contain large and bizarre nuclei, but this feature does not correlate with the likelihood of recurrence.[105] Immunocytochemical labeling for S-100 protein has been described in a few odontogenic myxomas and may lead to difficulty in distinguishing these lesions from nerve sheath tumors.[106]

Myxomas of the jaw bones are locally infiltrative neoplasms that may recur in up to 25% cases after curettage. Total local removal should be the therapeutic goal.[102]

Extragnathic Myxomas

Myxomas of bone other than the jaws are extremely rare, and most reports suggest an alternative primary diagnosis with secondary myxoid change. Three true myxomas of the femur[107] were bulky, expansile lesions in elderly patients that had aggressive radiologic features, histologic features as described earlier for the jaw lesions, and a benign clinical course. Some fibromyxoid tumors of the proximal femur may represent examples of the so-called polymorphous fibro-osseous lesion or liposclerosing fibromyxoid tumor[108, 109] described in Chapter 13.

Synovial Cysts

A synovial cyst is a continuation of the synovial membrane through the joint capsule or the expansion of a bursa. The fibrous wall has a lining of flattened synovial intimal cells. The cysts contain synovial fluid and may become infected. They are often associated with degenerative, traumatic, or an inflammatory process, of which rheumatoid disease is the most common.

Changes Associated with Inflammatory and Infectious Arthropathies

Rheumatoid Disease, Osteoarthrosis, Hemophilia, and Silicone Synovitis

The synovial changes in rheumatoid disease are discussed earlier. Similar histologic features can be seen in the tissue that characteristically erodes the subchondral and periarticular bone. MRI demonstrates these changes and has shown that subchondral cysts may contain synovial tissue and fluid. Some cysts may arise within bone rather than as extensions from the joint.[110]

In osteoarthrosis, cysts of the subchondral bone are a common feature, occurring where the articular cartilage has been denuded. The "cysts" are filled with fibrous tissue with foci of cartilaginous metaplasia, and sometimes with cartilage fragments and areas of edema.[111] They may arise through a combination of bone resorption around foci of necrosis and the penetration of synovial fluid through cracks in the denuded bone; the high pressure of the fluid leads to localized bone resorption, which is then replaced by fibrous tissue.[112] In the diagnosis of a subchondral bone cyst, examination of plain radiographs for evidence of osteoarthrosis is essential (Fig. 18–13). Occasionally, cysts may be associated with small areas of cartilage degeneration, whereas the majority of the joint is radiologically normal.[112]

Subchondral cysts containing altered blood can also occur as part of the spectrum of joint damage in hemophilia.[112]

In joints that have been replaced by a silicone prosthesis, degradation of the silicone may result in painful soft tissue swellings or subchondral bone cysts due to an inflammatory reaction to particles of silicone.[113] These particles are not birefringent, but they are refractile and can be identified in tissue spaces if the condenser in the microscope is lowered.

Granulomatous Infections of the Synovium

Tuberculous Arthritis

Tuberculous infection usually spreads to joints by the bloodstream, most commonly involving the hip and knee, and leads to a painful, swollen, tender, doughy joint, occasionally with a draining sinus tract.[114] The early radiographic features are relatively nonspecific, with soft tissue swelling due to synovial hypertrophy and effusion. Chronic synovitis leads to periar-

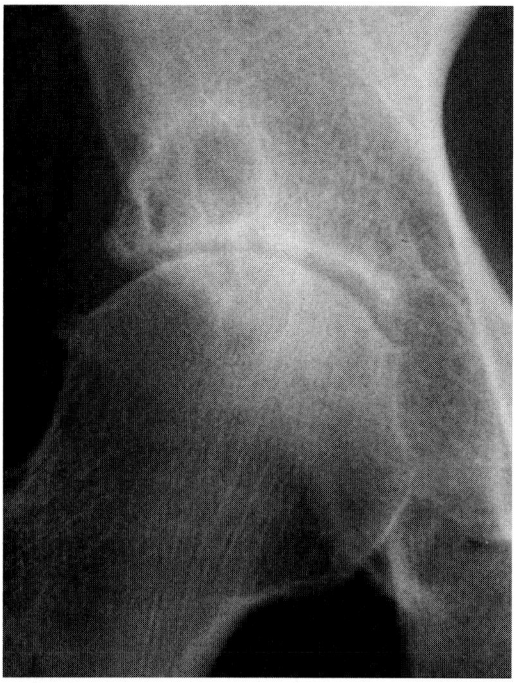

Figure 18–13. Osteoarthrosis of the hip joint. There is loss of joint space with periarticular sclerosis and a subchondral cyst in the acetabulum.

ticular osteoporosis with ill-defined cortical erosions at the articular margins and slowly progressive narrowing of the joint space (Fig. 18–14*A*). In children, the hyperemia leads to epiphyseal overgrowth and accelerated maturation of bone ends. Cartilage destruction is slow in comparison to pyogenic infection because of the lack of proteolytic enzymes within the tuberculous exudate.

The pathologic features are as seen in other tissues affected by tuberculosis, with epithelioid cell granulomas associated with multinucleate giant cells and central necrosis. Organisms are rarely demonstrable on Ziehl-Neelsen–stained tissue sections, and culture or polymerase chain reaction analysis of the tissue is required to confirm the diagnosis.

Atypical Mycobacterial Infection

Atypical mycobacterial infection in the immunocompromised patient may result in a diffuse synovial thickening, owing to the accumulation of sheets of histiocytes. These cells have ovoid, pale nuclei without mitotic activity and may be accompanied by a few lymphocytes (Fig. 18–14*B*). Ziehl-Neelsen staining of the sections reveals numerous intracellular bacilli (Fig. 18–14*C*).

Crystal Arthropathies

Gout

Clinical and Radiologic Features

Gout is synovial inflammation induced by crystals of monosodium urate (MSU). The disease occurs most commonly in middle-aged or elderly adult males, with a peak incidence in the fifth decade. Although many patients with hyperuricemia remain asymptomatic, some develop attacks of acute gouty arthritis that last 3 to 10 days if untreated. After many years of episodic acute arthritis and intervening periods of crystal deposition, localized accumulations of MSU may form tophi.

Early gouty arthritis is usually monoarticular, affecting the first metatarsophalangeal joint in approximately 75% of cases. Other joints that may be affected include the ankle, tarsus, and knee. The radiographic features at this stage are nonspecific, with soft tissue swelling, effusion, and preservation of joint space and bone density.[115]

Chronic tophaceous gout is characterized by asymmetrical polyarticular involvement of the feet, hands, wrists, elbows, and knees. The tophaceous deposits are found in the skin, kidneys, earlobes, nasal cartilages, and particularly in the periarticular ligaments and tendons, where they cause well-defined, "punched-out" erosions of the articular margins with an "overhanging" edge (Fig. 18–15*A*).[116] These erosions may produce large intraosseous cysts.[117] If an erosion extends into a joint, the cartilage damage tends to be localized, thus accounting for the preservation of the joint space until late in the disease. Calcification is uncommon within tophi, but its presence should suggest impaired calcium metabolism often related to underlying renal disease.

Pathogenesis and Pathologic Features

On polarizing microscopy of synovial fluid, MSU forms rod or needle-shaped crystals with negative birefringence when viewed with a first-order quartz plate. Crystals form in synovial fluid when the concentration of MSU rises. Acute arthritis occurs when the crystals are coated with plasma proteins, particularly IgG,

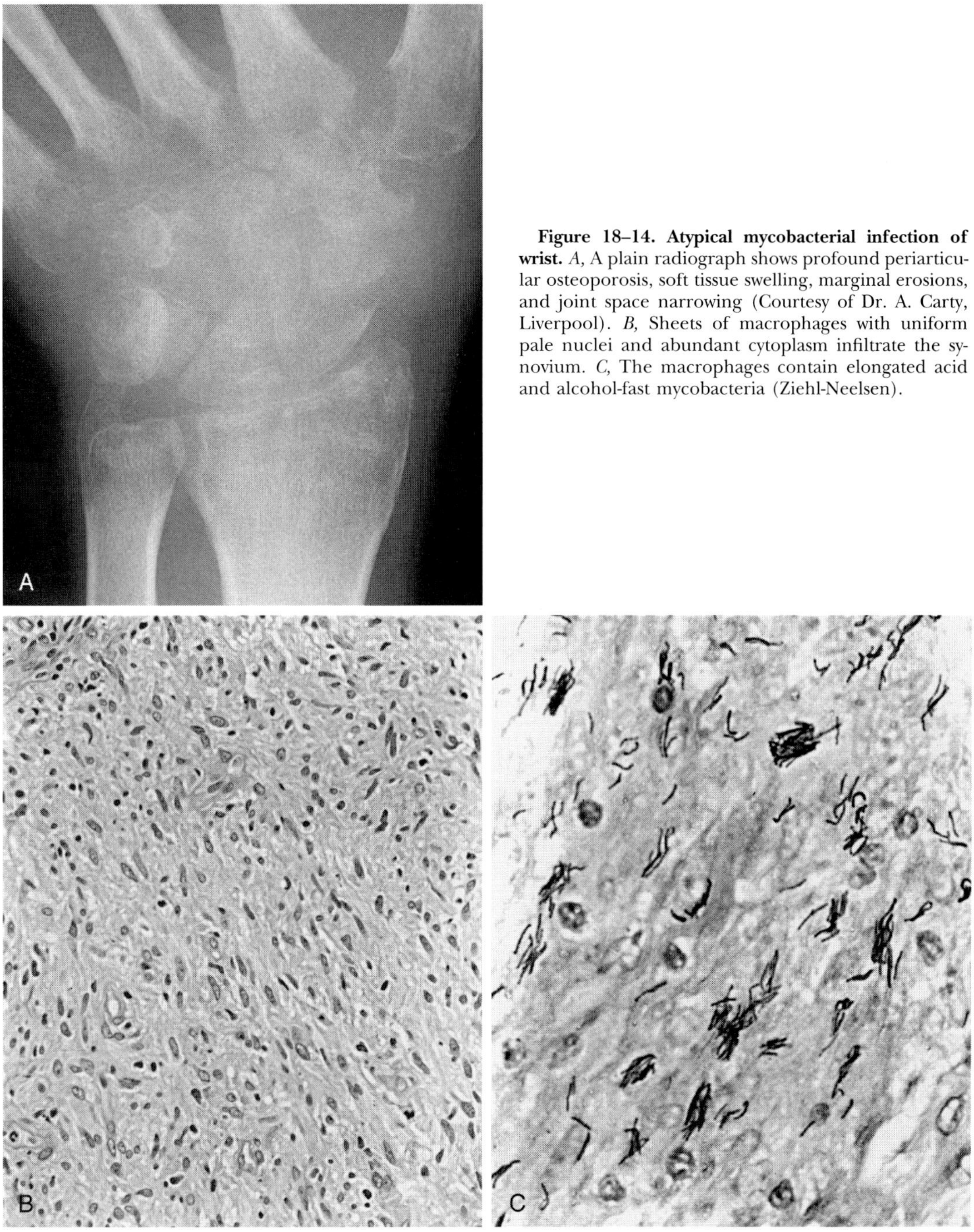

Figure 18–14. Atypical mycobacterial infection of wrist. *A,* A plain radiograph shows profound periarticular osteoporosis, soft tissue swelling, marginal erosions, and joint space narrowing (Courtesy of Dr. A. Carty, Liverpool). *B,* Sheets of macrophages with uniform pale nuclei and abundant cytoplasm infiltrate the synovium. *C,* The macrophages contain elongated acid and alcohol-fast mycobacteria (Ziehl-Neelsen).

which activates complement and attracts neutrophil polymorphs into the fluid.[118]

Tophi are masses of crystals surrounded by macrophages (Fig. 18–15*B* and *C*), presumably formed due to changes in the local tissue concentration of MSU related to trauma and temperature. It has been suggested that active cellular transport of MSU by macrophages may be an important factor in the development of tophi.[119]

Urate crystals are water soluble and tend to dissolve in aqueous fixatives such as formaldehyde. In routinely fixed, processed, and stained tissues, crystals may not be demonstrable in small tophaceous deposits, although in larger deposits some crystals usually remain.

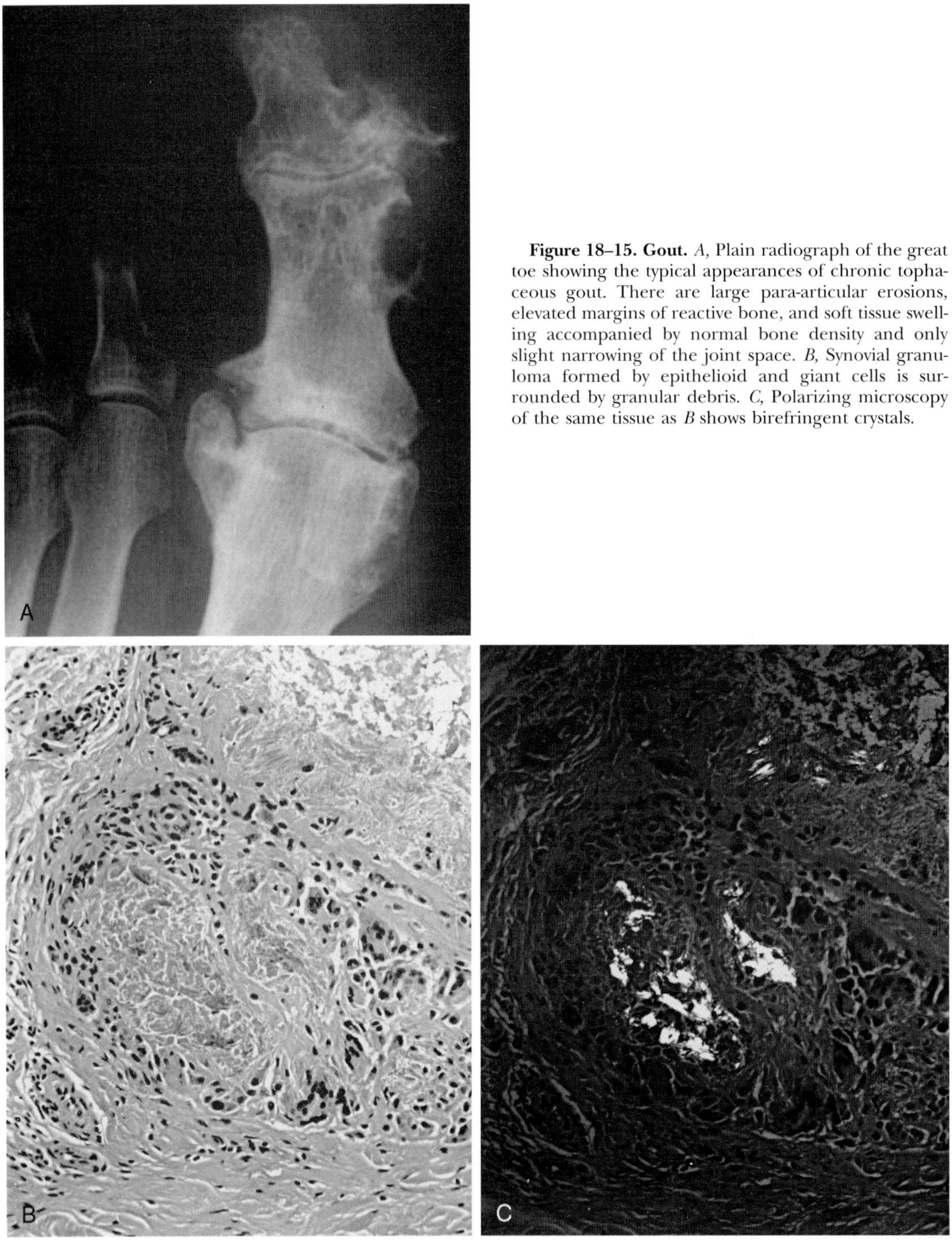

Figure 18–15. Gout. *A,* Plain radiograph of the great toe showing the typical appearances of chronic tophaceous gout. There are large para-articular erosions, elevated margins of reactive bone, and soft tissue swelling accompanied by normal bone density and only slight narrowing of the joint space. *B,* Synovial granuloma formed by epithelioid and giant cells is surrounded by granular debris. *C,* Polarizing microscopy of the same tissue as *B* shows birefringent crystals.

Alcohol fixation of tissue will preserve the crystals, which can also be demonstrated on frozen sections or touch preparations. If paraffin-embedded tissue is the only material available, it is worth examining dewaxed, unstained sections for crystals, because hematoxylin and eosin staining may remove crystals that have resisted fixation and processing.

Calcium Pyrophosphate Dihydrate Disease

Intra-articular calcium pyrophosphate dihydrate (CPPD) crystal deposition is a common idiopathic condition of the elderly, although it can also be associated with hereditary and metabolic disorders. Deposits of calcium-containing crystals are found in both hyaline and fibrocartilage as chondrocalcinosis,[118] and crystals may be deposited in the capsule, synovium, bursa, tendons, ligaments, and soft tissues.

The articular damage in CPPD disease may mimic osteoarthrosis, with cartilage loss, reactive sclerosis, osteophytosis, and extensive subchondral cyst formation.[118] However, the distribution of the joints affected by these diseases is often sufficiently distinctive to allow differentiation, because CPPD arthropathy tends to affect the second and third metacarpophalangeal, radiocarpal, elbow, and glenohumeral joints, joints not commonly involved in primary osteoarthritis. In the hip, if large subchondral cysts are seen, then pyrophosphate arthropathy should be considered even when chondrocalcinosis is not present.

Approximately 25% of patients present with pseudogout—acute self-limiting attacks simulating gout or infection.[120] A small number of patients may present with more continuous attacks simulating rheumatoid arthritis.

Pathologic Features

Crystals of CPPD are identified in synovial fluid by their square or rhomboidal shape and positive birefringence when viewed with a first-order quartz plate. The crystals are more resistant to formaldehyde fixation and processing than MSU, and crystal deposits in cartilage or soft tissues can be recognized as birefringent, weakly hematoxyphilic granular areas with or without a macrophage reaction (Fig. 18–16).[24]

Calcium Hydroxyapatite Deposition Disease

The deposition of calcium hydroxyapatite (CHA) has been implicated in the development of acute and chronic articular disease. Plain radiographs show CHA crystals varying from faint milky calcifications with ill-defined margins to dense calcifications with sharp margins.[121]

In periarticular disease, CHA crystals are deposited mainly in tendons or other structures around the shoulder and occasionally at the wrist, hand, and elbow. Although often asymptomatic, the CHA crystals can provoke an intensely painful inflammatory response.

The role of CHA crystals in producing articular disease is a subject of debate. Three clinical presentations may occur.[122] Acute synovitis is uncommon and believed to be due to intra-articular release of crystals triggering an acute inflammatory response. In osteoarthrosis, 50%

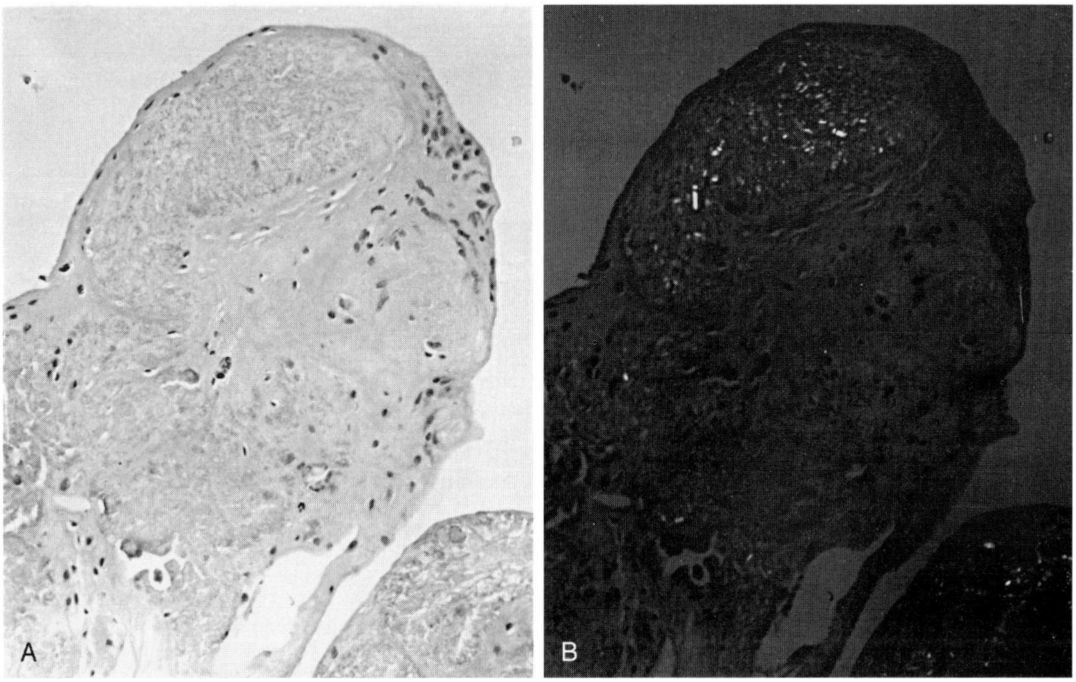

Figure 18–16. Calcium pyrophosphate deposition disease. *A,* Granular mass of calcium pyrophosphate crystals in subintimal synovial tissue. *B,* Polarizing microscopy of the same tissue as in *A* shows birefringent crystals.

of synovial fluid samples contain CHA crystals, the significance of which is uncertain.[123] Third, a destructive arthropathy may occur, most frequently in the shoulder (Milwaukee shoulder syndrome), in which there is cartilage loss, subchondral sclerosis, glenohumeral impaction, and an effusion that may contain calcific debris.

Amyloid

Amyloidosis is characterized by the abnormal extracellular deposition of autologous protein in the form of β-pleated sheets, a configuration that results in orange/apple-green birefringence when the tissue is stained with Congo red dye. Amyloid deposition may be localized or systemic and is classified according to the chemical nature of the fibril subunit proteins.[124] The deposition of amyloid in bones, joints, and soft tissues occurs predominantly in the AL (primary amyloidosis and myeloma) and Aβ2M (in chronic hemodialysis) forms of amyloidosis. The musculoskeletal changes are the same regardless of the type of amyloid, but imaging studies are important in diagnosis and management.

Synovial amyloidosis is usually bilaterally symmetrical, affecting the shoulders, hips, wrists, and knees.[113, 125] Involvement of the tendons at the wrist may result in palpable nodules and the carpal tunnel syndrome. Plain radiographs show nodular soft tissue swelling, marked periarticular osteoporosis, well-defined subchondral cysts, and preservation of joint space. Amyloid deposits have a low to intermediate signal on all MRI sequences.[126] In dialysis-associated amyloidosis, periarticular osteoporosis may be exacerbated by secondary hyperparathyroidism, osteomalacia, or aluminium toxicity. Subchondral "cysts" may be the result of infiltration by amyloid[125] or due to extrinsic pressure of the synovial and pericapsular material on intracapsular cortices.[126] When subchondral cysts are large, they predispose to pathologic fractures, especially around the hip.[127] Extensive joint destruction may result from subarticular osteonecrosis or a neuropathic arthropathy.

The diagnosis can be confirmed by the biopsy of synovial, rectal, or subcutaneous tissues in which deposition of amyloid in the walls of arterioles and venules may be observed. Noninvasive imaging of radioiodine-labeled amyloid P protein has been successful in confirming the diagnosis and monitoring progression of the disease.[128]

REFERENCES

1. Bauer TW, Zehr RJ, Belhobek GH, et al: Juxta-articular osteoid osteoma. Am J Surg Pathol 15:381, 1991.
2. Lever JD, Ford EHR: Histological, histochemical, and electron microscopic observations on synovial membrane. Anat Rec 132:525, 1958.
3. Barland P, Novikoff AB, Hamerman D: Electron microscopy of the human synovial membrane. J Cell Biol 14:207, 1962.
4. Schmidt D, Mackay B: Ultrastructure of human tendon sheath and synovium: Implication for tumor histogenesis. Ultrastruct Pathol 3:269, 1982.
5. Burmester GR, Dimitriu-Bona A, Waters SJ, et al: Identification of three major synovial lining cell populations by monoclonal antibodies directed to Ia antigens and antigens associated with monocytes/macrophages and fibroblasts. Scand J Immunol 17:69, 1983.
6. Freund E: Chondromatosis of joints. Arch Surg 34:670, 1937.
7. Lichtenstein L: Tumors of synovial joints, bursae, and tendon sheaths. Cancer 8:816, 1955.
8. Fechner RE, Mills SE: Lesions of the synovium. *In* Tumors of the Bones and Joints. Washington, DC, Armed Forces Institute of Pathology, 1993, p 279.
9. Steinberg GG, Desai SS, Malhotra R, et al: Familial synovial chondromatosis. J Bone Joint Surg 71B: 144, 1989.
10. Maurice H, Crone M, Watt I: Synovial chondromatosis. J Bone Joint Surg 70B:807, 1988.
11. Sim FH, Dahlin DC, Ivins JC: Extra-articular synovial chondromatosis. J Bone Joint Surg 59A:492, 1977.
12. Crooty JM, Monu JUV, Pope TL: Synovial osteochondromatosis. Radiol Clin North Am 34:327, 1996.
13. Leu J-K, Matsubara T, Hirohata K: Ultrastructural morphology of early cellular changes in the synovium of primary synovial chondromatosis. Clin Orthop Rel Res 276:299, 1992.
14. Milgram JW: Synovial osteochondromatosis: A histopathological study of thirty cases. J Bone Joint Surg 59A:792, 1977.
15. Kay PR, Freemont AJ, Davies DRA: The aetiology of multiple loose bodies: Snow storm knee. J Bone Joint Surg 71B:501, 1989.
16. Friedman B, Nerubay J, Blankstein A, et al: Case report 439: Synovial chondromatosis (osteochondromatosis) of the right hip: "Hidden" radiologic manifestations. Skeletal Radiol 16:504, 1987.
17. Kramer J, Recht M, Deely DM, et al: MRI appearance of idiopathic synovial osteochondromatosis. J Comput Assist Tomogr 17:772, 1993.
18. Blandino A, Salvi L, Chirico G, et al: Synovial chondromatosis of the ankle: MRI findings. Clin Imaging 16:34, 1992.
19. Edeiken J, Edeiken BS, Ayala AG, et al: Giant solitary synovial chondromatosis. Skeletal Radiol 23:23, 1994.
20. Sviland L, Malcolm AJ: Synovial chondromatosis presenting as painless soft tissue mass—a report of 19 cases. Histopathology 27:275, 1995.
21. Bertoni F, Unni KK, Beabout JW, et al: Chondrosarcomas of the synovium. Cancer 67:155, 1991.
22. Villacin AB, Brigham LN, Bullough PG: Primary and

secondary synovial chondrometaplasia: Histopathologic and clinicoradiologic differences. Hum Pathol 10:439, 1979.
23. Trias A, Quintina O: Synovial chondrometaplasia: Review of world literature and a study of 18 Canadian cases. Can J Surg 19:151, 1976.
24. Ishida T, Dorfman HD, Bullough PG: Tophaceous pseudogout (tumoral calcium pyrophosphate dihydrate crystal deposition disease). Hum Pathol 26:587, 1995.
25. Sariento A, Elkins RW: Giant intra-articular osteochondroma of the knee. J Bone Joint Surg 57A:560, 1975.
26. Kenan S, Abdelwahab IF, Klein MJ, et al: Case report 817: Synovial chondrosarcoma secondary to synovial chondromatosis. Skeletal Radiol 22:263, 1993.
27. Manivel JC, Dehner LP, Thompson R: Case report 460: Synovial chondrosarcoma of left knee. Skeletal Radiol 17:66, 1988.
28. King JW, Spjut HJ, Fechner RE, et al: Synovial chondrosarcoma of the knee joint. J Bone Joint Surg 49A:1389, 1967.
29. Ontell F, Greenspan A: Chondrosarcoma complicating synovial chondromatosis: findings with magnetic resonance imaging. Can Assoc Radiol J 45:318, 1994.
30. Rao AS, Vigorita VJ: Pigmented villonodular synovitis (giant cell tumour of the tendon sheath and synovial membrane): A review of 81 cases. J Bone Joint Surg 66A:76, 1984.
31. Enzinger F, Weiss S: Benign tumours and tumour-like lesions of synovial tissue. *In* Soft Tissue Tumours. Vol 3. St. Louis, CV Mosby, 1995, p 735.
32. Jaffe HL, Lichtenstein L, Sutro CJ: Pigmented villonodular synovitis, bursitis and tenosynovitis. Arch Pathol 31:731, 1941.
33. Byers PD, Cotton RE, Deacon OW, et al: The diagnosis and treatment of pigmented villonodular synovitis. J Bone Joint Surg 50B:290, 1968.
34. Goldman AB, DiCarlo EF: Pigmented villonodular synovitis: Diagnosis and differential diagnosis. Radiol Clin North Am 26:1327, 1988.
35. Granowitz SP, D'Antonio J, Mankin HL: The pathogenesis and long-term end results of pigmented villonodular synovitis. Clin Orthop Rel Res 114:335, 1976.
36. Docken WP: Pigmented villonodular synovitis: A review with illustrative case reports. Semin Arthritis Rheum 9:1, 1979.
37. Abdul-Karim FW, El-Nagger AK, Joyce MJ, et al: Diffuse and localized tenosynovial giant cell tumour and pigmented villonodular synovitis: A clinicopathologic and flow cytometric DNA analysis. Hum Pathol 23:729, 1992.
38. Choong PFM, Willen H, Nilbert M, et al: Pigmented villonodular synovitis: Monoclonality and metastasis—case for neoplastic origin? Acta Orthop Scand 66:64, 1995.
39. Ray RA, Morton CC, Lipinski KK, et al: Cytogenetic evidence of clonality in a case of pigmented villonodular synovitis. Cancer 67:121, 1991.
40. Mertens F, Orndal C, Mandahl N, et al: Chromosome aberrations in tenosynovial giant cell tumors and other nontumorous synovial tissue. Genes Chromosomes Cancer 6:212, 1993.
41. Rowlands CG, Roland B, Hwang WS, et al: Diffuse-variant tenosynovial giant cell tumor: A rare and aggressive lesion. Hum Pathol 25:423, 1994.
42. Halpern A, Donovan TL, Horovitz B, et al: Arthrographic demonstration of pigmented villonodular synovitis of the knee. AJR Am J Roentgenol 132:193, 1978.
43. Myers BW, Massi AT, Feigenbaum SL: Pigmented villo-nodular synovitis and tenosynovitis: A clinical epidemiological study of 166 cases and literature review. Medicine 19:223, 1980.
44. Butt WP, Hardy G, Ostlere SJ: Pigmented villonodular synovitis of the knee: Computed tomographic appearances. Skeletal Radiol 19:191, 1990.
45. Rosenthal DI, Aronow S, Murray WT: Iron content of pigmented villonodular synovitis detected by computed tomography. Radiology 133:409, 1979.
46. Jelinek JS, Kransdorf MJ, Utz RT, et al: Imaging of pigmented villo-nodular synovitis with emphasis on MR imaging. AJR Am J Roentgenol 152:337, 1989.
47. Poletti SC, Gates HS, Martinez SM, et al: The use of magnetic resonance imaging in the diagnosis of pigmented villo-nodular synovitis. Orthopaedics 13:185, 1990.
48. Nakashima M, Ito M, Ohtsuru A, et al: Expression of parathyroid hormone (PTH)-related peptide (PTHrP) and PTH/PTHrP receptor in giant cell tumour of tendon sheath. J Pathol 180:80, 1996.
49. Darling JM, Glimcher LH, Shortkroff S, et al: Expression of metalloproteinases in pigmented villonodular synovitis. Hum Pathol S25:825, 1994.
50. Ushijima M, Hashimoto H, Tsuneyoshi M, et al: Giant cell tumor of the tendon sheath (nodular tenosynovitis). Cancer 57:875, 1986.
51. Wyllie GC: The stromal cell reaction of pigmented villonodular synovitis: An electron microscopic study. Arthritis Rheum 12:205, 1969.
52. Ghadially FN, Lalonde A, Dick CE: Ultrastructure of pigmented villonodular synovitis. J Pathol 127:19, 1978.
53. O'Connell JX, Fanburg JC, Rosenberg AE: Giant cell tumor of tendon sheath and pigmented villonodular synovitis: Immunophenotype suggests a synovial cell origin. Hum Pathol 26:771, 1995.
54. Neale SD, Kristelly R, Gundle R, et al: Giant cells in pigmented villonodular synovitis express an osteoclast phenotype. J Clin Pathol 50:605, 1997.
55. Myers BW, Masi AT, Feigenbaum SL: Pigmented villonodular synovitis and tenosynovitis: A clinical epidemiologic study of 166 cases and literature review. Medicine 59:223, 1980.
56. Wright C: Benign giant cell synovioma. Br J Surg 38:257, 1954.
57. Ogilvie-Harris DJ, McLean J, Zarnett ME: Pigmented villonodular synovitis of the knee. J Bone Joint Surg 74A:119, 1992.
58. Flandry FC, Hughston JC, Jacobson KE, et al: Surgical treatment of diffuse pigmented villonodular synovitis of the knee. Clin Orthop Rel Res 300:183, 1994.
59. O'Sullivan B, Cummings B, Catton C, et al: Outcome following radiation treatment for high-risk pigmented villonodular synovitis. Int J Radiat Oncol Biol Phys 32:777, 1995.
60. Carstens PHB, Howell RS: Malignant giant cell tumor of tendon sheath. Virchows Arch (A) 382:237, 1979.
61. Collins DH: Haemosiderosis and haemochromatosis of synovial tissues. J Bone Joint Surg 33B:436, 1951.
62. France MP, Gupta SK: Nonhemophilic hemosiderotic synovitis of the shoulder. Clin Orthop Rel Res 262:132, 1991.
63. Martin DJ, Merenda G, McDonald DJ, et al: Recurrent hemarthrosis associated with gout. Clin Orthop Rel Res 277:262, 1992.

64. Hume RL, Short LA, Gudas CJ: Hemarthrosis: A review of the literature. J Am Podiatr Assoc 70:283, 1980.
65. Roy S, Ghadially FN: Pathology of experimental haemoarthrosis. Ann Rheum Dis 26:402, 1966.
66. Vigorita VJ: Pigmented villonodular synovitis-like lesions in association with rare cases of rheumatoid arthritis, osteonecrosis, and advanced degenerative joint disease. Clin Orthop Rel Res 183:115, 1984.
67. Fisher C: Synovial sarcoma. Curr Diagn Pathol 1:13, 1994.
68. Lee W, Han K, Harris CP, et al: Use of FISH to detect chromosomal translocations and deletions. Am J Pathol 143:15, 1993.
69. Helliwell TR, King A, Rarety M, et al: Biphasic synovial sarcoma arising in the small intestinal mesentery. Cancer 75:2862, 1995.
70. McKinney CD, Mills SE, Fechner RE: Intraarticular synovial sarcoma. Am J Surg Pathol 16:1017, 1992.
71. Devaney K, Vinh TN, Sweet DE: Synovial hemangioma: A report of 20 cases with differential diagnostic considerations. Hum Pathol 24:737, 1993.
72. Bennett GE, Cobey MC: Hemangioma of joints. Arch Surg 38:487, 1939.
73. Rao VK, Weiss SW: Angiomatosis of soft tissue: An analysis of the histologic features and clinical outcome in 51 cases. Am J Surg Pathol 16:764, 1992.
74. Forrest J, Staple TW: Synovial haemangioma of the knee: Demonstration by arthrography and arteriography. Am J Roentgenol 112:512, 1971.
75. Cotten A, Flipo RM, Herbaux B, et al: Synovial haemangioma of the knee: A frequently misdiagnosed lesion. Skeletal Radiol 24:257, 1995.
76. Eichhorn JH, Rosenberg AE: Intravascular papillary endothelial hyperplasia involving the synovium. Arch Pathol Lab Med 112:647, 1988.
77. Hill JA, Martin WR, Milgram JW: Unusual arthroscopic knee lesions: Case report of an intra-articular lipoma. J Natl Med Assoc 85:697, 1993.
78. Sullivan CR, Dahlin DC, Bryan RS: Lipoma of the tendon sheath. J Bone Joint Surg 38A:1275, 1956.
79. Strauss A: Lipoma of the tendon sheaths. Surg Gynecol Obstet 35:161, 1922.
80. Hallel T, Lew S, Israel K-S, et al: Villous lipomatous proliferation of the synovial membrane (lipoma arborescens). J Bone Joint Surg 70A:264, 1988.
81. Dawson JS, Dowling F, Preston BJ, et al: Lipoma arborescens of the sub-deltoid bursa. Br J Radiol 68:197, 1995.
82. Placeo F, Tassi D: Considerazioni cliniche su 62 osservazioni di lipoma arborescente posttraumatico del ginocchio come entita pataologica a se associata a lesione meniscale. Min Chir 8:316, 1953.
83. Armstrong SJ, Watt I: Lipoma arborescens of the knee. Br J Radiol 62:178, 1989.
84. Martinez D, Millner PA, Coral A, et al: Case report 745. Skeletal Radiol 21:393, 1992.
85. Hoffa A: The influence of adipose tissue with regard to the pathology of the knee joint. JAMA 43:795, 1904.
86. Madewell JE, Sweet DE: Tumors and tumor-like lesions in or around joints. *In* Resnick D (ed): Diagnosis of Bone and Joint Disorders. 3rd ed. Philadelphia, WB Saunders, 1995, p 3939.
87. Chaljub G, Johnson PR: In vivo MRI characteristics of lipoma arborescens utilising fat suppression and contrast administration. J Comput Assist Tomogr 20:85, 1996.
88. Feller JF, Rishi M, Hughes EC: Lipoma arborescens of the knee: MR demonstration. AJR Am J Roentgenol 163:162, 1994.
89. Grieten M, Buckwaleter KA, Cardinal E, et al: Case report 873. Skeletal Radiol 23:652, 1994.
90. Pudlowski RM, Gilula LA, Kyriakos M: Intra-articular lipoma with osseous metaplasia: Radiographic pathologic correlation. AJR Am J Roentgenol 132:471, 1979.
91. Arzimanoglu A: Bilateral arborescent lipoma of the knee. J Bone Joint Surg 39A:976, 1957.
92. Weitzman G: Lipoma arborescens of the knee. J Bone Joint Surg 47A:1030, 1965.
93. Steiner E, Steinbach LS, Schnarkowski P, et al: Ganglia and cysts around joints. Radiol Clin North Am 34:395, 1996.
94. Ferrer-Roca O, Vilalta C: Lesions of the meniscus: II. Horizontal cleavage and lateral cysts. Clin Orthop Rel Res 146:301, 1980.
95. Barrie HJ: The pathogenesis and significance of meniscal cysts. J Bone Joint Surg 61B:184, 1976.
96. Kenan S, Moseley K, Steiner GC, et al: Periosteal ganglion: Case report and review of the literature. Bull Hosp Joint Dis Orthop Inst 47:46, 1987.
97. Pope TL, Fechner RE, Keats TE: Intra-osseous ganglion: Report of four cases and review of the literature. Skeletal Radiol 18:185, 1989.
98. Schajowitz F, Clavel Saintz M, Slullitel JA: Juxta-articular bone cysts (intra-osseous ganglia): A clinicopathological study of eighty-eight cases. J Bone Joint Surg 61B:107, 1979.
99. Meis JM, Enzinger FM: Juxta-articular myxoma: A clinical and pathologic study of 65 cases. Hum Pathol 23:639, 1992.
100. Dutz W, Stout AP: The myxoma in childhood. Cancer 14:629, 1961.
101. Stout AP: Myxoma, the tumor or primitive mesenchyme. Ann Surg 127:706, 1948.
102. Allphin AL, Manigilia AJ, Gregor RT, et al: Myxomas of the mandible and maxilla. Ear Nose Throat J 72:280, 1993.
103. Ang HK, Ramani P, Michaels L: Myxoma of the maxillary antrum in children. Histopathology 23:361, 1993.
104. Shalev M, Murphy JC, Fox JG, et al: Myxoma of bone in a nonhuman primate. Cancer 45:2573, 1980.
105. Unni KK: Dahlin's Bone Tumors: General Aspects and Data on 11,807 Cases. 5th ed. Philadelphia, Lippincott-Raven, 1996, p 445.
106. Lombardi T, Lock C, Samson J, et al: S100, alpha smooth muscle actin and cytokeratin 19 immunohistochemistry in odontogenic and soft tissue myxomas. J Clin Pathol 48:759, 1995.
107. McClure DK, Dahlin DC: Myxoma of bone: Report of three cases. Mayo Clin Proc 52:249, 1977.
108. Ragsdale BD: Polymorphic fibro-osseous lesions of bone: An almost site-specific diagnostic problem of the proximal femur. Hum Pathol 24:505, 1993.
109. Gilkey FW: Liposclerosing myxofibrous tumor of bone. Hum Pathol 24:1264, 1993.
110. Gubler FM, Algra PR, Maas M, et al: Gadolinium-DTPA enhanced magnetic resonance imaging of bone cysts in patients with rheumatoid arthritis. Ann Rheum Dis 62:716, 1993.
111. Byers PD, Contepomi CA, Farkas TA: Post-mortem study of the hip joint: II. Histological basis for limited and progressive cartilage alterations. Ann Rheum Dis 35:114, 1976.

112. Bullough PG, Bansal M: The differential diagnosis of geodes. Radiol Clin North Am 26:1165, 1988.
113. Goldman AB, Bansal M: Amyloidosis and silcone synovitis: Updated classification, updated pathophysiology, and synovial articular abnormalities. Radiol Clin North Am 34:375, 1996.
114. Chapman M, Murray RO, Stoker DJ: Tuberculosis of bones and joints. Semin Roentgenol 14:266, 1979.
115. Bloch C, Hermann G, Yu T-F: A radiologic reevaluation of gout: A study of 2000 patients. AJR Am J Roentgenol 134:781, 1980.
116. Watt I: Radiology of the crystal-associated arthritides. Ann Rheum Dis 42(Suppl):73, 1983.
117. Cope R, Marsan R, Castelli MJ: Case report 732. Skeletal Radiol 21:269, 1992.
118. Uri DS, Dalinka MK: Crystal disease. Radiol Clin North Am 34:359, 1996.
119. Palmer DG, Highton J, Hessian PA: Development of the gout tophus: An hypothesis. Am J Clin Pathol 91:190, 1989.
120. McCarty DJ: Calcium pyrophosphate dihydrate crystal deposition disease. *In* Primer on Rheumatic Diseases, 10th ed. Atlanta, Arthritis Foundation, 1993, p 219.
121. Resnick D: Calcium hydroxyapatite disease. *In* Resnick D (ed): Diagnosis of Bone and Joint Disorders. 3rd ed. Philadelphia, WB Saunders, 1995, p 1615.
122. Dieppe PA: Apatites and miscellaneous crystals. *In* Primer on Rheumatic Diseases. 10th ed. Atlanta, Arthritis Foundation, 1993, p 222.
123. Dieppe PA, Watt I: Crystal deposition in osteoarthritis: An opportunistic event? Clin Rheum Dis 11:367, 1985.
124. Husby G: Nomenclature and classification of amyloid and amyloidosis. J Intern Med 232:511, 1992.
125. Sargent MA, Fleming SJ, Chattopadhyay C, et al: Bone cysts and haemodialysis-related amyloidosis. Clin Radiol 40:277, 1989.
126. Cobby MJ, Adler RS, Swartz R, et al: Dialysis-related amyloid arthropathy: MRI findings in four cases. AJR Am J Roentgenol 157:1023, 1991.
127. Tatzishi H, Maeda M, Yoh K, et al: Pathologic fracture associated with amyloid deposition in the bone of a chronic hemodialysis patient. Clin Orthop Rel Res 274:300, 1992.
128. Pepys MB: Amyloid P component and the diagnosis of amyloidosis. J Intern Med 232:519, 1992.

Index

Note: Page numbers in *italics* refer to illustrations; page numbers followed by t refer to tables.

ISBN 0-7216-6439-3
90038
9 780721 664392